METHODS
IN PHARMACOLOGY

Volume 4B
Renal Pharmacology

General Editor: **Arnold Schwartz**
Baylor College of Medicine, Houston, Texas

Volume 1
Edited by **Arnold Schwartz**

Volume 2: PHYSICAL METHODS
Edited by **Colin F. Chignell**

Volume 3: SMOOTH MUSCLE
Edited by **Edwin E. Daniel** and **David M. Paton**

Volume 4A: RENAL PHARMACOLOGY
Edited by **Manuel Martinez-Maldonado**

Volume 4B: RENAL PHARMACOLOGY
Edited by **Manuel Martinez-Maldonado**

A Continuation Order Plan is available for this series. A continuation order will bring delivery of each new volume immediately upon publication. Volumes are billed only upon actual shipment. For further information please contact the publisher.

METHODS IN PHARMACOLOGY

Volume 4B
Renal Pharmacology

Edited by
Manuel Martinez-Maldonado
*University of Puerto Rico School of Medicine
and Veterans Administration Center
San Juan, Puerto Rico*

PLENUM PRESS • NEW YORK AND LONDON

The Library of Congress Cataloged the First Volume in this Series as Follows:

Methods in pharmacology. v. 1—
   New York, Meredith Corp. [1971-   ]
   v. illus. 25 cm.
   Editor: 1971-   A. Schwartz.

   1. Pharmacology — Collected works. I. Schwartz. Arnold, ed.
QP905.M45   615'.7   70-92660

Library of Congress Catalog Card Number 74-34441

© 1978 Plenum Press, New York
Softcover reprint of the hardcover 1st edition 1978
A Division of Plenum Publishing Corporation
227 West 17th Street, New York, N.Y. 10011

ISBN 978-1-4615-8896-2   ISBN 978-1-4615-8894-8 (eBook)
DOI 10.1007/978-1-4615-8894-8

Preface

Frequently attempts to design experiments utilizing the methodology described in articles in trade journals can be frustrating. Description of procedures, because of space constraints, are not always complete. The present volume attempts to bring together in one reference source many of the techniques which are utilized in the study of the kidney. It provides a thorough compendium of research tools, framed by the critical analysis of the theoretical background of renal physiology, biochemistry, and pharmacology discussed in Volume 4A. Some areas previously dealt with are not covered from a methodological point of view since adequate information does exist elsewhere (e.g., methods of whole kidney ATPase isolation). Since drugs acting on the kidney may alter not only functional but anatomical integrity, a chapter on the preparation of tissue for morphological studies has been included. The important developments in analysis of minute (ultramicro) quantities of tissue and biological fluids, as well as methodological advances in studies of the isolated kidney, are thoroughly covered.

It is my hope that investigators, research fellows, and graduate students will benefit from the information contained in this volume and that, together with its companion tome, it will be a ready reference for the renal physiologist, the renal pharmacologist, and the nephrologist.

The contributors have provided painstaking descriptions and, when required, mathematical analyses of the techniques described herein. I wish to thank all of them for their enthusiasm and the excellence of their contributions. The organizations and choice of materials, however, has been my own doing and any omissions are my responsibility.

Once more I want to thank Ms. Consuelo López for her help with the manuscript and Ms. Lucy Bartolomei and Ms. Sonia Glicken for their help with proofreading and indexing.

Last, but not least, I want to dedicate this volume to my teachers. To Floyd E. Rector, Jr., for having taught me much of the renal physiology I know, and to Donald W. Seldin, on his 25th anniversary as Chairman of the Department of Medicine at Southwestern Medical School in Dallas, for everything else.

Manuel Martinez-Maldonado

San Juan

Contributors

ROLAND C. BLANTZ
Department of Medicine
School of Medicine and Nephrology Division
University of California, San Diego
and Veterans Administration Hospital
San Diego, California

EMILE L. BOULPAEP
Department of Physiology
Yale University School of Medicine
New Haven, Connecticut

ROGER H. BOWMAN
Veterans Administration Hospital
and Department of Pharmacology
State University of New York
Upstate Medical Center
Syracuse, New York

RUTH ELLEN BULGER
Department of Anatomy
University of Massachusetts
Worcester, Massachusetts

NORMAN W. CARTER
Department of Internal Medicine
University of Texas Health Science Center at
Dallas
Southwestern Medical School
Dallas, Texas

DANIELLE CHABARDES
Laboratoire de Physiologie Cellulaire
Collège de France
Paris, France

ARNOLD M. CHONKO
Department of Medicine, Division of
Nephrology
University of Kansas Medical Center College
of Health Sciences and Hospital
Kansas City, Kansas

ELAINE L. CHUANG
Department of Medicine
University of Texas Health Science Center
San Antonio, Texas

DENNIS DOBYAN
Department of Anatomy
University of Massachusetts
Worcester, Massachusetts

G. GIEBISCH
Department of Physiology
Yale University School of Medicine
New Haven, Connecticut

R. GREGER
Institute of Physiology
Innsbruck, Austria

MICHAEL HORSTER
Institute of Physiology
University of Munich
Munich, Germany

MARTINE IMBERT-TEBOUL
Laboratoire de Physiologie Cellulaire
Collège de France
Paris, France

JAMES M. IRISH III
Department of Medicine, Division of
Nephrology
University of Kansas Medical Center College
of Health Sciences and Hospital
Kansas City, Kansas

GEORGE J. KALOYANIDES
Division of Nephrology
UCLA San Fernando Valley Medical Program
Veterans Administration Hospital
Sepulveda, California

SAULO KLAHR
Renal Division, Department of Medicine
Washington University School of Medicine
St. Louis, Missouri

F. G. KNOX
Department of Physiology and Biophysics
Mayo Clinic and Mayo Foundation
Rochester, Minnesota

NORBERT H. LAMEIRE
Department of Medicine
University of Texas Health Science Center
San Antonio, Texas

F. LANG
Institute of Physiology
Innsbruck, Austria

C. LECHENE
Biotechnology Resource in Electron Probe
Analysis
Harvard Medical School
Boston, Massachusetts

MANUEL MARTINEZ-MALDONADO
Veterans Administration Center
and Departments of Physiology and Medicine
University of Puerto Rico School of Medicine
San Juan, Puerto Rico

FRANÇOIS MOREL
Laboratoire de Physiologie Cellulaire
Collège de France
Paris, France

ALPHONSE H. NIZET
Department of Medical Clinics and Semiology
Institute of Medicine
University of Liège
Liège, Belgium

RICHARD W. OSGOOD
Department of Medicine
University of Texas Health Science Center
San Antonio, Texas

LEO R. PUCACCO
Department of Internal Medicine
University of Texas Health Science Center at
Dallas
Southwestern Medical School
Dallas, Texas

UDO SCHMIDT
Enzyme Laboratory
Medical Polyclinic
Department of Internal Medicine
University of Basel
Basel, Switzerland
and Institute of Pathology
University of Tübingen
Tübingen, Germany

JAY H. STEIN
Department of Medicine
University of Texas Health Science Center
San Antonio, Texas

SUSAN OPAVA STITZER
Department of Physiology
University of Puerto Rico School of Medicine
San Juan, Puerto Rico

BRYAN J. TUCKER
Department of Medicine
School of Medicine and Nephrology Division
University of California, San Diego
and Veterans Administration Hospital
San Diego, California

DAN J. WELLING
Departments of Pathology and Physiology
University of Kansas Medical Center College
of Health Sciences and Hospital
Kansas City, Kansas

Contents

Chapter **1**

Morphological Techniques for Study of the Kidney

Ruth Ellen Bulger and Dennis Dobyan

Department of Anatomy
University of Massachusetts
Worcester, Massachusetts

I. INTRODUCTION

The structure and function of the kidney are inextricably related, not only on a gross organ level but on a tissue, cellular, subcellular, and atomic level as well. On a tissue level, the looping shape of the nephron is a clue to its countercurrent function. On a cellular level, the elaborate shape of the proximal convoluted tubular cells provides an increased surface area and an elaborate labyrinth of extracellular spaces to facilitate active sodium reabsorption. Even on a subcellular level, the morphology of cell junctions explains the specific and varying permeabilities for the various nephron segments (Schwartz and Venkatachalam, 1974; Whittembury and Rawlins, 1971). Hence, exploitation of anatomical techniques becomes an important if not obligatory component of pathophysiological studies of the kidney.

In order for morphological studies to have meaning, the structure of the living organ must be maintained as faithfully as possible and artifacts which have been created must be recognized. In the kidney, the morphology is extremely labile, and alterations in a number of factors can lead to immediate and dramatic changes in form. Hence, adequate fixation of kidney is particularly difficult to obtain.

A variety of kinds of morphological information may be obtained, depending on the nature of the investigations being performed. This chapter attempts to provide insight into the techniques available and the type of information obtainable by morphological procedures such as light microscopy (LM), trans-

1

mission electron microscopy (TEM), scanning electron microscopy (SEM), and X-ray microanalysis.

II. STUDY OF LIVING ORGANS

A. Examining the Kidney with Dissecting Microscope and Micropuncture Techniques

Wearn and Richards (1924) sampled fluid from nephrons on the surface of an amphibian kidney using a dissecting microscope in conjunction with delicate micromanipulators. The continued development of micropuncture techniques with microanalysis of the collected fluid has provided much data on tubular function. However, because of the low resolution of the dissecting microscope, there is not much information on the specific identification of the nephron region studied or on the degree of damage caused by micropuncture. TEM studies done in conjunction with micropuncture studies increase the information available. For example, Barratt et al. (1975) clearly demonstrated that differences in electrochemical potential measured in the distal nephron by micropuncture were related to the type of cells lining the nephron at the specific puncture site.

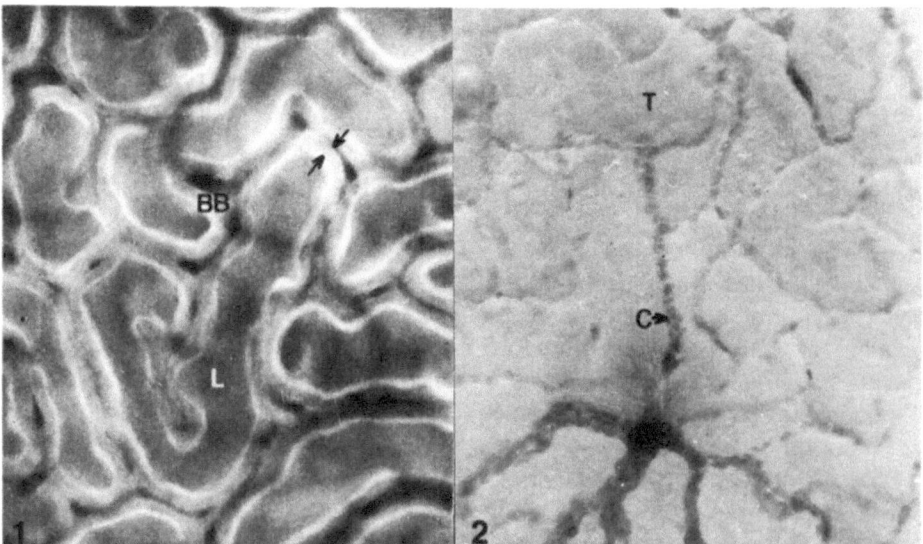

Figure 1. Appearance of the tubules from a living undisturbed kidney photographed using a light microscope and incident illumination. The brush border (BB) appears bright and separates the lumen (L) from the proximal tubular epithelium (arrows). 120×. (From Griffith et al., 1967.)

Figure 2. Appearance of the tubules from a living kidney immediately after occlusion of the renal artery. The tubules (T) now appear solid with no visible lumen. The capillaries (C) demonstrate stasis. 120×. (From Griffith et al., 1967.)

B. Incident-Light Illumination with a Light Microscope

The living, functioning kidney can be viewed *in situ* through a light microscope. This technique was first employed by Ghiron in 1912 when he observed mouse kidney *in vivo* utilizing incident light. Since then the utilization of microscopes equipped with incident-light illuminators has provided valuable information (Griffith *et al.*, 1967; Steinhausen, 1965; Swann, 1960, 1964). For example, when viewed this way, the lumen of the proximal tubule is normally widely patent (Figure 1), but a large decrease in the blood pressure can bring about rapid collapse on the tubule, with disappearance of the patent lumen (Figure 2) (Griffith *et al.*, 1967).

C. Use of Isolated Tubules

Individual tubular segments can be dissected from various kidneys, such as those from the rabbit (Burg *et al.*, 1966) or fish (Forster, 1948). These nephron segments can be incubated and/or perfused to study transport processes in the tubules from which the segments were derived. Although such studies impart important physiological information about these isolated segments, many influences found in the intact kidney are not being exerted in this simplified preparation.

III. STUDY OF CHEMICALLY FIXED TISSUE

A. Goal of Fixation

The major goal of fixation is to preserve structure in a state which most closely approximates the appearance of the living organ as is possible. It is therefore mandatory that a well-fixed kidney retain the features seen when viewed by incident light in the living state. It is well known that the kidney is a functionally distended organ (Swann 1960, 1964; Griffith *et al.*, 1967) which depends upon the maintenance of blood pressure for its normal appearance in which the tubular lumens and vessels are widely patent (Figures 1, 3, 6). The fixation procedure to be used must be determined by the goal of the study. The route of fixative application may vary, as may the fixative solution itself. It is therefore important to evaluate the structure in terms of the artifacts which are known to be produced by the type of fixation used.

Fixation also fills several important roles. It must rapidly stop autolytic processes, harden the tissue so that it is stable during further processing, and in the case of osmium tetroxide, the fixative also serves as an electron stain as well. Certain criteria can be used to help evaluate whether the fixation is adequate. The living tissue can be observed in the light microscope and the dimensions and general structure compared before or after fixation (Penttila *et al.*, 1975). In addition, one can fix the tissue with two or more different solutions and compare the ultrastructural appearance of the tissue in each. Alternatively, a physical method such as freezing can be used in addition to the chemical

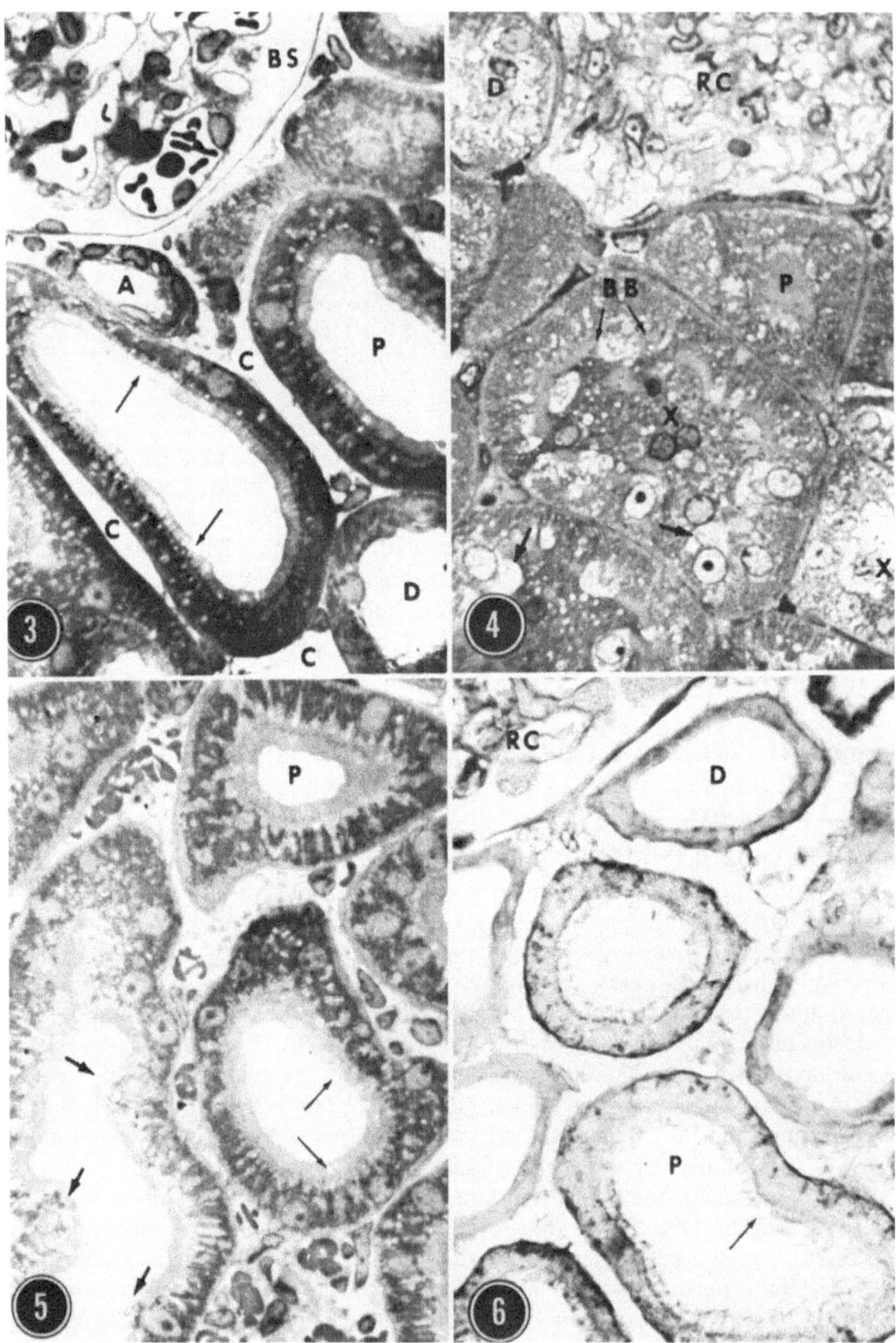

Figures 3-6. These four figures demonstrate the effect of the route of fixative application on renal morphology. Figure 3 represents tissue fixed by intravascular perfusion and embedded in plastic. Both proximal (P) and distal (D) tubule lumens are patent. Bowman's space (BS) is patent and both arterioles (A) and capillaries (C) are open. Figure 4 represents tissue fixed by excision and immersion. The lumens are filled with cell processes (X). The brush border (BB) is

procedures (Figure 6). In general, well-fixed tissue is characterized by continuity of cell membranes, and a lack of pale empty areas within organelles, or the cytoplasm.

B. Route of Fixative Application

1. Fixation by Immersion

Since the normal structure of the kidney is dependent on the maintenance of the blood pressure, it is no surprise that the common practice of removing an organ from an animal and dicing it into small pieces prior to immersion in a fixative solution produces dramatic and yet reproducible alterations in renal morphology. The cells lining the proximal tubules rapidly swell, take up the luminal fluid, and fill the once-patent lumen with large bulbous apical extensions (Figure 4). The nuclei move to a more apical position. Many of the cell organelles change in shape and position, and they in turn can swell. The lateral intercellular spaces vary in width, often demonstrating large accumulations of fluid. Immersion fixation, therefore, does not provide a faithful reproduction of the *in vivo* morphology and thus is generally not the best choice for experimental studies using animal models (Maunsbach *et al.*, 1962; Griffith *et al.*, 1967). In the study of human disease, however, tissue is obtained by open or percutaneous biopsy techniques and necessarily must be fixed by immersion procedures. The results of these studies must be analyzed in light of the known alterations seen when using immersion fixation. Some of these preservation artifacts are detailed in a study of renal morphology of *Macaca mulatta* (Tisher *et al.*, 1969).

Immersion fixation also would be a poor choice in the study of the position of vascular tracers because of the likelihood of tracer movement concomitant with the collapse of the kidney.

2. Vascular Perfusion of Fixative

Koenig *et al.* (1945) described an improved technique for fixation of the kidney which involved the vascular perfusion of fixative solution. Several methods of vascular perfusion of intact kidneys have now been described (Ericsson, 1966; Griffith *et al.*, 1967; Maunsbach, 1966a). These procedures can provide adequate maintenance of the gross and microscopic morphology of all regions of the kidney. The procedure by Griffith *et al.* (1967) includes the following steps: (1) Make a midline ventral incision through the skin and body wall. (2) Expose the descending aorta medial to the left adrenal gland and place a ligature under the vessel without occluding it. (3) Ligate the vessels to the gastrointestinal tract. (4) Expose the aorta between the renal artery and the

---

interrupted. The renal corpuscle (RC) is collapsed. Figure 5 represents tissue fixed by dripping fixative solutions on the renal surface. The proximal tubule lumens (P) are open. Some apical blebbing is occurring (thick arrows). The thin arrows demonstrate normal simplification of brush border. Figure 6 represents tissue prepared by freezing *in situ* followed by freeze-drying and vapor phase formaldehyde fixation. Both proximal (P) and distal (D) lumens are patent. The capillary lumens and interstitium are large. (These four figures are from Griffith *et al.*, 1967.)

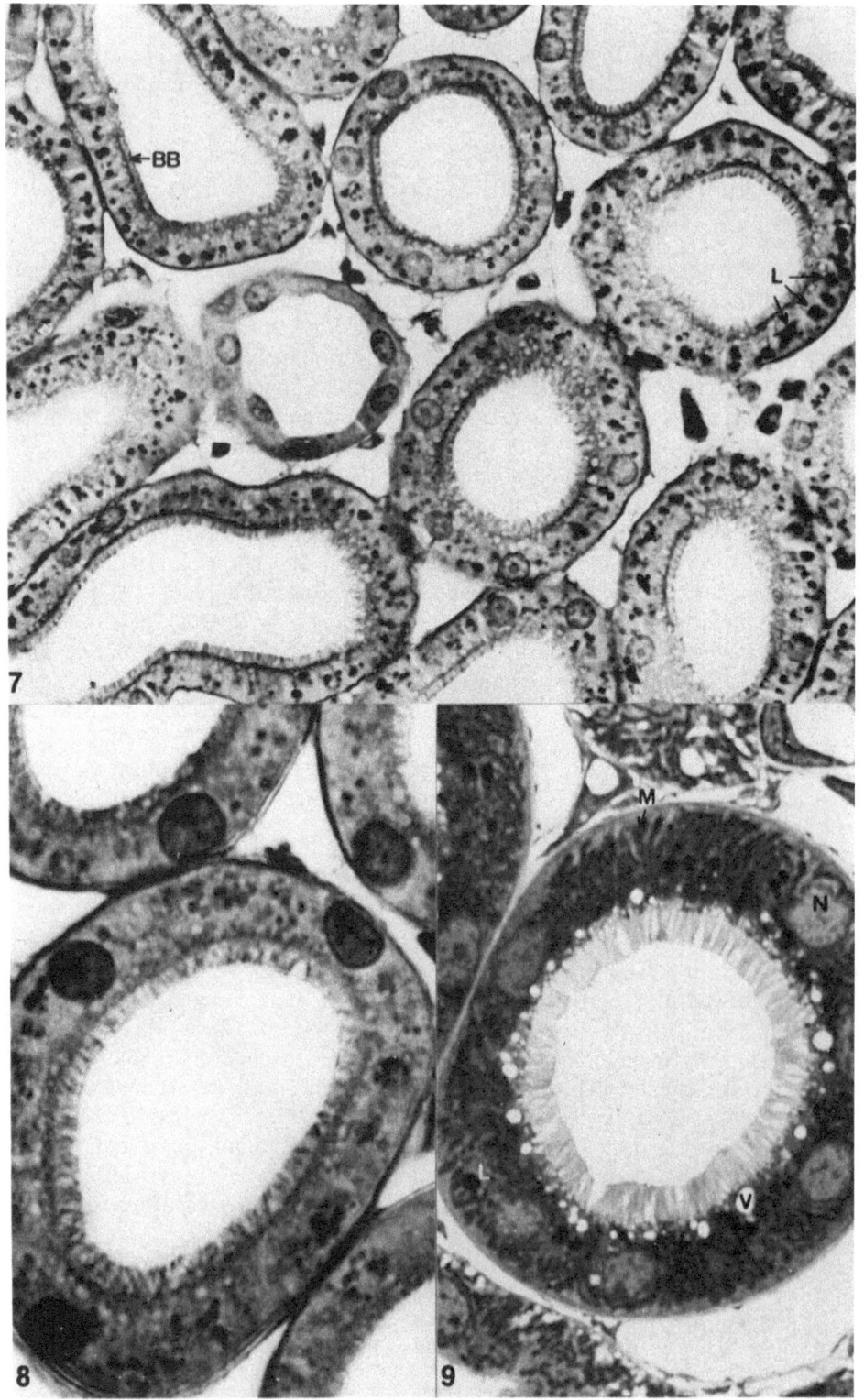

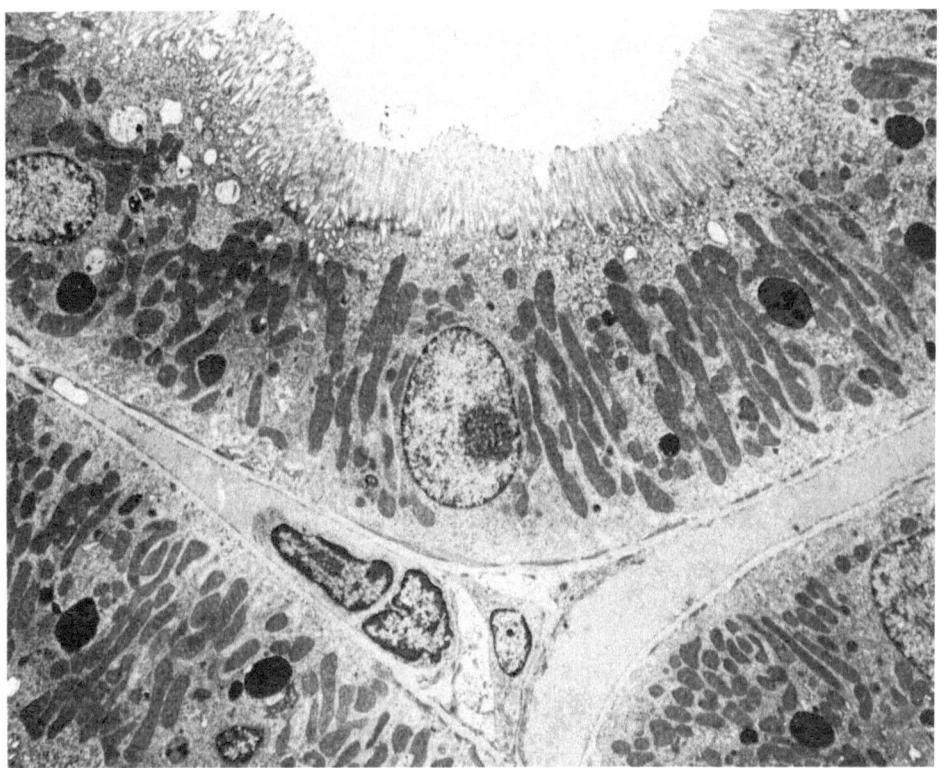

Figure 10. An electron micrograph taken at a somewhat greater magnification than Figures 8 and 9 clearly demonstrates the increased resolution of a TEM. Not only all the organelles but the suborganellar structure can now be seen. 3,300×.

aortic bifurcation and place two sutures under the aorta alone or under both the aorta and vena cava together. (5) Temporarily occlude the aorta below the level of the kidney with the upper of the two sutures from step 4. (6) Nick the wall of the aorta near the bifurcation and insert a cannula filled with heparinized saline. (7) Tie the cannula into place with the lower of the two sutures. (8) Release the occlusion of the upper suture. (9) Start the perfusion of fixative into the cannula,

←───

Figure 7. Low-magnification light micrograph of rat kidney cortex fixed by vascular perfusion, embedded in paraffin, and stained by hematoxylin and the periodic-Schiff's reaction. The dense lysosomes within the proximal tubular cells (L) and the brush border (BB) are easily identified due to their specific staining with these procedures. Most other cellular organelles are not resolved when tissue is prepared in this manner. 610×.

Figure 8. High-magnification light micrograph of the same tissue seen in Figure 7. The micrograph demonstrates that an increase in magnification does not increase the ability to resolve subcellular organelles. 1,000×.

Figure 9. High-magnification light micrograph of a proximal tubule from tissue which has been embedded in plastic and cut 1 μm in thickness. Processing tissue in this manner allows greater resolution of subcellular organelles. Nuclei (N), lysosomes (L), endocytic vacuoles (V), and mitochondria (M) can be identified. 1,000×.

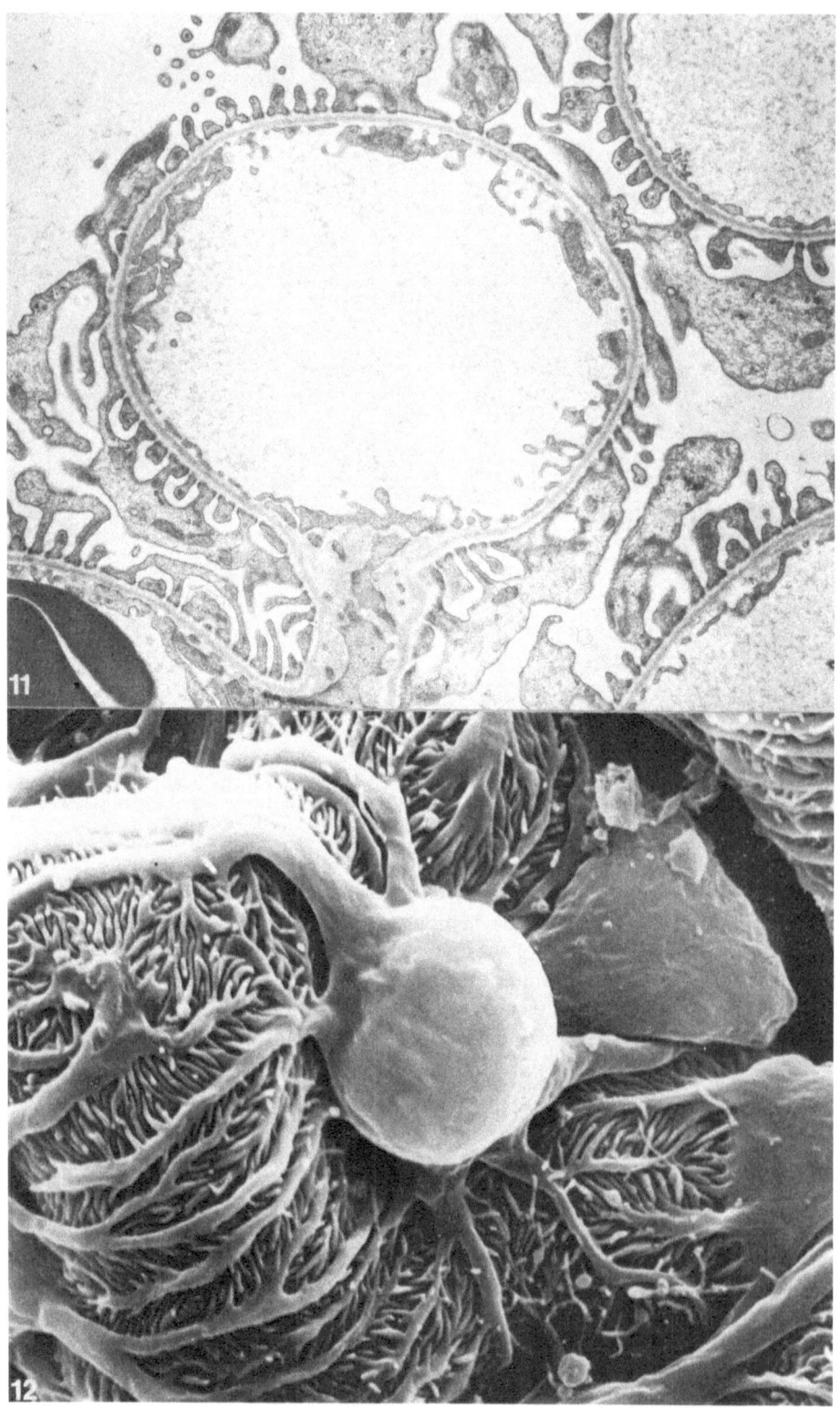

making sure not to exceed 180 mm of mercury. (10) After the perfusion has begun, occlude the aorta at the level of the adrenal. (11) Cut the renal vein to permit outflow of the fixative solution.

A modification of this basic perfusion technique (Griffith *et al.*, 1967) allows an animal to be perfused without handling at the time of perfusion. This procedure is more difficult technically and is necessary only if one wishes to prevent the secretion of antidiuretic hormone that occurs during surgery.

Perfusion fixation of the kidney is the method of choice for most studies in experimental animals (Figures 7–14). However, vascular perfusion would be an inappropriate procedure if one were interested in the position of vascular tracer particles previously given to the animal because the position of the tracer would be changed during the vascular perfusion.

Andrews and Porter (1974) demonstrated by scanning electron microscopy the presence of apical processes, which they called tendrils, after intravascular perfusion with two solutions—a rinse solution and the fixative. They postulated that the tendrils were rudimentary cilia. It now seems likely that these elongated apical processes were formed by the reexpansion of partially collapsed proximal tubules (Maunsbach, 1966a; Bulger *et al.*, 1976) (Figure 15).

3. Applying Fixative to the Kidney Surface in Vivo

In 1955 Pease dripped fixative on the surface of an *in situ* functioning kidney. Such a procedure provides adequate fixation for only a narrow zone of tissue from the outer cortex adjacent to the surface. These outer rows of tubules are fixed with patent lumens (Figure 5). The animal will continue to live for an extended period. However, in the normal experimental animal, only a very occasional renal corpuscle is superficial enough to be fixed by the dripping procedure. More recently, to study glomerular structure by dripping procedures, investigators have used the mutant strain of Wistar rats developed in Munich, which is characterized by the presence of superficial glomeruli. One must question whether these Wistar rats are truly normal or represent some type of developmental pathology. This question has not been carefully studied. If, instead of dripping fixative on the kidney, one fills the abdominal cavity with fixative solution, the animal lives for approximately 15 min and a larger area of superficial cortex from the upper half of the kidney (which can include a few renal corpuscles) is well fixed. However, if the fixative is dripped *in situ* onto only a small area of the lateral superficial cortex and then off of the animal and not allowed to enter the abdominal cavity, the animal will live for longer periods with no change in blood pressure (Tisher, personal communication). In this case, the zone of fixed tubules extends deeper into the cortex. The depth of

←——

Figure 11. A transmission electron micrograph of a rat glomerular capillary loop gives a two-dimensional image of a thin section of the kidney with a high resolution. 8,600×.

Figure 12. A scanning electron micrograph of a rabbit glomerular capillary loop gives a three-dimensional image with a resolution intermediate between LM and TEM. 6,500×.

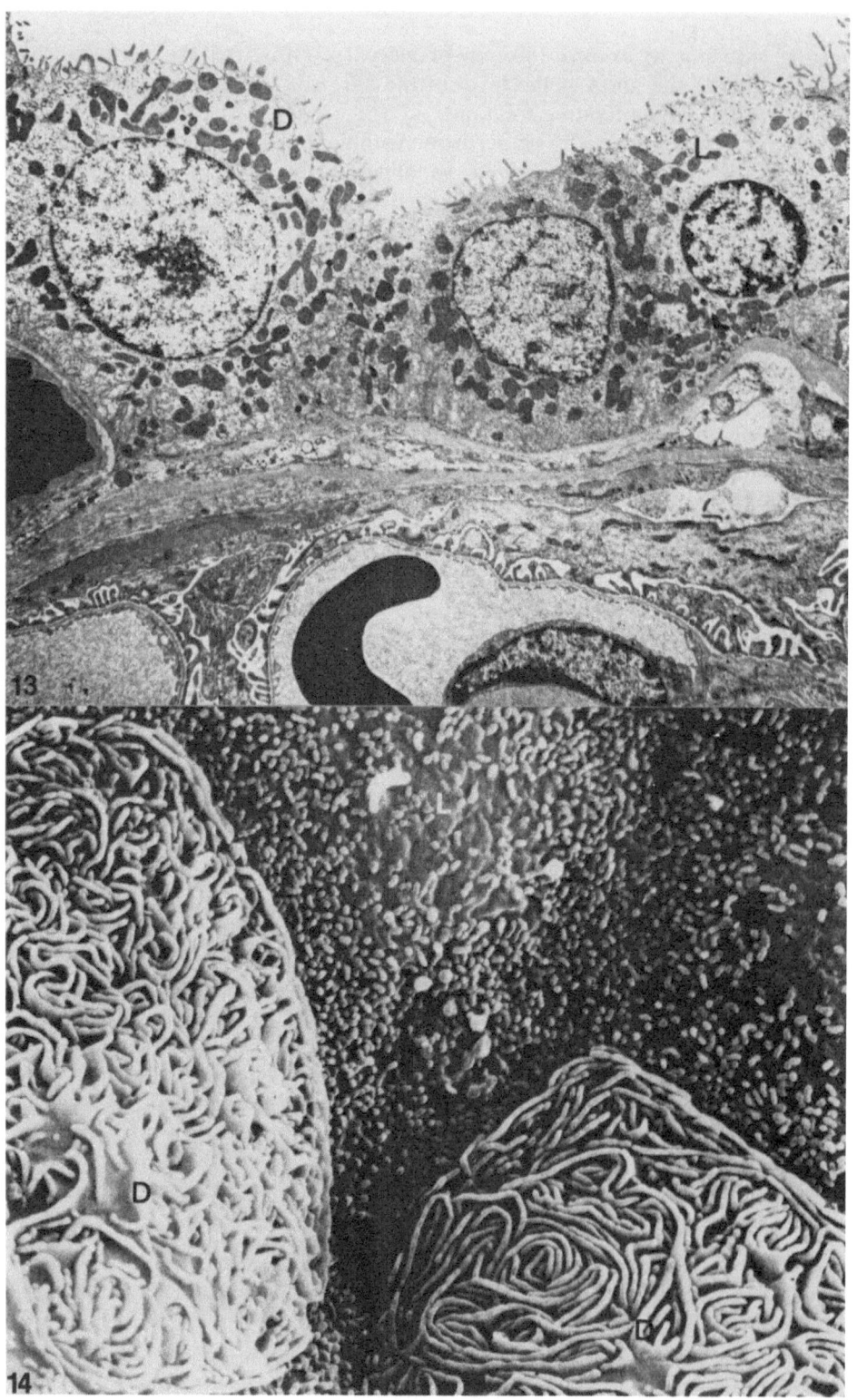

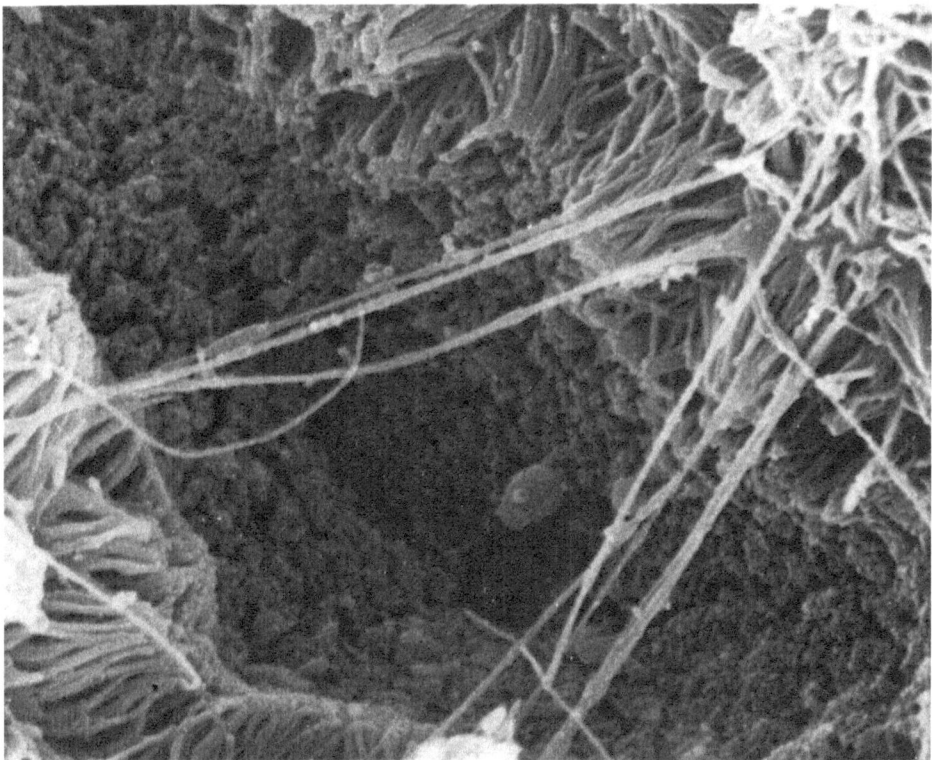

Figure 15. A scanning electron micrograph showing long extensions from the apical surface of a proximal tubule which is an artifact thought to be produced by the reexpansion of a partially collapsed tubule during perfusion fixation. 10,200×.

penetration is also increased by adding formaldehyde to the fixative or by decreasing the concentration of glutaraldehyde.

4. Microperfusion of a Tubule

Thoenes et al. (1965) developed a technique for the fixation of a renal tubule by microinjection of the fixative directly into the lumen of the tubule. With this procedure one gets rapid fixation of the perfused tubule because of the proximity of the fixative to the cells. In addition, one can fix a tubule previously studied by micropuncture. If one uses osmium tetroxide in the fixative, the fixed area turns brown and can be easily identified for processing. Alternately, a marker dye such as Lissamine green and/or a plastic can be microinjected into a tubule

←

Figure 13. A transmission electron micrograph of a rat collecting duct showing dark (D) and light (L) cells in section. 4,200×.

Figure 14. A scanning electron micrograph of a rat collecting duct showing a surface view of dark (D) and light (L) cells. 8,050×.

lumen which has been studied by micropuncture techniques. In the study of Barratt *et al.* (1975), the punctured tubule was fixed first by microinjection of the fixative, followed by a microinjection of latex to aid in identification of the puncture site.

5. Injection of Fixative

In specific instances, the injection of fixative directly into the kidney has been a useful fixation technique. For example, good fixation of the renal medulla has been obtained by this method (Bulger and Trump, 1966). In addition, injections were utilized by Farquhar *et al.* (1961) to obtain adequate fixation of injected vasculature tracer particles in glomeruli.

C. Chemical Fixatives

The composition of the fixative and the vehicle in which the fixing agent exists can profoundly affect the ultrastructural appearance of the kidney (Bulger, 1965; Maunsbach *et al.*, 1962; Maunsbach, 1966b, 1973; Trump and Ericsson, 1965). Buffered osmium tetroxide solutions were used as the fixative in the early ultrastructural studies (Palade, 1952). Osmium tetroxide reacts primarily with lipids, but appears also to fix some proteins. In spite of this, kidneys fixed initially with osmium tetroxide were not protected from osmotic stresses and the cells and organelles were characterized by swelling (Bulger, 1969). In addition, osmium tetroxide largely inactivates enzymes, which severely limits its use in studies involving histochemical reactions (Sabatini *et al.*, 1963). The introduction of aldehyde fixatives such as formaldehyde or glutaraldehyde (Sabatini *et al.*, 1963) or a combination of these (Karnovsky, 1965) has provided much new information because of the good quality of these solutions in stabilizing proteins. The glutaraldehyde cross-links proteins but is not a good fixative for lipids. When used at room temperature, it preserves the intracellular microtubules which are not preserved in cold osmium tetroxide. Maunsbach (1966b) demonstrated that the addition of varying amounts of sodium chloride to certain glutaraldehyde fixative solutions can change the ultrastructure of the tissue. Bohman and Maunsbach (1970) have shown that adding oncotically active substances such as dextran or polyvinylpyrrolidone to aldehyde fixatives utilized for intravascular perfusion prevents expansion of extravascular spaces in tissues, including the kidney.

Improved fixation of the renal medulla was obtained by Bohman (1974) by increasing the perfusion pressure, adding lidocaine chloride to the perfusion fluid, and using sodium chloride to adjust the final osmolality of the fixative to that found in the medullary zone to be fixed.

Aldehyde-fixed tissues are generally postfixed with osmium tetroxide, which not only stabilizes the lipid but also serves as an electron stain. Membranes which are not postfixed appear light in electron micrographs.

It has recently been found that injured cells can react significantly differently to fixation than normal cells (Penttila *et al.*, 1975). Therefore, more attention must be paid to the preservation of cellular volume during fixation if one is studying injured cells.

For kidney fixation on clinical services, it would be ideal to use the same fixative for both light and electron microscopy. Suitable fixatives have been developed for this purpose (Carson *et al.*, 1973; McDowell and Trump, in press). A fixative containing 4% commercial formaldehyde and 1% glutaraldehyde prepared in a 200 milliosmolar phosphate buffer provides adequate preservation for use with routine automated histologic processing, while the edge of the block is still satisfactory for electron microscopy, even after prolonged storage in the fixative solution (McDowell and Trump, in press).

D. Additives during the Fixation Procedure

Numerous histochemical procedures can be utilized on glutaraldehyde-fixed tissue for demonstration of enzymes at an electron microscope level (see review of Longley, 1969). In addition, a variety of chemical compounds have been added to fixatives in order to display certain morphological features not readily demonstrated by routine fixation procedures. Colloidal or ionic lanthanum salts have been used to demonstrate "tightness" of renal junctional elements (Revel and Karnovsky, 1967; Silverblatt and Bulger, 1970; Whittembury and Rawlins, 1971; Tisher and Yarger, 1973; Giacomelli and Wiener, 1976). Tannic acid added to the fixative delineates substructure of extracellular components such as the filtration-slit membrane (Rodewald and Karnovsky, 1974). The addition of lead citrate to the fixative will stain dextran particles which have been injected as a vascular tracer (Caulfield and Farquhar, 1974). The addition of cationized ferritin prepared at a variety of pH values can be used to study the location of charge in tissue (Rennke *et al.*, 1975).

E. Species Differences

Profound morphological differences are seen among kidneys of different species. The morphology of rat kidney has been studied most thoroughly (see review of Maunsbach, 1973; Trump and Bulger, 1968). A series of papers on the ultrastructure of human kidneys exists, but these kidneys were largely obtained many years ago and therefore were fixed with osmium tetroxide (Ericsson *et al.*, 1965; Tisher *et al.*, 1966, 1968; Bulger *et al.*, 1967; Myers *et al.*, 1966; Jorgensen and Bentzon, 1968; Trump and Bulger, 1968). These papers do show that human kidneys differ from rat kidneys in a number of important ways. Recent papers on the ultrastructure of rabbit proximal tubule (Wellings and Wellings, 1975, 1976) document important differences between rabbit and rat kidney as well. However, many of the physiological studies utilize rabbits and dogs as experimental animals. The morphology of these species has not been studied as thoroughly as is necessary for making good structural–functional correlations in these species. Because of the marked species variation in structure, it does not seem justifiable to refer to the structure found in the rat to explain functional studies obtained with other species.

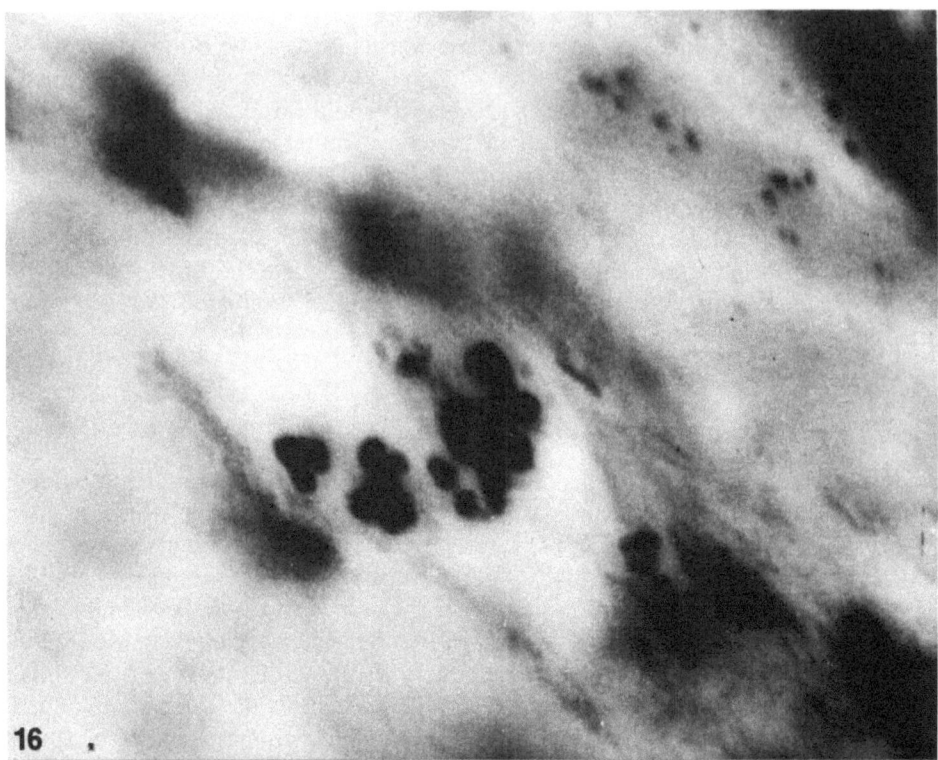

16

PHA22 ADD .020KEV/CH   100.5ECS
BUG= 3.700KEV,   170.

.000   10.220
                              100.
17

IV. AN ALTERNATE METHOD OF FREEZING

The adequacy of chemical fixation can be monitored by the use of alternate methods such as rapid freezing of tissue. Rebhun (1972) has written an excellent review on tissue freezing. (Figure 6 is an example of kidney which was rapidly frozen, dried at −40°C, fixed in formaldehyde vapor, vacuum-embedded, sectioned, and photographed (Griffith *et al.*, 1967). Frozen tissues can also be processed for viewing by substitution of solvents at low temperature, or they can be sectioned directly for viewing either at a light or electron microscope level (Christensen, 1971) (Figure 16).

Tissues which have been fixed with aldehyde can also be rapidly frozen and then fractured (with or without the removal of water by etching). A carbon and platinum replica is then prepared for viewing with an electron microscope (Friederici, 1969; Leak, 1968; Pricam *et al.*, 1974).

V. MORPHOLOGICAL PROCEDURES AVAILABLE FOR USE

A. Light Microscopy

The light microscope has provided much information about kidneys on a tissue and cellular level (Figures 3–10). Although the surface of living kidney can be viewed using a light microscope, most studies have relied on tissue which has been fixed, dehydrated, embedded in paraffin, sectioned, and stained (Figures 7, 8). Using these techniques, large areas of kidney can be studied. Numerous general staining and specific histochemical procedures have been utilized in describing renal morphology (see reviews of Mollendorff, 1930; Rouiller and Muller, 1969; Longley, 1969). The light microscope has limited usefulness in resolving subcellular organelles from kidney cells, although improved images are obtained if semithin (1 μm) plastic sections are used instead of the thicker paraffin ones (Figure 9). Any structure smaller than 0.2 μm cannot be resolved by the light microscope; therefore the study of renal morphology gained an enormous impetus when the transmission electron microscope with its vastly improved resolution was applied to renal research (Figure 10).

B. Transmission Electron Microscopy

The transmission electron microscope (TEM) utilizes the short wavelength associated with electrons to provide an image with high resolving power (3–5 Å)

Figure 16. A transmission electron micrograph of kidney which has been rapidly frozen and sectioned by cryoultramicrotomy. This micrograph shows granules in a kidney mitochondria. (Courtesy of Mr. Seung Chang.) 52,200×.

Figure 17. An energy dispersive spectrum taken from a dense granule in a kidney mitochondria from frozen material which demonstrates high concentrations of calcium and phosphorus. The two peaks on the right are derived from the titanium grid on which the section was placed.

(Figures 10, 11, 13). The tissues to be studied are all fixed, embedded in plastic, and sectioned very thinly (less than 1,000 Å) so that the slices can be penetrated by the electrons in the instrument's beam. Because of the thin sections, the images produced have a two-dimensional quality. The high resolution allows one to study the subcellular and suborganellar architecture, as well as that of large molecules in the kidney. Because of the technical difficulty encountered in processing material for electron microscopy, very small pieces of tissue must be examined. One must guard against the sampling error due to the small number of cells which are studied. A concomitant study of semithin plastic sections with a light microscope serves as a control for the TEM studies. The examination of any textbook on renal pathophysiology will demonstrate the enormous impact of TEM on the understanding of normal and abnormal structure.

C. Scanning Electron Microscopy (SEM)

The scanning electron microscope has recently been developed and applied to the study of renal morphology (Andrews and Porter, 1974; Arakawa, 1970, 1971; Arakawa and Tokunaga, 1972, 1974; Bulger *et al.*, 1974, 1976; Buss, 1970; Buss and Krönert, 1969; Spinelli *et al.*, 1972).

The scanning electron microscope produces a three-dimensional representation of surface structure (Figures 12 and 14). Although the resolution of this instrument (~70 Å) is not as high as in TEM, tissue processing is easy and large pieces of tissue can be scanned at magnifications equivalent to light microscopy, and then specific areas can be studied at this higher resolution. In a scanning electron microscope, a narrow beam of electrons scans across the specimen. As this occurs, a variety of radiations are reflected or produced. The secondary electrons given off by the atoms of the specimen are collected and used to produce the familiar secondary image. In addition, X-rays and electrons of specific types are given off which can be collected and analyzed to provide information on the kind and number of atoms present in the tissue (Figure 17). The morphology of the atoms of the kidney can now be studied (see below).

D. Microanalysis of Tissue Sections

The most exciting new technology now available for morphological study is that which allows one to identify the atoms in tissue in both a qualitative and quantitative manner. Some of the X-rays which are emitted from a tissue specimen when it is bombarded by an electron beam in an SEM or TEM have wavelengths and energies characteristic for the atoms from which they are derived. The X-rays can be collected and sorted on the basis of these wavelengths or energies. A typical electron energy spectrum from kidney can be seen in Figure 17. One can therefore identify elements with atomic numbers greater than and including sodium if they are present in the tissue at concentration levels of 0.1% or above. In addition to the characteristic X-rays, some nonspecific radiation occurs which is used to provide a guide to specimen thickness, thus allowing quantitative analysis of elements within the sections. When one is dealing with an insoluble precipitate, tissues can be processed using routine procedures. Osmium fixation and heavy metal staining should be avoided. However, if one is interested in soluble substances or ions, one must fix the tissue by shock freezing (Rebhun, 1972) and it must be sectioned using a freezing attachment on an ultramicrotome (Christensen, 1971) while the tissue is maintained at a temperature lower than that at which ice recrystallization occurs. The sections are dried before use. Many recent symposia, such as that published in the *Journal de Microscopie et de Biologie Cellulaire* (Vol. 22, pp. 121–493, 1975), have considered technical difficulties associated with microanalysis and should be consulted for more information. Dorge *et al.* (1975) have utilized kidney slices for microanalysis of ionic composition. Saubermann and Echlin (1975) have developed a technique to study frozen sections while they are still hydrated.

In addition to X-ray emission, Auger electrons are given off by the bombarded atoms and these electrons can be used for analysis by Auger spectroscopy. Electrons in the beam also undergo characteristic energy changes when interacting with the specimen, and some investigators are attempting to utilize this electron energy loss for elemental analysis. Although many technical difficulties are experienced in microanalysis, this area offers an exciting challenge for future research.

VI. PROCEDURES FOR ELECTRON MICROSCOPY OF KIDNEY

Although many variations in routine processing have been successfully utilized in renal research, the following procedures are those utilized in our laboratory.

A. Routine Procedures for Transmission Electron Microscopy

1. Fix tissue by method of choice (see earlier discussion on routes of fixative administration). The following are fixatives frequently used in studies of kidney tissue.

   a. Karnovsky's fixative (Karnovsky, 1965). Many investigators use this fixative, which consists of 5% glutaraldehyde and 4% formaldehyde, buffered either with phosphate or cacodylate and used either at full or half strength.

   b. McDowell–Trump fixative (McDowell and Trump, in press). These authors advocate the use of 4% formaldehyde–1% glutaraldehyde in 200 mOs*M* phosphate buffer which is made from commercial grade formaldehyde and is suitable for both routine light and electron microscopy.

   c. 2.5–4% glutaraldehyde in 0.1 *M* phosphate or cacodylate buffer (~pH 7.2–7.4). Various concentrations of glutaraldehyde have been used with success.

2. Quickly dice tissue into 1-mm cubes and place in fixative for 4 hr. (Tissue to be fixed by immersion can be diced in the fixative.)

3. Wash tissue by placing overnight in a solution of 0.1 M cacodylate buffer (pH 7.2) which contains 7% sucrose.

4. Postfix tissue for 1 hr at 4°C in 1–2% osmium tetroxide in 0.1 M s-collidine solution (pH 7.2–7.4) (Bennett and Luft, 1959).

5. If desired, stain in block with 0.5% uranyl acetate in veronal acetate buffer (pH 5.0) for 1 hr at room temperature (Farquhar and Palade, 1965). If phosphate buffer is used in step 4, the tissue must be rinsed in veronal acetate buffer (pH 5.0) prior to staining.

6. Dehydration. To dehydrate, decant the solution in the bottle and then add the next solution listed at 15-min intervals.

    a. Fixative
    b. 35% alcohol
    c. 70% alcohol
    d. 95% alcohol
    e. 100% alcohol
    f. 100% alcohol
    g. propylene oxide
    h. propylene oxide

7. Embedding. The Epon epoxy embedding procedure of Luft (1961) is generally used.

    a. Stock solutions

       1. Mixture A
           Epon 812   70 ml
           DDSA   100 ml

       2. Mixture B
           Epon 812 100 ml
           NMA   79 ml

       3. DMP-30   1½–2%

Stock solutions of mixtures A and B are kept in the refrigerator. They should be removed from the refrigerator in time for the mixtures to be at room temperature when opened. DMP-30 is used to catalyze the reaction. It should be mixed with solutions A and B in a ratio of 1.5% to 2% by volume. (Presently we are using 2%.) For usual hardness, a 1:1 ratio of A and B gives the desired result. Dodecenyl succinic anhydride (DDSA) makes the resin soft. Nadic methyl anhydride (NMA) is used for hardening. To vary the hardness, increase or decrease the amount of A with respect to B. This embedding medium must be well mixed before use (10–20 min of stirring).

8. Procedure for embedding

    a. After decanting the second change of propylene oxide, add a mixture of ½ propylene oxide and ½ Epon resin prepared from stock solutions A and B with catalyzer and leave for 1 hr.

    b. Add an additional volume of resin equal to the volume in the bottle and allow tissue to remain in this from 2 hr to overnight.

    c. Place gelatin or Beem capsules in embedding boards.

    d. Fill each capsule with a strip on which the sample number is typed and the resin mixture. The tissue is placed on the resin surface and allowed to settle. The embedding boards are placed in a 60°C oven for 2 days.

B. Rapid Procedures for Transmission Electron Microscopy

  1. Method (Bencosme and Tsutsumi, 1970; Johannessen, 1973):

    a. Fix tissues by the method of choice (cut not thicker than 0.5 mm) for 15 min.

    b. Rinse in three changes of 0.1 M sodium cacodylate with 7% sucrose (pH 7.4).

    c. Postfix in 1% O_sO_4 in 0.1 M s-collidine buffer for 15 min. The tissue may be stained in block with uranyl acetate for 20 min if desired.

    d. Place in 50% ethanol for 3 min.

    e. Place in 70% ethanol for 3 min.

    f. Place in 95% ethanol for 3 min.

    g. Place in two changes of 100% ethanol for 5 min each.

    h. Place in two changes of propylene oxide for 5 min each.

    i. Place in 1:1 mixture of complete Epon solution and propylene oxide for 5 min.

    j. Place in a mixture of 1 part propylene oxide to 3 parts Epon solution for 15 min.

Note: All the above steps are carried out at room temperature on a tissue rotor.

    k. Embed tissues in fresh Epon solution in Beem capsules.

    l. Place capsules with tissues in 70°C oven for 45 min.

    m. Transfer capsules to 95° oven for 45 min.

C. Routine Sample Preparation for Scanning Electron Microscopy

  1. Fix by the desired route using procedures as described for transmission microscopy. Larger pieces of tissue can be used but they must not exceed the size of the metal stub on which they are to be mounted.

  2. Postfix in a solution of 1% osmium tetroxide buffered with 0.1 M s-collidine (pH 7.2–7.4) for 90 min at room temperature.

  3. Dehydrate in a graded series of ethanol.

  4. The tissues are then dried in a critical point drying apparatus (Anderson, 1951).

  5. Mount the dried pieces of tissue on aluminum stubs using double-sided tape or conducting silver paint.

  6. The tissues are then coated with a thin coat of gold or gold–palladium using a sputtering device. The coating protects the tissue from charging when it is bombarded by the scanning electron beam.

  7. Examine.

REFERENCES

Anderson, T. F. 1951. Techniques for the preservation of three-dimensional structure in preparing specimens for the electron microscope. *Trans. N.Y. Acad. Sci., 13:*130.

Andrews, P. M., and Porter, K. R. 1974. A scanning electron microscopic study of the nephron. *Am. J. Anat., 140:*81.

Arakawa, M. 1970. A scanning electron microscopy of the glomerulus of normal and nephrotic rats. *Lab. Invest., 23:*489.

Arakawa, M. 1971. A scanning electron microscope study of the human glomerulus. *Am. J. Path., 64:*457.

Arakawa, M., and Tokunaga, J. 1972. A scanning electron microscope study of the glomerulus. Further considerations of the mechanism of fusion of podocyte terminal processes in nephrotic rats. *Lab. Invest., 27:*366.

Arakawa, M., and Tokunaga, J. 1974. Further scanning electron microscope studies of the human glomerulus. *Lab. Invest., 31:*436.

Barratt, L. J., Rector, F. C., Jr., Kokko, J. P., Tisher, C. C., and Seldin, D. W. 1975. Transepithelial potential difference profile in the distal tubule of the rat kidney. *Kidney Internat., 8:*368.

Bencosme, S. A., and Tsutsumi, V. 1970. A fast method for processing biologic material for electron microscopy. *Lab. Invest., 23:*447.

Bennett, H. S., and Luft, J. H. 1959. *s*-Collidine as a basis for buffering fixatives. *J. Biophys. Biochem. Cytol., 6:*113.

Bohman, S.-O. 1974. The ultrastructure of the rat renal medulla as observed after improved fixation methods. *J. Ultrastruct. Res., 47:*329.

Bohman, S.-O., and Maunsbach, A. B. 1970. Effects on tissue fine structure of variations in colloid osmotic pressure of glutaraldehyde fixatives. *J. Ultrastruct. Res., 30:*195.

Bulger, R. E., 1965. The fine structure of the aglomerular nephron of the toadfish, *Opsanus tau. Am. J. Anat., 117:*171.

Bulger, R. E. 1969. The use of potassium pyroantimonate in the localization of sodium ions in rat kidney tissue. *J. Cell Biol., 40:*79.

Bulger, R. E., and Trump, B. F. 1966. Fine structure of the rat renal papilla. *Am. J. Anat., 118:*685.

Bulger, R. E., Tisher, C. C., Myers, C. H., and Trump, B. F. 1967. Human renal ultrastructure. II. The thin limb of Henle's loop and the interstitium in healthy individuals. *Lab. Invest., 16:*124.

Bulger, R. E., Siegel, F. L., and Pendergrass, R. 1974. Scanning and transmission electron microscopy of the rat kidney. *Am. J. Anat., 139:*483.

Bulger, R. E., Siegel, F. L., and Pendergrass, R. 1976. Proximal tubule tendrils: Fact or artifact. *Am. J. Anat., 146:*323.

Burg, M., Grantham, J., Abramow, M., and Orloff, J. 1966. Preparation and study of fragments of single rabbit nephrons. *Am. J. Physiol., 210:*1296.

Buss, H. 1970. Die morphologische Differenzierung des Viscera en Blattes der Bowmanschen Kapsel. Raster-und durchstrahlungselectronenmikroskopische Untersuchungen am Nierenglomerulum der Ratte, *Z. Zellforsch., 111:*346.

Buss, H., and Krönert, W. 1969. Zur Struktur des Nierenglomerulum der Ratte, *Virchows Arch. Abt. B. Zellpath., 4:*79.

Carson, F. L., Martin, J. H., and Lynn, J. A. 1973. Formalin fixation for electron microscopy. A reevaluation, *Am. J. Clin. Path., 59:*368.

Caulfield, J. P., and Farquhar, M. G. 1974. The permeability of glomerular capillaries to graded dextrans. Identification of the basement membrane as the primary filtration barrier. *J. Cell Biol., 63:*883.

Christensen, A. K. 1971. Frozen thin sections of fresh tissue for electron microscopy, with a description of pancreas and liver. *J. Cell Biol., 51:*772.

Dorge, A., Rick, R., Gehring, K., Mason, J., and Thurau, K. 1975. Preparation and applicability of freeze-dried sections in the microprobe analysis of biological soft tissue. *J. Microscopie Biol. Cell, 22:*205.

Ericsson, J. L. E. 1966. Glutaraldehyde perfusion of the kidney for preservation of proximal tubules with patent lumens. *J. Microscopie 5:*97.

Ericsson, J. L. E., Bergstrand, A., Andres, G., Bucht, H., and Cinottii, G. 1965. Morphology of the renal tubular epithelium in young healthy humans. *Acta Path. Microbiol. Scand., 63:*361.

Farquhar, M. G., and Palade, G. E. 1965. Cell junctions in amphibian skin. *J. Cell Biol., 26:*263.

Farquhar, M. G., Wissig, S. L., and Palade, G. 1961. Glomerular permeability. I. Ferritin transfer across the normal glomerular capillary wall. *J. Exp. Med., 113:*47.

Forster, R. P. 1948. Use of thin kidney slices and isolated renal tubules for direct study of cellular transport kinetics. *Science, 108:*65.

Friederici, H. H. R. 1969. The surface structure of some renal cell membranes. *Lab. Invest., 21:*459.

Ghiron, M. 1912. Über eine neue Methode mikroskopischer Untersuchung am lebenden Organismus. *Zbl. Physiol., 26:*613.

Giacomelli, F., and Wiener, J. 1976. Specialized junction in the distal convoluted tubule of rat kidney. *Anat. Rec., 185:*197.

Griffith, L. D., Bulger, R. E., and Trump, B. F. 1967. The ultrastructure of the functioning kidney. *Lab. Invest., 16:*220.

Johannessen, J. V. 1973. Rapid processing of kidney biopsies for electron microscopy. *Kidney Internat., 3:*46.

Jorgensen, F., and Bentzon, M. W. 1968. The ultrastructure of the normal human glomerulus. Thickness of glomerular basement membrane. *Lab. Invest., 18:*42.

Karnovsky, M. J. 1965. A formaldehyde–glutaraldehyde fixative of high osmolality for use in electron microscopy. *J. Cell Biol., 27:*137A.

Koenig, H., Groat, A., and Windel, W. F. 1945. A physiological approach to perfusion-fixation of tissues with formalin. *Stain Technol., 20:*13.

Leak, L. V. 1968. Ultrastructure of proximal tubule cells in mouse kidney as revealed by freeze etching. *J. Ultrastruct. Res., 25:*253.

Longley, J. B. 1969. Histochemistry of the kidney. In: *The Kidney. Morphology, Biochemistry, Physiology,* Vol. I, pp. 157–259. Ed. by Rouiller, C., and Muller, A., Academic Press, New York.

Luft, J. H. 1961. Improvements in epoxy resin embedding methods. *J. Biophys. Biochem. Cytol., 9:*409.

Maunsbach, A. B. 1966a. The influence of different fixatives and fixation methods on the ultrastructure of rat kidney proximal tubule cells. I. Comparison of different perfusion fixation methods and of glutaraldehyde, formaldehyde and osmium tetroxide fixatives. *J. Ultrastruct. Res., 15:*242.

Maunsbach, A. B. 1966b. The influence of different fixatives and fixation methods on the ultrastructure of rat kidney proximal tubule cells. II. Effects of varying osmolality, ionic strength, buffer system and fixative concentration of glutaraldehyde solutions. *J. Ultrastruct. Res., 15:*283.

Maunsbach, A. B. 1973. Ultrastructure of the proximal tubule. In: *Handbook of Physiology,* Vol. 8, pp. 31–79. Ed. by Orloff, J., and Berliner, R. American Physiological Society, Washington, D.C.

Maunsbach, A. B., Madden, S. C., and Latta, H. 1962. Variations in fine structure of renal tubular epithelium under different conditions of fixation. *J. Ultrastruct. Res., 6:*511.

McDowell, E. M., and Trump, B. F. In press. Histological fixatives suitable for routine diagnostic light and electron microscopy. *Arch. Path.*

Mollendorff, W. V. 1930. Der Exkretionsapparat. In: *Handbuch der Mikroscopischen Anatomie des Menschen,* Vol. VII, Part I. Ed. by Mollendorff, W. V. Springer, Berlin.

Myers, C. E., Bulger, R. E., Tisher, C. C., and Trump, B. F. 1966. Human renal ultrastructure. IV. Collecting ducts of healthy individuals. *Lab. Invest., 15:*1921.

Palade, G. E. 1952. A study of fixation for electron microscopy. *J. Exp. Med. 95:*285.

Pease, D. C. 1955. Electron microscopy of the tubular cells of the kidney cortex. *Anat. Rec., 121:*723.

Penttila, A., McDowell, E. M., and Trump, B. F. 1975. Effects of fixation and postfixation treatments on volume of injured cells. *J. Histochem. Cytochem., 23:*251.

Pricam, C., Humbert, F., Perrelet, A., and Orci, L. 1974a. A freeze-etch study of the tight junctions of the rat kidney tubules. *Lab. Invest., 30:*286.

Rebhun, L. I. 1972. Freeze-substitution and freeze-drying. In: *Principles and Techniques of Electron*

Microscopy. Biological Applications, Vol. 2, pp. 3–53. Ed. by Hayat, M. A. Reinhold, New York.

Rennke, H. G., Cotran, R. S., and Venkatachalam, M. A. 1975. Role of molecular charge in glomerular permeability. Tracer studies with cationized ferritins. *J. Cell Biol., 67:*638.

Revel, J. P., and Karnovsky, M. J. 1967. Hexagonal array of subunits in intercellular junctions of the mouse heart and liver. *J. Cell Biol., 33:*C7.

Rodewald, R., and Karnovsky, M. J. 1974. Porous substructure of the glomerular slit diaphragm in the rat and mouse. *J. Cell Biol., 60:*423.

Rouiller, C., and Muller, A. 1969. *The Kidney. Morphology, Biochemistry, Physiology,* Vol. I, Academic Press, New York.

Sabatini, D. D., Bensch, K., and Barrnett, R. J. 1963. Cytochemistry and electron microscopy. The preservation of cellular ultrastructure and enzymatic activity by aldehyde fixation. *J. Cell Biol., 17:*19.

Saubermann, A. J., and Echlin, P. 1975. The preparation, examination and analysis of frozen hydrated tissue sections by scanning transmission electron microscopy and x-ray microanalysis. *J. Microscop., 105:*155.

Schwartz, M. M., and Venkatachalam, M. A. 1974. Structural differences in thin limbs of Henle: physiological implications. *Kidney Internat., 6:*193.

Silverblatt, F. J., and Bulger, R. E. 1970. Gap junctions occur in vertebrate renal proximal tubule cells. *J. Cell Biol., 47:*513.

Spinelli, F., Wirz, H., Brucher, C., and Pehling, G. 1972. *Fine Structure of the Kidney Revealed by Scanning Electron Microscopy* Ciba-Geigy, Basle, Switzerland.

Steinhausen, M. 1965. Microscopy and photomigrography of the living kidney with the ultropak incident-light illuminator. *Sci. Tech. Information* (Leitz) *1*(4):103.

Swann, H. G. 1960. The functional distention of the kidney: A review. *Texas Rep. Biol. Med., 18:*566.

Swann, H. G. 1964. Some aspects of renal blood flow and tissue pressure. *Circ. Res., 15*(Suppl. 2):115.

Tisher, C. C., and Yarger, W. E. 1973. Lanthanum permeability of the tight junction (zonula occludens) in the renal tubule of the rat. *Kidney Int., 3:*238.

Tisher, C. C., Bulger, R. E., and Trump, B. F. 1966. Human renal ultrastructure. I. Proximal tubule of healthy individuals. *Lab. Invest., 14:*1357.

Tisher, C. C., Bulger, R. E., and Trump, B. F. 1968. Human renal ultrastructure. III. The distal tubule in healthy individuals. *Lab. Invest., 18:*655.

Tisher, C. C., Rosen, S., and Osborne, G. B. 1969. Ultrastructure of the proximal tubule of the Rhesus monkey kidney. *Am. J. Pathol., 56:*469.

Thoenes, W., Hierholzer, K., and Wiederholt, M. 1965. Gezielte Fixierung von Nierentubuli *in vivo* durch Mikroperfusion zur licht- und elektronenmikroskopischen Untersuchung. *Klin. Wschr., 43:*794.

Trump, B. F., and Bulger, R. E. 1968. Morphology of the kidney. In: *Structural Basis of Renal Disease.* Ed. by Becker, E. L. Harper & Row, New York.

Trump, B. F., and Ericsson, J. L. E. 1965. The effect of the fixative solution on the ultrastructure of cells and tissues. A comparative analysis with particular attention to the proximal convoluted tubule of the rat kidney. *Lab. Invest., 14:*1245.

Valtin, H. 1967. Hereditary hypothalamic diabetes insipidus in rats (Brattleboro strain). A useful experimental model. *Am. J. Med., 42:*814.

Wearn, J. T., and Richards, A. N. 1924. Observations on the composition of glomerular urine with particular reference to the problem of reabsorption in the renal tubules. *Am. J. Physiol., 71:*209.

Wellings, L. W., and Wellings, D. J. 1975. Surface areas of the brush border and lateral cell walls in the rabbit proximal nephron. *Kidney Int. 8:*343.

Wellings, L. W., and Wellings, D. J. 1976. Shape of epithelial cells and intercellular channels in the rabbit proximal nephron. *Kidney Int., 9:*385.

Whittembury, G., and Rawlins, F. A. 1971. Evidence of a paracellular pathway for ion flow in the kidney proximal tubule: electronmicroscopic demonstration of lanthanum precipitate in the tight junction. *Pflugers Arch., 330:*302.

Chapter **2**

Clearance Methods in the Rat

Susan Opava Stitzer

Department of Physiology
University of Puerto Rico School of Medicine
San Juan, Puerto Rico

and

Manuel Martinez-Maldonado

Veterans Administration Center and
Departments of Physiology and Medicine
University of Puerto Rico School of Medicine
San Juan, Puerto Rico

I. INTRODUCTION

Prior to the advent of micropuncture and microperfusion techniques, clearance studies were the foundation of research in renal physiology. Even today, despite the availability of more sophisticated methods, they are still the mainstay of the renal investigator. Clearance studies continue to be the only method for observing effects on the function of the kidney as a whole *in vivo* and can be used to examine all of the major functions which the kidney performs, i.e., filtration, reabsorption, and secretion. Another obvious advantage of clearance methods over micropuncture or microperfusion techniques is that they are considerably easier and less costly to utilize.

Even a cursory review of the application of clearance techniques since the initiation of their use reveals that the vast majority of clearance studies have been carried out in the dog. No doubt this is because of the relative ease of surgical preparation and the lack of technical problems in the dog. Nevertheless, when one considers the advantages that the rat offers as a preparation for clearance studies, it is surprising that so few studies have been carried out in this species. Lately a number of studies from several laboratories have relied on clearance techniques in the rat, showing the suitability and reliability of this species for studies of concentrating and diluting ability (Martínez-Maldonado *et al.*, 1969, 1974; Eknoyan *et al.*, 1970; Wallin *et al.*, 1973; Emmanouel *et al.*, 1974; Michael *et al.*, 1972.)

One of the advantages which immediately comes to mind is that it is far less costly to perform experiments in the rat than in the dog. This is true not only because the animal itself is usually cheaper to obtain but also because the quantities of supplies which are used in each experiment are much smaller. This can be an important consideration if isotopes or expensive drugs are to be used. Aside from the cost factor, rats are clearly easier to maintain in large numbers and can actually be bred by the investigator without the need for elaborate facilities. From the point of view of experimental design also, the rat is sometimes the species of choice. In cases where it is necessary or advisable to carry out balance studies or manipulate dietary conditions prior to acute clearance studies, the rat is clearly easier to use than the dog. The same is true if the experimental protocol requires that the clearance study be performed in the awake animal. Although experiments can be performed in the conscious dog, this usually requires a period of training prior to the actual experiment. In contrast, untrained rats can be studied in the conscious state by the use of a restraining cage (Figure 1). One experimental situation in which the protocol requires that the animal be conscious and therefore one for which the rat is

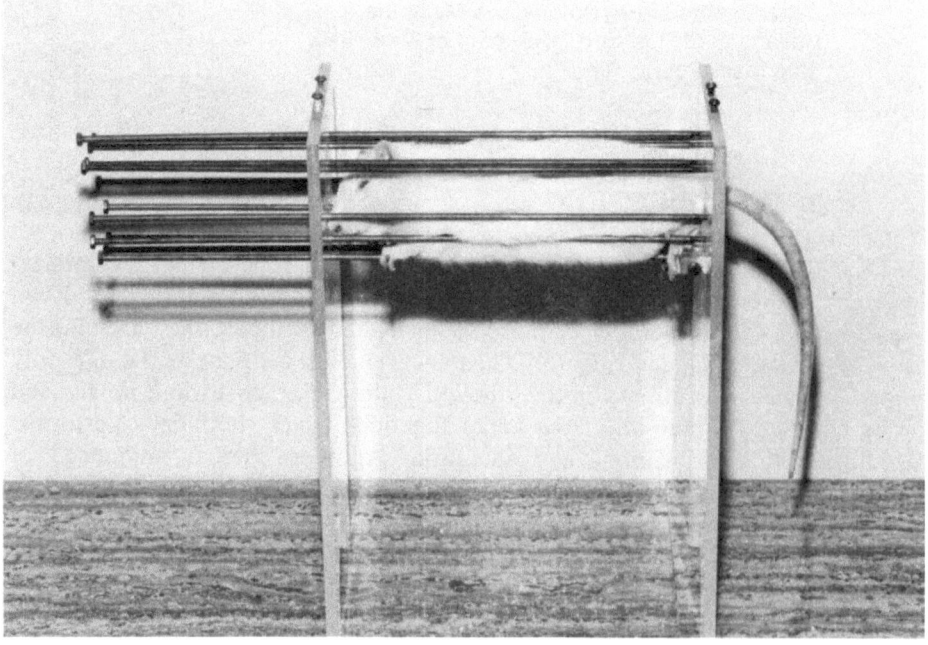

Figure 1. Restraining cage for use in studies in the conscious rat. For the photograph, the rat was not prepared surgically.

particularly suitable, is in the measurement of C_{H_2O}. Due to stimulation of ADH, maximal urine dilution can rarely be achieved under anesthesia. In contrast, the awake normal rat has a diluting ability not significantly different from the awake Brattleboro rat with its complete lack of endogenous ADH (Martínez-Maldonado and Opava Stitzer, unpublished observation.)

II. GENERAL CONSIDERATIONS

The clearance of any substance is the volume of plasma from which a substance is completely removed in a fixed period of time. The clearance of any compound may always be represented by the formula $U_X V/P_X$, where U_X and P_X are the urine and plasma concentrations of the substance, and V is the urine flow rate.

For most substances (the exceptions will be discussed below), the "clearance" is a theoretical volume, since there is no real volume of plasma from which all of the substance is removed. Rather the substance is "cleared" proportionally from each unit of plasma. Nevertheless, the clearance concept is a useful once since it simply represents the quantity of the substance that was excreted ($U_X V$) corrected for the plasma concentration (P_X).

The true value of the clearance is that in specific cases the theoretical volume (the clearance) also represents a real volume. This is true for substances which are only filtered by the kidney and for substances which are completely extracted from the plasma in one passage through the kidney. In the former case, the clearance is equal to the volume of plasma which is filtered at the glomeruli or the glomerular filtration rate (GFR). In the latter, the clearance is equal to the volume of plasma which perfuses the kidney or the renal plasma flow (RPF). These identities may be easily derived from mass balance equations as follows:

1. For a substance which is only filtered, the mass filtered *must* equal the mass excreted. An example of such a substance is inulin.

$$\underset{\text{(mg/min)}}{\text{Mass filtered}} = \underset{\text{(mg/min)}}{\text{Mass excreted}} \tag{1}$$

$$\text{GFR} \times P_{In} = U_{inulin} V \tag{2}$$

$$\text{GFR} = U_{In} V/P_{In} \tag{3}$$

$$\text{GFR} = \text{clearance of inulin} \tag{4}$$

2. For a substance which is completely extracted from the plasma in one passage through the kidney, the amount of the substance which entered the kidney *must* equal the amount excreted in the urine since there will be none of the substance remaining in the venous effluent. An example of such a substance is p-aminohippuric acid (PAH).

$$\underset{\text{(mg/min)}}{\text{Mass entering kidney}} = \underset{\text{(mg/min)}}{\text{Mass leaving kidney}} \tag{5}$$

$$\text{RPF} \times \text{PAH}_{artery} = (\text{RPF} \times \text{PAH}_{vein}) + U_{PAH} V \tag{6}$$

Since $PAH_{vein.} = 0$ and PAH_{artery} may be represented by P_{PAH}:

$$RPF \times P_{PAH} = U_{PAH}V \qquad (7)$$

$$RPF = U_{PAH}V/P_{PAH} \qquad (8)$$

$$RPF = \text{clearance of PAH} \qquad (9)$$

The above examples are valid only if the substances in question are not metabolized by the kidney. Inulin and PAH meet this requirement and for this reason their clearances are used routinely to calculate the GFR and RPF respectively.

The clearance of inulin is particularly useful since it can provide important information on the renal handling of other substances. The clearance of inulin does not vary as a function of the plasma concentration since the excretion rate varies proportionally with the plasma concentration. Any substance which is found to have a clearance greater than inulin ($C_X > C_{In}$) *must* be secreted in some part of the nephron. It may also be reabsorbed but if so, the secretory process exceeds the reabsorptive process. Conversely, when the clearance of a substance is found to be less than the clearance of inulin ($C_X < C_{In}$), the necessary conclusion is that the substance undergoes *net* reabsorption or is metabolized by the kidney. Likewise if $C_X = C_{In}$, or in other words C_X does not vary with P_X, the substance is most likely[1] neither reabsorbed nor secreted, but only filtered, as is inulin. It should be noted that if one is interested only in a comparison of the clearance of inulin with the clearance of another substance, it is unnecessary to measure V since it will contribute equally to both clearance values. The same conclusion can be drawn by comparing $(U/P)_{In}$ to $(U/P)_X$.

III. STANDARD CLEARANCE METHODS

Only three measurements need be made to calculate a clearance: U_X, P_X, and V. The method therefore, involves a timed collection of urine and the sampling of arterial blood, usually at the midpoint of the urine collection. To ensure that the arterial plasma concentration is unchanging throughout the period of urine collection, the substance to be measured should be infused intravenously at a constant rate. In the case of a compound which is to be administered as a single injection, plasma samples may be obtained instead, at the beginning and at the end of each urine collection. This will guarantee a value for the concentration in plasma which is representative of the real concentration in the plasma perfusing the kidney during the time in which the urine sample was produced.

The volume of the urine sample must be measured accurately and divided by the time over which the sample was collected (V). Sufficiently sensitive methods must be available for the assay of the substance in urine (U_X) and plasma (P_X). Plasma may require special treatment, such as precipitation of plasma proteins, to prevent interference in the required assay.

---

[1] If $C_X = C_{In}$ it is also possible that the substance is *equally* reabsorbed and secreted. It is unlikely, however, that this equality would hold over a wide range of plasma concentrations.

IV. APPLICATION OF THE CLEARANCE METHOD TO THE RAT

A. Anesthetized Rat

1. Sodium Pentobarbital

Clearance methods are conventionally used in the sodium pentobarbital anesthetized rat. A dose of 50 mg/kg of body weight intraperitoneally may be sufficient to induce and maintain deep anesthesia for as long as 8 hr without supplement. All rats which are to be anesthetized should be fasted overnight. Whether or not water is also to be removed will be determined by the protocol (e.g., antidiuresis or diuresis). When the rat is sufficiently anesthetized, a polyethylene tube (PE200) should be placed in the trachea. The length of this catheter should be no longer than approximately 3 cm to avoid respiratory acidosis caused by enlarged respiratory dead space. Polyethylene catheters (PE50) should be placed in both femoral veins and femoral arteries, and a polyethylene catheter (PE90) in the bladder. The bladder catheter may be inserted through the urethra in a female rat, or the bladder may be externalized through a short midline incision and the catheter inserted via a small incision in the bladder wall. If the latter method is used, the urethra must be ligated to ensure total urine collection through the bladder catheter. If the former, the urethra must be ligated around the catheter. If sampling of urine from each kidney separately is desired, the ureters must be catheterized instead of the bladder. PE50 tubing should be used, as PE10 has been shown to result in partial ureteral occlusion due to the small lumen (Cortell *et al.,* 1972). If GFR and/or RPF are to be measured, one venous catheter may be used for the constant infusion of inulin and/or PAH. The other venous catheter may be used for infusion or injection of other substances as the protocol demands. One arterial catheter may be connected to a blood-pressure transducer and recording apparatus for continuous monitoring of arterial pressure. The other arterial catheter is used to obtain plasma for calculation of clearances. Blood samples should be drawn into a heparinized syringe, centrifuged immediately, and the plasma separated. Each sample of arterial blood may be as large as 1 ml but should be replaced with an equal volume of whole blood from a donor rat. The donor rat may be anesthetized and prepared with an arterial catheter, or the blood may be obtained prior to the experiment by cardiac puncture or decapitation of the donor rat. If obtained in advance, the blood should be heparinized and stored on ice, and rewarmed to at least room temperature before transfusion. Donor rats should not be fasted because hypoglycemia may occur. This will result in hemolysis of the blood used for transfusion. If doubt exists about this point, we have circumvented the problem by adding enough glucose to the blood to maintain concentrations around 100 mg/100 ml. An alternative to whole blood transfusion from a donor rat is to resuspend the red cells, after plasma separation, in a Ringer's bicarbonate or Henseleit solution. A volume equal to extracted plasma should be used and the red cell suspension retransfused. This must be done rapidly lest hemolysis occur.

Urine is collected into preweighed tubes or bottles through the bladder or ureteral catheters. Urine must be collected for a period long enough to allow accumulation of a volume sufficient for analysis. The exact volume of urine obtained in a fixed period of time is determined by weighing. Frequently the container into which urine is collected contains paraffin oil to prevent sample evaporation. Should the volume be very small, it is frequently difficult to retrieve the sample for analysis. Because of this, we have opted for collection of urine samples directly into tuberculin syringes when the sample is anticipated to be small. This method is less accurate for volume determination than is the weight method. On the other hand, it allows accurate analysis without problems of oil contamination. The weight method, too, is subject to error since it assumes that 1 ml of urine weighs 1 g, yet the specific gravity of urine is always greater than 1 and may vary considerably during an experiment.

A sample experiment to determine the renal clearance of endogenous urea in the hydropenic and saline-loaded rat might be carried out as follows:

	Time (minutes)	
Clearance 1	0	Begin collection of urine into preweighed tube (No. 1).
	10	Obtain 0.5 ml of arterial blood in a heparinized syringe (P_1). Replace immediately with 0.5 ml of whole blood or resuspended cells.
	20	End collection of urine in tube 1. Begin collection in tube 2.
Clearance 2	30	Repeat blood sampling as at 10 min (P_2).
	40	End collection of urine in tube 2.
	42	Begin infusion of isotonic saline through venous catheter at a constant rate.
	42–80	Equilibration period.
Clearance 3	80	Begin urine collection into tube 3.
	85	Repeat blood sampling as previously (P_3).
	90	End collection of urine in tube 3. Begin collection in tube 4.
Clearance 4	95	Repeat blood sampling (P_4).
	100	End collection of urine into tube 4.

Four clearance values of urea can be calculated from this experiment. The four preweighed tubes containing urine are reweighed to determine the urine volume (1 ml is assumed to weigh exactly 1 g). For tubes 1 and 2 the volume obtained is divided by 20 min (the period of urine collection) to determine V (ml/min). For tubes 3 and 4 the volume is divided by 10 min. The urine, and the plasma samples obtained by centrifugation of the arterial blood, are analyzed for urea concentration. The clearances are then calculated as follows:

$$C_1 = \frac{(U_{\text{urea}}V)_1}{P_{\text{urea}_1}}, \quad C_2 = \frac{(U_{\text{urea}}V)_2}{P_{\text{urea}_2}}, \quad \text{etc.} \tag{10}$$

2. *Inactin*

Sodium pentobarbital is the most commonly used anesthetic in clearance studies. Nevertheless, mention should be made of another anesthetic, the thiobarbiturate inactin, because of its frequent use in the rat, particularly in micropuncture experiments. Effects on cardiovascular parameters may be expected from either barbiturate and it has recently been shown (Koeppen *et al.*, 1977) that renal blood flow is diminished under both pentobarbital and inactin anesthesia. In addition, pentobarbital resulted in a redistribution of blood flow away from the outer cortex.

A more recent study (Knight *et al.*, 1976) has demonstrated that inactin, in addition to its hemodynamic effects, may affect renal function in other ways. Rats under inactin anesthesia had a diminished ability to excrete an isotonic saline load when compared to pentobarbital-anesthetized or awake rats. Thus caution should be observed that the anesthetic chosen will not in itself influence the experimental results.

B. Unanesthetized Rat

In certain experiments anesthesia is undesirable. In this case clearance procedures may be applied to the conscious rat. The rat should be prepared surgically as described above but under ether anesthesia and without tracheal tube. When surgery is completed, the rat is placed in a restraining cage (Figure 1) and allowed to awaken. Clearance studies are then performed in exactly the same manner as in the anesthetized rat.

Rats may also be prepared for long-term study in a similar manner. It is preferable to catheterize the carotid artery and jugular vein in place of the femorals, however, so that the catheters may be externalized through an opening made in the skin at the back of the head. The catheters are then cut short and sutured to the scalp. In this location the rat is less able to damage the catheters. The catheters must be kept filled, and flushed at least once daily with heparinized normal saline, to prevent clotting. The open ends may be sealed by melting the tubing with an open flame. This method creates a polyethylene bubble which may be punctured with a hypodermic needle for flushing, infusions, and blood sampling, and resealed by burning. Such catheters may remain functional for several weeks.

If continuous measurements are to be made over an extended period of time, the same method may be adapted to allow the rat free access to food and water and free movement during the actual experiment. The catheters, instead of being shortened after externalization, are passed through a flexible spring, and brought out through the top of a regular housing cage. The spring is fixed snugly to the top of the rat's head and covers the entire length of catheter to which the rat may have access, thereby providing protection but at the same time allowing the rat normal mobility within the cage (Kleinman *et al.*, 1964).

V. DETAILS OF THE MEASUREMENT OF GLOMERULAR FILTRATION RATE AND RENAL PLASMA FLOW IN THE RAT

Measurement of GFR should be done routinely in any clearance study since alterations in GFR may affect the clearance of many substances. The measurement of RPF may also provide useful information. Because of the widespread use of these two clearance techniques in particular, they will be considered in detail.

A. Conventional Method for Measurement of Glomerular Filtration Rate[2]

As mentioned above, the clearance of inulin is equivalent to the GFR in most species, including the rat (Harvey and Malvin, 1965). The clearance of creatinine may also be used but is most accurate in the female, since the male rat secretes a small quantity of creatinine (Harvey and Malvin, 1965). If a chemical method of analysis is to be used, creatinine may be preferable to inulin because the method is simpler (Bonsnes and Taussky, 1945).

Because of the small samples which are obtained from the rat, it is always preferable to use a labeled compound, permitting analysis of very small samples. Labeled inulin is available commercially as [³H]inulin or [¹⁴C]inulin.

Inulin should be infused throughout the experiment to ensure a constant plasma concentration. The first step in determining the amount of inulin to be infused is to select a plasma concentration of inulin which will be great enough to be measured reliably in the volume of plasma and urine obtained in the experiment. In the case of chemical assay techniques (Walser *et al.*, 1955; Schreiner, 1950), this concentration should fall within the optimal range for the assay. The chosen plasma concentration can be attained by giving a priming dose of inulin sufficient to raise the plasma concentration to the desired level. This dose is calculated by assuming that the extracellular fluid volume (in which inulin is distributed) is equivalent in milliliters to 20% of the body weight of the rat. In the following example a plasma concentration of 250 μg/ml was selected. The priming dose for a 200-g rat would be

$$(20\%) \times (200 \text{ g}) \times (250 \ \mu\text{g/ml}) = \text{priming dose} \tag{11}$$

$$10 \text{ mg} = \text{priming dose} \tag{12}$$

In the case of labeled inulin, it might be desirable to have approximately 150 CPM/μl of plasma. In this case,

$$(20\%) \times (200 \text{ g}) \times (150 \text{ CPM}/\mu\text{l}) = \text{priming dose} \tag{13}$$

$$6 \times 10^6 \text{ CPM} = \text{priming dose} \tag{14}$$

To achieve this, 10 μCi might be administered (DPM/ml $\times$ % efficiency = CPM, 1.0 μCi = 2.2 $\times 10^6$ DPM).

---

[2] Although the examples used will apply specifically to the measurement of GFR, the principles involved are equally applicable to the determination of clearances, in general.

The priming dose may be administered intravenously in 0.1–0.2 ml of isotonic saline. Immediately following administration, a continuous infusion of inulin in isotonic saline should be begun at a rate designed to maintain the desired plasma concentration. Since the only route of excretion of inulin is the urine, and since the excretion rate is equal to the filtered amount, the correct rate of infusion can be calculated as follows, estimating a GFR of 2.0 ml/min.

$$\text{Excretion rate} = \text{infusion rate} \tag{15}$$

$$(P_{\text{In}}) \times (\text{GFR}) = X \tag{16}$$

$$(250 \ \mu\text{g/ml}) \times (2 \ \text{ml/min}) = X \tag{17}$$

$$0.5 \ \text{mg/min} = X \tag{18}$$

The maintenance infusion should be given in a volume compatible with the experimental protocol (e.g., at a rate of 0.01 ml/min in procedures where volume expansion is undesirable). The actual experimental procedure for determining GFR is identical to that described in the sample experiment in Section IV.

Because of the nature of the clearance calculation, it is unnecessary to obtain a standard curve each time an analysis of inulin concentrations in urine and plasma is made. Only the ratio of the concentrations in urine and plasma ($U_{\text{In}}/P_{\text{In}}$) is needed, not the actual concentration of inulin. In the case of tritiated or [^{14}C]inulin, the calculation of C_{In} might be made as follows:

$$\frac{(\text{CPM/ml}) \ \text{urine}}{(\text{CPM/ml}) \ \text{plasma}} \times V = C_{\text{In}} \tag{19}$$

$$\frac{3,000 \ \text{CPM/ml}}{150 \ \text{CPM/ml}} \times 0.05 \ \text{ml/min} = C_{\text{In}} = 1.0 \ \text{ml/min} \tag{20}$$

If a chemical analysis of inulin is made, it is not always feasible to omit the standard curve. If the standard curve is linear over the range of concentrations found in urine and plasma, it may be omitted without correction. For example, the U/P ratio of optical densities (OD) from a colorimetric reaction might be used directly.

$$\text{Example:} \quad \frac{\text{OD urine}}{\text{OD plasma}} \times V = C_{\text{In}} \tag{21}$$

Substituting actual figures:

$$\frac{0.400}{0.100} \times 0.05 \ \text{ml/min} = 2.0 \ \text{ml/min} \tag{22}$$

If the standard curve is *not* linear, it may still be omitted but the urine samples must be diluted to a concentration as close as possible to the concentration of inulin in the plasma. The assumption is then made that the standard curve is linear over this greatly reduced range. The proper dilution of each urine sample can only be estimated, according to the following reasoning. The inulin in urine has been concentrated with respect to the inulin in the plasma by a factor equal to GFR/V. [Inulin in the glomerular filtrate (GFR) was at a concentration equal to that in systemic plasma. All of that inulin was concentrated in the much smaller urine volume (V)]. Therefore, the proper dilution for each urine sample would be

$$\frac{\text{Estimated GFR}}{V} \times \text{plasma dilution}^3 \qquad (23)$$

Let us assume that, for one urine sample, V was 0.05 ml/min and the corresponding plasma sample was diluted 1:10. The correct urine dilution would be approximately

$$\frac{2.0 \text{ ml/min}}{0.05 \text{ ml/min}} \times 10 = 400, \quad \text{or } 1:400 \qquad (24)$$

In this case a 1:500 dilution might be used, since the calculation itself is an estimate. GFR might then be calculated as follows:

$$\text{Example:} \quad \frac{\text{OD urine}}{\text{OD plasma}} \times \frac{\text{urine dilution}}{\text{plasma dilution}} \times V = C_{\text{Inulin}} \qquad (25)$$

Substituting actual figures:

$$\frac{0.70}{0.100} \times \frac{500}{10} \times 0.05 \text{ ml/min} = 1.75 \text{ ml/min} \qquad (26)$$

B. Continuous Infusion Method for Measurement of Glomerular Filtration Rate

A variation of the standard clearance method which does not require the collection of urine may also be used for the measurement of GFR (Earle and Berliner, 1946). The method provides no real advantages over the standard clearance method except in cases where collection of urine is impossible for some reason or the available urine volume is insufficient for analysis. With the use of [^{3}H]inulin, the latter circumstance usually does not arise, as even 10 μl of urine may be sufficient for determination of U_{In}. It is possible, however, that under hydropenic conditions, so little urine may be produced that substantial renal dead-space errors may be introduced. In this case the continuous infusion method may yield more accurate measurements of GFR.

The method consists of giving an intravenous priming dose of inulin sufficient to raise the plasma inulin concentration to the desired level (see Section V,A). Immediately after the loading dose, an intravenous infusion of inulin, designed to maintain the desired plasma level, is begun. This infusion is continued throughout the experiment. After an equilibration period of 30–60 min, during which the concentration of inulin should become homogeneous throughout the extracellular fluid compartment, the experiment may begin. At any time during the experiment blood may be sampled and the GFR calculated

---

^{3} If the plasma has been diluted for the analysis.

as follows:

$$\text{Infusion rate of inulin} = \text{excretion rate of inulin} \tag{27}$$

$$\text{Perfusion rate} \times \text{In}_{\text{perfusate}} = U_{\text{In}} V \tag{28}$$

It is assumed that P_{In} does not change during the time of plasma collection. Therefore:

$$\frac{\text{Perfusion rate} \times \text{In}_{\text{perfusate}}}{P_{\text{In}}} = U_{\text{In}} V / P_{\text{In}} \tag{29}$$

$$\frac{\text{Perfusion rate} \times \text{In}_{\text{perfusate}}}{P_{\text{In}}} = C_{\text{In}} \tag{30}$$

It should be noted that this method does not detect abrupt changes in GFR. Such changes would alter P_{In}, but this method reveals only the GFR at the time the plasma sample was obtained. The standard clearance method is somewhat preferable when GFR is expected to be unstable since it involves collection of urine over an extended period of time. It too, however, is subject to error since the P_{In} of the single plasma sample may not be representative of the P_{In} throughout the entire clearance period.

C. Single-Injection Clearance Method for Measurement of Glomerular Filtration Rate

For short experimental procedures in which a rapid measurement of GFR is desired, the single injection method (Findley and White, 1940; Israelit *et al.*, 1973) may be used. This method is desirable because it requires virtually no surgical preparation. A needle may be inserted and left in the tail vein for sampling of venous plasma. The method consists of a single subcutaneous injection of the isotope ^{125}I or [131]I (inulin or iothalamate). After an equilibration period (~90 min), during which the iothalamate is absorbed and equilibrates in the extracellular fluid compartment, repeated plasma sampling yields a curve of disappearance of the compound from plasma. The disappearance rate is proportional to the GFR.

D. Conventional Method for Measurement of Renal Plasma Flow in the Rat

As has already been noted, the clearance of PAH is a suitable measurement of renal plasma flow in the rat. It has been suggested, however, that C_{PAH} is technically equivalent to the "effective" RPF or the plasma flow perfusing nephrons (Smith, 1951). In most situations, it is precisely this functional RPF which is of interest and the clearance of PAH may be used with confidence. It should not be used, however, for the calculation of total renal blood flow as it will result in an underestimate. The true renal plasma flow is usually about 10%

greater than the PAH clearance since part of the renal plasma flow perfuses regions of the kidney which do not participate in the elaboration of the urine, such as the renal capsule and the perirenal fat, and nephron segments not involved in the secretion of PAH. The PAH which is present in this blood exits from the kidney in the renal vein.

The actual measurement of the clearance of PAH is made in the same manner as for inulin. Labeled PAH is available commercially as [^{14}C]PAH and as [^{125}I]PAH. Unlabeled PAH may also be used and chemical analysis of the concentrations done (Smith *et al.,* 1945). It will be difficult, however, to obtain sufficient plasma and urine for chemical analysis of both inulin and PAH if other analyses are also to be made.

The priming dose of PAH may be calculated as for inulin except that the volume of distribution is assumed to equal 30% of body weight since some PAH also enters red blood cells. A second consideration must be made in selecting the plasma concentration of PAH. C_{PAH} will only equal the effective RPF if 100% of the PAH perfusing nephrons appears in the urine. This in turn, will only be true if the PAH concentration does not exceed the maximum tubular secretory rate for PAH ($T_{m_{PAH}}$). In the rat, the transport maximum is not reached until the plasma concentration is approximately 3 mg/100 ml (Kramp *et al.,* 1974). When labeled PAH is used, the plasma concentration of PAH is always far below this value. If a chemical analysis of PAH is to be made, however, the plasma concentration achieved by infusion should be kept well below 2 mg/100 ml.

The maintenance infusion rate of PAH is calculated in a manner similar to that for inulin except that the excretion rate will be equal to $P_{PAH} \times$ RPF. A RPF of 6.0 ml/min is used as an estimate.

$$\text{Example:} \quad \text{Infusion rate} = \text{excretion rate} \tag{31}$$

$$X = (P_{PAH})\,(\text{RPF}) \tag{32}$$

$$X = 50{,}000 \text{ CPM/ml } (6.0 \text{ ml/min}) \tag{33}$$

$$X = 300{,}000 \text{ CPM/min} \tag{34}$$

The clearance of PAH is then determined as for any other clearance. If a chemical analysis of PAH (or any other substance) is made, the same cautions apply to the omission of the standard curve as were described for inulin. If urine and plasma are to be diluted to the same approximate concentration, the urine dilution would be calculated as

$$\frac{\text{RPF}}{V} \times \text{plasma dilution} \tag{35}$$

Using as an example a urine sample in which V was 0.05 ml/min and the corresponding plasma sample was diluted 1:10, and assuming a RPF of 6.0 ml/ min:

$$\frac{6.0}{0.05} \times 10 = 1200 \tag{36}$$

A 1:1000 dilution might be made.

If the clearance of PAH is to be used as a measure of the effective renal plasma flow, care must be taken that no other substance used in the protocol interferes with the PAH secretory mechanism. The transport mechanism for PAH appears to be a general organic acid transport mechanism and many compounds have been found to compete with PAH for secretion. Among these are phenol red, hippurate, penicillin, chlorothiazide, and a number of urologic contrast agents (Pitts, 1974). If it is suspected that a substance is interfering with PAH transport or that the extraction of PAH is not constant throughout an experiment, the extraction ratio of PAH

$$E_{\text{PAH}} = \frac{(\text{PAH}_{\text{artery}} - \text{PAH}_{\text{vein}})}{\text{PAH}_{\text{artery}}}$$

may be determined by directly puncturing the renal vein (Arendshorst *et al.*, 1975), provided the rat is anesthetized during the experiment. From E_{PAH} the "true" RPF may be calculated as $C_{\text{PAH}}/E_{\text{PAH}}$.

VI. DETAILS OF THE MEASUREMENT OF $T^C_{\text{H}_2\text{O}}$ AND $C_{\text{H}_2\text{O}}$ IN THE RAT

Since the rat has been shown to be a particularly suitable model for the study of concentrating and diluting ability (Martínez-Maldonado *et al.*, 1969, 1974; Eknoyan *et al.*, 1970; Wallin *et al.*, 1973), we will consider in detail the methods for determining free water reabsorption ($T^C_{\text{H}_2\text{O}}$) and free water clearance ($C_{\text{H}_2\text{O}}$) in these species. Although neither $T^C_{\text{H}_2\text{O}}$ nor $C_{\text{H}_2\text{O}}$ is a true clearance according to the strict definition, the principles and techniques involved are similar enough to warrant inclusion in a discussion of clearance methods.

A. Free Water Reabsorption ($T^C_{\text{H}_2\text{O}}$)

For the measurement of $T^C_{\text{H}_2\text{O}}$ the rat may be anesthetized with sodium pentobarbital and prepared surgically as previously described. Both food and water should be removed the afternoon prior to the experiment. C_{In} or C_{Cr} must be measured because any variations in GFR will affect $T^C_{\text{H}_2\text{O}}$. The procedure for determination of GFR is the same as described in Section V. The volume in which creatinine or inulin is infused, however, should be kept small (e.g., 0.01 ml/min) to prevent infusion of large isotonic volumes.

When surgery is complete, 0.5 units of Pitressin tannate in oil should be administered intramuscularly or subcutaneously. ADH should not be given intravenously as it has been shown to alter renal sodium and H_2O handling and to have vasomotor effects (Martínez-Maldonado *et al.*, 1971). At least 30 min after Pitressin administration and after sufficient time has been allowed for inulin equilibration, an infusion of 2% saline is begun in a peripheral vein at a rate of 0.1 ml/min. After 10 min of infusion two or three clearances are done in the same manner as described in Section IV with a timed urine collection and blood sampling. The rate of infusion of 2% saline is then increased to 0.2 ml/min. After

10 min of infusion at the new rate, two or three clearance periods follow. The rest of the protocol consists of increasing the rate of infusion of 2% saline in a stepwise fashion (0.3, 0.4, 0.5, 0.75 ml/min). For each new rate of infusion a 10-min equilibration period is allowed and then two or three clearances are done. The infusion of hypertonic saline and the administration of Pitressin ensure that plasma levels of ADH will remain high throughout the experiment. The increasing rate of infusion of hypertonic saline provides an increasing delivery of sodium chloride to the sites in the distal nephron responsible for generation of the interstitial corticomedullary osmotic gradient.

In addition to inulin analysis, the osmolality of each plasma and urine sample must be determined. This is conventionally done by freezing point depression, but the relatively new vapor pressure osmometer allows measurement of the osmolality of much smaller samples. $T_{H_2O}^C$ is calculated according to the formula

$$T_{H_2O}^C = C_{osm} - V \tag{37}$$

where C_{osm} is the osmolar clearance and V is the urine volume in milliliters per minute. C_{osm} is a true clearance and has the units of all clearances, ml/min. It may be calculated from the formula

$$C_{osm} = \frac{U_{osm}V}{P_{osm}} \tag{38}$$

where U_{osm} and P_{osm} are the osmolalities of urine and plasma, respectively, and V is the urine volume in milliliters per minute.

For each experiment or group of experiments, a curve may be constructed depicting the amount of free water reabsorption corrected for the GFR ($T_{H_2O}^C$/GFR) as a function of distal delivery of sodium also corrected for the GFR (C_{osm}/GFR). C_{osm} is conventionally used as an index of distal delivery. A typical $T_{H_2O}^C$ curve is shown in Figure 2A. Since distal NaCl delivery is increasing due to the stepwise increases in infusion rate, free water reabsorption also increases. The effect of drugs or various physiological states on free water reabsorption may be studied by comparing the experimental $T_{H_2O}^C$ curves with control curves obtained in untreated rats.

Infusion of hypertonic mannitol has been used in place of hypertonic saline to increase distal NaCl delivery. This solute, however, has the disadvantage that although it does increase distal delivery of NaCl, it also lowers the luminal NaCl concentration. $T_{H_2O}^C$ curves obtained using hypertonic mannitol infusion consistently fall below $T_{H_2O}^C$ curves obtained under hypertonic saline infusion (Goldberg *et al.*, 1965; Brunner *et al.*, 1966; Martínez-Maldonado *et al.*, 1969), indicating less free water reabsorption at any rate of distal delivery.

B. Free Water Clearance (C_{H_2O})

The measurement of C_{H_2O} presents a special problem not characteristic of the measurement of $T_{H_2O}^C$. By its nature, the experimental protocol presumes minimal levels of ADH. Otherwise, free water would not be excreted but

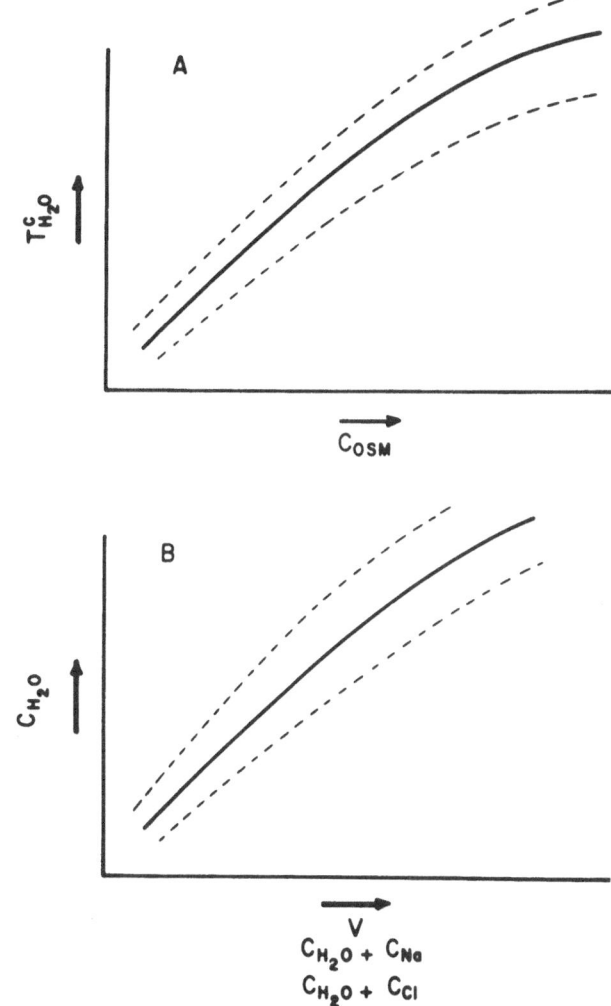

Figure 2. Generalized features of free water reabsorption and free water clearance. (A) Idealized curve depicting $T^C_{H_2O}$ as a function of C_{osm} in the rat. (B) Idealized curve depicting C_{H_2O} as a function of V, $C_{H_2O} + C_{Na}$, or $C_{H_2O} + C_{Cl}$. During hypotonic saline infusion, the curves resulting from use of any of these delivery terms are identical.

reabsorbed, i.e., C_{H_2O} would be negative. Although successful C_{H_2O} studies have been performed in anesthetized rats (Martínez-Maldonado *et al.,* 1972), it is usually very difficult to obtain positive free water clearances under anesthesia. For this reason, it is preferable to use the awake rat for studies of C_{H_2O}. It has been shown that in the awake rat one can obtain free water clearance curves which are not significantly different from those obtained in the anesthetized Brattleboro rat, indicating that in this model plasma ADH levels must be virtually zero (Martínez-Maldonado and Opava Stitzer, unpublished observations).

The afternoon before the experiment, food should be removed and drinking water replaced with a 5% glucose solution. This will, in itself, lower plasma osmolality and thereby inhibit ADH. On the morning of the experiment, the rat is given a total load of distilled water equal to 3% of body weight. This load is divided into three equal doses which are administered by gavage at 15-min intervals. While it has been previously recommended to add alcohol to the water load (Czackes and Kleeman, 1964), this is unnecessary and even undesirable as the alcohol may be measured as an osmotic particle in the plasma and urine. After the last water load, the rat is anesthetized with ether and prepared surgically as previously described. As soon as the surgery is completed, the rat is placed in a restraining cage as illustrated in Figure 1 and an infusion of 0.225% saline (1/4 isotonic) is begun into a peripheral vein at a rate of 0.1 ml/min. This infusion is continued until the osmolality of the urine (determined at regular intervals) has fallen to 200 mosm/liter or less. In this protocol also, the measurement of GFR is essential. The priming dose of inulin and the onset of inulin infusion should be timed so that the inulin equilibration period coincides with this period of hypotonic saline infusion.

When a U_{osm} of 200 mosm/liter or less has been achieved, the actual experiment is begun. A 0.45% saline solution is substituted for the 0.225% solution at the same rate of infusion (0.1 ml/min). From this point on, the protocol is identical to that for $T^C_{H_2O}$ except that the infusion solution is hypotonic instead of hypertonic saline. At each rate of infusion a 10-min equilibration period is followed by two or three clearance periods. The infusion rate is increased stepwise from 0.1 ml/min to 0.2, 0.3, 0.4, 0.5, and 0.75 ml/min. The infusion of hypotonic saline ensures that endogenous ADH will be inhibited throughout the experiment. The increasing rate of infusion provides an increasing delivery of sodium chloride to sites in the distal nephron responsible for free water generation. C_{H_2O}, or free water clearance, is calculated according to the formula

$$C_{H_2O} = V - C_{osm} \tag{39}$$

or

$$C_{H_2O} = V - \frac{U_{osm} V}{P_{osm}} \tag{40}$$

The terms of the equation and their units are the same as in Eqs. (37) and (38).

As in the case of $T^C_{H_2O}$, a C_{H_2O} curve may be constructed for each experiment or group of experiments. Free water clearance corrected for GFR (C_{H_2O}/GFR) is plotted as a function of distal delivery also corrected for GFR. The index of distal delivery which is conventionally used, however, is not C_{osm}, but V, C_{H_2O} + C_{Na}, or C_{H_2O} + C_{Cl}. For discussion of the relative merits of these various indices, the reader is referred to the original literature (Eknoyan et al., 1967; Seldin and Rector, 1973) or the recent review in Methods of Pharmacology, Vol. 4A, Chapter 4 (Eknoyan et al., 1976). Whichever distal delivery term is chosen, a C_{H_2O} curve will be obtained which is similar to that shown in Figure 2b. Fractional free water clearance increases as a function of increasing delivery of sodium chloride to the distal nephron. The effects of drugs or various physiological states on free water excretion may be studied by comparing the experimental C_{H_2O} curves with control curves obtained in untreated rats.

The effect of the infusion of hypotonic solutions other than hypotonic saline on free water clearances has been studied in detail (Martínez-Maldonado, 1975;

Martínez-Maldonado and Opava Stitzer, unpublished observations). A comparison of C_{H_2O} curves obtained during infusion of hypotonic solutions of saline, mannitol, urea, and glucose suggests that the most suitable solution for increasing the distal delivery of NaCl is a solution of NaCl itself.

REFERENCES

Arendshorst, W. J., Finn, W. F., and Gottschalk, C. W. 1975. Autoregulation of blood flow in the rat kidney. *Am. J. Physiol.*, *228:*127.

Bonsnes, R. W., and Taussky, H. H. 1945. On the colorimetric determination of creatinine by the Jaffe raction. *J. Biol. Chem.*, *158:*581.

Brunner, F. P., Rector, F. C., and Seldin, D. W. 1966. The mechanism of the urinary concentrating defect in potassium-deficient rats. *Pflügers Arch.*, *290:*202.

Cortell, S., Davidman, M., Gennari, F. J., and Schwartz, W. B. 1972. Catheter size as a determinant of outflow resistance and intrarenal pressure. *Am. J. Physiol.*, *223:*910.

Czackes, J. W., and Kleeman, C. R. 1964. The effect of various states of hydration and the plasma concentration on the turnover of antidiuretic hormone in mammals. *J. Clin. Invest.*, *43:*1649.

Earle, D. R., Jr., and Berliner, R. W. 1946. A simplified clinical procedure for measurement of glomerular filtration rate and renal plasma flow. *Proc. Soc. Exper. Biol. Med.*, *62:*262.

Eknoyan, G., Suki, W. N., Rector, F. C., Jr., and Seldin, D. W. 1967. Functional characteristics of the diluting segment of the dog nephron and the effect of extracellular volume expansion on its reabsorptive capacity. *J. Clin. Invest.*, *46(7):*1178.

Eknoyan, G., Martínez-Maldonado, M., Suki, W. N., and Richie, Y. 1970. Renal diluting capacity in the hypokalemic rat. *Am. J. Physiol.*, *219:*933.

Eknoyan, G., Martínez-Maldonado, M., and Suki, W. N. 1976. The use of clearance methods for the determination of sites of action of diuretics in the kidney. *In: Methods in Pharmacology*, Vol. 4A. pp. 99–119. Ed. by Martínez-Maldonado, M. Plenum Press, New York.

Emmanouel, D. S., Lindheimer, M. D., and Katz, A. I. 1974. Mechanism of impaired water excretion in the hypothyroid rat. *J. Clin. Invest.*, *54:*926.

Findley, T., and White, H. L. 1940. Measurement of diodrast and inulin clearances in man after subcutaneous administration. *Proc. Soc. Exper. Biol. Med.*, *45:*623.

Goldberg, M., McCurdy, D. K., and Ramirez, M. A. 1965. Differences between saline and mannitol diuresis in hydropenic man. *J. Clin. Invest.*, *44:*182.

Harvey, A. M., and Malvin, R. L. 1965. Comparison of creatinine and inulin clearances in male and female rats. *Am. J. Physiol.*, *209:*849.

Israelit, A. H., Long, D. L., White, M. G., and Hull, A. R. 1973. Measurement of glomerular filtration rate utilizing a single subcutaneous injection of ^{125}I-iothalamate. *Kidney Int.*, *4:*346.

Kleinman, L. I., Radford, E. P., and Torelli, G. 1964. Urea and inulin clearance in undisturbed, unanesthetized rats. *Am. J. Physiol.*, *207:*578.

Knight, T. F., Samson, S., Frankfurt, S. J., and Weinman, E. J. 1976. Effect of anesthesia on the excretion of an isotonic sodium load in the rat. In: *Proc. 9th Ann. Mtg. Am. Soc. of Nephr.*, p. 102.

Koeppen, B. M., Katz, A. I., and Lindheimer, M. D. 1977. Effect of general anesthesia on renal hemodynamics in the rat. *Clin. Res.*, *25:*438a.

Kramp, R. A., MacDowell, M., Gottschalk, C. W., and Oliver, J. R. 1974. A study by microdissection and micropuncture of the structure and the function of the kidneys and the nephrons of rats with chronic renal damage. *Kidney Int.*, *5:*147.

Martínez-Maldonado, M., Suki, W. N., and Schenker, S. 1969. The nature of the urinary concentrating defect in the Gunn strain of rat. *Am. J. Physiol.*, *216:*1386.

Martínez-Maldonado, M., Eknoyan, G., and Suki, W. N. 1971. Natriuretic effects of vasopressin and cyclic AMP: possible site of action in the nephron. *Am. J. Physiol.*, *220:*2013.

Martínez-Maldonado, M., Eknoyan, G., and Suki, W. N. 1972. Functional importance of thin limbs of Henle's loop in urine concentration and dilution. *Proc. Vth Intern. Cong. Nephr.*, p. 80.

Martínez-Maldonado, M., Eknoyan, G., and Suki, W. N. 1974. Influence of volume expansion on renal diluting capacity in the rat. *Clin. Sci. Mol. Med., 46:*331.

Martínez-Maldonado, M. 1975. Renal diluting capacity (C_{H_2O}) in the rat: Comparisons of infusion of saline with mannitol (M), glucose (G), and urea (U) solutions. (Abstr.) *Clin. Res., 23:*369a.

Martínez-Maldonado, M. and Opava Stitzer, S. Submitted. Evaluation of free water clearance curves during saline, mannitol, glucose, and urea diuresis.

Michael, U. F., Barenberg, R. L., Chavez, R., Vaamonde, C. A., and Papper, S. 1972. Renal handling of sodium and water in the hypothyroid rat. *J. Clin. Invest., 51:*1405.

Pitts, R. F. 1974. *Physiology of the Kidney and Body Fluids.* Yearbook Medical Publishers, Chicago.

Schreiner, G. 1950. Determination of inulin by means of resorcinol. *Proc. Soc. Exper. Biol. Med., 74:*117.

Seldin, D. W., and Rector, F. C., Jr. 1973. Evaluation of clearance methods for localization of site of action diuretics. In: *Modern Diuretic Therapy in the Treatment of Cardiovascular and Renal Disease,* p. 97. Ed. by Lant, A. F., and Wilson, G. M. Excerpta Medica, Amsterdam.

Smith, H. W. 1951. *The Kidney: Structure and Function in Health and Disease.* Oxford University Press, New York.

Smith, H. W., Finkelstein, N., Aliminosa, L., Crawford, B., and Graber, M. 1945. The renal clearances of substituted hippuric acid derivatives and other aromatic acids in dog and man. *J. Clin. Invest., 24:*388.

Wallin, J. D., Barratt, L. J., Rector, F. C., Jr., and Seldin, D. W. 1973. The influence of flow rate and chloride delivery on $T^C_{H_2O}$ formation in the rat. *Kidney Int., 3:*282.

Walser, M., Davidson, D., and Orloff, J. 1955. Renal clearance of alkali stable inulin. *J. Clin. Invest., 34:*1520.

Chapter **3**

Measurement of Intrarenal Blood Flow Distribution

Norbert H. Lameire,[1] Elaine L. Chuang,
Richard W. Osgood, and Jay H. Stein

Department of Medicine
The University of Texas Health Science Center
San Antonio, Texas

I. INTRODUCTION

Recent interest in evaluating the hemodynamic and functional characteristics of different nephron populations within the kidney has led to the development of a variety of methods to determine these parameters.

This chapter will discuss the theoretical and pragmatic aspects of a number of these methods which have been utilized to measure total renal blood flow and intrarenal blood flow distribution. A few introductory points should be made. First, for reasons of space, we have not attempted to discuss every method available. A complete list of these methods can be found in Table I. It was felt, however, that some discussion of the electromagnetic flowmeter and PAH clearance method was indicated since these two techniques are the standards of reference for the measurement of total blood flow in most experimental studies. Second, it is the opinion of the authors that the radioactive microsphere method is presently the most precise experimental method available for the measurement of intrarenal blood flow distribution. Therefore, this method will be discussed most extensively with the intent of giving the investigator a working knowledge of this technique. Third, the use of the albumin accumulation method for measuring plasma flow in the renal papilla will be discussed in detail. Although

---

[1] Present address of Norbert H. Lameire is Department of Medicine, University of Ghent Medical School, Ghent, Belgium.

Table I. Methods for Study of Intrarenal Blood Flow Distribution

A. Methods based on the quantitative uptake of an indicator in the kidney
    PAH-clearance and extraction[a]
    [42]K uptake (Sapirstein, 1958)
    [86]Rb uptake (Harving and Pelley, 1965)
    Radioactive microspheres[a]
    Antiglomerular basement membrane antibody method (Wallin *et al.*, 1971)
B. Methods based on the measurement of an indicator transit time
    1. External measurement of the indicator
        a. Highly diffusible indicators
            Inert gas (^{133}Xe, [85]Kr) washout[a]
        b. Intravascular indicators
            [^{131}I]albumin (Lilienfield *et al.*, 1961)[a]
            [^{51}Cr]red blood cells (Pedersen *et al.*, 1965)
            Dye-dilution curve[a]
    2. Intrarenal measurement of the indicator
        a. Highly diffusible indicators
            Thermodilution (Ochwadt and Schmier, 1954)
            Thermocouple (Gransjö, 1968)
            Hydrogen washout[a]
        b. Intravascular indicators
            Photoelectrical method (Kramer *et al.*, 1960)
            ^{32}P-labeled red blood cells (Gransjö *et al.*, 1966)

[a] These methods are discussed in the text.

the method has a number of practical problems, it is theoretically sound and has considerable promise in unraveling some of the mysteries of the renal medulla.

II. ELECTROMAGNETIC FLOWMETER

A. Theoretical Background

Measurement of blood flow by the electromagnetic method is based on the law of electromagnetic induction discovered by Faraday. This states that

$$E = (MLV) \times 10^{-8} \tag{1}$$

where E is the electromotive force (volts), M is the magnetic field (gauss), L is the lumen diameter (cm), and V is the velocity of the liquid (cm/sec).

The induced electromotive force (emf) observed by Faraday on solid bodies can also be obtained by permitting a conductive liquid (blood) to flow through a magnetic field in which it generates an electromotive force (volts) in a direction perpendicular to both the magnetic field and the direction of motion as illustrated in Figure 1.

In the diagram, two electrodes (e) are held rigidly at an angle of 180° from each other. As the conducting fluid (blood) is moved through the magnetic field at a given velocity, a voltage (emf) is produced directly proportional to the velocity. Therefore, a linear relationship exists between the velocity of the blood and the magnitude of the induced emf. Equation (1) is independent of velocity profile as long as the latter is axially symmetrical. It holds for laminar as well as turbulent flow. The blood does not need to be in direct contact with the electrodes as long as the tube in Figure 1 is electrically conductive, such as an artery, vein, or porous vascular prosthesis. Therefore, the electrodes need not pierce the artery wall; they can pick up the electric current flow merely by touching the outside of the intact vessel. The vessel can also be incised and cannulated so that the electromagnetic sensors are placed directly in the bloodstream.

The sensitivity of the electromagnetic blood flow transducer is affected significantly by the presence or absence of a vessel wall, but it is practically independent of the thickness of the wall, provided the outside diameter of the vessel remains constant. The electrodes are essentially nonpolarizable platinum and are fixed in a rigid ring, or probe, that maintains the diameter of the artery, secures the application of the electrodes, and immobilizes the blood vessel relative to the magnet.

The electromagnet located within the probe is excited by a current producing a magnetic field at right angles to the direction of flow. As the flowing blood cuts the magnetic lines of force, a pulsatile emf (voltage) is developed which is sensed by the electrodes. The signal flow voltage which is directly proportional to blood flow through the sensor is amplified, integrated, and displayed on the flowmeter.

Excitation of the magnet in the blood flow probe can be achieved by variations of the continuous or pulsed electrical wave forms. Sine-wave excitation is the simplest to generate, but it suffers from the disadvantage that the flow signal and the in-phase artifact are difficult to separate from each other. A sine-wave system, therefore, suffers from a certain degree of baseline instability. Square-wave excitation has an advantage in that the flow information and the

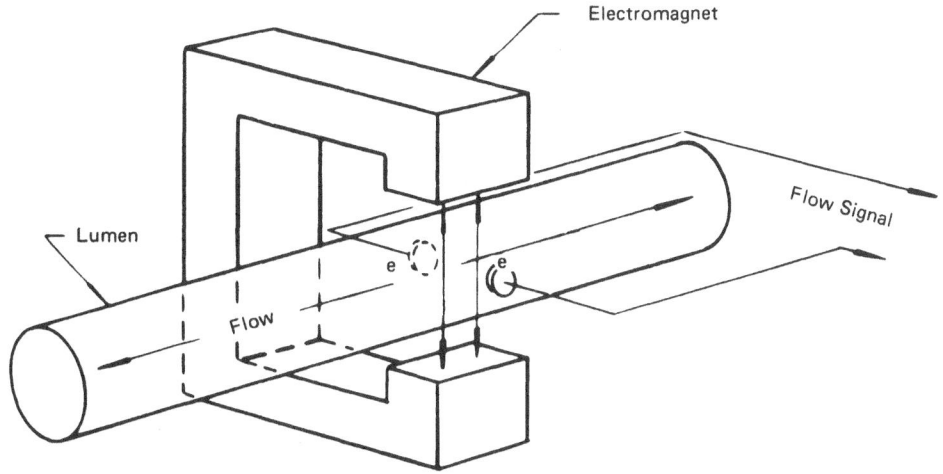

Figure 1. Illustration of electromagnetic induction (see text for explanation).

artifact signals have different wave shapes. Therefore, it is possible to discriminate against the artifact signals by sampling the flow signal at a time when the artifact signal has decreased to a lower value. The success of the square-wave principle is also related to its ability to reduce the effects of the environmental noise voltages.

A wide assortment of blood flow transducers are available. Most frequently, periarterial probes are used. Standard periarterial probes are provided with lumen diameters from 1 to 40 mm. Various configurations and widths are available to suit the specific needs of the user. Most of these blood flow transducers have a C-shaped lumen with a slotted cover which slides and/or snaps into place to complete encirclement of the vessel.

B. Procedure

There are a number of practical considerations prior to using probes for actual measurement of blood flow. These include: cleaning and soaking the probes, surgical exposure of the vessel, zero flow baseline reference, and calibration of flow probe.

1. Cleaning the Probes

All portions of the probes must be kept free of contamination. This applies particularly to the platinum electrode tips which make contact with the vessel wall or bloodstream. A thin oxide film readily forms over the metal and results in increased impedance. Prior to sterilization and use, the electrode surface should be carefully cleaned with commercial abrasive powders such as Ajax cleanser, Bon Ami, or comparable agents. Normal saline should be used instead of water. Cotton swabs (Q-tips) are satisfactory for probes with a diameter of 4.0 mm or larger. For accurate and optimum flow signals, it is recommended that the flow probes be recleaned every time they are removed and reapplied to a vessel.

2. Soaking the Probes

To assure better conduction and to keep the probes clean, it is important that they be placed in a container of saline for at least 10 min prior to actual use. Probes should be recleaned and soaked when they are removed and reapplied during the same study.

3. Surgical Exposure of the Renal Artery

Approach to the renal artery should take advantage of well-planned exposure via accepted surgical incisions. The vessel should be isolated from contiguous structures, removed from its sheath, and freed from adventitia. Any fat overlying or attached to the vessel should be removed. The incision should be large enough to permit clean dissection of the vessel and the length of vessel exposed and prepared should be sufficient to allow easy application of the flow probe without tension, twisting, or any distortion which might affect the flow pattern.

To ensure good electrode-to-vessel-wall contact for acute blood flow determination, the probe should be slightly constrictive on the artery, about 10% smaller than the diameter of the vessel. Since contact between electrode and vessel wall is responsible for detection and transfer of flow signal, proper probe size is of critical importance.

4. Baseline Reference

Mechanical occlusion of the renal artery is the method usually used to establish a baseline reference for zero flow. The preferred technique is to occlude the vessel with a vascular or bulldog clamp distal to and as far away from the electromagnetic flow probe as possible. If the artery is occluded proximal to the probe, the walls can collapse away from the electrodes, resulting in a positive or negative shift in the baseline.

5. Calibration

Electromagnetic blood flow transducers are calibrated by individual users according to their own techniques and standards.

The calibration system can be carried out completely (or partially) *in vivo* or *in vitro*. A completely *in vivo* system is one in which the probe is calibrated on the renal artery after each experiment. A completely *in vitro* study does not use normal tissues, such as blood and excised blood vessels.

The calibration system used in dog experiments by the authors is the direct "bleedout" method. After an experiment is completed, the renal artery is clamped distal to the flow probe and a PE240 tube is inserted into the renal artery in the direction of the flow probe. This outflow line is unclamped and the "bleedout" is begun with a graduated cylinder and is timed with a stopwatch over 30–40 sec. The potential errors of this technique include:

1. Incorrect reading of the graduated cylinder.
2. Incorrect timing of the bleeding period.
3. Fluctuations in flow as a result of reactive hyperemia when the vessel is unclamped and as a result of reductions in perfusion pressure during the test period if the bleeding continues for a reasonable period of time. These problems may be overcome by waiting for 1 min following unclamping before beginning to determine the mean flow.
4. Collapse of the vessel wall away from the probe.

An example of the results of an *in vivo* calibration of the flow probe on the renal artery of a dog is given in Figure 2.

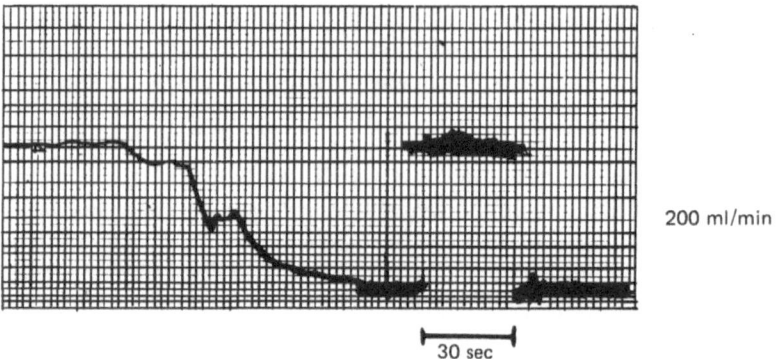

200 ml/min

30 sec

Figure 2. Recording of an *in vivo* calibration of the flow probe on the renal artery of the dog by direct bleedout.

III. PAH CLEARANCE AND EXTRACTION

A. Theoretical Background and Methodology

Another approach to the measurement of renal blood flow is the use of the Fick principle, which requires that the organ under study extract or add a measurable amount of a given substance to the bloodstream and that the arteriovenous concentration difference of this substance across the organ is known. Thus, if the amount of urine formed per unit time (V) and the content of a given substance per 100 ml of urine (U) are known, then the amount of substance excreted per unit time equals ($U/100$) $\times$ V. If the concentrations of the substance in arterial plasma (P_a) and in the plasma flowing from the renal veins (P_v) are known, the amount of substance extracted by the kidney per 100 ml of plasma equals $P_a - P_v$. Thus, by knowing the urinary excretion of the marker, and the arteriovenous difference across the kidney, renal plasma flow (RPF) may be calculated by the simple formula

$$\text{RPF} = UV/(P_a - P_v) \tag{2}$$

If the blood hematocrit (Hct) is known, renal blood flow (RPF) may also be calculated.

$$\text{RBF} = \frac{UV}{(P_a - P_v)} \times 1/(1 - \text{Hct}) \tag{3}$$

A radio-opaque catheter can be introduced into the inferior vena cava and from there the catheter can be maneuvered into the orifice of the renal vein in both animal and man to obtain renal venous blood for analysis.

The finding that some substances are almost quantitatively extracted by the kidney and excreted in the urine was a major advance in the development of methods for measuring renal blood flow. These substances include certain organic iodine compounds such as Diodrast and the closely related compounds

Hippuran (Landis *et al.*, 1936) and *p*-aminohippuric acid (Smith *et al.*, 1945). If the arteriovenous difference in renal blood is expressed as a percentage of the arterial concentration of the given substance, the extraction (*E*) is given by

$$E = (P_a - P_v)/P_a \times 100 \qquad (4)$$

If P_v of the given substance approximates zero, its extraction will be essentially 100%. Under these circumstances, Eq. (2) is reduced to

$$\text{RPF} = UV/P_a \qquad (5)$$

The quantities, *U*, *V*, and P_a can easily be determined. Renal blood flow can then be calculated by the formula,

$$\text{RBF} = \text{RPF}/(1 - \text{Hct}) \qquad (6)$$

Although this calculation will always underestimate the true renal blood flow, it is usually utilized in man to avoid renal vein catheterization. The value obtained is termed the effective renal blood flow.

Extraction of Diodrast and PAH depends on the integrity of the proximal tubular organic acid secretory pump, the transit time of blood through the kidney, and other factors. It has been clearly shown that PAH secretion has a rate limitation. Therefore, if the amount of the substance delivered to the tubular cells exceeds a certain transport capacity, renal extraction will begin to decline. Thus, it is important that renal plasma flow be determined at a low plasma concentration of the test substance. The optimum concentration of PAH is 1–2 mg/100 ml. Even at these low concentrations, however, the extraction of PAH is not equal to 100%. According to Phillips *et al.* (1946) and Earley and Friedler (1965a), PAH extraction in hydropenic dogs is 87 ± 9% and 78 ± 7% respectively. In cats, Nissen (1968) found a value of 95% in the outer cortex and 82% in the inner cortex. Reubi and Schroeder (1949) and Warren *et al.* (1944) found that PAH extraction in man ranged from 75 to 95%.

Certain criteria must be fulfilled in order for clearance measurements employing PAH to be valid:

1. Urine flow must be high enough for accurate and reproducible collections and should be stable throughout the collection period. Since there is a considerable dead space from renal pelvis to urinary bladder, a rapid increase in urine flow, as occurs with the administration of a diuretic agent, will cause spuriously high clearance values, the so-called washout phenomenon. When urine flow is more than 10% of the glomerular filtration rate, it is necessary to correct for urinary losses in the measurement of renal blood flow (Wolf, 1941). When urine flow is quite low, clearance measurements may be inaccurate and poorly reproducible. In anuric patients, clearances obviously cannot be obtained.

2. The plasma concentration of the marker should be stable throughout the period of study.

3. The marker should not be metabolized, stored, or formed within the kidney. In addition, when only effective renal plasma flow is measured, any factor that decreases the extraction of the marker will give an erroneously low measurement of plasma flow.

B. Use of PAH Extraction as an Index of Blood Flow Distribution

Reubi (1958) introduced the concept that noncortical blood flow can be calculated by the following formula:

$$\text{Noncortical blood flow} = (C_{\text{PAH}}/E_{\text{PAH}} - C_{\text{PAH}}) \times 1/(1 - \text{Hct}) \qquad (7)$$

where C_{PAH} is the clearance of PAH and E_{PAH} is the fractional extraction of PAH. A number of more recent observations, however, have indicated that this technique cannot be utilized to measure cortical and noncortical blood flow. Schnermann and Thurau (1965) found that the PAH concentration in vasa recta blood is 4–12 times that in arterial blood in hydropenic hamsters. These data suggest that PAH diffuses out of the loop of Henle and/or collecting duct into the vasa recta, thereby leading to a spurious overestimate of noncortical blood flow. Nissen (1968) measured the extraction ratio of PAH in the superficial and deep venous drainage areas of the cat kidney. In that species, the outer half of the cortex is drained by superficial cortical and capsular veins, and the inner half by a deep venous system. The extraction ratio of PAH (E_{PAH}) in the outer cortex averaged 0.95 in control experiments. During mannitol or saline diuresis, E_{PAH} in the outer cortex decreased to an average of 86%, indicating that E_{PAH} in the cortex was not complete in any of these conditions. Cortney *et al.* (1965) came to a similar conclusion in studies in the rat. Earley and Friedler (1965a,b) noted an E_{PAH} as low as 30–40% during massive saline loading or drug-induced renal vasodilatation. If these data were taken literally, this would indicate that 60–70% of blood flow was noncortical. Direct methods (McNay and Abe, 1970; Stein *et al.*, 1971) have shown that no more than 15% of blood flow enters juxtamedullary nephrons. Thus, E_{PAH} may grossly overestimate noncortical blood flow under certain circumstances. Since both saline loading and drug-induced renal vasodilatation are associated with a significant increase in total renal blood flow, the decrease in extraction may be related to the increased peritubular capillary blood flow, and hence, diminished contact time with the peritubular secretory pump which transports PAH into the renal cell (Tune *et al.*, 1969).

IV. DYE DILUTION

A. Theoretical Background and Procedure

If a substance which is not extracted by the renal parenchyma, such as Evan's blue or indocyanine green, is infused at a continuous rate (M) into the renal artery, and if complete and rapid mixing of the substance occurs before the renal artery divides into subbranches, the concentration of the substance in the renal vein (R) will be inversely proportionate to the amount of blood into which it is introduced per unit time (the renal blood flow). Because of recirculation of the indicator, the concentration of the test substance in the arterial blood (A) has to be subtracted from the concentration in the renal vein. Hence

$$\text{RBF} = M/(R - A)(1 - \text{Hct}) \qquad (8)$$

The primary technical difficulty of this method is the necessity of keeping the tip of the arterial catheter well within the main branch of the renal artery for a prolonged period. The advantage of the method, however, is that it allows continuous monitoring of renal blood flow.

If the test substance is introduced as a single injection (M) and the same type of sampling is performed from the renal vein, the sum of the renal venous concentrations per unit time (T) can be substituted for the single concentration (R) in Eq. (8):

$$\text{RBF} = M / \int_0^t c(dt) \tag{9}$$

The technique consists of the injection of a known amount of dye (cardio green or Evan's blue) into the renal artery, concomitant with the withdrawal of renal venous blood at a constant flow rate (15–30 ml/min). The renal venous blood is drawn into an oximetric cuvette and a dye dilution curve is obtained.

Practically, the Hamilton equation can be used instead of Eq. (8):

$$F = 60\, M/ct = 60\, M/S \tag{10}$$

where F is renal blood flow, c is mean dye concentration during the recording of the curve, t is duration of the curve in seconds, and S is area of the recorded curve as measured by planimetry. The area S must be compared with a calibration area s obtained after the injection of a known amount of dye m injected directly into the recording system. If S is area of the calibration curve and f is flow rate of the withdrawal pump, then

$$F = Mfs/Sm \tag{11}$$

Mean transit time ($\bar{t}$) can be calculated as the ratio of the area under the indicator dilution curve to the cumulative concentration according to the equation

$$\bar{t} = \int_0^t Rdt/\Sigma R \tag{12}$$

Intrarenal blood volume can be calculated as the product of flow (F) and mean transit time ($\bar{t}$) according to an equation of the general form

$$V = \bar{t} \times F \tag{13}$$

B. Use of the Method for Intrarenal Blood Flow Distribution

If tissue is homogeneous and the indicator substance arrives in or disappears from all parts of the tissue at the same rate, the concentration-time curve can be described by a one-term exponential; that is, a straight line corresponding to the exponential coefficient of a monoexponential curve can be fitted exactly to the declining values for concentration plotted semilogarithmically against time. A deviation from a monoexponential curve may indicate the presence of two or more regions with different rates of blood flow (Dobson and Warner, 1957).

The late part of a normal renal dye-dilution curve deviates from the form described by a single-term exponential. Reubi *et al.* (1966) found recirculation to be negligible and attributed the second curve obtained to be a function of medullary blood flow. They reported that cortical blood flow in the normal human kidney ranged from 80 to 93% of the total flow at a rate of 334–548 ml/ min and vascular volume ranged from 60 to 109 ml. Noncortical blood flow ranged from 13 to 43 ml. Effros *et al.* (1967) reported that recirculation of cardio green was the source of the deviation of the late part of the dye dilution curve and Ofstad *et al.* (1967a,b) presented evidence that inadequate mixing of indicator in renal arterial blood may cause similar deviations of the terminal part of the curve. Although there is good correspondence between the measurement of total renal blood flow obtained by the indicator-dilution technique and values obtained by other methods, it is doubtful that this procedure can be utilized to differentiate cortical and medullary blood flow.

V. INERT GAS WASHOUT METHOD

A. Theoretical Background

The theory of the inert gas washout techniques is discussed by Kety (1951). They are based on the assumption that the diffusibility of an inert gas is sufficiently high to maintain equilibrium under all physiological conditions between tissue and venous blood leaving the tissue.

Application of the Fick principle leads to the following relation:

$$dQ/dt = F(C_a - C_v) \tag{14}$$

where dQ/dt is the amount of gas leaving the tissue per unit time, F the total blood flow, and C_a and C_v the concentration of the gas in the arterial and venous blood.

If C_i is the concentration of the gas in the tissue with volume V, we have

$$V dC_i/dt = F(C_a - C_v) \tag{15}$$

Assuming that equilibrium of the gases is extremely rapid, then

$$C_v = C_i/\lambda \tag{16}$$

where λ is the partition coefficient of the indicator between tissue and blood (in ml tissue/ml blood). After a single injection of an inert gas, it can be assumed that $C_a \simeq 0$, since the recirculation of the inert gas is small, because of the very effective elimination in the lungs. Thus,

$$dG_i/dt = F/V \times C_i/\lambda \tag{17}$$

Integrating this equation between the limits $t = 0$ and $t = t$

$$C_i = C_0 \times e^{-kt} \tag{18}$$

where C_0 is the concentration in the tissue at $t = 0$ and

$$k = F/V \times \lambda \tag{19}$$

or for the total amount of tracer in the tissue, multiplying Eq. (18) by V,

$$Q_i = Q_0 \times e^{-kt} \tag{20}$$

On semilogarithmic paper, a plot Q_i/Q_0 versus t gives a straight line with the slope k. From this plot k can be obtained:

$$k = 0.693/T_{1/2} \tag{21}$$

where $T_{1/2}$ is the time in minutes for Q_i/Q_0 to be reduced to half of its numerical value. The general form of Eq. (25) for a heterogeneously perfused tissue is given by

$$Q_i = Q_{1,0} \times e^{-k_1 t} + Q_{2,0} \times e^{-k_2 t} + Q_{3,0} \times e^{-k_3 t} + \cdots + Q_{n,0} \times e^{-k_n t} \tag{22}$$

where n is the number of different perfused tissue zones.

For application to the kidney, the washout curves are subjected to a conventional graphical analysis on semilogarithmic paper. The procedure is illustrated in Figure 3 which demonstrates a curve obtained in a conscious dog. The data are plotted on a semilogarithmic scale and four compartments determined by graphic analysis.

The blood flow in each compartment in ml/g/min is calculated from the half-

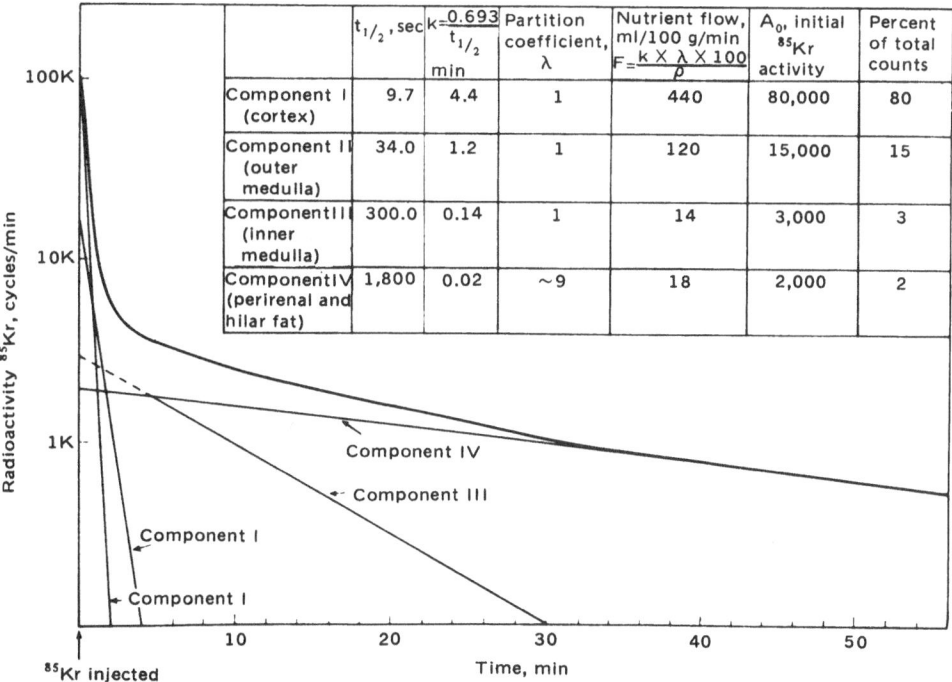

Figure 3. A typical ^{85}Kr washout curve in a normal conscious dog. Also represented is the compartmental analysis dividing the washout curve into four components. I, cortex; II, outer medulla; III, inner medulla; and IV, perirenal and hilar fat. (Reprinted from Thorburn *et al.*, 1963, with permission.)

time $(T_{1/2})$ of each component according to Eqs. (19) and (21) as

$$\text{Flow/volume} = \frac{0.693 \times T}{T_{1/2} \times P} \qquad (23)$$

where P denotes the specific weight of kidney tissue (≈ 1). Andersen and Ladefoged (1965) found the value of λ to be 0.7 at hematocrit 50% and it was linearly dependent on the hematocrit as follows:

$$\lambda \times \text{Hct}_x = \lambda \times \text{Hct}_{50} (1.69/1.05 \times 0.013 \text{ Hct}) \qquad (24)$$

B. Procedure

Measurement of the renal blood flow with the washout technique has been carried out with either ^{133}Xe or ^{85}Kr as the indicator. About 2 mCi of the indicator dissolved in 2–5 ml saline are injected within a few seconds into the renal artery. The disappearance of the gas from the kidney can be followed with a scintillation detector located over the kidney in a cylindrical collimator, allowing measurement of radioactivity from the whole kidney. The detector is connected to a linear rate meter and a linear recorder.

C. Validity of the Method

There are a number of considerations concerning the washout method which are worthy of further examination. From a purely technical standpoint, Mowat *et al.* (1972) have found a variable fall in renal blood flow after a bolus injection of ^{133}Xe via a small plastic catheter into the renal artery. This obviously would complicate any interpretation of washout measurements. However, this disturbance in renal hemodynamics after the bolus injection has not been found to be a problem in other laboratories.

With regard to more theoretical considerations, there are three principal reservations. First, these methods do not provide measurements of blood flow, but rather of flow per unit of renal volume. If renal volume is not constant, K may be unchanged in spite of significant changes in flow. Examples of this possibility include saline diuresis and elevated ureteral pressure where renal volume increases significantly.

Second, the use of a given partition coefficient λ in various experimental conditions has not been validated rigorously. Whether changes in tissue-water content could alter this value or whether a single index of solubility can be applied in all areas of the kidney are questions that have never been studied. Carrière (1970) has shown that blood flow rates are greater with the use of ^{85}Kr then with ^{133}Xe, a gas with a lower partition coefficient. This suggests that the partition coefficient utilized may not necessarily be accurate in a given *in vivo* circumstance.

Third, there is little evidence that complete equilibration of the gas occurs during the time of the washout curve. If complete equilibration does not occur, K will be determined by the diffusional characteristics of the gas as well as by the capillary removal rate. Bolme and Edwall (1970) found that the disappearance rate of ^{133}Xe increased faster than the change in blood flow rate in the gastrocnemicius muscle during maneuvers that caused vasodilatation. This dissociation of disappearance rate and directly measured blood flow rate was due to the increase in surface area available for tissue-blood exchange during vasodilatation. A similar phenomenon could possibly occur under specified conditions in the kidney.

Although these theoretical objections are important, the crucial problem with the inert gas method relates to the inability to define which component of the multiexponential washout curve is related to blood flow in a given anatomical area of the kidney. Although autoradiography has been used in an attempt to solve this problem, it is quite subjective, and does not clearly delineate specific anatomic areas of the kidney. As shown in Figure 3 (Thorburn *et al.*, 1963), the washout curve is divided into four components, I through IV, which purport to represent the cortex, the outer medulla, the inner medulla, and the perirenal and hilar fat, respectively. Investigators (Slotkoff *et al.*, 1971; Lameire and Ringoir, 1975) utilizing other techniques have found a fairly good correlation between component I, the most rapid component, and cortical blood flow, but further differentiation is not possible. In addition, measurement of medullary blood flow with diffusible gas indicators is not possible because of countercurrent exchange and the alterations that occur with changes in urinary flow rate. In addition, a component may not represent the same anatomical area in a given control and experimental period. For example, Carrière and Friborg (1969) found that component II represented outer medullary flow in a control period but corresponded to a slower component of cortical flow during the infusion of angiotensin. Thus, while it seems that component I may be a valid index of total cortical flow, it is difficult to interpret the remaining components of the washout curve.

To obviate the problem of localization, Aukland and Berliner (1964) and Aukland (1967) have used a hydrogen-sensitive platinum electrode implanted into the kidney parenchyma at a given depth. They obtained washout curves at varying depths of cortex and outer medulla after giving hydrogen either through an intratracheal tube or into the renal artery. Although this method obviates the problems of localization, there are still several major disadvantages. First, the technique necessitates considerable manipulation and stabilization of the kidney during placement of electrodes. Second, tissue damage at the site of implantation of the electrode must occur, and its effects on the desaturation curves are not clear. Third, in various experimental maneuvers where renal volume was increased or decreased, only an approximation of the site of previous implantation could be obtained. If the electrodes were left in place, its localization might also be altered by a given experimental maneuver.

VI. RADIOACTIVE MICROSPHERE METHOD

Particulate matter injected into the bloodstream has been used to measure total organ flow, regional flow within an organ, and the flow through an arteriovenous fistula. The distribution and fate of a particle injected into the bloodstream depends primarily upon particle size, the site of injection, and the hemodynamic characteristics of the system. Radiolabeled spheres have been developed which, after injection into the arterial circulation, will embolize in vessels of arteriolar or capillary caliber, depending upon the size of sphere utilized. The radiolabel is quite stable and there is no substantial evidence that the microsphere can be dislodged from the site of embolization. Thus, these radiolabeled particles can be utilized in both acute and chronic hemodynamic studies.

A. Theoretical Background

In utilizing a particulate marker to measure total or regional blood flow to a given organ, there are certain assumptions which must be justified:

1. The particle must be uniformly mixed during injection and follow the distribution of red blood cells.
2. The injection must not alter systemic hemodynamics.
3. The injection must not alter local organ hemodynamics.
4. The particle is totally extracted by the organ under study.

All of these assumptions have been adequately validated as discussed by Stein *et al.* (1973a).

The particles are usually injected through a catheter placed in the left atrium or left ventricle. The number of particles entering each organ during the first transit is proportional to the blood flow to that organ. If the blood flowing through the organ is completely cleared of the particles during a single passage, the number of particles in the organ is given by

$$q = f \int_0^\infty C(t) \, dt \tag{25}$$

where q is the number of particles in the organ under study, f is blood flow (ml/min) to the organ, and C is the concentration of particles in the blood (particles/ml).

According to the principle of Stewart-Hamilton, cardiac output (CO) is expressed as follows:

$$\text{CO} = Q / \int_0^\infty Cd(t) \, dt \tag{26}$$

where Q is the amount of indicator injected. The following equation is obtained from Eqs. (25) and (26):

$$f/\text{CO} = q/Q \quad \text{or} \quad f = \text{CO} \times q/Q \tag{27}$$

Accordingly, the fractional distribution of cardiac output to various organs can be obtained by measuring the radioactivity of each organ and the injected dose of particles. If cardiac output is measured independently at the time the particles are injected, blood flow to each organ in milliliters per minutes can be obtained using Eq. (27). Regional blood flow in a given organ can also be measured with this method. In the kidney, virtually all of the spheres are trapped with glomerular capillaries. Therefore, the measurement of regional blood flow with microspheres would provide an index of glomerular perfusion into different areas of the renal cortex.

B. Validation of Microsphere Techniques

Adequate mixing of the spheres after left ventricular injection has been tested in the dog. In thirteen experiments no significant difference in distribution of total radioactivity between the two kidneys could be detected (Lameire, 1975). Warren and Ledingham (1975) confirmed these results in the rabbit. This provides strong evidence that adequate mixing of the spheres occurs.

The effects of increasing doses of microspheres on renal functions in the dog have been examined by several investigators (Slotkoff *et al.*, 1971; Stein *et al.*, 1971; Lameire, 1975). Total glomerular filtration rate, renal blood flow, and sodium excretion are not altered in the dog provided the investigator does not utilize a cumulative dose greater than the equivalent of 2 million 15-μm microspheres. Some discrepancy has been observed in the rabbit. Injection of more than 200,000 microspheres resulted in a 50% fall of kidney GFR in one study (Warren and Ledingham, 1975) while in the other (Bankir *et al.*, 1973), administration of up to 6 million spheres in the same species did not influence this parameter. The reason for this major discrepancy is not clear. In our hands, injection of 100,000 spheres does not influence the total kidney GFR in the rat.

Studies from this (Stein *et al.*, 1971; O'Dorisio *et al.*, 1973; Lameire, 1975) and other laboratories (Slotkoff *et al.*, 1971) have indicated virtually total extraction of the 15-μm microspheres in one circulation through the kidney, with over 99% of the counts localized in cortical tissue. Upon microscopic examination, the 15-μm sphere is usually found to have lodged in a peripheral loop of a glomerular capillary (Figure 4).

Several investigators have compared the measurement of total renal blood flow obtained with microspheres with other techniques such as electromagnetic flowmeter over a wide range of blood flows (Lameire, 1975). Arruda *et al.* (1974) also obtained excellent agreement between the results obtained with the microsphere method and PAH clearance measurements.

Even if radioactive microspheres can be validly used for the measurement of total renal blood flow, other assumptions must be considered before these particles can be utilized to measure regional blood flow in the kidney. First, measurement of blood flow in small portions of the renal cortex introduces the problem of sample size. It is necessary to have at least 400 microspheres per cortical tissue slice in order to reduce the sample counting error to less than 5% (Buckberg *et al.*, 1971). Therefore, a balance must be reached between the statistical error of low bead counts versus renal functional impairment induced by the injection of a larger number of spheres.

In this regard, we developed a method of cutting the renal cortex into four equidistant sections which were designated zones 1 through 4, going from outer to inner cortex, respectively (Stein *et al.*, 1971). Our intention was to divide the cortex into areas that would be representative of superficial nephrons (zone 1), midcortical nephrons (zones 2 and 3), and juxtamedullary nephrons (zone 4). To

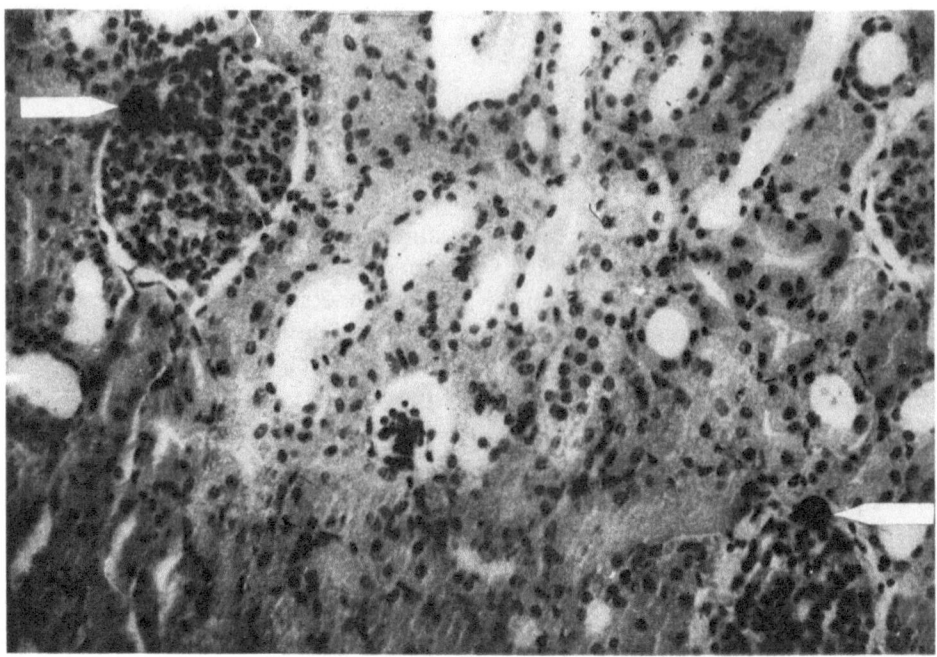

Figure 4. Localization of 15-μm microspheres in a peripheral glomerular capillary loop.

determine whether any consistent differentiation in flow rate was present in the four cortical zones, as well as to evaluate the replication of this technique, initial studies were performed in which sections from the cortical zones were obtained from different portions of the kidney after a single injection of microspheres. As shown in Figure 5, definite differences in flow were present in the various cortical zones, with over two-thirds of the cortical flow occurring in the two outer zones. When simultaneous glomerular counts were performed, it was found that this greater flow in outer cortical nephrons was due both to a greater number of glomeruli per gram of cortex as well as to a greater flow per glomerulus. Additionally, as shown in Figure 5, sections cut in two different areas of the kidney had quite similar percentage flows in each cortical zone. Similar results were found when indexes of absolute flow (the counts/min/g in each section) were compared.

These data indicate that a consistent pattern of flow distribution is found with the microspheres and that the cutting technique is quite reproducible. Figure 6 shows data comparing the fractional distribution of flow obtained with two different injections of microspheres given 30 min apart. There was no significant difference in the percentage distribution in any of the four cortical zones. Therefore, a consistent pattern of blood flow distribution was found in different portions of the same kidney after a single injection of spheres and in the same portion of the kidney after separate injections of microspheres.

Similar findings have been noted when the cortex was divided into two sections—outer and inner cortex. A consistent pattern of blood flow distribution

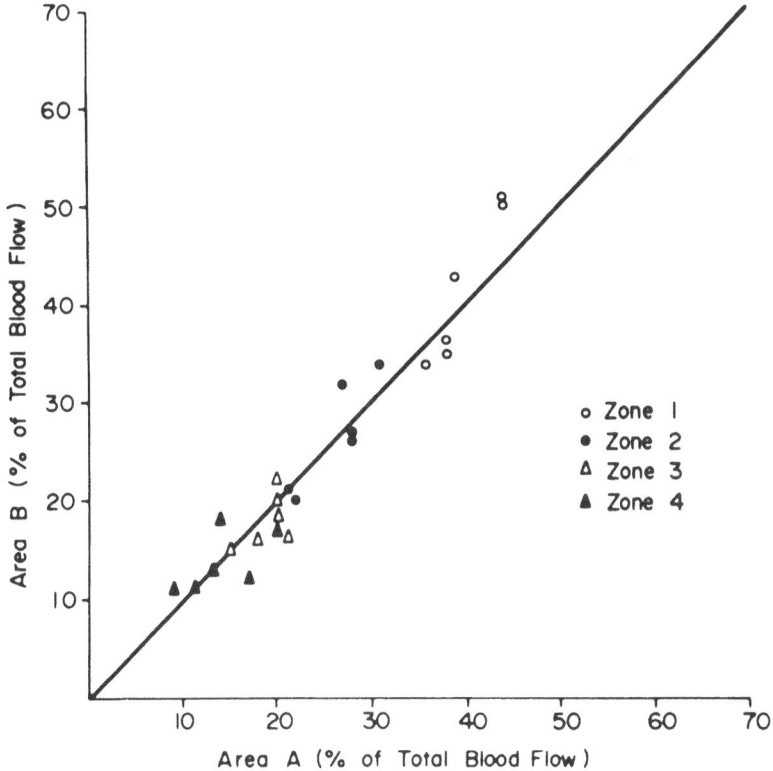

Figure 5. Comparison of the fractional distribution of blood flow between two different areas of the renal cortex after a single injection of radioactive microspheres. (Reprinted from Stein *et al.*, 1971 with permission.)

was present in hydropenic dogs, with definite differences between the outer (6.82 ml/min/g) and the inner cortex (3.85 ml/min/g) (Lameire, 1975). Tissue sections obtained from two different kidney areas (upper pole versus lower pole) had a similar radioactivity, indicating homogeneous flow characteristics in the dog kidney (Lameire, 1975).

In addition, the rheologic characteristics of microspheres must be considered. The principal criticism of the method has been related to the possible rheologic differences between a rigid sphere and the red blood cell of the species under investigation. In the dog, the red blood cell is spherical, has a diameter of 7 μm and a density of 1.10. The microsphere has a mean diameter of 15 μm and a density of 1.35.

Because of the unique arborization of the renal circulation, the possible significance of "streaming artifacts" must be considered. Pappenheimer and Kinter (1956) suggested that the hematocrit in the interlobular artery should progressively increase as blood flows toward the outer cortex because of the tendency for particles to congregate in the center of the vessel while plasma was being concentrated along the vessel wall (so called plasma skimming). Micro-

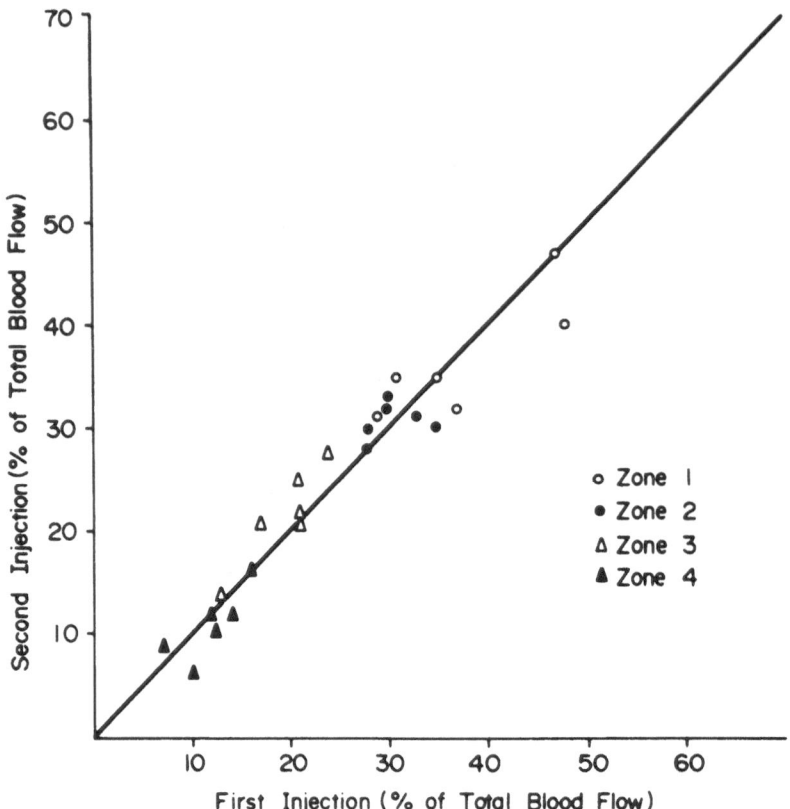

Figure 6. Comparison of the fractional distribution of blood flow in the same area of the cortex after the injection of two different radioactive microspheres. (Reprinted from Stein *et al.*, 1971 with permission.)

puncture studies in both dog (Stein *et al.*, 1972) and rat (Brenner and Galla, 1971), however, indicated no significant difference in the filtration fraction of superficial nephrons calculated from either efferent arteriolar hematocrit or protein concentration. If significant axial streaming of red cells had been present, a higher value should have been obtained with the hematocrit method. Even if streaming of red cells does not occur, it is still possible that "streaming" may be a factor in the intrarenal distribution of spheres. There is, however, strong evidence against intrarenal streaming of the beads. Much of this evidence has been discussed previously (Stein *et al.*, 1973a).

Baehler *et al.* (1973) compared the fractional distribution of renal cortical blood flow with radioactive microspheres and labeled frog red cells. The frog red cell has the same density as a dog red cell, approximately 1.08. The erythrocytes are elliptical in shape with dimensions of approximately $18 \times 10 \ \mu$m. After fixation in glutaraldehyde, they were coated with radioactive technetium. Histologic studies revealed that the frog red blood cells were localized totally in glomerular capillaries. No difference in fractional cortical blood flow distribution between the frog red cell and 15-μm microspheres could be observed in various models in the dog. Therefore, these results clearly demonstrate that the density of the microspheres does not artifactually alter the distribution of renal cortical blood flow obtained with this method.

C. Description and Handling of Tracer Microspheres

1. Physical and Chemical Properties

Radioactive microspheres are available from the 3M Company, St. Paul, Minnesota, U.S.A. or as Tracer Sephadex Microspheres from Pharmacia Fine Chemical, Upsala, Sweden. The 3M microspheres are labeled by the manufacturer and the isotope is incorporated into the matrix of the particles. In contrast, the Sephadex microspheres must be labeled immediately before use by the investigator himself and the particle is "coated" with the metallic nuclide. From information obtained by Pharmacia, the density of these Sephadex particles is 1.12 ± 0.02 g/ml, their diameter has a narrow size distribution, and they do not aggregate, eliminating the necessity for pretreatment of the particles with detergents or by sonication. Their sedimentation rate in 10% Ficoll 70 solution is 2.0 mm/min and they can be labeled with six different nuclides: ^{46}Sc, ^{51}Cr, ^{58}Co, ^{141}Ce, ^{160}Tb, and ^{169}Yb.

In the past 7 years, the authors have had extensive experience with the 3M microspheres but have not utilized the Sephadex product. Therefore, the following description is based exclusively on the experience with 3M microspheres.

The 3M microspheres, sometimes referred to as "carbonized microspheres," are black in appearance and consist of carbon, oxygen, hydrogen, and a trace amount of the nuclide of interest. The nuclide is incorporated into the microsphere and is not merely a coating on the surface. The microspheres have an absolute density of approximately 1.3 g/cc. They resist temperatures up to 400°C, above which they begin to disintegrate. They are fairly hard but are readily cut when making tissue slices.

The microspheres themselves are quite insoluble in all common organic or inorganic solvents at room temperature, but can be dissolved by boiling in concentrated acids or bases. The "leachability" of the tracer nuclide from the microsphere depends on both the nuclide and the solvent. However, in the solvents utilized in most studies (dextran, saline, water, blood, or body fluids) no significant leaching is observed, even over prolonged periods.

Microspheres labeled with six different nuclides are available: ^{169}Yb, ^{51}Cr, ^{85}Sr, ^{141}Ce, ^{125}I, and ^{46}Sc. These nuclides can be purchased with a specific activity as high as 10 mCi/g. Microsphere preparations ranging in size up to 50 μm in diameter are available. The variation in size in a given batch is quite substantial and will be discussed subsequently. For studies of the renal circulation, spheres with a mean diameter of 15 μm are most frequently utilized.

Suspending Medium. The medium chosen will depend on the needs of the experiment and the settling rate of microspheres. Since the microspheres are more dense than the suspending medium, they will tend to sediment. The

Table II. Approximate Settling of 3M Brand Tracer
Microspheres in Suspending Agents (cm/min)

Size	Saline	10% Dextran	20% Dextran
15 ± 5	0.4	0.04	0.008
25 ± 5	1.0	0.1	0.02
35 ± 5	2.0	0.2	0.04
50 ± 10	4.0	0.4	0.08
80 ± 10	10.0	1.0	0.2

increased viscosity of dextran will retard such settling (Table II). It has been demonstrated repeatedly that no settling effects are demonstrable *in vivo*.

Isotope Selection. Gamma-emitting isotopes which cover a broad range of energy peaks are utilized. The standard nuclides available are summarized in Table III. The isotope that is most often chosen when only one nuclide is needed is strontium-85. This isotope has pure gamma emission, a long half-life and a relatively strong energy peak. Any of the other isotopes can be used with strontium for dual isotope studies. As many as six isotopes have been used in individual studies.

Specific Activity. To determine what level of specific activity (mCi of the isotope/g of microspheres) is to be chosen, two factors must be considered. The virtue of using a larger number of microspheres, each emitting a lower level of radiation, is balanced against the use of a smaller number of microspheres, each containing a higher concentration of nuclide. Table IV demonstrates the number of microspheres per milligram of preparation as a function of the size of microsphere utilized. In most situations, it is optimal to utilize a preparation with high specific activity (10 mCi/g of microspheres) and to give as few spheres as are necessary for adequate counting statistics and valid measurement of flow. In this regard, it should be emphasized, however, that at least 400 microspheres are

Table III. Radioactive Characteristics of Available
Nuclides

Nuclide	Half-life (days)	Principal gamma radiation (keV)
^{125}I	60	35
^{169}Yb	31	63
^{141}Ce	32.5	145
^{51}Cr	27.8	320
^{85}Sr	65	514
^{46}Sc	83.8	890

Table IV. Number of Microspheres per
Milligram vs. Mean Diameter

Standard size (μm)	Approximate number of microspheres/mg
0.5 − 10	—
15 ± 5	440,000
25 ± 5	85,000
35 ± 5	35,000
50 ± 10	12,000

needed in a given tissue section to allow for a 5% error in flow measurement (Buckberg *et al.*, 1971).

2. Handling of Microspheres

Microspheres are packaged either in the dry form or as an autoclaved suspension in 10 or 20% dextran or isotonic saline solution. Under certain conditions, the microspheres have a tendency to aggregate. In order to avoid this problem, and to provide a homogeneous dispersion, a few drops of 5% Tween (polyoxyethylene sorbitan monooleate) are injected into each ampule. Should the microspheres be obtained in powder form, it is recommended that a few drops of 5% Tween be added (1 drop/10 ml) and the suspension be subjected to ultrasonic treatment, which also disperses any aggregates.

3. Determination of Diameter Distribution

It is recommended that the investigator determine the frequency distribution of the batch of microspheres utilized. The following procedure can be followed:

1. Place a drop of a homogeneously mixed microsphere suspension into a hemocytometer.
2. Project the microscopic picture of this preparation (magnification 270) by means of a drawing mirror onto millimeter paper.
3. Trace 400–600 microspheres on the paper and measure them using an eyepiece micrometer.

The results of such measurements in six different microsphere batches are given in Table V.

D. Method of Microsphere Injection

A microsphere injectate which is well mixed and homogeneous and a patent arterial catheter are essential for reproducible studies. In our laboratory, we have utilized a Goodale–Lubin catheter threaded into the left ventricle, but left

Table V. Diameter Size Distribution of Six Different Batches
of 15-μm Microspheres

Number of spheres	Mean diameter (μm)	Standard error (μm)
121	15.2	2.71
470	14.7	2.07
639	15.0	2.00
364	15.0	1.94
717	14.6	2.45
675	14.7	2.52

atrial placement is also satisfactory for proper mixing. The catheter may be passed through the right carotid artery or either femoral artery into the left ventricle. The catheter placement is considered satisfactory only when a typical left ventricular pressure pulse tracing has been obtained.

The standard injectate utilized for dog experiments in this laboratory contains 20 μCi of high specific activity 15-μm spheres (approximately 400,000 spheres per injection). From the standard 10-ml vial of 3M spheres, 200 μl of well-mixed solution are drawn into a 1-ml syringe that already contains 800 μl of 10% dextran. Just prior to injection, the syringe containing the injection material should be placed in an ultrasonic cleaner for at least 2 min to break down any aggregates of microspheres that may have formed. After air is purged from the syringe, it is connected to the left ventricular catheter. The spheres are then injected into the catheter, which has a dead space greater than the volume of the 1-ml injectate. The stopcock is closed, the small syringe is removed and replaced with a syringe containing 10–15 ml of saline solution. The stopcock is then opened and the saline solution is injected over a 20-sec period. Systemic blood pressure should be monitored during the microsphere injection to be certain that some type of alteration in systemic hemodynamics does not occur during this period. If the injection technique was properly performed, this should not occur.

E. Measurement of Cardiac Output

In numerous studies, it is quite advantageous to be able to measure cardiac output along with the determination of renal hemodynamics. This parameter can be obtained with the microsphere method if the total number of counts injected is known and a reference sample is collected.

There are several possible ways of determining the number of counts injected, but we have found that this can be done most accurately using a method in which the weight of the sphere solution in a standard mixture and in the injectate are compared.

1. Method

A microhematocrit tube is placed in a small test tube and the total contents are weighed. A 1-ml tuberculin syringe is also weighed and approximately 0.2 ml of the well-mixed stock sphere solution is added to the syringe, which is reweighed. Using forceps, the microhematocrit tube is removed and placed at the surface of the stock solution of spheres. The solution of spheres will enter by capillary action. The microhematocrit tube is then immediately placed back in the test tube and reweighed. Three to five measurements should be obtained for each injection. After the test tube and microhematocrit samples are weighed, the radioactivity is measured in a gamma counter and counts per minute (CPM) per milliliter of sample determined. If properly performed, the coefficient of variation of five samples should be 5% or less. The amount of CPM injected is then determined from the relationship between the CPM/mg in the aliquot to the total weight of the injectate in the syringe. In initial studies, an investigator should also determine the radioactivity left in the injection syringe. With practice, this amount is usually quite small.

While this method is reasonably simple and accurate, there are some pitfalls to be avoided. In weighing the aliquots, the time between sampling and the second weighing should be as short as possible to reduce evaporation of the small quantity of solution taken. The activity of the aliquots must also be considered as they may exceed the upper limit (250,000–300,000 CPM) of accuracy of the gamma counter.

In addition to knowing the total CPM in the injectate, a reference sample is needed to determine cardiac output. This is obtained from a peripheral vessel such as the brachial or femoral artery. Ten seconds before injecting the spheres into the animal, a withdrawal pump is started at a known rate from this peripheral vessel. We use a Harvard infusion pump (Harvard Apparatus Co., Millis, Mass.) and withdraw at a rate of 25 ml/min. The pump is continued for the 20-sec period of injection and 25–30 sec thereafter. The pump is then stopped, and the blood samples are spun down. The reference blood sample is then transferred to counting tubes and the collection syringe is rinsed with Haemo-Sol (Meinecke and Co., Baltimore, Md.). This rinse is added to a counting tube. The tubes are then centrifuged for 5 min to sediment the microspheres and subsequently counted.

2. Calculations

$$\text{CPM injected} = \text{CPM/mg aliquot} \times \text{Wt}_I \qquad (28)$$

where Wt_I is the weight of the injectate in milligrams.

$$\text{Cardiac output} = \text{CPM injected} \times \frac{\text{blood withdrawal rate (ml/min)}}{\text{CPM reference sample}} \qquad (29)$$

F. Measurement of Total Renal Blood Flow

Total renal blood flow can be measured with microspheres in a manner quite similar to cardiac output. In this case, however, the total CPM of a nuclide in the kidney must be measured.

1. Method

At the conclusion of the experiment, the kidney under study is removed, decapsulated, and then dissolved in approximately 100 ml of concentrated hydrochloric acid for 24 hr. After the kidney is totally dissolved, the exact volume of the hydrochloric acid mixture is determined in a graduated cylinder. The solution is then thoroughly mixed and five 1-ml aliquots are withdrawn and placed in separate counting tubes. The mean CPM/ml is multiplied by the total volume of the homogenate mixture to obtain the total CPM in the kidney.

Otherwise, the same procedure is utilized for sphere injection and reference sample collection as for cardiac output measurement.

2. Calculations

$$\text{Total renal blood flow} = \text{CPM}_{\text{kidney}} \times \frac{\text{blood withdrawal rate (ml/min)}}{\text{CPM reference sample}} \quad (30)$$

G. Measurement of Cortical Blood Flow Distribution

1. Method

At the end of the experiment, the kidney is removed and decapsulated. The poles of the kidney are cut off with a sharp razor blade and the remaining kidney is bisected. The remaining kidney exposed in this manner has a clear demarcation between cortex and medulla. Three or more sections 1 cm in thickness are then obtained. From each of these sections, approximately a 1-cm cube is removed with a fresh razor blade with the depth of these cuts extending from the outer cortex to the outer medulla. The cortical thickness is then measured and the tissue sample is placed in a metal kidney cutter (Figure 7). These cutters are of varying lengths with four equidistant grooves on each side of the housing of the apparatus. For example, if the cortical thickness is 8 mm, the grooves are 2 mm apart. The section is placed in the cutter so that the outer cortical zone is

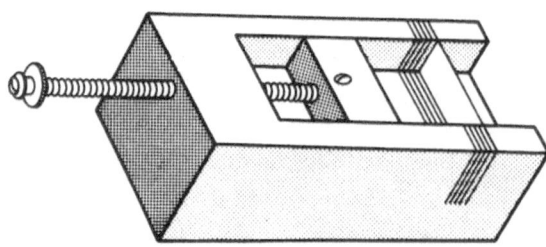

Figure 7. Schematic drawing of apparatus used to cut cortical kidney slices in the dog. Note the series of equidistant grooves on the housing of the cutter.

juxtaposed to the end of the holder and the medullary zone is kept under constant pressure by a screw clamp. Four equal sections are then cut with a fresh razor blade placed in each of the four grooves. It has been found that the entire cortex is obtained with these four sections and that a small area of medulla is usually also present in the inner portion of the last section. However, it is felt necessary to include this area to be certain that all juxtamedullary nephrons are counted.

These sections have been designated zones 1–4, with zone 1 being the most outer cortical zone and zone 4 the most inner cortical zone. Each section is placed in a preweighed counting tube, reweighed, and counted in a gamma counter.

2. Calculations

The uncorrected percent of renal blood flow per cortical zone (P_z), percent of flow per gram, is determined by dividing the counts per minute per gram of tissue in the respective zone (CPM_z) by the total for all the measured cortical zones (CPM_t).

The corrected percent of renal blood flow per cortical zone can be determined by the following formula:

$$\text{Corrected percent zonal blood flow } (P_z') = CPM_z \times Wt_z/CPM_t' \qquad (31)$$

where Wt_z is the weight of the zone and CPM_t' is the total counts per minute per gram times the zonal weight for all zones. Wt_z is obtained by using the derivation of the volume of four cortical zones obtained by McNay and Abe (1970) in which the percent of renal volume was found to be 27, 22, 17, and 12% in zones 1–4 respectively.

Therefore,

$$Wt_z = V_z \times Wt_T \qquad (32)$$

where V_z equals the volume of the respective zone and Wt_T equals the kidney weight.

Zonal blood flow (BF_z) is estimated by the following formula:

$$BF_z = P_z' \times RBF \qquad (33)$$

Zonal perfusion rate is determined by dividing BF_z by Wt_z.

H. Measurement of Radioactivity

Once the tissue and blood samples have been properly collected, there still remains the task of counting the various radioactive specimens. All of the nuclides utilized are gamma emitters and their activity can be determined with any of several commercially available gamma counters. Since the nomenclature and operational aspects vary from machine to machine, it would not be feasible to discuss the specific details of operating each of these gamma counters. The major unique problems involved with counting of radioactive microspheres relate to the use of multiple nuclides in a given experiment. Thus, to perform this type of study, one must be able to differentiate the energy spectrum of each nuclide and to correct for any overlap in the spectrum between nuclides.

1. Determining the Energy Spectrum of a Nuclide

Most gamma counters have two basic settings necessary to determine the photopeak of a given nuclide: the power setting and the window. The power setting controls an energy range for the pulse high analyzer and may vary from 0 to 1000 keV. This setting can be adjusted. The window setting defines the discrete portion of the energy range set by the power control in which pulses are accepted.

There are multiple ways in which the energy spectrum of a given nuclide can be determined. In our laboratory, we have utilized a Packard autogamma counter. The window setting has an upper level (base) and lower level (window) adjustment. Since the window range is relative to the base setting, the base may be changed arbitrarily and the window interval will change with it. Therefore, if the sample of isotope is placed in the counter, the window can be set at some interval (e.g., 5%) and the base at 0%. By repeating the measurement by adding 5% to the base setting while keeping the window constant, the entire energy spectrum for that isotope can be scanned. The results are then plotted on rectilinear graph paper (counts vs. base setting) for interpretation. Figure 8 shows the spectrum for ^{85}Sr. As can readily be seen, the major photopeak for ^{85}Sr is clearly defined and the base and window settings required to include only the major photopeak can be determined directly.

Any isotope will produce a spectrum of energy which covers more area than just the defined limits of the window setting. If another window is set for a lower energy isotope, there will be a percentage of the counts of the higher energy nuclide detected in the channel of the lower energy isotope. The obvious problem that will arise from such a phenomenon is that more counts will be recorded for an isotope that receives this crossover than are produced by the isotope alone.

As can be noted from Figure 9, there is some ^{85}Sr radioactivity present in the spectrum of the ^{141}Ce. Therefore, the amount of radioactivity obtained in the ^{141}Ce spectrum must be corrected for this "crossover." The technique to correct for this problem is straightforward. A sample of each nuclide is counted and the percentage of the total counts in each specific channel is determined for each nuclide. The crossover of radioactivity of one nuclide into the channel of another nuclide is then determined. Figure 9 demonstrates the pulse height analysis of ^{141}Ce and ^{85}Sr. As can be noted, there is no crossover of ^{141}Ce in the ^{85}Sr spectrum, but the reverse is not true.

In this example, there are approximately 100,000 CPM of either ^{141}Ce or ^{85}Sr when they are counted separately. When both nuclides are counted together, however, there are significantly more than 100,000 CPM detected in the ^{141}Ce channel. To correct, a standard solution containing only ^{85}Sr is utilized and the ratio of ^{85}Sr in the ^{141}Ce to ^{85}Sr channel is determined. If this crossover ratio

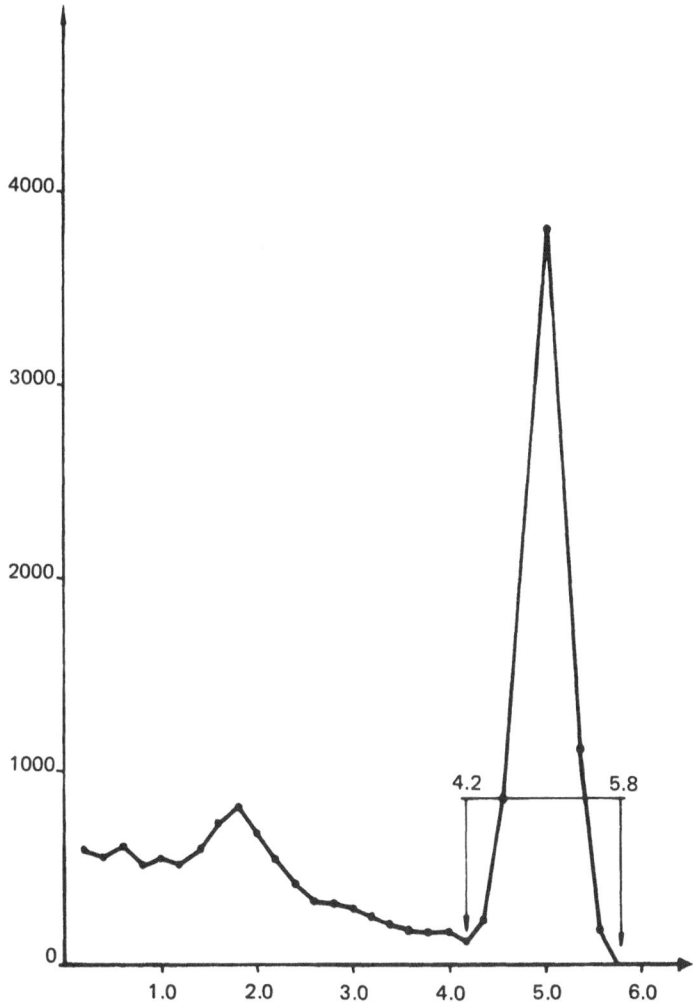

Figure 8. The energy spectrum of ^{85}Sr. Horizontal axis, MEV; vertical axis, CPM of the nuclide.

equals 15%, then the true ^{141}Ce CPM will be equal to the measured ^{141}Ce CPM -0.15 (^{85}Sr CPM). Similar but somewhat more complex corrections are necessary when three or more nuclides are utilized.

VII. ALBUMIN ACCUMULATION METHOD FOR MEASUREMENT OF PAPILLARY PLASMA FLOW

A. Theoretical Background

Papillary blood flow represents a small but highly significant fraction of total renal blood flow. Estimated to comprise approximately 1% of total flow

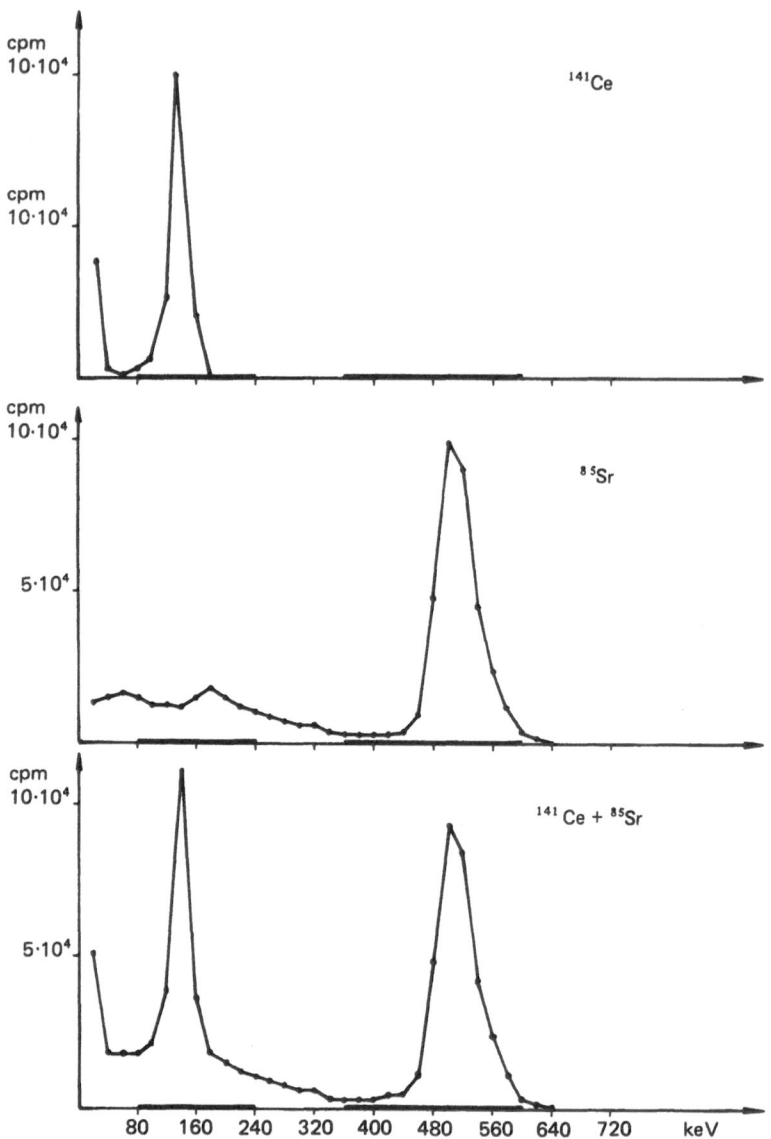

Figure 9. Demonstration of crossover of ^{85}Sr into the energy spectrum of ^{141}Ce. There are approximately 10×10^4 CPM when ^{141}Ce is counted above (upper panel). The peak spectrum of ^{85}Sr is 420–580 keV but there is significant activity in the spectrum of ^{141}Ce. This can be noted by the increase in radioactivity in the ^{141}Ce channel when the two nuclides are counted together (lower panel).

(Lilienfield *et al.*, 1961), papillary flow undoubtedly influences the regulation of the renal countercurrent mechanism. In addition to this role in water balance, interrelationships between papillary flow and other renal functions remain to be investigated. With such questions in mind, various techniques have been devised to attempt to measure papillary flow. One method, based on the original work of Lilienfield *et al.* (1961), and modifications by Ganguli and Tobian (1974) and

Solez *et al.* (1974) will be discussed here. This method measures the accumulation rate of a plasma marker, radioactive albumin, in the papilla.

Postglomerular blood from juxtamedullary nephrons is the principal if not the sole source of blood flow to the papilla. Within the long, small-caliber vasa recta, blood would be expected to travel in rather orderly fashion, entering blood steadily displacing that already present, with little mixing. Given a slow rate of flow, there exists a relatively long period during which the accumulation rate of a vascular label would be constant. For any time interval which does not exceed this transit time, it is possible to calculate papillary flow by relating the amount of marker in the tissue to the concentration of the label in the circulating blood. Radioactive albumin has been utilized as a plasma marker and its accumulation rate is measured over a period less than one transit time through the papilla. In order to translate tissue radioactivity into plasma flow, it is necessary to know the concentration of radioactive albumin in plasma entering the papilla. Plasma from a sample of arterial blood is counted for this purpose. Furthermore, since the labeled albumin is given as a constant infusion, the reference blood sample is withdrawn during the entire period of perfusion so the changes in the plasma concentration of albumin will be taken into consideration.

B. Method

Rats are anesthetized with inactin (100 mg/kg) and an airway is established. Body temperature is maintained on a heated platform at 37–38°C. Blood pressure is monitored through the right femoral artery. Two catheters are placed into the right jugular vein. Through one, Ringer solution is infused at 20 μl/min during the remainder of the procedure. The other catheter is utilized for subsequent infusion of a solution containing 6.6 μCi/ml [^{125}I]albumin in 2.3% FDC green dye. The dye provides a means of detecting the point at which labeled blood begins to enter the kidney (time zero). The left femoral artery is cannulated with PE50 tubing of sufficient length to contain the entire reference blood sample. A bidirectional Harvard pump is readied to infuse the albumin-FDC and withdraw the blood sample at the same rate so as to cause minimal disturbance in blood volume and systemic hemodynamics. An opening in the abdominal wall approximately 3 cm in diameter is made. The viscera are gently retracted and both kidneys are carefully freed laterally from peritoneal attachments. A loose tie is placed around each renal pedicle and a secondary branch of the left renal artery is visualized with a dissecting microscope. When possible, no dissection is done in the hilar region to avoid disruption of renal nerves and lymphatics. At this point, the infusion mixture is advanced behind a small air bubble into the second jugular catheter to a point where the meniscus is just visible. The femoral catheter is then prepared by positioning a small air bubble followed by a drop of mercury in the PE tubing into which the arterial sample will be drawn. The mercury allows the blood sample to be partitioned from the fluid which initially occupies the polyethylene tubing. After a short equilibration period, the albumin infusion is begun at 0.37 ml/min. At the appearance of dye in the left renal artery branch, the timing period (circulation time) and arterial collection are simultaneously begun. At the conclusion of the time interval under study, both pedicle ligatures are tightened and the arterial collection is terminated so that the blood sample obtained closely corresponds to blood which has perfused the kidneys.

The kidneys are removed with the ties intact and are chilled at −20°C for a period sufficient to partially freeze them. This step aids in the subsequent dissection. Each kidney is cut from pole to pole into slightly unequal halves so that the papilla lies undisturbed in one half. Adjacent tissue is carefully removed with a razor blade so that the papilla, still attached to the medulla, is completely exposed. Adherent blood is gently wiped off and then small dissecting scissors are used to sever most of the papilla from its attachment. A rim of papilla is always left behind so that only papillary tissue is analyzed. The severed portion is placed on a preweighed piece of paper, weighed, and then transferred to a glass counting tube.

The blood sample is allowed to run from the PE tubing in which it was collected into a microcentrifuge tube previously heparinized and dried. The sample is centrifuged and aliquots of plasma are counted in triplicate.

Because the method affords only one measurement of flow per animal, it is necessary to perform a series of experiments at different circulation times. The times utilized here are 8, 16, 24, and 30 sec. By dividing counts per 100 g papilla by counts per milliliter plasma, the vascular volume occupied by labeled plasma at each time interval is obtained. Plotting this volume of distribution (V_t) against the circulation time for each experimental measurement, a line is constructed which is linear up to a given point (Figure 10). It is at this point that, for the existent blood flow rate, labeled plasma has begun to exit the papilla; thus, the relationship between plasma radioactivity and tissue radioactivity changes. For circulation times less than this transit time, papillary plasma flow can be calculated by using the formula

$$PPF = \frac{CPM_{tissue}}{CPM_{plasma}} \times \frac{60 \text{ sec/min}}{\text{circulation time (sec)}}$$

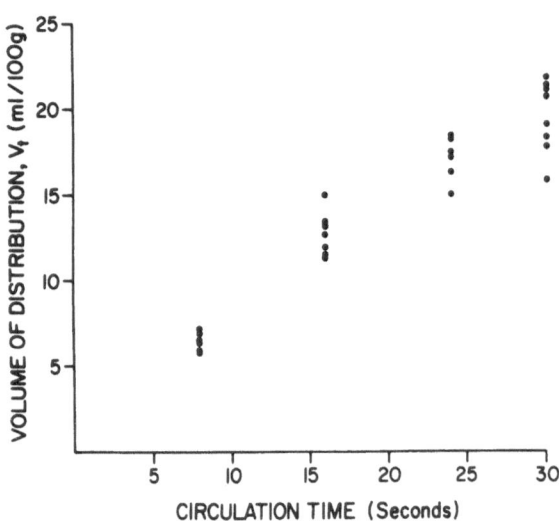

Figure 10. Volume of distribution of radioactive albumin in the papilla of the rat as a function of time after infusion. Volume of distribution increases linearly for at least the first 25 sec, suggesting that little radioactive albumin leaves the papilla during this time.

C. Discussion

The apparent plasma flow obtained by this technique requires qualification on several points. The method is based on the assumption that systemic concentrations of the radioactive albumin represent the concentration entering the papilla. Two inaccuracies of the present technique are recognized. First, the blood entering the vasa recta is postglomerular and has already been subjected to filtration so that the albumin concentration in entering papillary blood is higher than the systemic concentration. Actual flow is therefore overestimated. Since nearly 70% of glomerular filtrate is returned to the blood before it enters the papilla (Stein *et al.* 1973b), this overestimate is on the order of 30% of the filtration fraction. Therefore, at a filtration fraction of 0.20, this error is approximately 6%. Theoretically, for any given model, this error will be consistent but for conditions in which the filtration fraction and reabsorption proximal to the papilla are altered differently, the error will vary. In general, apparent flow will approach actual flow in states in which the filtration fraction is quite low. Second, the arterial reference sample will not be totally representative of the blood reaching the papilla during the interval of study since the final portion of the arterial sample will consist of blood which has not had adequate time to enter the papilla.

Since values are expressed as plasma flow per unit weight, states in which the degree of hydration and therefore the weight of tissue is altered may also introduce some error. Greater accuracy might be obtained by using desiccated tissue weights instead. It is not proper to convert the calculated plasma flow into blood flow using the systemic hematocrit since this latter value is much lower in the papilla (Wolgast, 1968).

ACKNOWLEDGMENTS

This work was supported in part by NIH program project grant AM-17387-03.

REFERENCES

Andersen, A. M., and Ladefoged, J. 1965. The relationship between hematocrit and solubility of ^{133}Xe in blood. *J. Pharmacol. Sci., 54:*1684.

Arruda, J. A. L., Boonjarern, S., Westenfelder, C., and Kurtzman, N. A. 1974. Measurement of renal blood flow with radioactive microspheres. *Proc. Soc. Exp. Biol. Med., 146:*263.

Aukland, K. 1967. Study of renal circulation with inert gas: measurements in tissue. In: *Proceedings of the Third International Congress of Nephrology,* 1966, Vol. 1, *Physiology.* Ed. by Schreiner, G. E., S. Karger, Basel, Switzerland.

Aukland, K., and Berliner, R. W. 1964. Renal medullary counter-current system studied with hydrogen gas. *Circ. Res., 15:*430.

Baehler, R. W., Catanzaro, A. J., Stein, J. H., and Hunter, W. 1973. The radio-labelled frog red blood cell: a new marker of cortical blood flow distribution in the kidney of the dog. *Circ. Res., 32:*718.

Bankir, L. F., Farman, N., Grunfeld, J. P., Huet de la Tour, E., and Funck-Brentano, J. L. 1973.

Radioactive microsphere distribution and single glomerular blood flow in the normal rabbit kidney. *Pflugers Archiv. 342:*111.

Bolme, P., and Edwall, L. 1970. Disappearance of Xe^{133} and I^{125} from skeletal muscle of the anesthetized dog during sympathetic cholinergic vasodilatation. *Acta Physiol. Scand., 78:*28.

Brenner, B. M., and Galla, J. H. 1971. Influence of postglomerular hematocrit and protein concentration on rat nephron fluid transfer. *Am. J. Physiol., 220:*148.

Buckberg, G. D., Luck, J. C., Payne, B. D., Hoffman, J. I. E., Archie, J. P., and Fixler, D. E. 1971. Some sources of error measuring regional blood flow with radioactive microspheres. *J. Appl. Physiol., 31:*598.

Carrière, S. 1970. A comparison of the disappearance curves of ^{133}Xe and ^{85}Kr for the measurement of the intrarenal distribution of blood flow. *Can. J. Physiol. Pharmacol., 48:*834.

Carrière, S., and Friborg, J. 1969. Intrarenal blood flow and PAH extraction during angiotensin infusion. *Am. J. Physiol., 217:*1708.

Cortney, M. A., Mylle, M., Lassiter, W. E., and Gottschalk, C. W. 1965. Renal tubular transport of water, solute and PAH in rats loaded with isotonic saline. *Am. J. Physiol., 209:*1199.

Dobson, E. L., and Warner, G. F. 1957. Measurement of regional sodium turnover rates and their application to the estimation of regional blood flow. *Am. J. Physiol., 189:*269.

Earley, L. E., and Friedler, R. M. 1965a. Changes in renal blood flow and possibly the intrarenal distribution of blood during the natriuresis accompanying saline loading in the dog. *J. Clin. Invest., 44:*929.

Earley, L. E., and Friedler, R. M. 1965b. Studies on the mechanism of natriuresis accompanying increased renal blood flow and its role in the renal response to extracellular volume expansion. *J. Clin. Invest., 44:*1857.

Effros, R. M., Lowenstein, J., Baldwin, D. S., and Chinard, F. P. 1967. Vascular and extravascular volumes of the kidney of man. *Circ. Res., 20:*162.

Ganguli, M., and Tobian, L. 1974. Does the kidney autoregulate papillary plasma flow in chronic postsalt hypertension? *Am. J. Physiol., 226:*330.

Gransjö, G. 1968. Variations in the cortical and medullary blood flow through the dog kidney measured with treated thermocouples. Ph.D Thesis, University of Upsala.

Gransjo, G., Ulfendahl, H. R., and Wolgast, M. 1966. Determination of regional blood flow by means of small semiconductor detectors and red cells tagged with phosphorus.^{32} *Nature (Lond.), 211:*1411.

Harving, L., and Pelley, K. 1965. Die Bestimmung der Nierenmark Durchblutung auf Grund der Ablagerung und Verteilung von ^{86}Rb. *Arch. ges. Physiol., 285:*302.

Kety, S. S. 1951. The theory and applications of the exchange of inert gas at the lungs and tissues. *Pharmacol. Rev., 3:*1.

Kramer, K., Thurau, K., and Deetjen, P. 1960. Hämodynamik des Nierenmarks. 1. Capillare Passagezet, Blutvolumen, Durchblutung, Gewebshamatokrit und O_2—Verbrauch des Nierenmarks *in situ. Pflügers Arch., 270:*251.

Lameire, N. H. 1975. Onderzoekingen over de aanpassingen van de doorbloedingsverdeling in de nierschors, Ph.D. Thesis, University of Ghent.

Lameire, N. H., and Ringoir, S. 1975. Comparison of the xenon washout method, the electromagnetic flowmeter and radioactive microspheres for the measurement of renal blood flow. *Rein et Foie, Maladies de la Nutrition, 16:*107.

Landis, E., Elsom, K. A., and Shiels, E. H. 1936. Simultaneous plasma clearances of creatinine and certain organic compounds of iodine in relation to human kidney function. *J. Clin. Invest., 15:*397.

Lilienfield, L. S., Maganzani, H. C., and Bauer, M. H. 1961. Blood flow in the renal medulla. *Circ. Res., 9:*614.

McNay, J. L., and Abe, Y. 1970. Pressure-dependent heterogeneity of renal cortical blood flow in dogs. *Circ. Res., 27:*571.

Mowat, P., Lupu, A. N., and Maxwell, M. H. 1972. Limitation of ^{133}Xe washout technique in estimation of renal blood flow. *Am. J. Physiol., 223:*682.

Nissen, O. I. 1968. The extraction fraction of *p*-aminohippurate in the superficial and deep venous drainage area of the cat kidney. *Acta Physiol. Scand., 73:*329.

Ochwadt, B., and Schmier, J. 1954. Über Temperatur- und Kreislaufzeit-messungen in verschiedenen Abschnitten der Hundenniere. *Pflügers Arch., 258:*261.

O'Dorisio, T. M., Stein, J. H., Osgood, R. W., and Ferris, T. F. 1973. Absence of aglomerular blood flow during renal vasodilatation and hemorrhage in the dog. *Proc. Soc. Exp. Biol. Med., 143:*612.

Ofstad, J., Lund-Johansen, P., and Kolsaker, L. 1967a. Dye dilution measurement of renal blood flow *in vivo* and in glass models. *Scand. J. Lab. Clin. Invest., 20:*281.

Ofstad, J., Lund-Johansen, P., and Kölsaker, L. 1967b. Dye dilution measurement of renal blood flow: observations of the down slope of the dye-dilution curve. *Scand. J. Lab. Clin. Invest., 20:*289.

Pappenheimer, J. R., and Kinter, W. B. 1956. Hematocrit ratio of blood within mammalian kidney and its significance for renal hemodynamics. *Am. J. Physiol., 185:*377.

Pedersen, F., Ladefoged, J., Doutheil, U., and Selkurt, E. E. 1965. Circulation times in the dog measured by an external counting technique and by a dye dilution method. *Arch. ges. Physiol., 286:*36.

Phillips, R. A., Dole, V. P., Hamilton, P. B., Emerson, K., Archibald, P. M., and Van Slycke, D. D. 1946. Effect of acute hemorrhagic and traumatic shock on renal functions of dogs. *Am. J. Physiol., 145:*314.

Reubi, F. 1958. Objections à la théorie de la séparation intrarénale des hématies et du plasma (Pappenheimer). *Helv. Med. Acta, 25:*516.

Reubi, F. C., and Schroeder, H. A. 1949. Can vascular shunting be induced in the kidney by vasoactive drugs? *J. Clin. Invest., 28:*114.

Reubi, F. C., Gossweiler, N., and Gurtler, R. 1966. Renal circulation in man studied by means of a dye-dilution method. *Circulation, 33:*426.

Rudolph, A. M. and Heymann, M. A. 1967. The circulation of the fetus *in utero*. Methods for studying distribution of blood flow, cardiac output and organ blood flow. *Circ. Res., 21:*163.

Sapirstein, L. A. 1958. Regional blood flow by fractional distribution of indicators. *Am. J. Physiol., 193:*161.

Schnermann, J., and Thurau, K. 1965. Micropunctionsversuch zum Verhalter der PAH-konzentration im Vasa Recta Blut Goldhamsterniere. *Arch. ges. Physiol., 283:*171.

Slotkoff, L. M., Logan, A., Jose, P., d'Avela, J., and Eisner, G. M. 1971. Microsphere measurement of intrarenal circulation of the dog. *Circ. Res., 28:*158.

Smith, H. W., Finkelstein, N., Aliminosa, L., Crawford, B., and Graber, M. 1945. The renal clearances of substituted hippuric acid derivatives and other aromatic acids in dog and man. *J. Clin. Invest., 24:*388.

Solez, K., Kramer, E. C., Fox, J. A. 1974. Medullary plasma flow and intravascular leukocyte accumulation in acute renal failure. *Kidney Intern., 6:*24.

Stein, J. H., Ferris, T. F., Huprich, J. E., Smith, T. C., and Osgood, R. W. 1971. Effect of renal vasodilatation on the distribution of cortical blood flow in the kidney of the dog. *J. Clin. Invest., 50:*1429.

Stein, J. H., Congbalay, R. C., Karsch, D. L., Osgood, R. W., and Ferris, T. F. 1972. Effect of bradykinin on proximal tubular sodium reabsorption in the dog: evidence for functional nephron heterogeneity. *J. Clin. Invest., 51:*1709.

Stein, J. H., Boonjarern, S., Wilson, C. B., and Ferris, T. F. 1973a. Alterations in intrarenal blood flow distribution: Methods of measurement and relationship to sodium balance, *Circ. Res.,* Suppl. *23:*I-61.

Stein, J. H., Osgood, R., Boonjarern, S., and Ferris, T. F. 1973b. A comparison of the segmental analysis of sodium reabsorption during Ringer's and hyperoncotic albumin infusion in the rat. *J. Clin. Invest., 52:*2313.

Thorburn, G. D., Kopald, H. H., Herd, J. A., Hollenberg, M., O'Morchoe, C. C. C., and Barger, A. D. 1963. Intrarenal distribution of nutrient blood flow determined with krypton[85] in the unanesthetized dog. *Circ. Res., 13:*290.

Tune, B. M., Burg, M. B., and Patlack, C. S. 1969. Characteristics of *p*-aminohippurate transport in proximal renal tubules. *Am. J. Physiol., 217:*1057.

Wallin, J. D., Rector, F. C., Jr., and Seldin, D. W. 1971. Measurement of intrarenal plasma flow with antiglomerular basement membrane antibody, *Am. J. Physiol., 221:*1621.

Warren, D. J., and Ledingham, J. G. G. 1975. Measurement of intrarenal blood flow distribution in the rabbit using radioactive microspheres. *Clin. Science & Mol. Med., 48:*51.

Warren, J. V., Brannon, E. S., and Merrill, A. J. 1944. Method of obtaining renal venous blood in unanesthetized persons with observations of the extraction of oxygen and sodium para-amino-hippurate, *Science, 100:*108.

Wolf, A. V. 1941. Total renal blood flow at any urine flow or extraction fraction (abstract). *Am. J. Physiol., 133:*496.

Wolgast, M. 1968. Studies on the regional renal blood flow meter P^{32} labelled red cells and small beta-sensitive semi-conductor detectors, *Acta. Physiol. Scand.,* Suppl. 313:1.

Chapter **4**

Micropuncture Techniques

F. Lang and R. Greger

Institute of Physiology
Innsbruck, Austria

C. Lechene

Biotechnology Resource in Electron Probe Microanalysis
Harvard Medical School
Boston, Massachusetts

and

F. G. Knox

Department of Physiology and Biophysics
Mayo Clinic and Mayo Foundation
Rochester, Minnesota

I. INTRODUCTION

In the 1920s Richards and co-workers introduced the idea of collecting fluid from single nephrons in the frog to gain insight into the formation of urine (Wearn and Richards, 1924; Richards and Schmidt, 1924). Since 1941, when Walker *et al.* first applied this technique to the mammalian kidney, the use of micropuncture has increased markedly. The development of stationary micro-perfusion (Richards and Walker, 1937), shrinking droplet (Gertz and Ullrich, 1961), microinjection (Gottschalk *et al.*, 1965), microcatheterization (Jarausch and Ullrich, 1956), microperfusion (Sonnenberg and Deetjen, 1964), and peritu-bular microperfusion and injection techniques (Lechene and Morel, 1965; Frömter *et al.*, 1968; Windhager, 1968b) proved to be important sophistications of the micropuncture technique. Although free-flow micropuncture remains the basic tool, all of the above techniques have found widespread use and have contributed considerably to the knowledge of current nephrology.

This chapter will deal with the advantages, applications, and limitations of micropuncture procedures. Measurement of pressures has been dealt with in Chapter 3 of Volume 4A in this series (Knox and Marchand, 1976) and measurement of pH and potentials are dealt with in a separate chapter of this book.

In general, the techniques and materials will be described as they are used in our laboratories. Accordingly, the techniques are described as they are applied to the rat, small rodents, or dog, although micropuncture has been applied to a variety of mammalian and nonmammalian animals.

II. PREPARATION FOR MICROPUNCTURE

The most commonly used strains of rats are the Wistar and the Sprague–Dawley. Munich–Wistar rats have the advantage of superficial glomeruli accessible to micropuncture. For micropuncture of the cortex, the most convenient body weight is 200–250 g. The papilla protrudes into the ureter and is accessible to micropuncture in rats below 150 g.

For anesthesia, thiobarbital (Inactin, 720–140 mg/kg, BW) or pentobarbital (Diabutal, 50 mg/kg BW) are injected into the peritoneal cavity. Inactin has the advantage of sustained anesthesia for hours, whereas pentobarbital usually requires further application of the drug. Inactin, on the other hand, has been claimed to interfere with some parameters of renal function (Elmer *et al.*, 1972; Steinhausen *et al.*, 1976). Other investigators did not find any differences between some renal functions under Inactin or pentobarbital (Dev *et al.*, 1973). A tracheostomy should be performed to avoid aspiration. Care must be taken not to damage the thyroid gland, and the sternohyoid muscles should be separated with blunt forceps. If a PE250 tracheal catheter is used, it should not exceed 1 cm in order to limit dead space. A jugular vein is cannulated for infusions. A catheter in the femoral or carotid artery is used to obtain blood. The arterial catheter should contain heparinized solution (5 IU/liter).

Either both ureters or one ureter and the bladder are catheterized to collect urine. For the bladder, a funnel-shaped catheter is introduced into a hole in the tip of the bladder. Catheterization of the ureter is best made with PE50 tubing (Cortell *et al.*, 1972) which is pulled slightly for moderate diameter reduction and softening.

For the preparation of the kidney, either abdominal (Windhager, 1968a) or flank approaches are used. For example, in the flank approach, a 3-cm cut is made at the left subcostal margin. The abdominal cavity is filled with oil at 37°C to prevent heat and water losses. The oil should cover the kidney during the preparation. The kidney is dissected free from its surrounding fat tissue, leaving a small fringe of tissue for subsequent fixation. This can be done either with fine forceps or by cutting. Care must be taken not to damage the adrenal gland or major vessels. When the kidney is mobile and attached only at the pedicle, it is placed in an appropriate cup. A thin layer of cotton wool should cover the bottom of the cup. The kidney is fixed in the cup, and the fringe is pushed into the cup with cotton wool. During preparation and fixation of the kidney, no tension should be applied to the pedicle, which could cause vasoconstriction of the renal artery.

If collecting ducts, loops of Henle, or vasa recta are to be punctured, the kidney papilla must be exposed by removing the fat that covers the papilla. Lateral and perpendicular incisions are made in the ureter to cut both circular and longitudinal muscle fibers.

Dogs are prepared in a similar fashion, with the following exceptions. First, Inactin has not been satisfactory for dogs and therefore pentobarbital remains the drug of choice for anesthesia. During surgery, the renal vein must be freed carefully from all surrounding tissue to avoid constriction of the vessel when the kidney is placed in the holder. A portion of the capsule must be removed to visualize the renal tubules.

A. Materials

In addition to the usual equipment for surgery in animals, a few tools are required for the performance of micropuncture.

1. Microscope

A stereomicroscope and light source are required for visualization of the kidney surface during micropuncture and during some of the surgical procedures. The essential features of the microscope are the magnification range (10–100× without exchange of eyepieces would be ideal), the field diameter (not less than 2 mm at 100×), and the quality of the image with special respect to the stereoscopic view. The minimal working distance is about 4 cm. The most

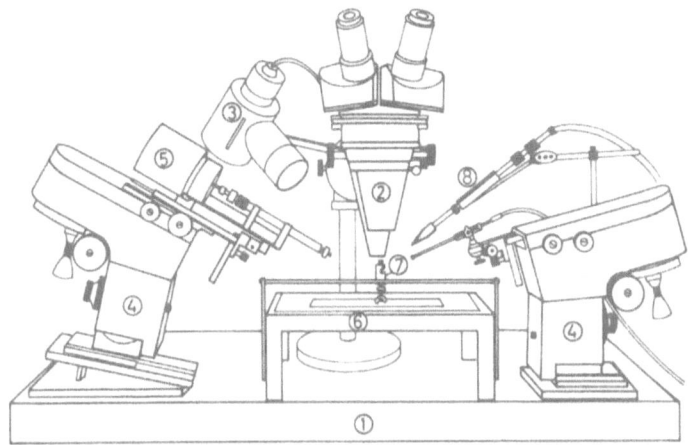

Figure 1. Experimental setup for micropuncture in the rat. Stone plate (1), microscope (2), illumination (3), manipulators (4), microperfusion pump (5), operating table (6) with holder for kidney cup (7), heatable oil supplier (8).

convenient system for changing magnification is the use of a zoom-optic. However, stereomicroscopes with separate optical pathways have better stereoscopic resolution. Dual view stereomicroscopes are available for teaching purposes or for experiments requiring two operators. The light should be cool and can be brought to the kidney surface with fiber optics (Figure 1).

2. Manipulation

The most commonly used micromanipulators are the De Fonbrune, which works with pneumatic transmission, and the Leitz, which operates with mechanical transmission. The advantage of the former is that the head of the manipulator is separate from the controls, which is especially convenient for micropuncture of dogs. The advantage of the latter is that it has a mechanical drive that will support electrical and perfusion systems.

3. Preparation of Micropipets

Glass capillaries of 0.8–1 mm outer diameter are used for the preparation of pipets. To produce tips, the pipets are heated in the middle by a heatable coil and pulled apart (Figure 2). The heat and the strength of the pulling force are adjusted until the pipet tip is appropriate. Vertical and horizontal pullers are available. A grinding device is required for sharpening the pipet. The pipet is lowered via a manipulator onto a rotating grinding stone which is constantly superfused with water. The angle of the pipet to the grinding stone should be about 30°. The procedure is controlled with a stereomicroscope (magnification 10–20×). Figure 3 illustrates the setup. The tip of the pipet should be beveled 30° and should be free of irregular edges. After grinding, the pipet is cleaned by rinsing with distilled water and acetone. For the preparation of double-barreled micropipet, two pipets are fused together with sealing wax. Then they are melted together with a microflame and twisted and pulled slightly (Ullrich *et al.*, 1969). The rest of the procedure (pulling and sharpening) is the same as for single-barreled pipets.

The outer diameter of the pipet tip depends on the tubule site or animal

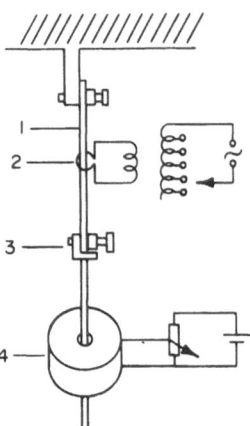

Figure 2. Vertical pipet puller. Pipet (1), heating coil (2), mobile magnet fixed only to the pipet (3), electromagnet fixed to the apparatus (4).

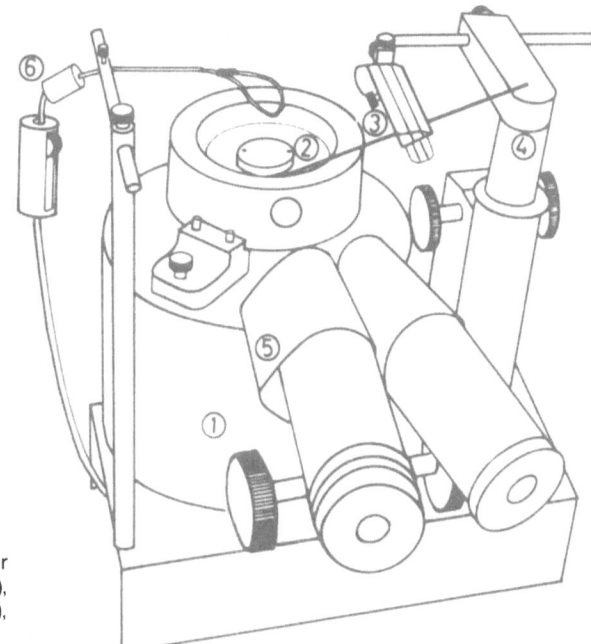

Figure 3. Pipet sharpener. Motor (1), grinding stone (2), pipet (3), manipulator (4), microscope (5), water rinsing (6).

under study. Pipets with tips of 10 μm may be used for micropunctures in the proximal tubule of the rat, 8 μm in the distal convoluted tubule, 12 μm for the injection of latex (see below), and 6 μm for loops of Henle.

4. Microperfusion Pump

A microperfusion pump is used for microperfusion of tubules and for microinfusion. This can be done with a microsyringe connected to the pipet with hard wall tubing. The microperfusion pump developed by Sonnenberg and Deetjen (1964) originally delivered perfusion rates of 10–40 nl/min but is now available for a range of 1–40 nl/min and allows both pumping and suction. In this pump, the piston is pushed forward into the pipet, which minimizes dead space and increases accuracy. A modification allows for recording pressures in the pipet during operation (Hierholzer *et al.*, 1972; Lohfert *et al.*, 1971). A microfusion pump can be employed for peritubular perfusion or injection. Figure 4 shows a simple device which is used for peritubular microperfusion when an area of several tubules is to be completely circumfused.

5. Temperature Control

After anesthesia, body temperature must be monitored by a thermometer and kept constant at its normal level by a heatable operating table. Furthermore, the oil superfusing the kidney must be kept at 37°C, which is accomplished by a heating coil wound around the supply tube.

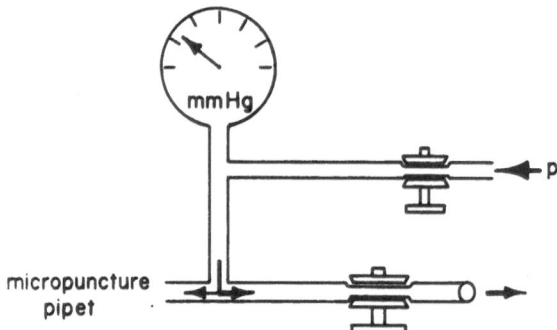

Figure 4. Setup for peritubular perfusion. Opening of the upper valve increases and opening of the lower valve decreases the pressure at the micropuncture pipet. The upper valve is connected to a gas system with high, constant pressure (e.g., gas bottle). The valves are adjusted until the perfusate completely pushes the blood away from the area under study.

6. *Tubule Blockage*

Castor oil is used for blockage of tubular flow and isolation of collected samples from air. It is not taken up by cells, in contrast to mineral oil which has been abandoned for that reason (Langer *et al.,* 1968; Wiederholt *et al.,* 1968). The castor oil is stained with Sudan black and filtered before use. Gutsche *et al.* (1975) used solid paraffin for blockage of nephrons. The stability of the paraffin block constitutes an advantage in some experiments (e.g., stop-flow pressure determinations).

III. MICROPUNCTURE PROCEDURES

After exposure of the kidney surface, the nephron segment under study must be identified. At the surface of the cortex only proximal or distal tubules can be identified. The distal tubules have thinner walls, which is a useful distinctive mark. The lumen, on the other hand, is quite an unreliable feature. Although it is usually clearly smaller in distal tubules, the reverse might prove true at increased pressure in the distal nephron, e.g., under forced diuresis. In the renal papilla the loops of Henle are thin, white loops which have very small lumens. Collecting ducts, on the other hand, have very large lumens and are easily identified.

A very convenient and reliable way to identify tubule segments is the use of dye. Lissamine green has been introduced for this purpose by Steinhausen (1963). After intravenous injection (0.05 ml 10% solution), Lissamine green appears first in the capillaries of the kidney surface. In the rat it reaches the last loops of the superficial proximal tubules in 10 sec. It completely disappears from the surface and after 20 sec it reappears in distal tubules. Since passage time in an intact kidney is virtually the same in all nephrons, the passage time is a reliable measure for the approximate puncture site in the nephron. Whereas a tubule, stained with Lissamine green 30 sec after first appearance in an intact kidney, can be clearly identified as distal (*cave*: previously punctured tubules), use of the time of appearance of Lissamine green to determine the site within the distal tubule is debatable. Lissamine green has been shown to interfere with electrolyte transport (Roch-Ramel and Jotterand, 1970; Heller, 1971). Furthermore, a change of the potential reading with the antimony electrode was observed when Lissamine green passed the puncture site in the proximal tubule and loop of Henle (Quehenberger *et al.*, 1974). However, this change was completely reversible within 1 min. Similarly, up to ten injections of Lissamine green failed to result in sustained natriuresis (Lynch *et al.*, 1973) and can be considered safe as long as after each injection the dye is allowed to completely disappear before micropuncture sampling is begun. Preferably, all injections should be completed ½ hr prior to micropuncture.

When the tubule segment to be studied is identified, the puncture pipet is advanced so that the angle to the kidney surface is 10–30°. Then the tip is lowered until it produces a shallow indentation on the tubule surface. The pipet is pushed forward to penetrate into the tubule along its long axis. During sampling, the pipet tip should be located in the middle of the tubule lumen without deforming the tubule.

Before collection is begun, an oil droplet is introduced which is 100–200 μm in length. A larger oil block may allow the tubule pressure to increase without oil movements, whereas a small oil block may allow retrograde tubule fluid contamination. The collection is started immediately after injecting the oil droplet by gentle suction. During the collection procedure care must be taken that the diameter of the punctured tubule remains similar to that of the adjacent tubules and the oil block is kept in place.

The collection time should exceed 2 min. Errors introduced during the blockage of tubular flow in the beginning of collection and due to handling of the minute volumes increase markedly if the sampling time is shortened. Before withdrawal of the sampling pipet, suction must be discontinued. The tip is withdrawn and a small drop of oil from the surface is used to seal the tip.

The accurate determination of the puncture site and the measurement of the length of perfused segments requires the use of latex casts. After completion of fluid collection, the nephron segment is repunctured with a pipet containing the latex solution (latex and Aquarex 1:4, Windhager, 1968a) through the hole left from the collection pipet. The diameter of the pipet tip with the latex should be 2 μm larger than the micropuncture pipet so that it completely seals the opening. The latex is injected into the tubule by gentle pressure. In micropuncture of late proximal tubules, repuncture at a more proximal site for further filling might prove necessary until the whole nephron is filled, including the glomerulus. A careful map of the tubule is drawn to help in subsequent microdissection. The site of micropuncture may be marked with a spot of India ink by using a third pipet.

After completion of the experiment, the kidney is cut out, the capsule is removed, and the kidney macerated in 6 M HCl for 90 min at 37°C. After the kidney is rinsed with water, the latex casts are dissected free under the microscope with the use of microdissection tools under water.

First, a large hole is made beside the latex casts. The tubule cast is then dissected, beginning from the collection site and working upstream guided by the map. For proximal tubules, measurements of tubule length are made with the glomerulus as a reference point using either a micrometer or a calibrated grid. For distal tubules, the macula densa and the joining of two tubules are used as reference points; however, this definition includes different histologic segments of nephrons. In microperfusion experiments, the microperfusion segment is known from the map.

In free-flow recollection micropuncture experiments, the exact tubule site is frequently not crucial. For a given physiologic condition, the TF/P inulin may be used as a rough indicator of puncture site. However, the TF/P inulin is not a useful measure for tubule length when function is changed, as it is following the administration of diuretics.

1. Advantages and Limitations

The advantages of micropuncture techniques in general are that they allow localization and analysis of renal transport processes *in vivo*. This advantage is weighed against limitations common to all micropuncture techniques. These are that micropuncture studies can be done only in certain species and extrapolation to other species and in particular to man might be inappropriate. Furthermore, micropuncture is necessarily preceded by anesthesia and extensive surgery. In addition, the exposure of the nephron for micropuncture might alter its function. Eventually, micropuncture involves perforation of the tubular wall, the introduction of oil, and possibly changes in luminal pressure. Some damage usually occurs in the vicinity of the micropuncture site, leading to increased permeability to various substances, as disclosed by microperfusion studies (Frömter *et al.*, 1973; Morel and Murayama, 1970). An important pitfall is the formation of fistulas against adjacent tubules, which has been shown to occur in some 10% of all micropunctures (Andreucci *et al.*, 1971, 1972). Increases of luminal pressure might result in decreases of glomerular filtration (Schnermann, 1972), whereas decreases in luminal pressure appear to be less critical (Brenner and Daugharty, 1972; Davidman *et al.*, 1971; Rector *et al.*, 1972).

A. Free-Flow Micropuncture

In free-flow micropuncture, fluid is collected from defined sites in the nephron. Analysis of the fluid for volume and concentrations of given substances allows conclusions to be made regarding net tubular transport.

The procedure is essentially as described in the preceding section. When single nephron filtration rate (SNGFR) is determined, the time is taken from the introduction of the oil block (Andreucci *et al.*, 1971). A critical discussion of the measurement of single nephron filtration rate can be found in Chapter 3 of Volume 4A in this series (Knox and Marchand, 1976).

1. Advantages and Limitations

Free-flow micropuncture values represent the cumulative results of tubular function. However, pitfalls might arise if free-flow studies are used for the analysis of the contributing mechanisms. Localization of transport processes with the use of free-flow micropuncture is based on the comparison of recoveries of the substance under study at various sites. The differences in recovery at early and late distal tubules, for example, could be used as an indicator of transport in the distal convoluted tubule. However, the comparison suffers from variance among different nephrons. This is a problem if the magnitude of the transport at the site under study is small compared with the transport in the preceding segments. The random variation of the latter might completely obscure transport in the successive segments. A more serious pitfall arises from the comparison of functionally different nephrons. Such a comparison is the calculation of collecting duct transport from the subtraction of recoveries in superficial distal nephrons and urine. The urine is a mixture of both superficial and deep nephrons which show definite differences in function (Jamison, 1973). Even though some 80% of the nephron population is cortical, it must be kept in mind that the cortical nephrons are not necessarily homogeneous. Therefore, as a rule, only qualified information can be gained by the comparison of distal and urinary recoveries in regard to collecting duct function. Similarly, interpretation of data from collecting duct punctures and microcatheterizations is hampered by the confluence of the collecting duct tree.

Distal tubule collections are particularly prone to the artifacts of accelerated anterograde flow or to contamination by fluid from downstream. Retrograde contamination occurs even though the collections are made proximal to an oil block, particularly during osmotic diuresis when the collection pipet constitutes a low resistance pathway compared to the high resistance to flow in the collecting duct system. To avoid these pitfalls, it has been proposed to collect a sample in the picoliter size range and subsequently analyze by electron probe microanalysis. An alternative technique is to collect two samples, one very small, then a larger sample for analytical determinations; the larger sample will be retained when its osmotic pressure is identical to that of the small sample.

In both proximal and distal tubule micropuncture, it is advisable to determine single nephron GFR from the sampling time, TF/P inulin, and sampled volume. If it is outside the range of 20–50 nl/min in the rat, it is an indicator of sampling errors such as reflux, fistula formation, or stopped flow.

Free-flow micropuncture is the most commonly applied micropuncture technique. It is the method of choice to determine the concentration profile along the nephron. Micropuncture can be done in superficial proximal and distal convoluted tubules, papillary descending and ascending limbs of loops of Henle, and collecting ducts. An important modification of the method is the recollection micropuncture; the same nephron site is punctured before and after administration of a substance, allowing for paired comparisons.

B. Microcatheterization

The microcatheterization (Jarausch and Ullrich, 1956) technique is similar to that of free-flow micropuncture in regard to the description of concentration profiles, but its use is limited to the collecting system.

An oil-filled PE catheter is fixed to a heatable platin loop with a melting fat droplet. The catheter is advanced into a collecting duct at the tip of the papilla. When the catheter is in the proper position, it is maintained in place by cooling and fixed to the tip of the papilla with the droplet of fat. Then the pressure in the catheter is lowered and urine collection begun.

1. Advantages and Limitations

Microcatheterization has advantages and limitations similar to those of free-flow micropuncture of the collecting duct. The unique features are that the tubule epithelium is not punctured, the central collecting ducts are accessible as well as superficial, and the proximal portions of the collecting tree can be sampled.

C. Microinjection and Microinfusion

In microinjection (Gottschalk *et al.,* 1965; Gottschalk and Lassiter, 1974), a small fluid volume containing ^{3}H- or ^{14}C-labeled inulin and labeled tracer of the substance under study is injected into segments of superficial nephrons. The urinary recovery of the tracer is compared to the recovery of inulin and allows estimation of the fractional reabsorption of the injected substance beyond the site of microinjection.

After insertion of the pipet in a proximal or distal tubule, approximately 30 nl of the tracer-containing solution are injected over a period of 15–30 sec (Gottschalk *et al.*, 1965). Urine is collected every 30 sec and the tracer recovery in the urine is determined by light scintillation counting. Microinfusion is a modification of the microinjection technique in which the pipet is mounted on a microperfusion pump. Microinfusion is made then at a very low flow rate (down to 1 nl/min) for several minutes. After completion of the microinfusion period (some 10 min), the pipet is left in place so that tubule fluid cannot escape from the hole and the tracer is washed out of the nephron. During microinfusion and for an additional 20 min, urine is collected every 2 min and the cumulative recovery utilized as an index of reabsorption (Figure 5). To correct for

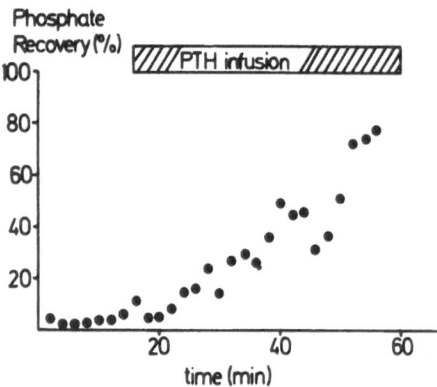

Figure 5. Continuous microinfusion experiment, where ^{32}phosphate and [^{3}H]inulin were infused into a late proximal tubule. Phosphate recovery in urine, relative to that of inulin, is plotted versus time. Intravenous infusion of parathyroid hormone (PTH) during microinfusion leads to increased phosphate recovery due to decreased reabsorption. In this experiment the tubule was blocked proximal to the microinfusion pipet.

recirculation of the injected substance, the activity in contralateral urine must be subtracted from that of ipsilateral urine. Such a correction is valid only if both kidneys behave identically in regard to the substance under study.

To reduce flow rate and to eliminate the influence of filtrate, microinfusion can be done in tubules blocked with oil proximal to the microinfusion pipet. The procedure is similar to microperfusion of loops of Henle (see below).

1. Advantages and Limitations

The microinjection technique is relatively simple. Furthermore, since appearance of labeled inulin in the contralateral kidney indicates a leaky impalement, it is better controlled than free-flow micropuncture. An important advantage for the pharmacologist is the fact that the microinjection pipet can be left in place and a control microinjection can be followed by a microinjection after application of the drug under study. The microinfusion modification has the further advantage that the drug can be applied during uninterrupted microinfusion (Figure 5). The modification with the oil-blocked tubule can serve to determine if the drug has to be filtered in order to be effective. Microinjection is the method of choice for the evaluation of reabsorption in the collecting duct.

A limitation of the technique is that it can be used only for the determination of unidirectional reabsorption. Even this must be qualified, since part of the reabsorbed substance might undergo subsequent secretion before being cleared from the kidney. Although discriminating between early and delayed recovery might indicate whether the substances recovered in the urine has escaped unidirectional reabsorption or was subjected to subsequent secretion, the delayed recovery might include a substance which has mixed with the cellular pool without being reabsorbed, and the direct recovery might include a substance being reabsorbed in the descending limb of the loop of Henle and secreted into the collecting duct. Furthermore, Kramp *et al.* (1971) found that urate has a different flow behavior than inulin in PE catheters. Therefore, interpretation of the appearance time in microinjection experiments might give rise to incorrect conclusions. Because of the variability of flow behavior of different substances, total rather than fractional inulin and substance recoveries should be used for evaluation. The application of the technique is limited to those substances which are available in labeled form. Although many of the substances of interest to the renal pharmacologist are available in a labeled form, sometimes the specific activities are too low to allow study without increasing tubular concentration or flow rates considerably above the physiologic range. The use of tracer warrants the control of purity (Greger *et al.*, 1977) and the possibility of intrarenal conversion must be kept in mind. Systemic conversion is not a problem, as long as the activity in the contralateral kidney is subtracted (Lang *et al.*, 1974).

Because of the relatively large urinary volumes undergoing subsequent analysis, the quenching of the scintillation cocktails should be corrected.

Another important limitation of the technique is that with the injection of large volumes, considerable change in intratubular flow dynamics could occur, which may considerably alter transport. In this respect, the continuous microinfusion of minute volumes is preferred to the rapid injection of large volumes.

D. Microperfusion

The method of continuous microperfusion as distinct from stationary microperfusion (see below) was developed by Sonnenberg and Deetjen (1964). Microperfusion involves the perfusion of a tubule segment. The decrease or increase in concentration of substances under study indicates influx or outflux. Water reabsorption is monitored with labeled inulin.

An oil-filled pipet is inserted in an early proximal tubule and an oil droplet injected for identification of the subsequent loops of the nephron. The microperfusion pipet is inserted in one of the successive loops; and in the last accessible loop an oil-filled collection pipet is inserted. The microperfusion is initiated (Figure 6) after introduction of a proximal and distal oil block.

For microperfusion of the loop of Henle, the following modification is necessary (Figure 7): A pipet, filled with Lissamine green-stained fluid, is inserted into an early to midproximal tubule. Injection of Lissamine green (oil would block the loop of Henle) allows identification of the remaining proximal tubule and the corresponding distal tubule of that segment. An oil-filled pipet is inserted into the next loop and the microperfusion pipet is inserted into the last accessible loop of the proximal nephron. The microperfusion pump is switched on and an oil block introduced with the second pipet. Care must be taken that no oil passes the microperfusion pipet. The oil block is kept in place by the pipet containing Lissamine green which collects the tubular fluid proximal to the oil

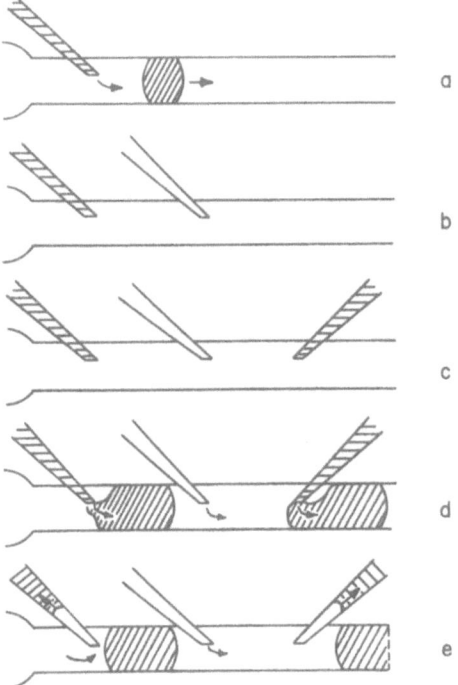

Figure 6. Microperfusion of proximal convoluted tubules. (a) Identification of the proximal nephron by injection of oil droplets. (b) Micropuncture of successive loops with the microperfusion and sampling (c) pipet. (d) Introduction of oil blocks. (e) Sampling.

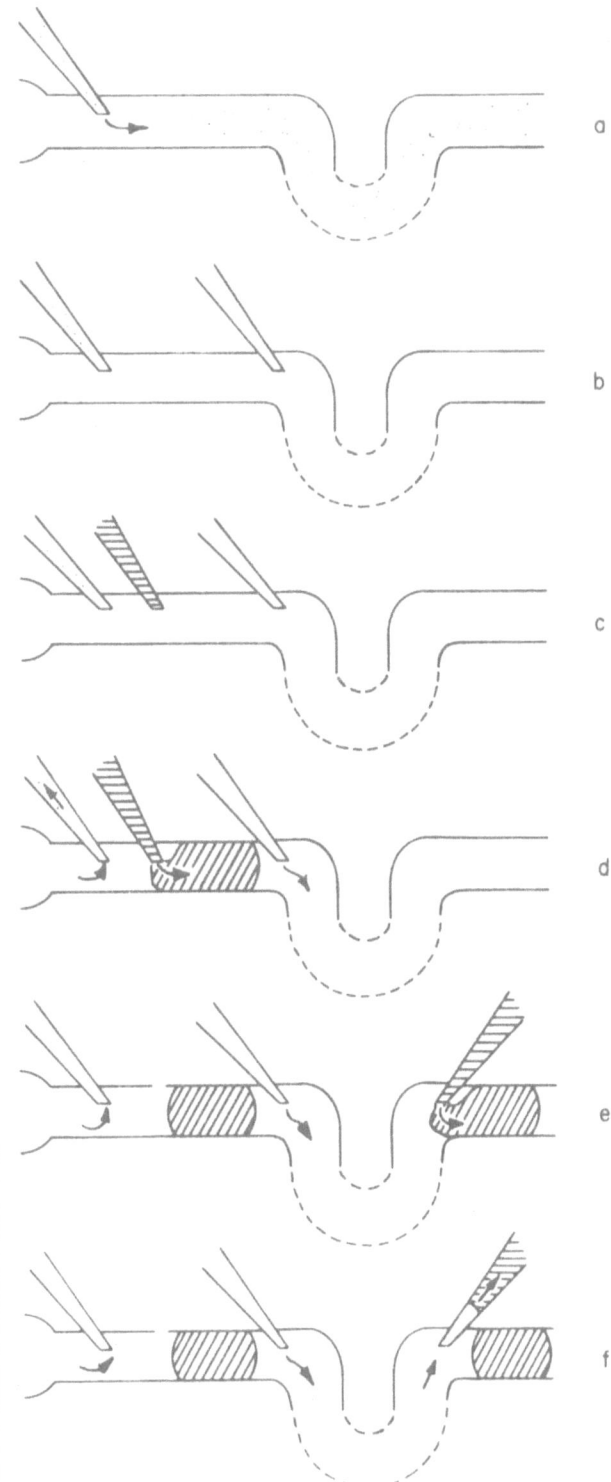

Figure 7. Microperfusion of loops of Henle. (a) Identification of the nephron with Lissamine green-containing fluid. (b) Insertion of microperfusion pipet in the last proximal loop. (c) Puncture of a proximal loop close to the first pipet with the collection pipet. (d) Introduction of proximal oil block. (e) Withdrawal of collection pipet from the proximal tubule and reinsertion in the distal tubule. (f) Injection of distal oil block and sampling.

block. The oil-containing pipet is withdrawn and reinserted into the distal tubule. After introduction of a distal oil block, sampling is begun.

Microperfusion of the distal tubule is similar to that for the loops of Henle (Figure 8). A Lissamine green-filled pipet in the proximal tubule is again used for identification of the subsequent nephron. If a sufficiently long distal tubule is found, a microperfusion pipet is inserted in an early segment and an oil-filled pipet in the late segment of the distal tubule. Then suction is applied to the Lissamine green-filled pipet and oil is injected into the distal tubule, which extends both upstream and downstream. When sufficient oil has passed proximal to the microperfusion pipet, the pump is switched on and gentle suction is applied to the sampling pipet. The perfusion fluid then pushes the oil out of the segment to be perfused and sampling is begun.

After completion of microperfusion, the length of the segment can be determined with the use of latex and microdissection.

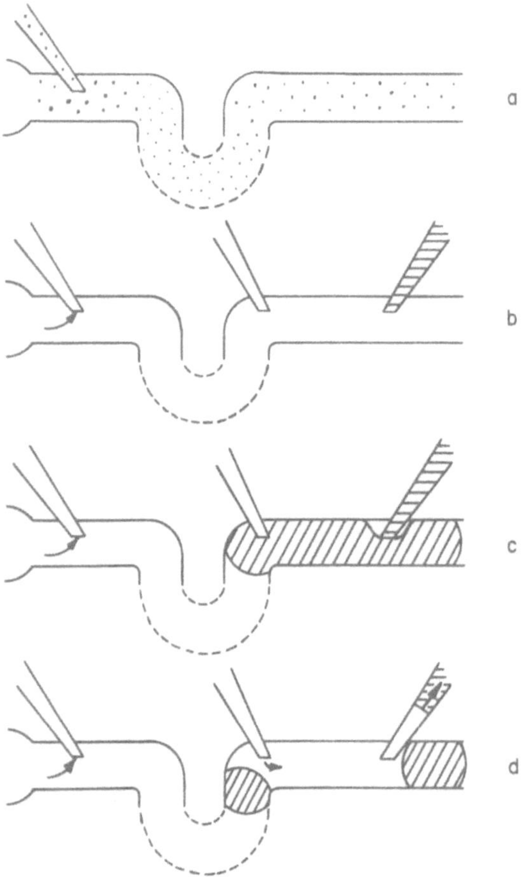

Figure 8. Microperfusion of distal convoluted tubules. (a) Identification of the nephron with Lissamine green-containing fluid. (b) Puncture of the distal tubule with microperfusion and collection pipet. (c) Introduction of an oil column. (d) Microperfusion.

1. Advantages and Limitations

This technique has the advantage of discriminating between efflux and influx, i.e., reabsorption and secretion. The efflux can be defined as unidirectional transport across the cell into the peritubular capillaries, but not simply disappearance from the lumen. In evaluation of the data from microperfusion, mixing with the cellular pool is usually not a problem as long as perfusion times exceed 2 min, since the perfused volume is at least 20 times larger than the cellular volume. Substances reaching the peritubular capillaries are rapidly carried away and secretion in the same tubule segment is highly unlikely. On the other hand, net secretion cannot be determined directly but can be calculated only after consideration of coexistent reabsorption since a secreted substance might undergo subsequent reabsorption (Lang *et al.,* 1972). The main disadvantage of the technique is that it is prone to technical pitfalls such as leaks. Furthermore, an altered permeability close to the micropuncture site has been demonstrated by the relatively sharp decline of recovery at short perfusion distances compared with the decline in the subsequent segments (Morel and Murayama, 1970). Accordingly, it is preferable to calculate transport rates from the decline as a function of perfused length. This possibility renders the microperfusion technique superior to microinjection or infusion, where this leakage cannot be corrected. In microperfusions of loops of Henle, samples should be collected from the proximal tubule close to the microperfusion pipet, in addition to the sampling in distal tubules, to detect initial leaks.

Leaks are a major source of error, particularly when the influx of a substance is to be studied. Systemic inulin can be used to check for contamination of the collected fluid when the microperfusate is inulin free. For accurate estimates of transport, a minimal length of tubule must be perfused and in proximal tubules, the difference between short and long perfusion distances should exceed 1 mm. If, on the other hand, the tubule segment under study is not homogeneous in regard to the transport of the given substance (Lingard *et al.,* 1973), this might be overlooked by the microperfusion technique. Microperfusion involves the introduction of artificial fluid into the tubule. The composition of the fluid may alter transport characteristics. On the other hand, variations in the composition of tubule fluid may allow identification of parameters influencing the transport system.

Microperfusion is the method of choice to study bidirectional transport of a substance as long as the transport coefficients or permeabilities are sufficiently high. It is a valuable tool for discriminating between luminal and peritubular action of a drug since the drug can be added to the perfusate only or to the systemic circulation. In recollection microperfusion, the perfused segment might serve as its own control.

E. Stationary Microperfusion and Shrinking Droplet

Richards and Walker (1937) described a method for studying an isolated fluid droplet in a tubule segment of *Necturus*. A very similar method, the stationary microperfusion technique, was described by Shipp *et al.* (1958). The technique of stationary microperfusion includes collection and analysis of the injected fluid droplet. Fluid reabsorption is retarded or prevented by the addition of unreabsorbable solute, and alterations in the concentration of the substance under study are used as an indicator of tubule transport. In 1961 Gertz and Ullrich developed the shrinking droplet method for the determination of isotonic fluid reabsorption in the mammalian kidney. A droplet of isotonic saline was injected into an oil droplet and the subsequent reabsorption of the droplet was recorded by microphotometry.

In the shrinking droplet technique, a double-barreled micropuncture pipet is filled with oil on one side and isotonic saline on the other side (Gertz, 1963). After insertion of the pipet, a large oil block is expelled into the tubule lumen (Figure 9). The oil droplet should extend about 200 μm proximally from the micropuncture pipet. Then fluid is injected and the fluid droplet is separated from the pipet by an additional injection of oil. The subsequent reabsorption of the saline droplet by the tubule results in the convergence of the two oil droplets. The proximal oil block should not exceed 300 μm in length to maintain mobility for convergence of the two oil blocks. For accurate measurements, the initial length of the fluid droplet should be at least 50 μm (Nakajima *et al.*, 1970). The progressive decrease in the distance between the oil droplets is monitored by serial photography and is taken as a measure of fluid reabsorption.

Shrinking of the droplet can be prevented by the addition of nonreabsorbable solutes in the test fluid. In stationary microperfusion the procedure is similar to that outlined above with the exception that the fluid is withdrawn by a single-barreled micropuncture pipet. Instead of a double-barreled pipet, two pipets may be used (Figure 10). An oil-filled pipet is inserted into an early proximal tubule and the direction of flow and subsequent nephron convolutions are identified by injection of small oil droplets. Then the pipet with the test fluid is inserted into the next loop most proximal to the first pipet and an additional oil-filled pipet into one of the later convolutions of the proximal tubule. An oil column is now

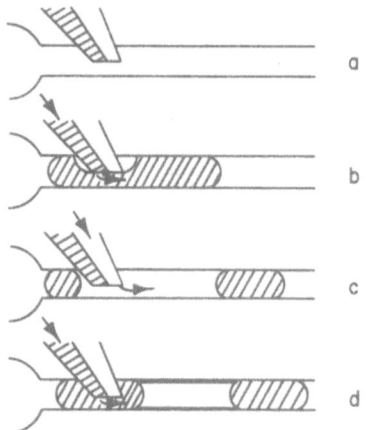

Figure 9. Shrinking droplet technique. (a) Puncture with double-barreled pipet. (b) Injection of oil. (c) Injection of test fluid. (d) Additional injection of oil. This is followed by serial photography of the shrinking fluid droplet.

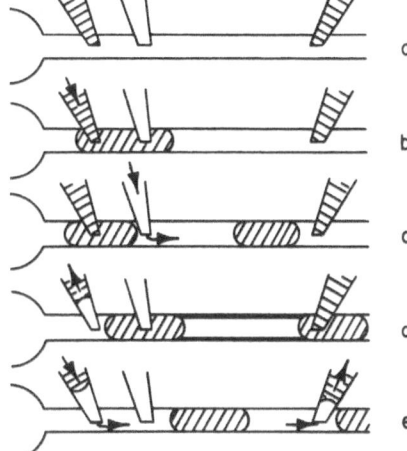

Figure 10. Stationary microperfusion of the proximal tubule. After identification of an early proximal tubule loop, this is punctured with an oil-filled pipet. (a) Injection of small oil droplets allows identification of the following loops which are punctured with a pipet containing the test fluid and a pipet filled with oil. (b) Introduction of oil block. (c) Splitting with test fluid. (d) Exposure of the fluid droplet. (e) Collection through the oil-filled pipet.

injected from the first pipet. When sufficient oil has passed the second pipet, fluid is injected to split the oil column. The fluid is then pushed downstream by additional injection of oil by the first pipet. After elapse of a given contact time, the fluid-containing oil column is pushed downstream by the first pipet and the test fluid aspirated into the collection pipet.

The application of the stationary microperfusion method to segments beyond the proximal convoluted tubule accessible to micropuncture requires use of three pipets. A first is filled with a Lissamine green-colored saline, a second with oil; a third is first filled with oil, then a 1–3 nl fluid droplet is introduced and the tip sealed with castor oil. The first pipet is inserted in any proximal tubule and the rest of that nephron identified by injection of stained solution. For study of the descending segments of that particular proximal convoluted tubule (Figure 11), the second pipet is inserted into one of the following convolutions and the third pipet into the last accessible portion of the proximal tubule. Oil is injected into the proximal tubule by the second pipet and kept in place by the first pipet, which collects the fluid proximal to the oil block. When a small segment of the injected oil has passed the third pipet, the test droplet is injected into the tubule and pushed downstream by injection of additional oil by the second pipet. The droplet is pushed downstream until it remains just visible at the end of the last superficial loop of the proximal tubule. After elapse of the contact time, the fluid droplet is aspirated into the third pipet. For study of the distal convoluted tubule and the connecting ascending segment of the nephron, a second and third pipet are inserted into the distal convoluted tubule. An oil block is introduced by the more distal second pipet. At the same time suction is applied to the first pipet, so that the oil block is moved upstream. When it passes the third pipet, the test fluid is expelled, and if the ascending segment is to be studied, the fluid is pushed upstream by additional injection of oil through the second pipet. After elapse of a given contact time, the droplet is collected by the third pipet (Lang *et al.*, 1977).

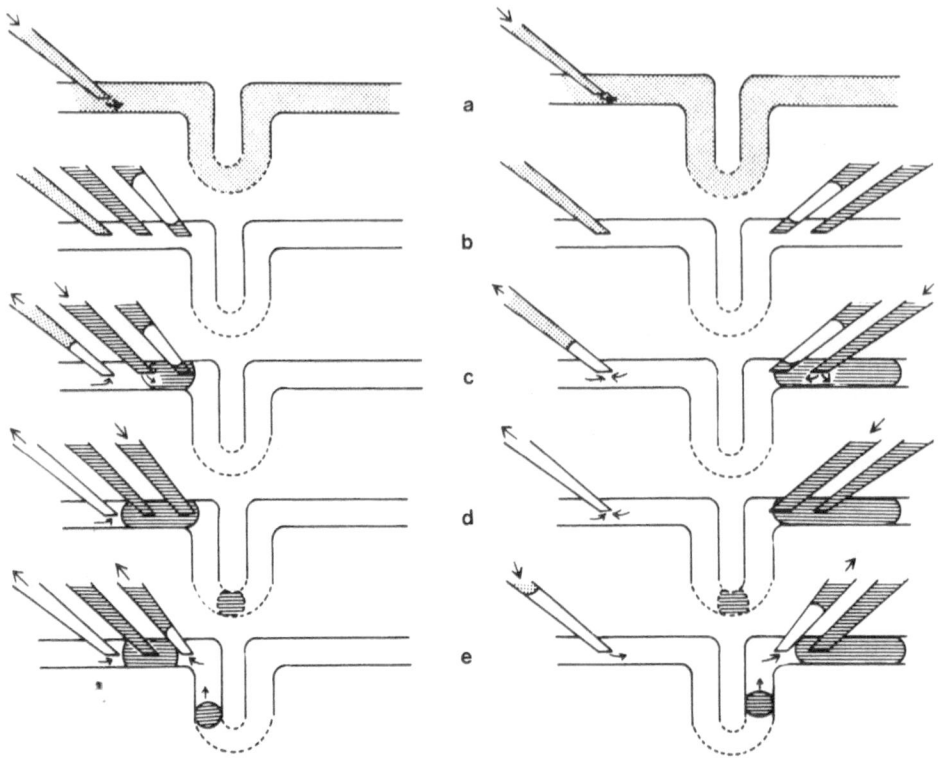

Figure 11. Stationary microperfusion in descending (left panel) and ascending (right panel) segments between late proximal and early distal tubules, accessible to micropuncture. (a) Identification of nephron with Lissamine green. (b) Puncture. (c) Introduction of oil block. (d) Injection of test droplet. (e) Recovery of test droplet. (From Lang et al., 1977).

1. Advantages and Limitations

The pitfalls of the shrinking droplet technique have been discussed in detail (Grandchamp and Boulpaep, 1972; Györy, 1971; Nakajima et al., 1970; Weinmann et al., 1972). A criticism is that the tubule is not a rigid tube and therefore the luminal diameter is not constant. Therefore, the distance between the oil menisci is a poor indicator of the volume of the remaining fluid. Another problem is whether the oil menisci or the base of the oil menisci should be taken as borders of reabsorbing epithelium. If the oil menisci are half globes, the surface of the reabsorbing epithelium must extend at each side one luminal diameter beyond the tip of the meniscus. Györy (1971) proposed to add two luminal diameters to the distance between the oil menisci.

The shrinking droplet has the advantage that the examination of the same tubule can be repeated. Furthermore, effects of changes in fluid delivery to the nephron by changing filtration rates are avoided with this technique. Therefore the technique may be useful for testing diuretics. On the other hand, diuretics might influence intrarenal pressure and alter the compliance of the tubule under study (Rector *et al.,* 1966).

Stationary microperfusion shares many of the advantages and limitations of continuous microperfusion. The most important advantage of the technique is that relatively long contact times can be used, which allow the determination of equilibrium concentrations. Stationary microperfusion has the disadvantage that the volume of the test droplet is only in the range of 1 nl whereas the microperfused volume might be as high as 100 nl. Therefore, the split droplet technique is applicable only when analytic techniques are sufficiently sensitive, or the specific activity of labeled substance is sufficiently high.

The small size of the samples poses another problem in that the cellular volume and hence the cellular pool of the substance under study is not negligible compared with the volume or amount of substance injected. Therefore, considerable alterations in luminal concentration might reflect mixing with the cellular pool. On the other hand, it may be possible to study the intracellular pool size or the differential permeabilities at the luminal and peritubular membranes. However, in this context another limitation should be mentioned. The prolonged exposure of fluid droplets to the tubule cells might result in altered transport of the substance under study due to local metabolic changes.

One of the advantages of the split droplet technique is that given segments of the proximal tubule can be studied separately, e.g., the early or late proximal tubule. Inhomogeneity of the proximal convoluted tubule could therefore be demonstrated by the use of split droplet experiments (Baumann *et al.,* 1975; Lingard *et al.,* 1973), whereas such an inhomogeneity was not apparent from microperfusion studies.

IV. MICROPUNCTURE OF PERITUBULAR CAPILLARIES AND VASA RECTA

The puncture of the peritubular capillary network is best accomplished at the "vascular star" in the rat or in relatively large capillaries in the dog. When the pipet penetrates into a capillary, blood enters the tip without the application of suction. Care must be taken not to perforate an adjacent tubule. For micropuncture of vasa recta, the papilla is exposed. The micropuncture pipet is best positioned such that the puncture is coaxial to the vasa recta.

1. Advantages and Limitations

The most important pitfalls are introduced with the further handling of the small samples. Damage of the blood cells can cause considerable errors in estimation of concentrations if the substance is accumulated in the cells.

The technique was applied to the determination of protein concentration in the efferent arteriole for estimating the force involved in glomerular filtration or the determination of pH and CO_2 concentrations in the kidney papilla. Renin and angiotensin concentrations have been determined in efferent arterioles.

A. Peritubular Microinjection

This technique was first introduced by Lechene and Morel (1965). The design is very similar to that for intratubular microinjection. Test fluid is injected into the vasa recta capillaries and the appearance of radioactive labeled substance is monitored in the urine.

A pipet with the test fluid is inserted into a vascular star and 100 nl injected within a half minute. The correct position of the pipet is indicated by reflux of blood into the tip of the pipet. After injection, urine is collected serially and the tracer recovery of the substance and inulin recorded.

1. Advantages and Limitations

The advantage of the technique is that influx into the lumen can be studied without the use of chemical methods or large amounts of radioactive material for systemic infusion. However, the short contact with tubule epithelium and the effect of postsecretory reabsorption lead to underestimation of secretory processes. In the case of *p*-aminohippurate, only some 10% of the injected tracer was recovered in the urine (Kramp, 1976). Therefore, the technique is useful only for the qualitative demonstration of influx. In addition, it may serve as a model for demonstrating inhibition of secretion by drugs.

B. Peritubule Perfusion

The technique of peritubule perfusion has been developed independently in several laboratories (Frömter *et al.*, 1968; Windhager, 1968b; Silbernagl and Deetjen, 1969; Spitzer and Windhager, 1970). The combination of peritubule and

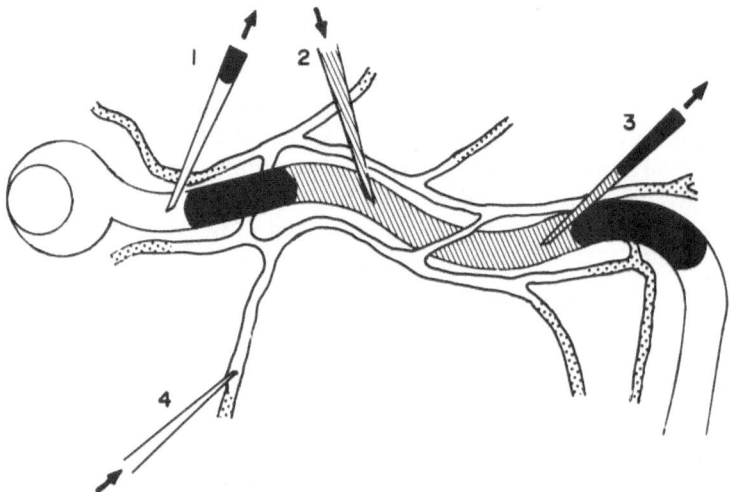

Figure 12. Combined peritubular and luminal microperfusion. Pipet collecting fluid proximal to the perfused segment, for stabilization of proximal oil block (1), luminal microperfusion pipet (2), collection pipet (3), and peritubular microperfusion pipet (4).

tubule perfusion makes it possible to vary both the composition of the peritubule and tubule fluid.

A pipet filled with a test fluid is inserted into a vascular star or one of the superficial capillaries (Figure 12). A correct puncture is indicated by erythrocytes entering the tip of the pipet. The pressure in the pipet is raised until the test fluid pushes the peritubular blood away from an area encompassing about five tubules. Split droplet, microperfusion, or micropuncture may be performed in the corresponding tubule segments.

1. Advantages and Limitations

The combined peritubule and tubule perfusion might be considered an alternative to the isolated tubule, with the advantage that the preceding manipulations are minimal and damage to tubule cells less likely. The limitations of the technique include the necessity to push away the peritubular blood with a pressure in the perfused capillary which is considerably higher than the usual hydrostatic pressure in the capillaries. Transport may be sensitive to the increased peritubule hydrostatic pressure (Bank *et al.*, 1972). Second, the tubules under study might not be completely circumfused with the test fluid. This is especially true if peritubular perfusion is combined with free-flow micropuncture or microperfusion. Therefore, if omission of a substance (e.g., Na^+) is desired, or if the concentration of the substance under study is a crucial parameter, peritubular perfusion should probably be combined only with the split droplet technique where the whole segment under study is on the surface. Another important drawback of the technique is the possible alteration of tubule function by exposure to artificial peritubular fluid. The alteration might be caused not only by the parameter under study, but by any other constituent in the test fluid compared with peritubule blood. Therefore, conclusions can be drawn from responses to alterations in the perfusate but not from responses to the replacement of peritubule blood with perfusate.

The question of whether drugs are effective when offered only from the peritubular side can be approached by applying peritubular perfusion. Peritubular infusion of only small volumes (10 nl/min in a vascular star) with a solution containing the drug at very high concentrations has the advantage that the peritubular fluid is virtually unaltered with the exception of the drug.

2. Evaluation

In the following discussion a few examples are given for the mathematical evaluation of tubule transport. Net fractional transport (T) of a substance in a given tubule segment may be calculated from

$$T = \frac{(S_0/In_0) - (S/In)}{(S_0/In_0)} \tag{1}$$

where S_0 and In_0 are the concentrations of substance and inulin at the beginning and S and In the concentrations at the end of the tubule segment under study.

Calculation pitfalls might arise because of deviation of the experimental reality from the assumption made. Use of radioactively labeled inulin, e.g., that which is contaminated with equally labeled permeating substance, might result in considerable underestimation of reabsorption. The investigator should bear in mind that alterations in tubule concentrations might be due to factors other than transport, e.g., leak, fistulas, confluence of tubule fluid from different nephrons, etc.

The Mass Constancy of the Tubule Segment. The concept was originally applied to the evaluation of data from continuous microperfusion (Fuchs, 1965). It is similarly applicable to the quantitative description of data from other micropuncture techniques, such as stationary microperfusion, free-flow micro-puncture, and microinjection. The concept is based on the assumption that under steady state, input and output of substance and volume into a given tubule segment should be equal (Figure 13). This is true if the concentration of substance and flow rate in the given tubule segment remain constant and substance or volume do not disappear by pathways other than transport (e.g., metabolism). Volume reabsorption is then defined by

$$\dot{V}_{(x)} - \dot{V}_{(x+\Delta x)} = I_w \Delta x \tag{2}$$

or

$$dV = I_w \times dx \tag{2a}$$

I_w can be determined from the luminal concentrations of inulin (In). If, for example, luminal concentrations of inulin increase in linear proportion to tubule length, $In_x = In_0(1 + mx)$, it follows that

$$\dot{V} = V_0/(1 + mx) \tag{2b}$$

and

$$d\dot{V}/dx = -V_0 m/(1 + mx)^2 \tag{2c}$$

The reabsorption of substance may be described as

$$d(c\dot{V}) = (I_{in} - I_{out})\, dx \tag{3}$$

If $\dot{V}$ is kept constant by means of an equilibrium solution,

$$dc = (I_{in} - I_{out})/\dot{V}\, dx \tag{3a}$$

However, if $\dot{V}$ is a function of tubule length itself, it follows that

$$\dot{V}dc + cd\dot{V} = (I_{in} - I_{out})\, dx \tag{4}$$

In the following examples, $\dot{V}$ shall be assumed constant.

A. I_{out} might be considered to be in linear proportion to the luminal concentration. If I_{in} is zero (at tracer experiments), it follows that

$$dc = -(k_{out}/\dot{V})c\, dx \tag{5}$$

Integration from $x_0 \rightarrow x$ and $c_0 \rightarrow c$ results in

$$c = c_0 e^{-(k_{out}/\dot{V})x} \tag{5a}$$

where k_{out}, the transport coefficient, is a measure for the "permeability" of the tubule in an outward direction, $k_{out} = I_{out}/c$.

Figure 13. Diagram of tubular transport. (The dimensions are given as
usually encountered in nephron
transport.) I_w = volume transport (nl/
min/mm); I_{in} = substance influx
(pmol/min/mm); I_{out} = substance outflux (pmol/min/mm); $\dot{V}$ = tubular flow
rate (nl/min); c = luminal concentration of substance (mmol/liter); x =
tubule length (mm).

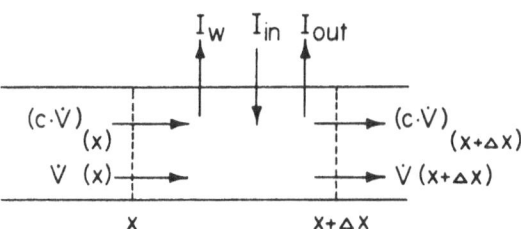

B. As a second example, if both influx and outflux occur, reabsorption is in
linear proportion, and secretion is independent from luminal concentration, we
can write

$$dc = \frac{(I_{in} - k_{out}c)\,dx}{\dot{V}} \tag{6}$$

or integrated from $x = 0$ to $x = x\ (c_0 \rightarrow c)$,

$$c = \frac{I_{in}}{k_{out}} + \left(c_0 - \frac{I_{in}}{k_{out}}\right) e^{-(k_{out}/\dot{V})x} \tag{6a}$$

If I_{in} is in linear proportion to the plasma concentration,

$$I_{in} = k_{in}c_{pl}$$

Eq. (6a) changes to

$$c = \frac{k_{in}}{k_{out}}\,c_{pl} + \left(c_0 - \frac{k_{in}}{k_{out}}\,c_{pl}\right) e^{-(k_{out}/\dot{V})\,x} \tag{6b}$$

Eqs. (6a) and (6b) can be written as well in the form

$$c = c_\infty + (c_0 - c_\infty)e^{-(k_{out}/\dot{V})x} \tag{6c}$$

where c_∞ is the luminal concentration in equilibrium $(x = \infty)$

C. A further example is given, when only reabsorption occurs which is
saturable following a Michaelis–Menten kinetic:

$$I_{out} = \frac{cI_{max}}{K_m + c}\,dx$$

In this case, we can write

$$dc = -[cI_{max}/(K_m + c)\dot{V}]\,dx \tag{7}$$

or integrated from $x = 0$ to $x = x\ (c_0 \rightarrow c)$,

$$c = c_0 - (I_{max}/\dot{V})x + K_m \ln (c_0/c) \tag{7a}$$

If in the preceding examples, volume reabsorption is allowed to occur, Eqs.
(5), (6), and (7) $[dc = f(c)\,dx]$ have to be changed to

$$dc = f(c)\,dx - c\,d\dot{V}/\dot{V}$$

where $d\dot{V}$ has to be expressed according to the volume reabsorption in the corresponding experiments [e.g., Eq. (2c)]. If integration in a closed form proves to be not possible, the concentration profile can be calculated from the differential equations in multiple steps, each step involving only minute segments (Δx). Δc is calculated from the initial c, $\dot{V}$, and $d\dot{V}$ and subtracted from c to yield the new c. The new $\dot{V}$ is similarly calculated from $V - \Delta V$ and the procedure repeated. In split droplet experiments analogous formulas can be used with the exception that tubular volume flow rate ($\dot{V}$) is replaced by the tubular volume per unit length ($V/x = \pi r^2$) and the tubule length (x) by contact time (t). Therefore, Eq. (5a) changes to

$$c = c_0 e^{-(k_{out}/\pi r^2)t}$$

Eq. (6c) to

$$c = c + (c_0 - c_\infty)e^{-(k_{out}/\pi r^2)t}$$

and Eq. (7a) to

$$c = c_0 - (I_{max}/\pi r^2)t + K_m \ln(c_0/c)$$

A special situation occurs in the shrinking droplet since reabsorption results in shrinking and subsequent reduction of the reabsorbing epithelium. If volume reabsorption is in linear proportion to the surface of reabsorbing epithelium, $I_w = +k'_w 2\pi rx$, where k'_w is the transport coefficient, r the luminal radius, and x the length of the tubule segment. [As mentioned before $x = 2r + l$, if l is the distance of the menisci of the opposing oil droplets (Györy, 1971)]. Therefore it follows that

$$dV/dt = -k'_w 2\pi rx \qquad (8)$$

or since $dV = d\,(\pi r^2 x)$

$$dx = -(2/r)k'_w x\,dt \qquad (8a)$$

and integration from $x = x_0$ to $x = x$ gives

$$x = x_0 e^{-(2k'_w/r)t} \qquad (8b)$$

The transport coefficients (k_{out}, k_{in}, k_w) can be determined using the appropriate regressions for the corresponding equations. They should be identical as determined from microperfusion or split droplet data. k_{out} allows the calculation of an apparent permeability (P_a), which is the transport coefficient per unit surface area instead of per unit tubule length. Therefore it follows that

$$P_a = k_{out}/2\pi r \qquad (9)$$

P_a allows comparison with membranes other than tubules. However, since the real surface of the luminal membrane is certainly far larger than $2\pi rx$, the numbers calculated are quite artificial. It must be pointed out that P_a calculated with this formula is not confined to passive but may include active transport (see below). The application of the mass constancy principle has many advantages: Comparisons can be made between results obtained at different tubular flow rates, substrate concentrations, and even between data from different techniques; e.g., split droplet, microperfusion, and free-flow micropuncture (Lang *et al.*, 1973; Young and Zingard, 1976). The effects of drugs on transport coefficients, maximal transport rates, or affinities of the transport system can be better defined and comparisons made between the efficiency of different drugs.

Application of Irreversible Thermodynamics to the Tubule Transport. A theoretical derivation of the equation(s) used in the application of the principles of irreversible thermodynamics to the renal tubule is given in the handbook of renal physiology (Sauer, 1973). However, some comments can be made on the practical impact of evaluating the application of irreversible thermodynamics to micropuncture data. The basic principle of the approach is that the observed fluxes are related to the driving forces. By this means the flux of a substance (J) across the tubular wall could be described as

$$J = (1 - \sigma)J_v \bar{c} + P(\Delta c + (zF\Delta E/RT)\bar{c}) + J_{\text{act}} \tag{10}$$

where J is the reflection coefficient, J_v the volume flux, $\bar{c}$ the arithmetic mean, Δc the difference of the peritubular and luminal concentration of the substance under study, ΔE the transcellular electrical potential, and J_{act} the active component of the transport. P, zF, R, and T stand for permeability, valence of the substance, the Faraday and gas constant, and the absolute temperature. The transport is therefore considered as the sum of solvent drag $(1 - \sigma)J_v \bar{c}$ "diffusion" driven by chemical ($P\Delta c$) and electrical ($P(zF\Delta E/RT)\bar{c}$) gradients and active transport.

Determination of σ, P, and J_{act} would allow complete description of the transport in regard to the driving forces, when $\bar{c}$, Δc, ΔE, and J_v are known. It must be pointed out, however, that P and J_{act} need not be constants. J_{act} would be constant only as long as the active transport process is completely saturated and independent from any of the other variables. P is a measure of passive transport, not of simple diffusion only. Therefore, it might well involve a carrier-mediated transport. Under this condition, P is a constant only as long as the transport is far from saturated. The possible variability of J_{act} and P imposes considerable problems on the analysis of data, because for determination of both P and J_{act}, at least two experimental designs are necessary, which obviously cannot be identical. This will be apparent from the following examples: The experimental design is directed to gain information from borderline situations, where Eq. (10) is simplified: If, e.g., volume reabsorption is prevented by intraluminal nonreabsorbable solutes and the substance under study is allowed to reach a luminal equilibrium concentration, we can write, since $J = 0$ and $J_v = 0$,

$$J_{\text{act}} = -P[\Delta c + (zF\Delta E/RT)\bar{c}] \tag{11}$$

All values except J_{act} and P might be determined in this experimental situation (if the substance is nonionic: $z = 0$ and $J_{\text{act}} = -P\Delta c$). From the fluxes before the equilibrium is reached,

$$J = P[\Delta c + (zF\Delta E/RT)\bar{c}] + J_{\text{act}} \tag{12}$$

and the corresponding ΔE, $\bar{c}$ and Δc, J_{act} and P can be determined, if they are identical to those in Eq. (11), since J_{act}/P is—under this condition—known from the equilibrium situation. However, this assumption might be erroneous since J_{act} or P might change with changing luminal or peritubular concentrations. Another approach is to use additional luminal tracer substance under the condition of equilibrium of the chemical substance. Under this circumstance, J_{act} is that of Eq. (11) and the tracer outflux may be described as

$$J^* = P[\Delta c^* + (zF\Delta E/RT)\bar{c}^*] + (\bar{c}^*/\bar{c})J_{act} \tag{13}$$

We assume that $\Delta c^* = c^*$, $\bar{c}^* = c^*/2$ and that the specific activity at the active transport carrier is $\bar{c}/\bar{c}$ (c^* = luminal tracer concentration). Then the apparent permeability $P_a = J^*/c^*$ yields the "true" permeability,

$$P = P_a/(1 - \Delta c/2\bar{c}) \tag{14}$$

However, the assumptions are somewhat random. The specific activity at the rate-limiting step of the active transport could be anything from 1 to 0, depending on the location. Therefore this correction factor and the whole approach are only justifiable when $\Delta c/2\bar{c}$ is very small compared with 1, which means that J_{act} is small compared with passive transport. If P is known, J_{act} can be calculated from Eq. (11). Additional experiments at various degrees of volume reabsorption allow estimation of the reflection coefficient. The advantage of the approach is that the driving forces of tubular transport are better defined and, as a matter of fact, the input of this approach has proved to be tremendous for the description of tubular transport (Ullrich, 1973). However, the example above demonstrates that interpretation of the results may be extremely hazardous because the "constants" P and J_{act} might be considerably different with alteration of the experimental situation and cannot be transferred from one experimental situation to another. Similarly, calculation of reflection coefficients may involve gross errors when J_{act} or P are influenced by the presence or absence of impermeant solutes.

On the other hand, the use of more than two series may allow calculation of J_{act} and P in different ways. Coincidence of the values is then a strong argument for the accuracy of the values. Furthermore, sometimes maximal errors can be estimated and allow the definition of the values by a range. A more serious limitation is that only extracellular events can be described, and the cell is considered a black box. If, e.g., a muscle is a black box, an isometric contraction has to be considered merely a passive event. In the tubule, a symmetrical bidirectional transport consuming energy is not recognized as such but labeled passive, since it does not operate against an electrochemical gradient. A bidirectional active transport occurs when a substance, e.g., amino acids (Foulkes, 1976) is accumulated in the cell from both peritubular and luminal sides.

REFERENCES

Andreucci, V. E., Rector, F. C. 1972. Some artifacts in measuring single-nephron glomerular filtration rate. *Yale J. Biol. Med.*, 45:217.
Andreucci, V. E., Herrera-Acosta, J., Rector, F. C., Jr., and Seldin, D. W. 1971. Measurement of

single-nephron glomerular filtration rate by micropuncture: analysis of error. *Am. J. Physiol.,* *221*:1551.

Bank, N., Aynedjian, H. S., and Wada, T. 1972. Effect of peritubular capillary perfusion rate on proximal sodium reabsorption. *Kidney Intern., 1*:397.

Baumann, K., deRouffignac, C., Roinel, N., Rumrich, G., and Ullrich, K. J. 1975. Renal phosphate transport: Inhomogeneity of local proximal transport rates and sodium dependence. *Pflügers Arch., 356*:287.

Brenner, B. M., and Daugharty, T. M. 1972. The measurement of glomerular filtration rate in single nephrons of the rat kidney. *Yale J. Biol. Med., 45*:200.

Cortell, St., Davidman, M., and Gennari, F. J. 1972. Catheter size as a determinant of outflow resistance and intrarenal pressure. *Am. J. Physiol., 223*:910.

Davidman, M., Lalone, R. C., Alexander, E. A., and Levinsky, N. G. 1971. Some micropuncture techniques in the rat. *Am. J. Physiol., 221*:1110.

Dev, B., Häberle, D., Schnermann, J., and Wunderlick, P. 1973. Effect of barbiturates on GFR and fluid reabsorption along proximal convoluted tubules and loops of Henle in rats. *Pflügers Arch., 344*:21.

Elmer, M., Eskildsen, P. C., Kristensen, L. O., and Leyssac, P. P. 1972. A comparison of renal function in rats anesthetized with inactin and sodium amytal. *Acta Physiol. Scand., 86*:41.

Foulkes, E. C. 1976. Peritubular transport of urate and amino acids in rat kidney. In: *Amino Acid Transport and Uric Transport,* pp. 211-216. Ed. by Silbernagl, S., Lang, F., and Greger, R. Thieme Verlag, Stuttgart.

Frömter, E., Rumrich, G., and Ullrich, K. J. 1973. Phenomenologic description of Na^+, Cl^- and HCO_3^- absorption from proximal tubules of the rat kidney. *Pflügers Arch., 343*:189.

Frömter, E., Müller, C. W., and Knauf, H. 1968. Fixe negative Wandladungen im proximalen Konvolut der Rattenniere und ihre Beeinflussung durch Calciumionen. In: *VI Symposium der Gesellschaft für Nephrologie,* Wien.

Fuchs, G. 1965. Stochastische Modelle in der Nierenphysiologie. *Biometr. Zschr., 2*:25.

Gertz, K. H., and Ullrich, K. J. 1961. Methode zur Analyse des Stofftransportes am einzelnen Tubulus der intakten Rattenniere, *Pflügers Arch., 274*:61.

Gertz, K. H. 1963. Transtubuläre Natriumchloridflüsse und Permeabilität für Nichtelektrolyte im proximalen und distalen Konvolut der Rattenier. *Pflügers Arch., 276*:336.

Gottschalk, C. W., and Lassiter, W. E. 1974. The intratubular microinjection technique. In: *Proc. 5th Int. Congr. Nephrol.,* Mexico, Vol. 2, pp. 116-123, Karger, Basel.

Gottschalk, C. W., Morel, F., and Mylle, M. 1965. Tracer microinjection studies of renal tubular permeability. *Am. J. Physiol., 209*:173.

Grandchamp, A., and Boulpaep, E. L. 1972. Effect of intraluminal pressure on proximal tubular sodium reabsorption. A shrinking drop micropuncture study. *Yale J. Biol. Med., 45*:275.

Greger, R., Lang, F., Marchand, G., and Knox, F. G. 1977. Site of renal phosphate reabsorption in rat kidney—micropuncture and microinfusion study. *Pflügers Arch., 369*:111.

Gutsche, H. U., Müller-Suur, R., Hegel, U., Hierholzer, K., and Lüderitz, S. 1975. A new method for intratubular blockade in micropuncture experiments. *Pflügers Arch., 354*:197.

Györy, A. Z. 1971. Reexamination of the split oil droplet method as applied to kidney tubules. *Pflügers Arch., 324*:328.

Heller, J. 1971. The influence of Lissamine green on tubular reabsorption of electrolytes and water in rats. *Pflügers Arch., 323*:27.

Hierholzer, K., Butz, M., Müller-Suur, R., and Lichtenstein, I. 1972. Pressure measurements in proximal surface tubules of the rat—single nephron filtration rate and tubuloglomerular feedback. *Yale J. Biol. Med., 45*:224.

Jamison, R. L. 1973. Intrarenal heterogeneity. The case for two functionally dissimilar populations of nephrons in the mammalian kidney. *Am. J. Med., 54*:281.

Jarausch, K. H., and Ullrich, K. J. 1956. Zur Technik der Entnahme von Harnproben aus einzelnen Sammelrohren der Säugetierniere mittels Polyäthylen-Capillaren. *Pflügers Arch., 264*:88.

Knox, F. G., and Marchand, G. R. 1976. Study of renal action of diuretics by micropuncture techniques. *In: Methods in Pharmacology,* Vol. 4A, *Renal Pharmacology,* pp. 73-98. Ed. by Martinez-Maldonaldo, M. Plenum Press, New York.

Kramp, R. A. 1976. Urate transport in the rat nephron: a microinjection study. In: *Amino Acid Transport and Uric Acid Transport*, pp. 201–211, Ed. by Silbernagl, S., Lang, F., and Greger, R. Thieme Verlag, Stuttgart.

Kramp, R. A., Lassiter, W. E., and Gottschalk, C. W. 1971. Urate-2-^{14}C transport in the rat nephron. *J. Clin. Invest., 50:*35.

Lang, F., Greger, R., and Deetjen, P. 1972. Handling of uric acid by the rat kidney. II. Microperfusion studies on bidirectional transport of urate in the proximal tubule. *Pflügers Arch., 335:*257.

Lang, F., Greger, R., and Deetjen, P. 1973. Handling of uric acid by the rat kidney. III. Microperfusion studies on steady state concentration of uric acid in the proximal tubule. Consideration of free flow conditions. *Pflügers Arch., 338:*295.

Lang, F., Greger, R., and Deetjen, P. 1974. *In vivo* studies on uricase activity in the rat. *Pflügers Arch., 351:*323.

Lang, F., Greger, R., Marchand, G., and Knox, F. 1977. Stationary microperfusion study of phosphate reabsorption in proximal and distal nephron segments. *Pflügers Arch., 368:*45.

Langer, K. H., Thoenes, W., and Wiederholt, M. 1968. Licht- und elektronenmikroskopische Untersuchungen am proximalen Tubuluskonvolut der Rattenniere nach intraluminaler Ölinjektion. *Pflügers Arch., 302:*149.

Lechene, C., and Morel, F. 1965. Microinjections de sodium et d'inuline marques dans les capillaires du rein de Hamster. I. Permeabilité au sodium des segments tubulaires corticaux. *Nephron, 2:*207.

Lingard, J., Rumrich, G., and Young, J. A. 1973. Reabsorption of L-glutamine and L-histidine from various regions of the rat proximal convolution studied by stationary microperfusion: Evidence that the proximal convolution is not homogeneous. *Pflügers Arch., 342:*1.

Lohfert, H., Lichtenstein, I., Butz, M., and Hierholzer, K. 1971. Continuous measurement of renal intratubular pressures with a combined pressure transducer microperfusion system. *Pflügers Arch., 327:*191.

Lynch, R. E., Schneider, E. G., Strandhoy, J. W., Willis, L. R., and Knox, F. G. 1973. Effect of Lissamine green dye on renal sodium reabsorption in the dog. *J. Appl. Physiol., 35:*169.

Morel, F., and Murayama, Y. 1970. Simultaneous measurement of unidirectional and net sodium fluxed in microperfused rat proximal tubules. *Pflügers Arch., 320:*1.

Nakajima, K., Clapp, J. R., and Robinson, R. R. 1970. Limitations of the shrinking-drop micropuncture technique. *Am. J. Physiol., 210:*345.

Quehenberger, P., Lang, F., Greger, R., and Deetjen, P. 1974. pH measurements in the loops of Henle of the rat kidney. *Pflügers Arch., 347:*R 68 (Abstract).

Rector, F. C., Andreucci, V. E., Herrera-Acosta, J., and Seldin, D. W. 1972. Potential sources of error in measuring single nephron filtration rate. *Yale J. Biol. Med., 45:*193.

Rector, F. C., Jr., Brunner, F. P., Sellman, J. C., and Seldin, D. W. 1966. Pitfalls in the use of micropuncture for the localization of diuretic action. *Ann. N.Y. Acad. Sci., 139:*400.

Richards, A. N., and Schmidt, C. F. 1924. A description of the glomerular circulation in the frog's kidney and observations concerning the action of adrenalin and various other substances upon it. *Am. J. Physiol., 71:*178.

Richards, A. N., and Walker, A. M. 1937. Methods of collecting fluid from known regions of the renal tubules of amphibia and of perfusing the lumen of a single tubule. *Am. J. Physiol., 118:*111.

Roch-Ramel, F., and Jotterand, N. 1970. Natriuretic effect of lissamine green. *Experientia, 26:*683.

Sauer, F. 1973. Nonequilibrium thermodynamics of kidney tubule transport. In: *Handbook of Physiology*, Vol. VIII, *Renal Physiology*, pp. 399–414. Ed. by Orloff, J. and Berliner, R. W. American Physiological Society, Washington, D.C.

Schnermann, J. 1972. Methodological aspects of filtrate determination by the micropuncture technique. *Yale J. Biol. Med., 45:*211.

Shipp, J. C., Hanenson, I. B., Windhager, E. E., Schatzmann, H. J., Whittembury, G., Yoshimura, H., and Solomon, A. K. 1958. Single proximal tubules of the *Necturus* kidney. Methods for micropuncture and microperfusion. *Am. J. Physiol., 195:*563.

Silbernagl, S., and Deetjen, P. 1969. Micropuncture studies of proximal tubular reabsorption of glycin. *Pflügers Arch., 312:*82 (abstr.).

Sonnenberg, H., and Deetjen, P. 1964. Methode zur Durchströmung einzelner Nephronabschnitte. *Pflügers Arch., 278:*669.

Spitzer, A., and Windhager, E. E. 1970. Effect of peritubular oncotic pressure changes on proximal tubular fluid reabsorption. *Am. J. Physiol., 218:*1188.

Steinhausen, M. 1963. Eine Methode zur Differenzierung proximaler und distaler Tubuli der Nierenrinde von Ratten in vivo and ihre Anwendung zur Bestimmung tubulärer Strömungsgeschwindigkeiten. *Pflügers Arch., 277:*23.

Steinhausen, M., Hill, E., and Parekh, N. 1976. Intravital microscopical studies of the tubular urine flow in the conscious rat. *Pflügers Arch., 362:*261.

Ullrich, K. J. 1973. Permeability characteristics of the mammalian nephron. In: *Handbook of Physiology,* Vol. VIII, *Renal Physiology,* pp. 377–398. Ed. by Orloff, J. and Berliner, R. W. American Physiological Society, Washington, D.C.

Ullrich, K. J., Frömter, E., and Baumann, K. 1969. Micropuncture and microanalysis in kidney physiology. In: *Laboratory Techniques in Membrane Biophysics,* pp. 106–129. Ed. by Passow, H. and Stämpfli, R. Springer Verlag, Berlin.

Walker, A. M., and Oliver, J. 1941. Methods for the collection of fluid from single glomeruli and tubules of the mammalian kidney. *Am. J. Physiol., 133:*562.

Walker, A. M., Bott, P. A., Oliver, J., and McDowell, M. C. 1941. The collection and analysis of fluid from single nephrons of the mammalian kidney. *Am. J. Physiol., 134:*580.

Wearn, J. T., and Richards, A. N. 1924. Observations on the composition of glomerular urine, with particular reference to the problem of reabsorption in the renal tubules. *Am. J. Physiol., 71:*209.

Weinmann, E. J., Hardy, R. J., Kashgarian, M., and Hayslett, J. P. 1972. Examination of the Gertz technique as applied to the proximal tubule of the rat kidney. *Yale J. Biol. Med., 45:*289.

Wiederholt, M., Langer, K. H., Thoenes, K., and Hierholzer, K. 1968. Funktionelle und morphologische Untersuchungen am proximalen und distalen Konvolut der Rattenniere zur Methode der gespaltenen Ölsäule, *Pflügers Arch., 302:*166.

Windhager, E. E. 1968a. *Micropuncture Techniques and Nephron Function.* Butterworth, London.

Windhager, E. E. 1968b. Peritubuläre Kontrolle der Natriumresorption im proximalen Tubulus. In: *VI Symposium der Gesellschaft für Nephrologie, Wien.*

Young, J. A., and Lingard, J. M. 1976. Handling of neutral amino acids by the proximal tubule of the rat nephron. In: *Amino Acid Transport and Uric Acid Transport,* pp. 86–95. Ed. by Silbernagl, S., Lang, F., and Greger, R. Thieme Verlag, Stuttgart.

Chapter **5**

Analysis of Tubule Fluid

R. Greger and F. Lang

Institute of Physiology
Innsbruck, Austria

F. G. Knox

Department of Physiology and Biophysics
Mayo Clinic and Mayo Foundation
Rochester, Minnesota

and

C. Lechene

Biotechnology Resource in Electron Probe Microanalysis
Harvard Medical School
Boston, Massachusetts

I. INTRODUCTION

The analysis of tubule fluid includes the measurement of the concentration of one or more substances and the measurement of the volume of the sample. The concentration measurement either employs microadaptations of macrochemical methods or radioactive tracers. In recent years the absolute sensitivity of elemental determinations has been increased by orders of magnitude with the application of electron probe analysis to liquid samples.

In this chapter the general equipment and the preparations necessary for ultramicroanalysis are described.

II. SETUP FOR MICROCHEMISTRY

In most of the microchemistry methods a small droplet of tubule fluid is diluted or mixed with reagent. Since the volumes are small, the procedure is

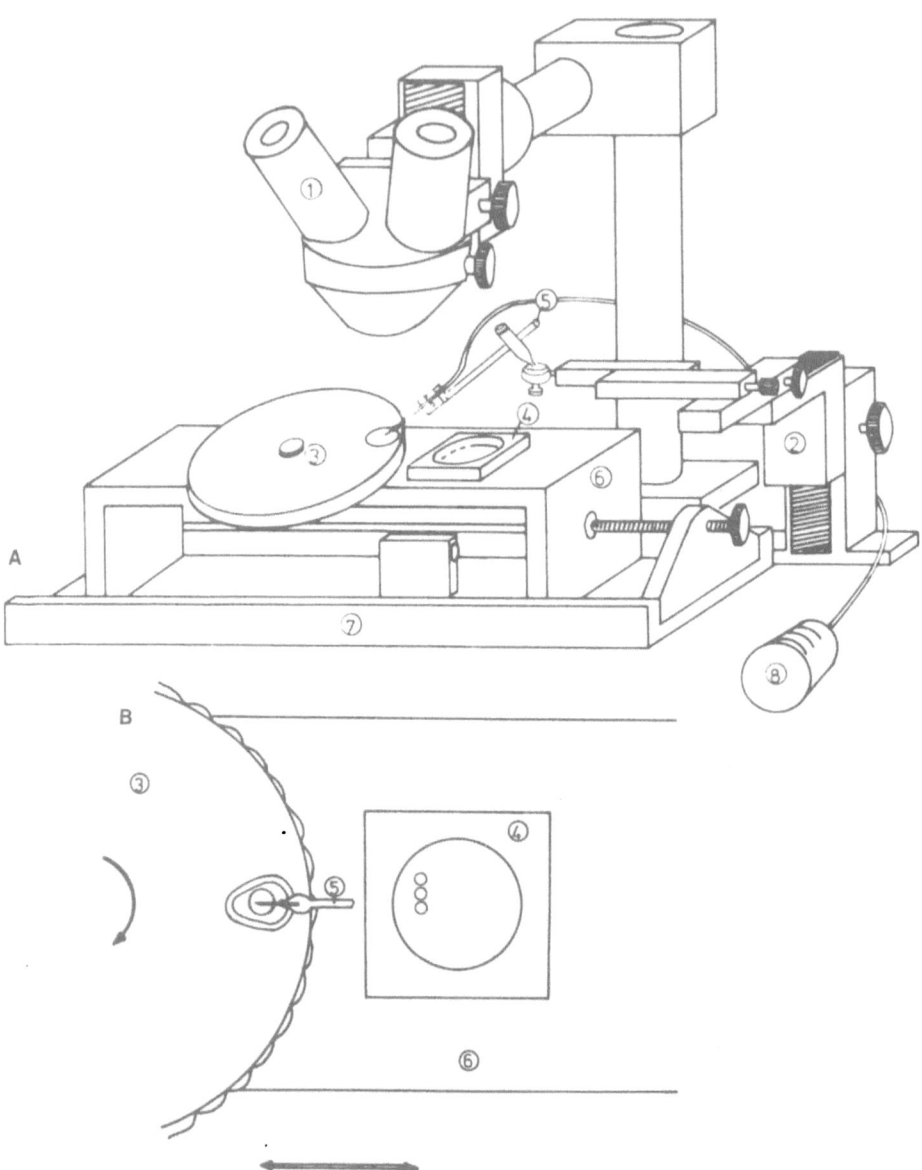

Figure 1. (A) Horizontal setup for microchemistry: (1) Stereo zoom microscope. (2) Right-hand micromanipulator with three drives. (3) Teflon disk with 20–30 grooves protected against dust by a plastic disk with an opening for sample placement. (4) Glass dish for storing samples under oil. (5) Micropipet holder with a self-filling pipet (Figure 3). (6) Bench made from stainless steel or brass. (7) Track for moving between sample dish and Teflon disk. (8) Syringe (preferably whole glass) attached to the micropipet by a PE catheter. (B) Detail of (A) as seen from above.

carried out under microscopic control. Two different types of microchemistry setups are in common use: in one the plane of focus of the microscope is horizontal, and in the other it is perpendicular.

The horizontal setup (Figure 1) incorporates a stereo zoom microscope with a magnification range of 10–100×. The microscope is mounted on a solid stand. The focus drive is perpendicular. A right-hand micromanipulator with three drives is used. A pipet holder is mounted to the micromanipulator. The disk and sample dish are attached to a solid bench. This bench is shifted from the sample dish to the Teflon disk on the table track with an adjustable screw. The filling and emptying of the pipet is controlled by a glass syringe. Diluent or reagent is pipeted into a Teflon disk which has 20–30 grooves of ellipsoidal shape. After placing each sample, the disk is rotated to the next groove. To protect the grooves from dust, the whole disk is covered by a Plexiglas plate, leaving one opening right above the groove used. Samples are stored in a glass dish and covered by saturated oil. Freshly saturated oil is made by having paraffin oil continuously emulsified with saline by a magnetic stirrer. The volume of oil needed for a day is centrifuged 20 min and kept under a humid atmosphere. It should be noted that nanoliter and picoliter volumes of samples are not fully protected from concentration, even in freshly prepared saturated oil. However, no concentration of samples occurs when samples are stored frozen at −80°C either in micropuncture pipets or in dishes covered with oil (Lechene, unpublished observations). Therefore, it is important to use identical timing for a given set of sample manipulations of droplets at room temperature and to reduce the time spent at room temperature as much as possible.

The procedure is as follows: First, samples are transferred from the micropuncture pipets to the glass dish. This may be done manually or by the use of the micromanipulator. Second, the reagent or diluent is pipeted into one groove of the Teflon disk. Third, a standard volume of sample is transferred with the micropipet to the droplet of reagent or diluent. Finally, the mixed fluids are placed in a capillary tube for subsequent steps in analysis.

The perpendicular setup also incorporates a stereo zoom microscope with a magnification range of 10–100× (Figure 2). The microscope is mounted on a solid perpendicular drive. A micropipet is attached to the microscope and remains fixed in focus. A plastic screw is mounted on a right-hand manipulator with three drives. The slit of this screw holds a Plexiglas block. The Plexiglas block is cylindrical and has a perpendicular groove on the front. This groove is filled with water-saturated oil. Samples are transferred to this groove so that they stick to the Plexiglas surface and are covered by oil. A left-hand micromanipulator with three drives carries the sample pipet and reagent tube holder. This holder has approximately six perpendicular grooves, each with a width of 1.0 mm and a depth of 0.8 mm. Sample pipets and reagent capillaries are fixed in position by springs made from steel wire of 0.3 mm diameter. The sample pipet and micropipet are each attached to glass syringes with PE tubing.

The procedure is as follows: First, a reagent capillary is prepared and fixed in the holder. Then the sample is transferred to the Plexiglas block. Now the focus drive of the stereomicroscope is used to drive the micropipet through the oil and to merge it into the sample. The micropipet is filled and then the Plexiglas

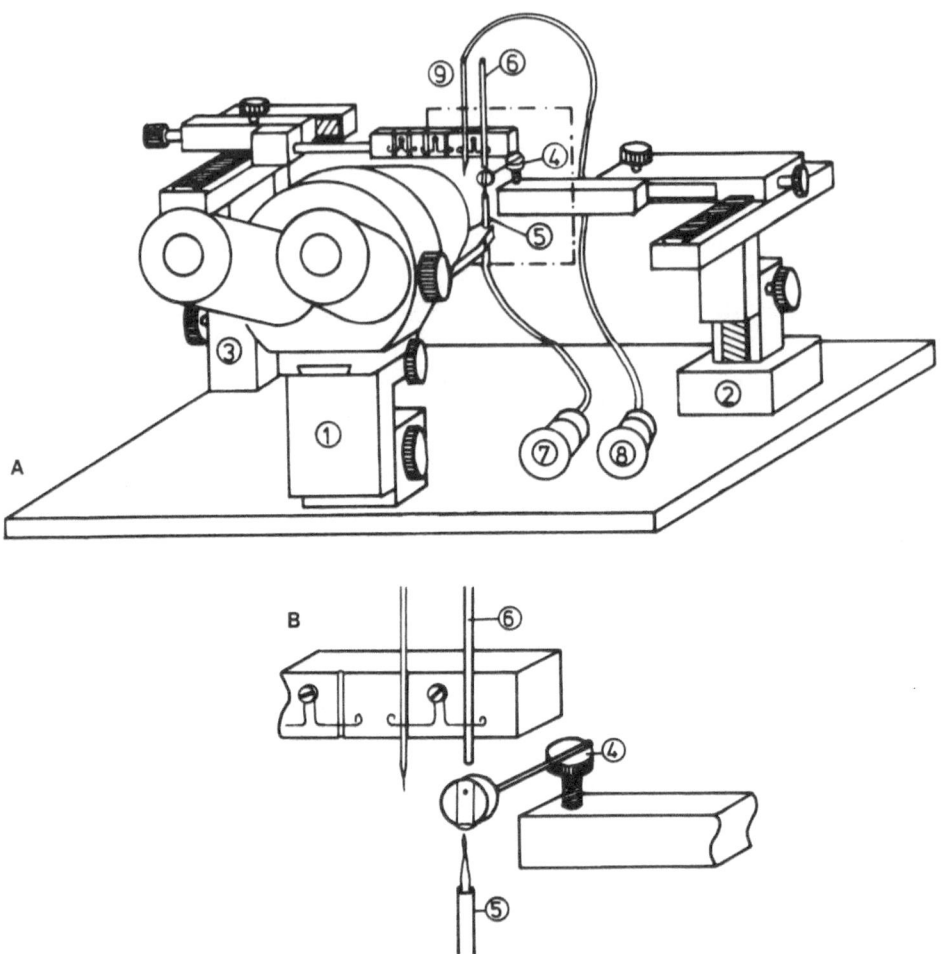

Figure 2. (A) Perpendicular setup for microchemistry: (1) Stereo zoom microscope mounted on
a perpendicular drive. (2) Right-hand micromanipulator. (3) Left-hand micromanipulator. (4)
Plastic screw (M4–M5) which holds the sample block. The sample block is made from a round
Plexiglas material (4 mm diameter). (5) Steel tubing which carries the micropipet. (6)
Incubation capillary. (7) Glass syringe attached to the micropipet (Figure 4). (8) Glass syringe
attached to the sample capillary (9). (9) Sample capillary = micropuncture capillary. Sample
capillary and incubation capillary (6) are both fixed in a holder. The holder has perpendicular
grooves in which both capillaries are fixed by steel springs (0.3 mm diameter). (B) Detail of the
area surrounded by a dashed line in (A).

block is moved back. The reagent capillary is brought into position over the
micropipet. The sample is injected into the reagent and both fluids are mixed by
slowly agitating the fluid column up and down in the reagent capillary.

   This setup, although more complicated than the horizontal one, has the
advantage that most steps are done using micromanipulator drives. The micropipet is in focus all the time.

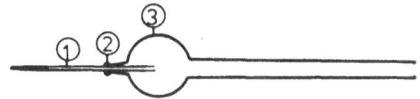

Figure 3. Production of self-filling pipets: (1) Capillary serving as pipet. (2) Seal between capillary and housing (3) made from epoxy glue. (3) Capillary housing. The table below the figure gives approximate inside diameters of capillaries with a length of 10 mm.

CAPILLARY RADIUS						
Volume (nl)	100	50	20	10	5	2
RADIUS (μm)	56	40	25	18	13	8

A. Production of Pipets

Two size categories of pipets are necessary for microchemistry: A reagent pipet in the microliter range and a sample pipet in the nanoliter range. A commercially available microliter pipet or a self-filling type of pipet is used to pipet reagents. The nanoliter pipets are made as constriction or as self-filling types. The constriction type of pipet is more convenient for the perpendicular microchemistry setup whereas the self-filling type of pipet is more convenient for the horizontal setup. The self-filling pipets can be constructed without any special tools. A microforge is necessary for the constriction type of pipet. Both types of pipets are made from flint glass.

A self-filling pipet consists of a capillary and a capillary housing, which are sealed with epoxy glue (Figure 3). The capillary may be pulled in a capillary puller or pulled manually. The distal tip of the capillary is narrowed to increase outflow resistance. In the table below Figure 3, the inside diameters are listed for pipets of given volumes and a capillary length of 10 mm. The capillary should not be longer than 10 mm to avoid unnecessary focusing of the microscope, or smaller than 10 mm to avoid immersion of the pipet housing in the oil in the sample dish. The pipet housing is made from a glass tube of approximately 2.0 mm outside diameter. One end of the tube is sealed and a small sphere is blown with constant twisting above a low flame. The tube is pulled close to the sphere to form a cone which is broken to accommodate the capillary. The capillary is sealed in the sphere with epoxy glue so that the proximal end of the capillary is in the middle of the sphere. The production of a similar type of pipet with volumes in the picoliter range has recently been described (Quinton, 1976).

A constriction pipet is made from flint glass tubing of 1.0 mm diameter. The tube is pulled in a capillary puller to give a long tip (Figure 4). A hook is formed at the tip of the pipet with a microforge [Figure 5(A)]. A small weight is hung on this hook [Figure 5(B)]. A constriction is formed with the heating coil of the

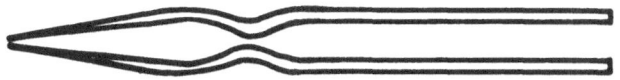

Figure 4. Schematic view of a constriction pipet. The inside diameter of the constriction is larger than the inside tip diameter to avoid air bubbles in the sample.

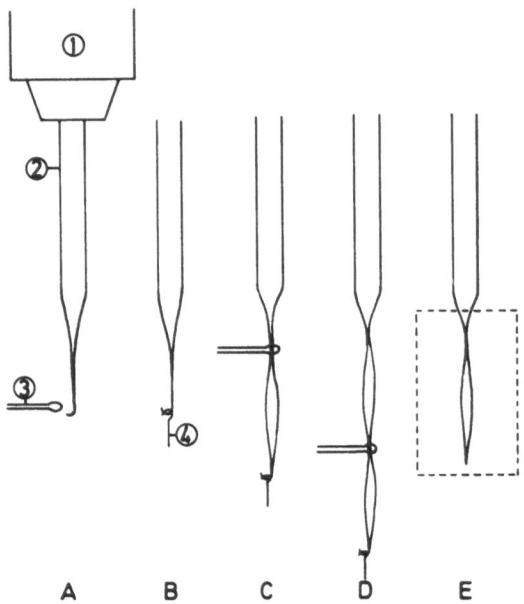

Figure 5. Production of constriction pipets. (1) Auger bit to hold the capillary (2). (3) Platinum wire connected to the power supply of the microforge. (4) Metal hook to put defined traction on the heated glass capillary (2). (A–C) Single steps of pipet production. (See text.)

microforge [Figure 5(C)]. A second constriction is formed at the pipet tip [Figure 5(D,E)]. The tip diameter should be smaller than the constriction so that air bubbles are not blown into the reagent when the pipet is emptied.

A constant-bore pipet for volume measurement is constructed similar to the self-filling type. The glass capillary is 20 mm of constant inside diameter and the maximum volume is 100 nl. The capillary has a fine tip which is necessary to completely collect samples.

For pipets in the picoliter range, containing multiple samples as used in electron probe analysis, two pullings are necessary. In order to make a second pulling of the capillary, the filament is held at one spot until the capillary has heated through enough to begin to narrow. Once a narrowing appears, the filament must be moved down the capillary just at the lower shoulder of the narrowing. The distance of the filament from the capillary must be continually adjusted in order to keep a constant diameter for the length of the second pulling. The capillary should be drawn out to a length at least the diameter of the field of vision of the microforge. Once the second pulling has been drawn out to a sufficient length, a tip is made on the pipet by heating through the end of the second pulling. A narrowing is then made in the pipet small enough to sufficiently slow any fluid being drawn up into the pipet, making it easy to stop at exactly the same point every time. A good pipet should be able to hold about 30 drops without developing too much resistance.

Pipets are mounted, siliconized, and calibrated. They are best siliconized by first saturating the glass with OH⁻ by leaving the pipet for 24 hr in an atmosphere saturated with water. The inside and outside of the pipets are exposed briefly to silicone (G.E. SC87, 7% solution in chloroform) and rinsed in toluene (E. Rochow, personal communication). No wet or dry heating steps are necessary. All pipets are calibrated using an aqueous radioactive tracer solution. For the constant-bore pipet, a standard curve is obtained by plotting the length versus the volume.

Cleaning the volumetric micropipet, especially when clogged with organic material, is best done by heating the tip of the pipet at 550°C in a specially built oven for several minutes. The pipet is then rinsed in acetone and chloroform.

The small glass capillary is the test tube of microchemistry. Samples and reagent are mixed in the capillary by gentle agitation or in some cases by centrifugation of sealed capillaries. The capillaries are sealed with an oxygen-gas microflame from a point source burner. Care must be taken to avoid charring samples in the capillary and this is best done by sealing some distance from liquid samples.

B. Microphotometry

Several of the analytical methods described in this chapter utilize colorimetric procedures. The amount of color produced in microprocedures is small compared with the macro procedures. Since according to the Lambert–Beer law $OD = c \cdot d \cdot \epsilon$ [OD = optical density, c = concentration (mmol/liter), d = optical path length (cm), ϵ = extinction coefficient], the cuvette must have both a small volume and a relatively long optical path length.

Vurek and Bowman (1969) designed a fiber optic instrument in which a small capillary serves as a cuvette. Fiber optic rods are inserted into the open ends of the capillary. One fiber optic is connected to a light source and the other to a photo tube. In a modified type which is commercially available, the reagent capillaries are broken at both ends and may be used as cuvettes. However, this modification requires 5–8 μl, volumes which are too high for some colorimetric procedures. Ullrich and Hampel (1958) and Ullrich et al. (1969) designed a cuvette which can be used with most sensitive photometers; however, most of the volume used for filling remains in the nozzles and only a fraction of the volume is utilized for the photometric measurement. Another type of cuvette has been designed by Schneider and Greger (1969). This cuvette consists of a black glass capillary mounted into a holder and sealed with two glass windows. Almost the whole filling volume is used for the photometric measurement. Cuvettes in the submicroliter range can be produced. The design of the cuvette is further shown in Figure 6. To fill the cuvette, first one of the glass windows is removed [Figure 6(A)]. The capillary containing the reagent is held obliquely to the open bend of the black glass capillary and then the reagent is blown out of the capillary. The black glass capillary will fill by capillary action. After the black glass capillary is filled, the opposite end of the cuvette is closed. Next the cuvette is turned to shift the fluid column so that it completely wets both windows. The filled capillary is checked for air bubbles and dust with a microscope. The cuvette is inserted in a photometer which is equipped with an adapter to fit the cuvette holder for an accurate positioning of the capillary in the light beam. After reading, the cuvette is cleaned by removing both windows, rinsed, and dried with compressed air or preferably with dry CO_2.

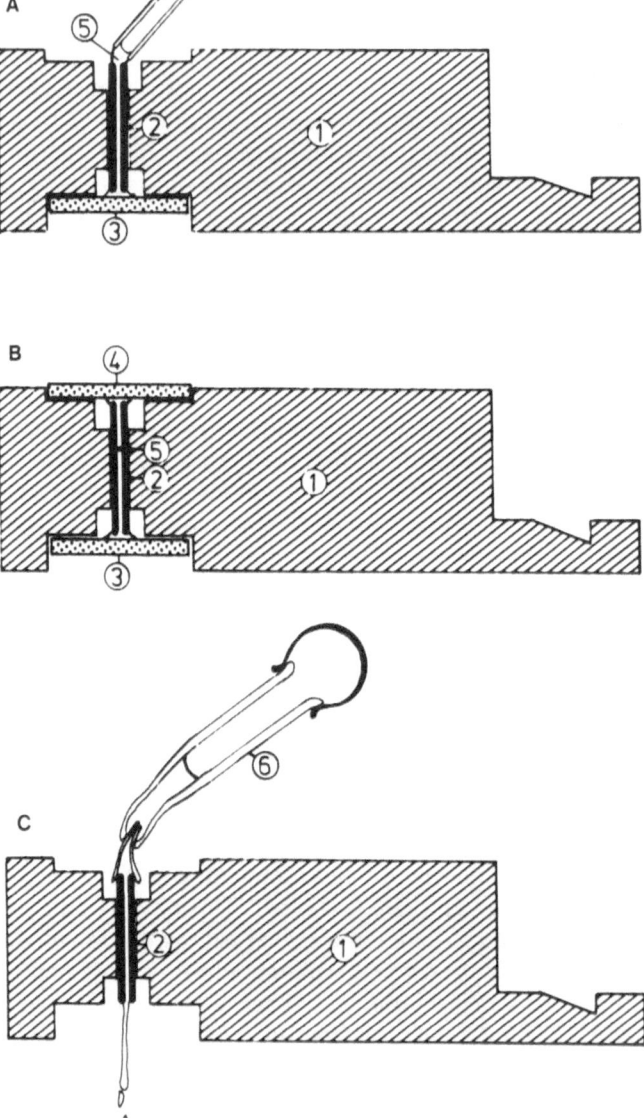

Figure 6(A–C). Steps in the use of a microphotometric cuvette. (1) Capillary holder made from polyvinyl chloride or brass. (2) Black glass capillary, length 9.9 mm, inside diameter, depending on volume, between 0.15–0.3 mm, which corresponds to a filling volume of 200–1000 nl. (3) Bottom window made from a 1-mm thick circular glass (or quartz glass plate for UV use) plate. (4) Top glass plate. (5) Fluid sample to be measured. (6) Eye dropper used for rinsing the cuvette.

Figure 7. Adapter for fluorometric analysis (kindly provided by Dr. Roch-Ramel, Lausanne, Switzerland). The adapter may be made from brass or polyvinyl chloride. The excitation and emission boring are cone shaped. They both have a small inside diameter of approximately 0.5 mm. The axes of the two drill holes are exactly at right angles to each other. The perpendicular boring for the sample capillary is adjusted to the outside diameter of the capillary glass so that the capillary fits snugly into the boring.

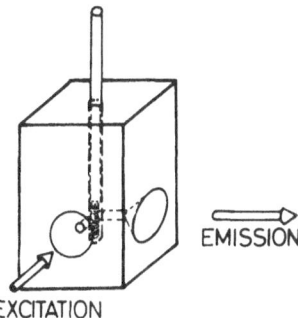

EMISSION

EXCITATION

C. Microfluorometry

Fluorometry is substantially more sensitive than absorption photometry and therefore fluorometric methods are increasingly utilized for analysis of tubular fluid. For most methods, simple filter fluorometers or spectrofluorometers are adequate. A typical cuvette adapter is shown in Figure 7. The adapter is placed in the macrocuvette space of the fluorometer. The reagent capillary containing the fluorescing solution is inserted into the perpendicular boring of the adapter. To obtain reproducible measurements, the reagent capillaries must be of constant diameter.

A special type of fluorometric cuvette holder with a lens on the excitation boring has been described by Vurek and Pegram (1966). It is commercially available for a filter fluorometer and utilizes standard capillaries.

D. Handling Radioactively Labeled Compounds

To determine the concentration of a radioactively labeled compound in tubule fluid or collected perfusate, a small accurate volume is transferred into 10 ml of scintillation cocktail (β-counting). This usually is done by first diluting the nanoliter sample volume with approximately 10–20 μl of bidistilled water. The volume of bidistilled water is not critical and will not produce significant quenching with the usual scintillation cocktails. Care must be taken that this transfer procedure does not leave any aqueous solution in the transfer capillary. The scintillation cocktail should dissolve at least 50 μl of water per 10 ml. Such scintillation cocktails are commercially available or can be prepared with special recipes (Bray, 1960; Truniger and Schmidt-Nielsen, 1964).

The total amount of radioactivity in tubule fluid samples is often very low. Radioactive inulin may give unstable or decreasing counts with the long counting times which are necessary to compensate for the low radioactivity. Accordingly, it is necessary to maximize the efficiency of counting and to optimize the signal-over-background ratio. Techniques that can be used to increase the counting efficiency include the use of plastic rather than glass vials to lower the background, use of scintillation media without alcohol or any other diluent for better counting efficiency, and drying samples on glass fiber filters to avoid quenching. To stabilize inulin counts, a suspending gel in the scintillation medium or fiber filters can be used to avoid decreasing count signal as a function of counting time.

The scintillation counting of tubule fluid frequently involves counting of two tracers. Details of scintillation counting methodology have been described (Bransome, 1970; Hendee, 1973; Rapkin; Horrocks and Peng; Schram; and Birks, 1963).

The chemical purity of the tracer should be validated at intervals when using radioactively labeled compounds. For inulin, one of the most frequently used radioactively labeled compounds, a simple thin-layer chromatographic separation procedure may be carried out as follows. Approximately 1 μl of an aqueous solution of labeled inulin is spotted on the starting point of a cellulose plate. A chamber is filled to a depth of 1 cm with a solvent system consisting of 10 volumes *n*-butanol, 6 volumes pyrimidine, 1 volume acetic acid, and 3 volumes bidistilled water. The chromatogram can be evaluated with a scanner or in a liquid scintillation counter. In the latter case, a chromatogram measuring 10 $\times$ 1.5 cm is cut into 20 segments, each 0.5 $\times$ 1.5 cm. Each segment is transferred in a counting vial filled with scintillation cocktail. The cellulose layer is separated from the plastic foil by exposing the counting vial to an ultrasonic cleaner. For [^{3}H]inulin, the pure tracer will stay at the starting point; subfractions of the inulin molecule travel to an R_f value of 0.38. Analogous procedures for testing the purity of ^{14}C-labeled purines, uric acid, allantoin, allantoic acid, and urea have been described elsewhere (Lang *et al.*, 1974; Friedman and Merril, 1973).

III. CATIONS Na$^+$, K$^+$, Ca^{2+}, Mg^{2+}

The alternatives to electron probe analysis for cations include (*a*) fluorometric methods as in the case of Mg^{2+} (Gomori, 1941–42; Brunette *et al.*, 1969; Schachter, 1959); (*b*) flame photometric methods as extensively applied to the determination of Na$^+$ and K$^+$ (Bott, 1960; Malnic *et al.*, 1964; Ramsay *et al.*, 1953; Mueller, 1958); (*c*) helium glow photometry which has been used for the determination of all four cations (Vurek and Bowman, 1965; Burg and Green, 1973; Edwards *et al.*, 1973; Holzer and Hohenegger, 1974). The principle of simultaneous micro flame-photometric determinations of Na$^+$ and K$^+$ was first described by Ramsay *et al.* (1953) and was further modified by Bott (1960). The current methodology is described by Malnic *et al.* (1964). The basic difference between flame photometry and helium glow photometry is in the mode of ion excitation. Whereas a gas flame is used in the first approach, a glow discharge is used in the latter. The principle of helium glow analysis was first described by Vurek and Bowman (1965): an energy transfer takes place between a helium discharge and cations which in turn emit their characteristic radiation (Figure 8). The helium discharge is produced in a quartz flow cell containing two electrodes to which a voltage oscillating in the radio frequency range is applied. The cation-containing sample is transferred to an inverted U-shaped lower electrode made from 0.2 mm iridium wire. In the operating cycle, 5 nl of diluted sample are placed on the lower electrode. The chamber is closed, purged with helium, and the discharge started. Simultaneously, a voltage is applied to the iridium wire loop to heat it. In the discharge, the vaporized ions emit characteristic radiation.

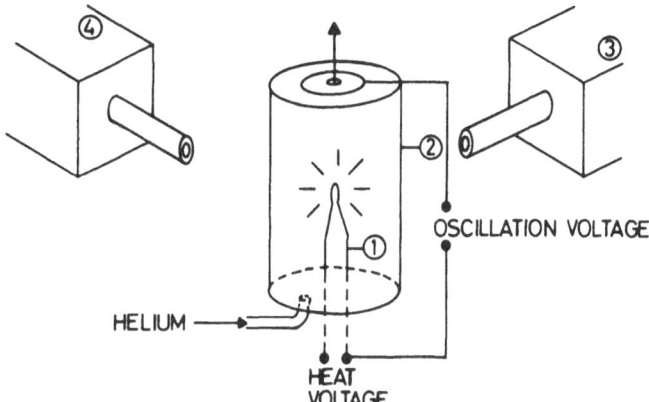

Figure 8. Helium glow: (1) Iridium wire 0.2 mm diameter, length about 1 inch. (2) Glow chamber made from quartz glass with two openings for the helium gas flow. The chamber can be opened for loading the iridium wire. In the chamber there are two electrodes for the oscillation voltage. One is on the top of the chamber and the other is the iridium wire. The iridium wire is connected to an adjustable heating voltage. (3) and (4) Photomultipliers for Na^+ and K^+ (or if equipped with special filters, for other cations).

The two photomultipliers independently record the radiation of two different ion species. The impulses are integrated over a preset time period and the sums are shown by a readout device.

Procedure: For Na^+ and K^+ determinations, 5 nl of the tubule fluid sample are diluted with 100 nl of an aqueous solution containing 5 mmol/liter NH_4 (H_2) PO_4 and 30 mmol/liter $CsNO_3$ (dilution ratio approx. 1:20). Standard solutions covering the expected concentration range of Na^+ and K^+ are diluted in the same way. The transfer pipet mounted in the helium glow photometer is a constriction pipet of approximately 5 nl. The loading of the iridium wire is achieved by moving the transfer pipet to the upper bend of the wire such that the pipet tip just touches the wire. It is important to always load at the same site on the wire. The pipet should have a small tip to allow reproducible transfer of the diluted sample to the iridium coil. Now the pipet is withdrawn, the chamber closed, and the cycle started. Constant timing of the steps is important. Triplicates should be made from standards and samples.

IV. CHLORIDE

The principle of the electro-titrimetric method for chloride has been described by Ramsay *et al.* (1955). If chloride is removed specifically from the solution, a corresponding drop in an electrical PD between two electrodes can be recorded. Chloride is removed by precipitating AgCl in an acid solution. The necessary amount of silver ions is either added stepwise by titrating with silver nitrate or produced electrically from a silver electrode by an external current source. In the modified version of Ramsay's method, the measured parameter is the time it takes to decrease the PD to the value of 240 mV. The basic design of a slightly modified system is shown in Figure 9. The microchemistry setup used for this method is shown in Figure 2. A plastic block described for the microchemistry setup is modified to include a horizontal boring and a horizontal groove. The groove of this block is filled with water-saturated oil. Through the horizontal boring, a 32-gauge (0.008 inch) silver wire enters the oil-filled groove and its end just touches the sample H_2SO_4 mixture. Opposite to the silver wire, a reference electrode is located which consists of an agar–$NaNO_3$-filled micropipet fixed in Teflon tubing. Both electrodes are connected to the electrical unit. The sample is transferred to the block and mixed with an equal volume of H_2SO_4 with a 300-pl constriction pipet. A schematic view of the reference electrode is given in Figure 9(B). The materials necessary for the method include: (*a*) 2% agar in 1 *N* $NaNO_3$ for filling the pipet of the reference electrode; (*b*) 1 *N* $AgNO_3$ to fill the chamber of the reference electrode; (*c*) 1 mm Ag wire for the reference electrode; (*d*) 32-gauge Ag wire for the titrating electrode; (*e*) dry film 1:2 in toluene to coat the tip of the thin wire; (*f*) 1.3 *N* H_2SO_4 to be used for diluting the sample; (*g*) 0.1 *N* HCl for coating the reference electrodes. The procedure is done in the following steps: (1) The agar-filled, air bubble-free micropipet is prepared daily. (2) The 1-mm silver wire of the reference electrode is cleaned either mechanically or electrolytically by connecting it to a battery. Thereafter, silver chloride coating is obtained by connecting this wire to the positive pole of a 3-V battery and immersing it in 0.1 *N* HCl. The reference electrode is now completed by filling it with 1 *N* $AgNO_3$ and thereafter it is connected to the electrical unit. (3) The thin silver wire is now coated with dry film toluene solution for a few seconds and dried and fixed in the block and wired to the

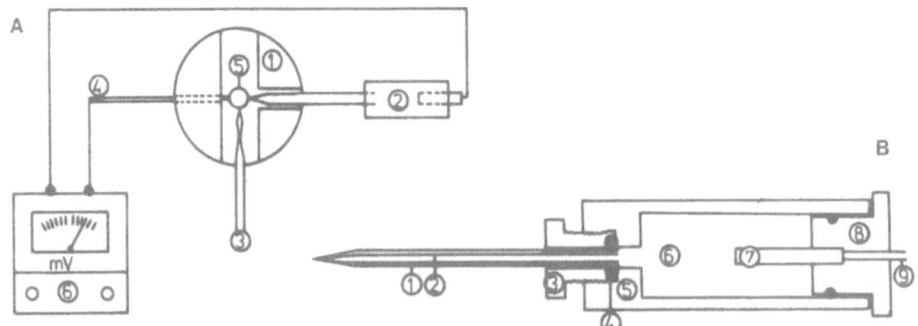

Figure 9. Micro chloride titrator. (A) (1) Plexiglas block for chloride measurements. (2) Reference electrode with an agar/$NaNO_3$-filled micropuncture pipet. The reference electrode is shown in detail in (B). (3) Sample pipet (constriction type) with a volume of 0.3 nl. (4) 32-gauge (0.008 inch) silver wire touching the sample/H_2SO_4 mixture. (5) Sample/H_2SO_4 mixture (1:1). Titrator with an mV meter and an external battery. (B) Reference electrode: (1) Micropuncture pipet, tip 7 μm filled with agar/$NaNO_3$ (2). (3) Front screw of Teflon tubing (5) sealed by a rubber ring (4). (5) Teflon tubing, approx. 2 inches long, inside diameter 10 mm, filled with 1 *N* $AgNO_3$ (6). (7) Silver wire 1 mm diameter coated by silver chloride. (8) Rear stopper with a rubber ring seal. (9) Plug for connection to titrator.

electrical unit. (4) When both electrodes are positioned, the sample is transferred from the sample block [Figure 2(B)] and diluted with the same volume of H_2SO_4. Now the electrodes touch the diluted sample droplet. (5) The titrator is switched on; a stopwatch is used to record the time necessary to decrease the voltage to 240 mV.

V. BICARBONATE, CARBON DIOXIDE

Several approaches have been taken for the microanalysis of CO_2 and bicarbonate; these include using pH electrodes (Caflisch and Carter, 1974; Karlmark and Sohtell, 1973), conductometric microanalysis (Maffly, 1968), and measuring pressure change in a closed system (Hevert, 1973). Very recently a new approach has been taken by Vurek *et al.* (1975) and by Warnock and Burg (1975). This method utilizes the heat which is produced when CO_2 reacts with

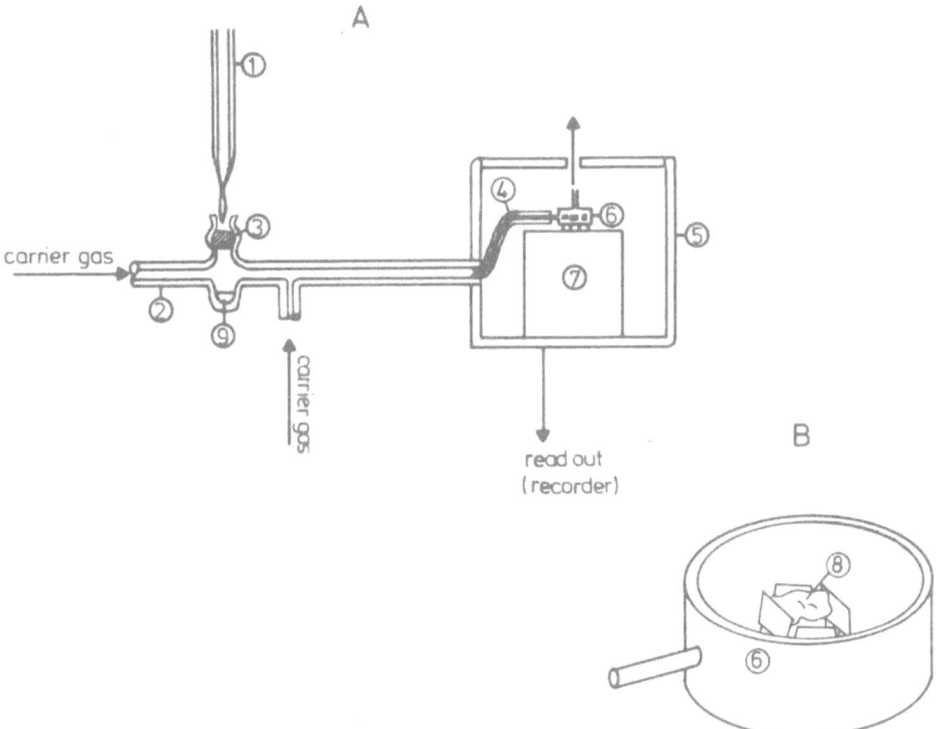

Figure 10. (A) Microcolorimetric setup for CO_2 measurement from Vurek *et al.* (1975): (1) 10–20 nl constriction pipet for transferring sample. (2) Quartz glass CO_2 release well made from quartz tubing 2.5 mm outside diameter. The release well is sealed by a mercury drop (3), the well is filled with phosphoric acid (9), and is purged by a constant carrier gas flow (4). Box (5) carrying preamplifier (7) and thermistor box (6). The thermistor box (6) is shown in detail in (B) with the cover removed. Between two thermistors an LiOH crystal is fixed (8); the carrier gas with the CO_2 enters from the opening at the left-hand side; the gas leaves the box through an opening in the top.

LiOH. The heat produced is measured by a thermistor bridge. The layout of the system is schematically shown in Figure 10. The system is best used in the perpendicular microchemistry setup. The sample is pipetted from above with a 10–20 nl pipet into a well filled with phosphoric acid and sealed by a small drop of mercury. The well is constantly perfused with a carrier gas (dichlorodifluoromethane) at a flow rate of 0.1 ml/min. The carrier gas will deliver the liberated CO_2 to the thermistor chamber where it reacts with a dried LiOH crystal mounted between two thermistors. This signal is amplified and recorded. The integral of the curve obtained is proportional to the CO_2 concentration. The materials necessary for the method include: (a) the well in which CO_2 is liberated, which is made from quartz tubing 2 mm outside diameter; (b) the thermistor chamber [Figure 10(B)] which measures about 5 mm outside diameter, has a removable cover, and carries matched thermistors of approximately 1 mm size and 2 MΩ resistance; (c) a preamplifier and amplifier; (d) a carrier gas (dichlorodifluoromethane); (e) granular lithium hydroxide, kept dry over silica gel; (f) mercury; (g) 85% phosphoric acid.

Procedure: (1) An appropriate LiOH crystal of about 0.5–1.0 mg is mounted between two thermistors and held in position by a little grease. The thermistor chamber is closed and fixed in the system. (2) The carrier gas is switched on and its flow rate adjusted. (3) The well is coated with a halocarbon film to prevent the acid from climbing out of the well. The mercury drop is inserted in the upper valve and the phosphoric acid is transferred into the well. Now the well is attached to the system. (4) Amplifiers and recorder are adjusted and a baseline is obtained. (5) Sample or standard solutions are pipetted using a 10–20 nl pipet in the well and a corresponding signal is recorded. The integral of the baseline difference of this recording is proportional to the CO_2 concentration. (6) When the baseline has stabilized again, a new sample can be measured. The crystal may be used several days; the phosphoric acid has to be changed every 30th measurement.

VI. PHOSPHATE

The colorimetric procedures for phosphate usually employ the reduction of phosphomolybdate to a blue-colored complex in conjunction with a reducing substance such as stannous chloride or ascorbic acid (Fiske and SubbaRow, 1925; Chen et al., 1956; Gomori, 1941–42). A modification of this method uses malachite green to produce a colored complex (Boudry et al., 1975; Bastiaanse and Meijers, 1968; Itaya and Ui, 1966). The method usually employed for ultramicrocolorimetric phosphate measurements is the one described by Chen et al. (1956) which uses ascorbic acid as the reducing substance. Recently (Greger et al., 1977b) this method has been applied with the microcuvette (Figure 6) and validated for micropuncture samples. Materials for that method include: (a) 20 mmol/liter ammonium molybdate solution; (b) 8 N H_2SO_4; (c) 568 mmol/liter ascorbic acid; (d) Drummond 100-μl microcaps; (e) PE50 tubing. The procedure preferably is done with the perpendicular microchemistry setup. It involves (1) preparation of the reagent: 7 volumes bidistilled water are mixed with 1 volume of the above ammonium molybdate solution, 1 volume of the 8 N H_2SO_4, and 1 volume of the ascorbic acid. This reagent is stable for up to 6 hr. (2) Incubation capillaries are made from a 2-inch piece of a Drummond 100-μl cap in which a piece of PE tubing is inserted so that it protrudes a few millimeters at either end. (3) Approximately 1 μl of the reagent is pipeted into an incubation tube and 10-nl sample or standard are added (for a concentration range of 1–6 mmol/liter). Both fluids are mixed by slowly agitating the fluid column up and down in the capillary. (4) The capillary is sealed on either end using an oxygen-gas flame. (5) After an incubation of 90 min in a water bath of 37°C, the optical density reading is done using an ultramicrocuvette (Figure 6) at 820 nm in a spectrophotometer.

This method is sufficiently sensitive to measure phosphate in the 10^{-12} mol range. The error should be below 5%. It is not influenced by Lissamine green, inulin, or mannitol up to 1 mol/liter. Organic phosphorus compounds are usually not picked up with this method, and no nonphosphate chromagens exist in urine and plasma.

VII. GLUCOSE

Earlier methods for glucose determination made use of its reducing ability (Hagedorn and Jensen, 1923). A microdetermination based on that principle has been described by Brown and Boston (1961) and was modified by Baumann and Huang (1969). Since this reaction is not specific, recent ultramicromodifications are based on an enzymatic method as described by Barthelmai and Czok (1962) and by Schmidt (1961). The chemical reaction involves two enzymatic steps of which the latter is highly specific. In the first step, glucose is converted to glucose-6-phosphate in the presence of ATP by the enzyme hexokinase. In the second step glucose-6-phosphate is oxidized to 6-phosphogluconate and simultaneously the coenzyme NADP is reduced to NADPH by glucose-6-dehydrogenase. The amount of NADPH produced is measured photometrically.

The materials necessary for this method include: (*a*) 12 mmol/liter NADP; (*b*) 16.5 mmol/liter ATP; (*c*) 0.7 mol/liter $MgCl_2$; (*d*) glucose-6-dehydrogenase, 500 mg/liter; (*e*) triethanolamine–HCl buffer, 0.1 mol/liter, pH 7.6; (*f*) hexokinase, 1 g/liter. The substances necessary may be obtained in a reagent kit.

Procedure: (1) A comixture is made from solutions (*a*–*e*): 0.1 ml (*a*) + 0.1 ml (*b*) + 0.1 ml (*c*) + 0.1 ml (*d*) + 5.0 ml (*e*). This solution can be kept in the refrigerator for several days. (2) Before starting the analysis, 1 μl of solution (*f*) is added to this mixture. (3) The analysis can be done with either microchemistry setup. Pipets necessary are 1 μl for the reagent and 20–40 nl for the standard or sample. The mixture of sample/standard and reagent is transferred into incubation capillaries and the optical density is measured at 334 nm in the ultramicrocuvette illustrated in Figure 6 after a minimum incubation of 10 min.

The above method has been successfully applied in the 10^{-11} mol range (Rohde and Deetjen, 1968; Loeschke and Baumann, 1969; Loeschke *et al.*, 1969). The use of the above microcuvette increases sensitivity by a factor of 2–5

(Baeyer et al., 1973). The method is specific for glucose. However, if high concentrations of fructose are present in the sample, contamination of the enzymes with hexophosphate isomerase might produce additional amounts of glucose-6-phosphate (Rohde and Deetjen, 1968). The error introduced by this enzyme impurity is negligible since fructose concentrations are low compared with glucose concentrations. Furthermore, inulin is not hydrolyzed significantly under the above conditions and therefore it does not liberate fructose.

The same method has been used fluorometrically by Zwiebel et al. (1968). Using a microcuvette with a volume of 10 μl, the fluorescence of NADPH produced (exc. 350 nm/emission 450 nm) is sufficient to measure glucose in the nanogram range. The same authors described a modification of this reaction system (Zwiebel et al., 1968) in which the amount of NADPH produced by glucose (or fructose) is used in an enzymatic cycling system as originally described by Lowry et al., (1961). After an incubation of 30 min, 1 mol of NADPH will produce 5000 mol of 6-phosphogluconate. Finally, the amount of this compound is measured enzymatically by adding NADP and 6-phosphogluconate dehydrogenase. Using this system, less than 1 ng of glucose can be measured in a final volume of 0.25 ml. This method has been applied to micropuncture samples (Frohnert et al., 1970).

VIII. UREA

Two types of chemical reactions are used in the analysis of urea in micropuncture samples. The first has been described by Marsh et al. (1965). It utilizes the reaction of urea with diacetyl monoxime. The principle of the reaction has been described by Beale and Croft (1961). The reagents necessary for this method include: (a) 18 N H_2SO_4; (b) NaH_2PO_4; (c) $MnCl_2$, 2.0 mol/liter; (d) $NaHCO_3$; (e) $NaNO_3$, 0.05 mol/liter; (f) conc. HCl; (g) diacetyl monoxime (butanedione monoxime)=DAM, 0.1 mol in 1 liter of 3.5 mM acetic acid; (h) phenylanthranilic acid (PAA). Dissolve 0.45 mmol PAA in 60 ml of 20% ethanol (volume/volume), and add 12 mmol $NaHCO_3$. After dissolving, add sufficient 20% ethanol solution to make 100 ml. (i) Acid phosphate stock reagent: dissolve 1 mol NaH_2PO_4 in 125 ml distilled water, add 615 ml sulfuric acid, add 50 ml manganous chloride, and 20 ml HCl and dilute to 1000 ml after mixing. (j) Activated phosphate reagent: whereas all above reagents are stable, this reagent has to be made fresh. One milliliter of the sodium nitrate reagent is mixed with 125 ml of the acid phosphate reagent. (k) Before the analysis equal volumes of DAM solution and PAA solution are mixed.

Procedure: One nanoliter of sample or standard solution is mixed first with 100 nl of bidistilled water, 100 nl of the mixture DAM and PAA (k), and 1 μl of the activated phosphate reagent is added (j). The droplet is mixed in a reagent capillary. For the pipetting procedure, either of the two microchemistry setups may be used. The incubation capillary is sealed and exposed to a boiling water bath for 11 min. Thereafter the capillaries are cooled to room temperature in a water bath and protected from light until photometric readings are done in a microcuvette (Figure 6) at 535 nm.

This method has been tested for specificity in samples of proximal, loop, and collecting duct fluid (Marsh *et al.*, 1965) and has been used to analyze tubular fluid (Joppich and Deetjen, 1971; Armsen *et al.*, 1969; Ullrich *et al.*, 1967; Clapp, 1966).

A fluorometric method for urea has been developed by Roch-Ramel (1967). This method is highly specific and its sensitivity is high enough to allow even a semimicro final volume (1.0 ml) for a sample of only 1 nl. The principle of the reaction involves splitting urea by urease. The ammonia produced is used to produce NADP in the reaction system: ketoglutarate + H^+ + NH_4^+ + NADPH glutamate + H_2O + NADP. The reaction is catalyzed by glutamate dehydrogenase. The amount of NADP produced is stoichiometrically proportional to the amount of urea present. Whereas the usual urea methods measure the decrease in NADPH photometrically at 340 nm, in this method the amount of NADP produced is measured fluorometrically. A highly fluorescing compound is produced from NADP by either exposing it to sodium hydroxide or by condensation to methyl ethyl ketone. The reagents necessary include: (*a*) urease, (2500 Sumner units/g), 10 mg/ml Tris maleate buffer (see below); (*b*) ketoglutarate, 0.08 mol/liter; (*c*) glutamate dehydrogenase (free of ammonia); (*d*) NADPH preweighed in 1-mg vials; (*e*) Tris maleate, 0.2 mol/liter, pH 8.6; (*f*) substrate–enzyme–NADPH buffer solution prepared from the above reagents (to be mixed immediately before beginning the analysis): 3.5 ml of buffer (*e*) + 0.1 ml (*b*) + 0.075 ml of (*c*) + 0.02 ml of the urease solution (*a*); (*g*) methyl ethyl ketone; (*h*) 1.0 N NaOH; (*i*) 0.17 N HCl; (*j*) freshly prepared for the assay: 9 ml 8 N NaOH + 1 ml 30 mmol/liter H_2O_2 in aqueous solution.

Procedure: Common step: 2–20 nl of sample or standard are mixed with 5 μl solution (*f*). The mixture is kept at 20°C for 40 min. Thereafter fluorescence is obtained with the methyl ethyl ketone reagent: 5 μl of the above mixture are mixed with 5 μl of the methyl ethyl ketone reagent (*g*). 20 μl NaOH (*h*) are added. The fluids are mixed and incubated for 6 min at room temperature. Thereafter 200 μl HCl (*i*) are added and the mixture exposed to a boiling water bath for precisely 3 min. The fluorescence is read in a semimicrocuvette after diluting with 700 μl of bidistilled water (excitation: 340 nm, emission: 450 nm). The alternative method for obtaining a fluorescent compound is less sensitive but more reproducible: The sample reagent mixture (see above) is mixed with 5 μl of HCl (1 N). This step destroys remaining NADPH. This mixture is mixed with 100 μl of solution (*j*). The mixture is kept at 20°C for 1 hr. Thereafter 700 μl bidistilled water are added and fluorescence is measured as described above. Since endogenous NH_4^+ concentrations are small compared with endogenous urea concentrations, this reaction can be used as a single-step system for the usual samples (Roch-Ramel *et al.*, 1968, 1970). If, however, high concentrations of NH_4^+ are expected, the reaction may be separated in a determination before and after destruction of urea with urease and by this means the ammonia concentration will be measured first and in the second determination the sum of ammonia and urea will be determined. The two methods described here measure urea in the 10^{-11} mol range. The latter, however, can be scaled down further since the final volume is still in the milliliter range.

IX. INULIN

Although a variety of methods have been used to measure inulin in tubule fluid samples, only two of these methods are in common use. One is a colorimetric procedure in which inulin is hydrolyzed to fructose and reacts with anthrone to form a green-colored complex. The color intensity is measured photometrically (Fuehr et al., 1955; Hilger et al., 1958; Holzer et al., 1973). The other method is fluorometric. It was developed for use in micropuncture by Vurek and Pegram (1966), although the chemical procedure itself was first described by Adachi (1964). Again, inulin is hydrolyzed to fructose and fructose reacts with dimedone to form a fluorescing compound. As an alternative to the chemical determination of inulin, radioactively labeled inulin has been widely used.

The anthrone method for microsamples is basically the same procedure as the one described by Fuehr et al. (1955) for "macro" samples. Materials necessary include: (a) 36 N H_2SO_4; (b) anthrone; (c) anthrone solution: to 150 ml bidistilled water add 350 ml sulfuric acid slowly in a water bath; 5.1 mmol anthrone are dissolved in the diluted acid. The solution should be clear and have a bright yellow color. This solution is stable for 1 week when stored in a brown bottle in a refrigerator.

Procedure: A 2-nl sample or standard is mixed with 1 μl of the anthrone reagent in either of the microchemical setups. The mixture is transferred into an incubation capillary which is sealed on either end. After an incubation period of 10 min in a 56°C water bath, the optical density is measured in the microcuvette (Figure 6) at 620 nm. Although this method, as the one described below, is not specific for inulin, interference with other carbohydrates, mainly glucose, is not a serious problem. The relative specificity is determined by the temperature and duration of the incubation (Nagel et al., 1967).

For the fluorometric method, the following reagents are necessary: (a) dimedone, 5.5 dimethyl-1.3-cyclohexanedione; (b) phosphoric acid (85%); (c) dimedone reagent: 0.7 mmol dimedone is dissolved in 10 ml of phosphoric acid. This reagent is stable for 12 hr.

Procedure: 5–15 nl of sample are mixed with 8 μl of dimedone reagent in precleaned capillaries. The capillaries are sealed on both ends and exposed to a boiling-water bath for about 15 min. Then they are cooled to room temperature in another water bath. Measurements are done fluorometrically (excitation 360 nm and emission 400 nm). An adapter like the one described in Figure 7 may be used with any spectrofluorometer. The sensitivity of the method is limited by the fluorescence of the blank, which depends critically on the cleanliness of the incubation capillaries. In our laboratory the following cleaning procedure has become standard. First, the capillaries are boiled 4 times with a detergent for 10 min. Second, the capillaries are boiled 6 times with quartz-distilled water. Third, the capillaries are dried in an oven and thereafter stored in closed tubes to prevent any contamination with dust. Another problem inherent to this method, and one caused by the hygroscopy of the dimedone reagent, has been discussed extensively by Conger et al. (1975). If capillaries containing dimedone reagent are prepared in advance, they must be stored in a dish containing a desiccant to prevent water uptake by the reagent.

Both of these methods are satisfactory for the routine measurement of inulin with an error of less than 5% in samples smaller than 10 ml. For even smaller amounts of inulin, the method described by Zwiebel et al. (1968) may be used.

X. p-AMINOHIPPURATE (PAH)

For the colorimetric measurement of PAH, the method of Bratton and Marshall (1939) has been used. Deetjen and Sonnenberg (1965) have adapted this method to micropuncture samples. The materials necessary include: (a) 0.1 N HCl; (b) 0.01 mol/liter sodium nitrite, $NaNO_2$ (prepared daily); (c) ammonium sulfamate ($NH_2-SO_3-NH_4$), 0.044 mol/liter (stable for 2 weeks when stored at 4°C in a dark bottle); (d) N-(1-naphthyl)-ethylenediamine HCl, 4.0 mmol/liter; (e) the mixture of 9 aliquots of hydrochloric acid and 1 aliquot of sodium nitrite must be made immediately prior to the analysis.

Procedure: Either microchemistry setup might be used. (1) A sample volume to contain approximately 10^{-12} to 10^{-11} mol PAH, i.e., 5 nl for a concentration of 1 mmol/liter, is mixed with 1 μl of solution (e) (2) One hundred nanoliters of solution (c) are added with thorough mixing. (3) One hundred nanoliters of solution (d) are added. The contents of the incubation capillary are mixed once again and the capillary is sealed. After an incubation of 30 min at room temperature, the optical density is measured in the cuvette (Figure 6) at 546 nm. The color should stay stable for at least 1 hr.

The error of the above method should not exceed 5%. A slightly modified version has been successfully applied to micropuncture samples of vasa recta blood (Schnermann and Thurau, 1965). The reaction of Bratton and Marshall is not specific for PAH but will also measure sulfonamides and related p-amino compounds.

Systemic infusion of ^{3}H-labeled PAH has been used in micropuncture studies (Cortney et al., 1965; Haeberle, 1975).

XI. URIC ACID

The endogenous urate concentration in plasma is relatively low, i.e., approximately 250 μmol/liter in man and lower (10–100 μmol/liter) in other mammals with the enzyme uricase. As a result of these low concentrations, relatively large volumes (approx. 50 nl or more) are necessary for the chemical analysis of urate in tubule fluid. Alternatively, plasma urate concentration may be increased by systemic infusion of urate.

Three different methods have been used to analyze tubule fluid for urate: (*a*) a colorimetric method utilizing essentially Folin's method (Folin and Denis, 1912–1913; Caraway, 1955), which is based on the reduction of phosphotungstic acid to a blue color by urate, (*b*) a fluorometric method which is based on the reaction first described by Bloch and Lata (1970) in which urate delays the oxidation of scopoletin by peroxide (catalyzed by horseradish peroxidase), and (*c*) radioactive methods with infusion of [^{14}C]urate. Since most animals possess a high activity of hepatic uricase (Lang *et al.*, 1974), this activity must be blocked prior to the tracer infusion either by hepatectomy or by administering oxonate (Greger, 1976). Alternatively, large amounts of tracer may be infused constantly and the samples then analyzed for [^{14}C]urate by chromatographic separation (Abramson and Levitt, 1975; Friedman and Merril, 1973; Lang *et al.*, 1974).

For the colorimetric procedure, the following materials are necessary: (*a*) sodium tungstate (Na_2WO_4); (*b*) 85% phosphoric acid; (*c*) boric acid, 0.4 mol/ liter; (*d*) 0.4 *N* NaOH. (*e*) Phosphotungstic acid is prepared from sodium tungstate and phosphoric acid by dissolving 0.3 mol of sodium tungstate in 800 ml of bidistilled water and adding 80 ml phosphoric acid. The mixture is kept in a boiling water bath for 2 hr. After cooling, the volume is filled up to 1 liter with bidistilled water. This reagent has a yellowish color. It must be stored in a dark bottle and will be stable for at least 1 month. (*f*) Buffer is prepared from boric acid and sodium hydroxide. Fifty milliliters of the boric acid solution are mixed with approximately 44 ml of sodium hydroxide solution. The chemicals used for this buffer solution must be free of potassium chloride. The buffer is stable.

Procedure: (1) For each sample a new reagent has to be prepared by mixing 16 volumes of buffer (*f*) with 1 volume of phosphotungstic acid (*e*). The dispenser must be made of glass or plastic since no metal parts should come into contact with the reagent. (2) One microliter of this alkaline reagent is immediately mixed with 30–50 nl of tubule fluid or standard. The perpendicular microchemistry setup is adequate for this procedure. The incubation capillary is sealed and stored at room temperature. After 20 min but not later than 60 min, optical density is read at 755 nm using a microcuvette (Figure 6). This method is sensitive enough to measure as little as $5 \cdot 10^{-12}$ mol of urate with an error of less than 10% (Greger *et al.*, 1971). However, several critical points must be considered: (1) The time between preparation of the alkaline reagent and the mixing of sample and reagent must be as short as possible (2 min) and the time must be identical for all samples and standards. (2) The pH of the alkaline reagent should be between 8.7 and 8.9. If the dispenser delivers a volume ratio slightly different from 16:1, one of the solutions has to be diluted so that the mixture meets the pH optimum. (3) As already pointed out above, the reagent must not have contact with any metal. (4) The reaction is not strictly specific for urate: in highly concentrated antidiuretic urine, the reading may be high due to the presence of unidentified reducing compounds (Roch-Ramel *et al.*, 1976a; Greger, 1976). However, the values for plasma and nonantidiuretic urine are comparable to the values obtained by a uricase method.

The reagents necessary for the fluorometric method (Roch-Ramel and Weiner, 1973) include: (*a*) scopoletin, 0.13 mmol/liter; (*b*) H_2O_2 solution, 8.82

mmol/liter; (c) phosphate buffer, pH 7.0, 0.1 mol/liter; (d) horseradish peroxidase, 0.25 mg/ml–1 mg/ml, made half hourly and kept on ice; (e) diluted scopoletin: 1 vol. scopoletin stock solution (a) + 150 vol. buffer (c), made daily, kept on ice; (f) diluted peroxide: 1 vol. 8.82 mmol/liter H_2O_2 (b) + 50 vol. buffer (c).

Procedure: Immediately prior to the analysis equal volumes of solution (e) and (f) are mixed. (1) Four microliters of this mixture are transferred into a capillary (150 μl). (2) Using the perpendicular setup, 20–80 nl of sample are added. The fluids are mixed, the capillary sealed at one end, and the fluorescence is set at 100% at excitation 348 nm and emission 465 nm using the cuvette holder (Figure 7). (3) Five hundred nanoliters peroxidase solution are added, the solutions are immediately mixed and fluorescence recorded. The time lag until decrease in fluorescence starts is proportional to the amount of urate present in the sample (Bloch and Lata, 1970).

This method has been successfully applied to micropuncture samples in a variety of species (Roch-Ramel et al., 1976b; Roch-Ramel and Weiner, 1973, 1975; and Roch-Ramel et al., 1976c). Critical points about this method are that (1) it is not strictly specific for urate (Bloch and Lata, 1970). (2) In urines of nonfasted Cebus monkeys, some unknown substances may produce low readings (Roch-Ramel and Weiner, 1973). It is essential to work fast and reproducibly in step (c). (3) The glass capillaries must be precleaned (Roch-Ramel and Weiner, 1973). (4) The fluorescence time curves must be extrapolated to obtain the lag time.

The use of radioactively labeled uric acid necessitates chromatographic separation of allantoin and urate in the different fluids. A thin-layer chromatographic procedure has been described by Lang et al. (1974). Using this method, micropuncture data on urate transport have been recently reported (Greger et al., 1977a,b).

XII. AMINO ACIDS

The usual column chromatography of amino acids with the detection of the ninhydrin derivatives is much too insensitive for samples of tubule fluid. A different approach has been developed by Neuhoff et al. (1969) and Briel and Neuhoff (1973) and applied to micropuncture samples by Eisenbach et al. (1975). In this method the sample is mixed with radioactively labeled dansyl chloride. The dansylated amino acids now carrying a ^{14}C label are separated by two-dimensional thin-layer chromatography. The single spots are identified under ultraviolet light, punched out, and transferred into counting vials. The counts are now directly proportional to the amino acid concentration. The following amino acids have been measured (Eisenbach et al., 1975) using this approach in the 10^{-11} to 10^{-10} mol range: alanine (Ala), glycine (Gly), leucine (Leu), lysine (Lys), isoleucine (Il), tyrosine (Tyr), glutamate (Glu), phenylalanine (Phe), proline (Pro), taurine (Tau).

Not all amino acids have defined spots in the chromatogram and some therefore cannot be measured satisfactorily with this method. One further disadvantage of this method is that the approximate amount of amino acid present in the sample has to be known in order to choose the amount of dansyl chloride that is necessary for complete amino acid dansylation (Briel and Neuhoff, 1973). The relatively low sensitivity of 10^{-10} to 10^{-11} mol is caused by the specific radioactivity of the commercially available dansyl chloride.

Instead of using ninhydrin, amino acids can be identified by *o*-phthalaldehyde (Roth, 1971; Roth and Hampai, 1973; Benson and Hare, 1975) which produces highly fluorescing compounds. A column chromatographic separation procedure followed by the above fluorescence detection has been described by Roth (1971); Roth and Hampai (1973); and Benson and Hare (1975). An ultramicro version of this method is currently being developed by Silbernagl[1] and Bayliss (personal communication). The principle of this method is described in Figure 11(A). The sample is sucked into the system through a valve (8). Buffer A is delivered at a flow rate of 0.5 ml/hr by pump (1). The stream is either directed into the main circulation or to any one of the cylinders (2, 3, 4) which are filled with buffers B and C and with NaOH. The direction of the stream is determined by a five-way valve (6) which is connected to a programmable timer (7). The respective buffer solution drags the sample through the resin-filled coil (5). This coil (length 0.7 m, inside diameter 0.7 mm) is thermostatically maintained at 45°C. The eluate meets the *o*-phthalaldehyde reagent which is delivered at 0.5 ml/hr by pump (9). Within a few seconds the fluorescing compounds are generated. Fluorescence (excitation 340 nm, emission 455 nm) is constantly recorded by an on-line fluorometer equipped with a flow-through cell. The outflow is fractionally collected by an automatic sample changer (12) for further analysis of the fluid (e.g., scintillation counting, if there are labeled compounds in the sample).

The column chromatograph, including the fluorometer, is commercially available. The reagents necessary include: (*a*) resin, Durrum DC6A; (*b*) buffers A, B, C; (*c*) *o*-phthalaldehyde; (*d*) 0.2 *N* NaOH; (*e*) borate buffer: boric acid, 1.0 mol/liter, KOH 0.5 mol/liter; (*f*) mercaptoethanol; (*g*) ethanol; (*h*) *o*-phthalaldehyde reagent: 0.15 mmol *o*-phthalaldehyde is dissolved in 1 ml mercaptoethanol, 5 ml ethanol, and 94 ml borate buffer are added. The pH is checked and if necessary adjusted to 10.4 by additional KOH. This solution must be prepared weekly.

Procedure: (1) All solutions (*b*, *d*, *g*) must be filtered through a Millipore filter to prevent contamination. (2) The chromatograph is loaded with the above solutions. (3) The resin is regenerated using buffer "A" and the system is equilibrated for approximately 4 hr. (4) The diluted sample (some 10–100 µl) is now sucked into the main stream. The sample volume necessary for this method depends on the amino acid under study. Five nanoliters of a proximal "free-flow" micropuncture sample would be sufficient for Gly or Ala but 50–100 nl are necessary for aspartate (Asp); it mainly depends on the plasma concentration of the respective amino acid. (5) Buffer "A" will wash out over the next 4–5 hr the following amino acids [Figure 11(B)]: cysteic acid, taurine, aspartic acid, threonine, serine, homoserine, glutamic acid, citrulline, glycine, alanine, and valine.

---

[1] The authors are indebted to Dr. S. Silbernagl who helped with this section.

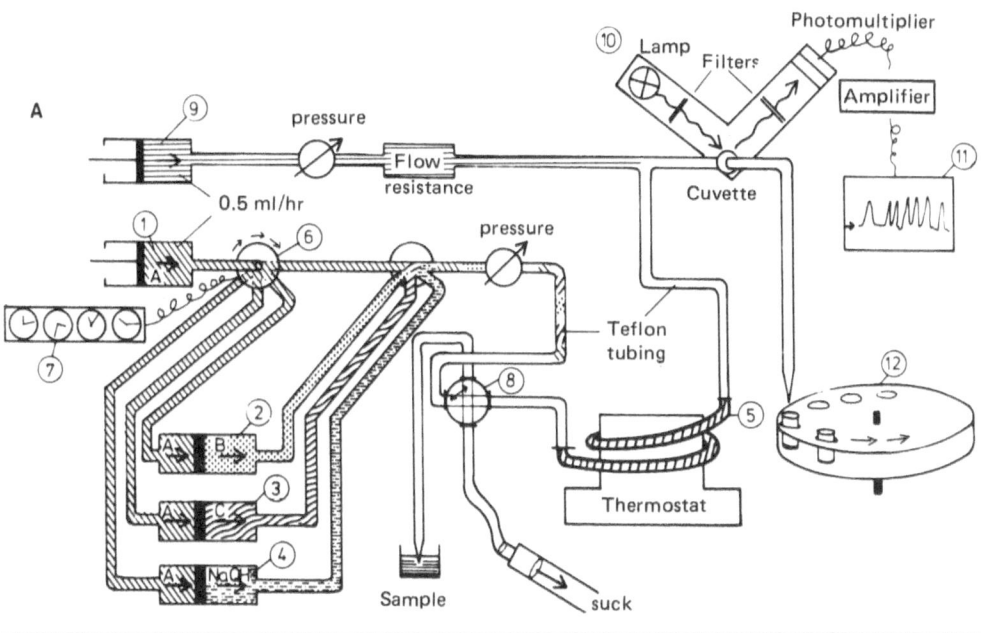

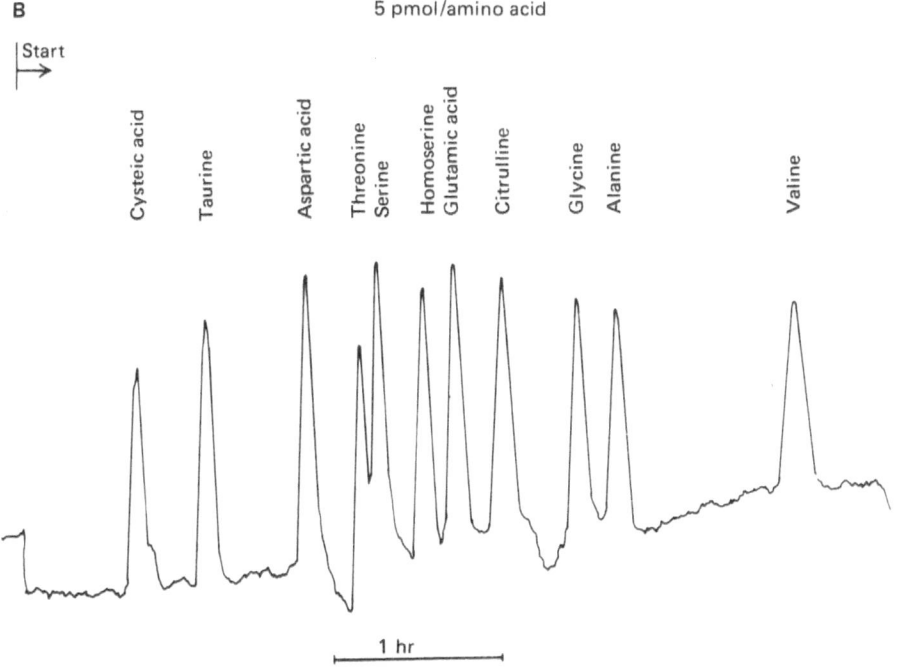

Figure 11(A). Scheme of an ultramicro column chromatograph for detection of amino acids in picomole quantities. (1) Pump for buffer "A." (2) Cylinder filled with buffer "B." (3) Cylinder filled with buffer "C." (4) Cylinder filled with NaOH. (5) Resin coil. (6) Five-way valve. (7) Timer. (8) Sample valve. (9) Pump for o-phthalaldehyde reagent. (10) On-line fluorometer. (11) One-axis recorder. (12) Automatic sample changer for fractional collection of outflow. (B) Ultramicro column chromatography of amino acids: Typical outflow pattern using buffer "A."

(6) After regeneration with NaOH for 1 hr and equilibration with buffer "B" for 4 hr, a new dilution of the same sample is injected. Buffer "B" will wash out methionine, isoleucine, and leucine. (7) Regeneration with NaOH for 1 hr and equilibration with buffer "C" for 4 hr. The third fraction of the sample is injected. Buffer "C" eluates tyrosine, phenylalanine, histidine, lysine, and arginine.

The sensitivity of this method is 0.5×10^{-12} mol and the error below 10%. Several critical points, however, have to be considered: (1) Not all amino acids can be measured by this method: e.g., proline (it first has to be oxidized by sodium hypochlorite), cysteine, ornithine. (2) At present, best results are obtained for the amino acids which are eluated by buffer "A" since with this buffer the noise at the fluorometer readout is minimal. (3) Free-flow micropuncture samples contain different amino acids in concentrations which are different by orders of magnitude. This must be considered for adjustment of sample size and amplification.

XIII. PROTEIN

Microanalytical methods for protein have been applied to micropuncture samples of tubule fluid (Walker *et al.*, 1941; Liew *et al.*, 1970; Dirks *et al.*, 1964) and plasma from vasa recta (Ullrich *et al.*, 1961) and peritubular capillaries (Brenner *et al.*, 1969; Knox *et al.*, 1972). A semiquantitative precipitation method was first described by Walker *et al.* (1941). Recently, the colorimetric determination by Lowry *et al.* (1951) was modified for micropuncture samples (Chou and Goldstein, 1969). Alternatively, the biuret reaction was used (Ullrich *et al.*, 1961). Since the protein concentration in tubule fluid is lower by at least two orders of magnitude, the reagent sample volume ratios have to be adjusted for plasma as compared to tubule fluid samples. Methods for both will be given below.

The materials necessary include: (*a*) sodium tartrate ($Na_2C_4H_4O_6$), 0.087 mol/liter; (*b*) copper sulfate ($CuSO_4$), 0.063 mol/liter; (*c*) sodium carbonate (Na_2CO_3), 0.19 mol/liter, 0.1 *N* NaOH. All three stock solutions are stable. (*d*) Reagent I: 0.1 ml of (*a*) + 0.1 ml of (*b*) + 9.8 ml of (*c*), mixed on the day of analysis. (*e*) Reagent II: 1 *N* phenol reagent (Folin Ciocalteau).

Procedure for the tubule fluid: Either microchemistry setup may be used. (1) Fifty to 100 nl of tubule fluid are mixed with 1 μl of reagent I. The incubation capillary is kept in a moist chamber for precisely 8 min. (2) After this interval, 100 nl of reagent II are added and both fluids mixed instantaneously. (3) The optical density at 750 nm is read after 30 min in a microcuvette (Figure 6).

Procedure for plasma samples: (1) The micropuncture pipet (tip inside diameter 15 μm, siliconized but not heparinized) is filled with the blood sample and sealed on both ends. To prevent the sample from being heat destroyed, oil is sucked into the tip first. Sample capillaries are centrifuged and broken close to the supernatant. (2) One nanoliter sample is mixed with 3 μl reagent I. (3) After an incubation of 8 min in a moist chamber, 0.3 liter of reagent II is added and both fluids mixed instantaneously. (4) Readings of optical density are obtained as mentioned above.

The above method has the advantage of being more sensitive compared with the biuret method (Ullrich *et al.*, 1961). It is, however, less specific: (1) polypeptides other than proteins, tryptophan, tyrosine, and cysteine can enhance the reading (Liew *et al.*, 1970); (2) Lissamine green interferes with the color reading (Brenner *et al.*, 1969); and (3) heparin interferes with the method (Knox *et al.*, 1972).

XIV. OSMOTIC PRESSURE

Osmotic pressure is measured in nanoliter or picoliter volume samples using the microcryometric method of Ramsay (1949). The sample contained in the tip of a micropipet is frozen and then observed through a microscope immersed in a temperature-controlled bath. The temperature of the bath is slowly raised and the temperature at which the last ice crystal melts is recorded using a mercury thermometer with a 1/100°C sensitivity. The osmotic pressure is calculated from the melting point. The mercury thermometer can be replaced by a quartz thermometer which is more accurate and sensitive and whose display can be stopped at will, allowing for more precise readings.

XV. ELECTRON PROBE ANALYSIS

Electron probe microanalysis is an X-ray spectrometric method. The principle of the method is as follows: The atoms contained in a sample are excited by high energy radiation from an electron beam. During the bombardment, two kinds of X-rays are emitted, a continuum emission due to the deceleration of electrons in the sample and a characteristic X-ray emission. Above the continuum emission, the characteristic X-rays are caused by the ionization of the inner shells (K, L, M) of electrons of the atoms constituting the sample. They are at very well-defined wavelengths. By measuring the wavelength of the characteristic lines, elements contained in the sample are recognized. By measuring the intensity of the characteristic line (subtracting the intensity of the continuum at the wavelength of the characteristic line, from the total intensity), the amount of element contained in the sample is quantitated. Several references to the general and biological applications and principles of the electron probe are available (Goldstein and Yakowitz, 1975; Coleman and Terepka, 1974; Chandler, 1975; Birks, 1963; Beaman and Isasi, 1971; Lechene and Warner, 1977; Castaing, 1951).

This method of elemental analysis has unique features which make it one of the most powerful analytical tools available. Practically any element of the periodic table above the low atomic number of carbon (6) can be analyzed. The characteristic X-ray lines are well separated, i.e., there is no interference from one element to another, and therefore an element can be recognized and quantitated whether isolated or mixed in the sample with any combination of other elements. The method is nondestructive so that the same sample can be reanalyzed and all the constituting elements can be measured. The amount of material needed for the analysis is extremely small: volumes of the order of a few femtoliters (1×10^{-15} liter) are currently analyzed in some kinds of samples. The absolute sensitivity of the method is enormous; 1×10^{-16} g of any element is easily quantifiable and, in special conditions, 10^{-18} g has been measured (Shuman and Somlyo, 1976).

The relative sensitivity, of minimum concentration measurable, is of the order of 100 ppm; electron probe microanalysis is not the method of choice compared with absorption spectrophotometry to detect trace elements in samples with large volumes.

X-ray spectrometry by electron beam excitation is the method of choice for unambiguous quantitative analysis of any number of elements in extremely small samples. The elements Na, Mg, K, Ca, P, S, and Cl can be routinely analyzed in 20–60 pl samples of tubule fluid.

Electron probe microanalysis can analyze several kinds of biological samples: liquid droplets of the order of 10–100 pl (1 picoliter = 1×10^{-12} liter = 1×10^3 μm^3); isolated cells of the order of 100 fl (1 femtoliter = 1×10^{-15} liter = 1 μm^3); biological tissues where the volumes excited are of the order of the femtoliter to the attoliter (1 al = 1×10^{-18} liter = 1000 $\mathring{A}^3$). The remainder of this chapter will describe electron probe microanalysis of liquid droplets. Analysis of liquid droplets is a well-established method for electron probe analysis of picoliter volumes of biological samples. It was initiated independently by Ingram and Hogben (1967) and Morel et al. (1969). The preparation of liquid samples for routine electron probe analysis was developed by Lechene (1970, 1974).

A. Choice of the Instrument

In choosing the instrument, several things must be kept in mind. An optical microscope incorporated in the column, allowing one to view the beam and center and focus the droplets under the electron beam, is of invaluable help. Wavelength dispersive spectrometers (WDS) are the spectrometers of choice. Compared to WDS, energy dispersive spectrometers (EDS) have very poor X-ray resolution and high background collection; spurious signals are detected and the stripping of the background is a complex and still uncertain procedure. The consequences are that P/B ratio is at least one order of magnitude smaller and the minimum concentrations detectable are much higher when using EDS than when using WDS for liquid droplets. Although all elements are detected simultaneously, there is no reduction in counting time because it takes approximately 10 times longer to count each sample with an EDS than with a WDS system. In the present state of the art, roughly the same precision is obtained but fewer elements are quantifiable. For example, a concentration of 2 mM/liter of Mg, Ca, S, and P in biological fluids that is easily measurable with a WDS system could be practically nondetectable with an EDS system.

The samples are excited with a stationary beam, enlarged to cover and excite the entire sample spot. Analysis with a focused beam and scanning over the sample will result in an increase in background of at least 27% due to scan of areas outside of the circular drop. Though the manipulation of the instrument and subsequent calculations can be performed manually, there are marked advantages in automation of both steps to increase the efficiency of the technique.

Picoliter volumes of liquid samples are deposited on a support under oil. After placement of all the samples, the oil is washed off by an organic solvent. The preparation is freeze-dried so that the salt content of each droplet forms a dried spot on the support. Hundreds of samples can be placed on the same support to be analyzed in the electron probe. During the analysis, each dried spot is placed successively under the electron beam and the characteristic X-ray intensity of the elements of interest is measured. Standards of known composition are prepared and measured under the same conditions and concentrations in the unknowns are calculated. The aim of the preparation is to obtain circular dried spots of identical diameter from the liquid droplets. Further, the salt crystals should be homogeneously spread within each spot and the salt crystals should not be larger than 2 μm.

The different steps of the preparation and analysis are as follows. Picoliter volume micropipets are made with a de Fonbrune microforge similar to the method for nanoliter constriction micropipets (Lechene et al., 1969). The micropipets (see page 110) are calibrated by using tritiated water. Separated by oil, 20–40 droplets of liquid without organic components could be loaded in a good micropipet which is siliconized.

The liquid droplets are deposited on a support covered by a layer of filtered paraffin oil. The support should assure good thermal and electrical conductivity. It should have surface properties such that the droplets do not spread and stick on the surface so that they are not washed off with the oil. The support should contribute minimally to the background, i.e., be very thin and/or have a low atomic number. Vitreous carbon etched in an oxygen plasma or a collodion film can be used in some circumstances. Silicon disks have the disadvantage of contributing to relatively high background. The best support is a block of beryllium with a highly polished face. The blocks can be reused for long periods if they are cleaned. The beryllium blocks are cleaned by polishing (autopolish Buchler) with a polishing cloth and 3-μm diamond paste for 6 min at low speed and using lapping oil. After polishing, the block is washed 3 times in trichloroethylene, absolute alcohol, and acetone, using high power ultrasonication in each bath. Blocks are dried with compressed CO_2. Due to the toxicity of beryllium, polishing and cleaning are done under a hood, wearing a mask and gloves. No other precautions are required for any other manipulation of the beryllium except to treat the beryllium wash like radioactive waste. Placement of liquid droplets on the beryllium block is done as follows. Three or four drops of saturated light paraffin oil are filtered onto the block through Millipore filters. A calibrated pipet, to contain multiple samples of approximately 50 pl each, is used for the transfer. Oil is first pulled into the pipet to slow down the uptake of the sample to facilitate accurate sample filling. The tip is then inserted into the drop of standard. It is important to have as little contact between the pipet and the drop as possible so that the pipet does not become sticky and the subsequent drops adhere to the pipet rather than to the beryllium block. The standard solution is then drawn into the pipet, the pipet is pulled out of the standard solution drop and placed into the oil, and a small amount of oil is drawn up behind the standard aliquot. This procedure is repeated for the samples with the pipet remaining under oil for the entire procedure. A good pipet should be able to pick up approximately 30 samples and standards. When placing drops on the block, it is often better to have the pipet tilted at a somewhat greater angle than was necessary for picking up the drops [Figure 12(A)]. With the tip of the pipet resting lightly on the surface of the block, gentle pressure is applied to the syringe to force the first drop onto the block. The pipet is then withdrawn from the drop with great care to avoid smearing it. Drops are deposited in rows such that approximately 100 drops are placed in each 2-mm square surface of block [Figure 12(B)].

During long preparation, droplets can slowly concentrate, although under oil, with ensuing formation of large salt crystals unfit for analysis. Concentration under oil can be avoided or slowed by using freshly saturated oil, cooling the beryllium droplet preparation in a refrigerator during successive loadings of the volumetric pipet, and exposing the preparation in a water-saturated atmosphere when the droplets are deposited on the support.

Once all the samples have been deposited on the beryllium block, the oil covering the drops must be washed off without disturbing the samples. This is accomplished by washing the block in spectrograde *m*-xylene. In order to wash with *m*-xylene (Eastman Spectrograde), the block must be placed in a large glass petri dish. The *m*-xylene is held in a 30-ml glass syringe with a swinny adapter. The adapter holds a Millipore filter. An 18-gauge needle is attached to the adapter with a small piece of polyethylene tubing over the end of the needle. The tubing acts as a cushion and can be rested on the edge of the block as the *m*-xylene is squirted over the surface of the block. A steady, even flow of the *m*-xylene should be maintained and it should be directed first to one side of the block and then to the other; this makes the mixture of oil and *m*-xylene swirl both clockwise and counterclockwise. When the swirling is no longer apparent, and the surface appears to undulate in wavelets, the oil is gone. This washing procedure must proceed very quickly (no more than 30 sec) in order to avoid evaporation. As soon as the oil appears to be gone, the block must be shock frozen. Immediately after washing, the preparation is shock-frozen by dipping in a quenching medium. Isopentane (m.p. = 160°C, b.p. = 28°C) cooled at −160°C in liquid nitrogen is convenient. Using the long forceps again, the block is removed from the isopentane and placed in the precooled freeze-drier, always with the sample side facing up. The faster the freezing rate, the smaller will be the ice and salt crystals.

Freeze-drying should be done at approximately −70°C since at warm temperatures recrystallization with large crystal growth could become a significant problem. A vacuum of 10^{-5} mm Hg is utilized (the ice vapor pressure at −70°C is 2×10^{-3} mm Hg) to avoid contaminating the preparation with oil vapor from the vacuum system (mechanical pump, diffusion pump) acting as a cold trap. A liquid nitrogen baffle may be necessary.

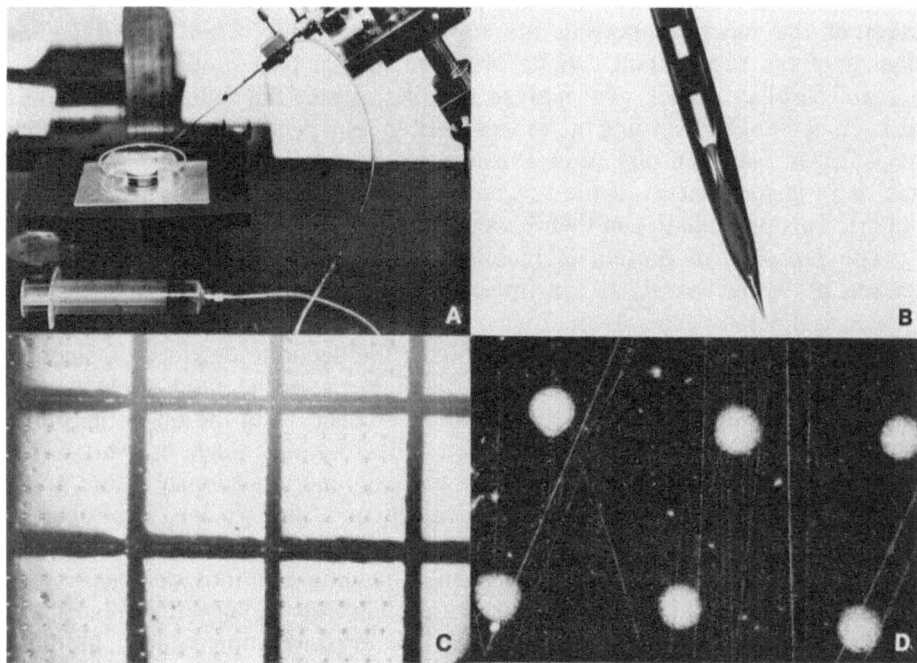

Figure 12. Electron probe microanalysis, (A) Pipetting samples on the beryllium block showing angle of pipet. (B) Magnification of the pipet. (C) Low-power view of liquid droplet samples on the block. (D) High-power view of dried samples.

Lyophilization usually takes several hours. However, after a few minutes under vacuum the frozen isopentane and xylene have disappeared and it is very likely that by this time the liquid droplets are dried.

The preparation is warmed above room temperature under vacuum to avoid trapping moisture when returned to ambient air. The preparation can be immediately analyzed and/or kept for months under vacuum.

The analytical conditions are chosen to maximize the peak over background ratios (P/B) while keeping the counting time within practical limits and avoiding loss of the sample by too intense radiation. For X-ray analysis of the usual biological elements in liquid droplets, accelerating voltage of 11 kV to 15 kV and an electron beam density of 0.4 nA/μm^2 (or 100 nA for an electron beam of 80 μm in diameter) provide the best P/B and no measurable mass loss, as ascertained by the absence of any decrease in count rate for any elements during the counting period.

X-ray analysis measures the total elemental content in the sample independent of the chemical state. To recognize between bound and ionized forms for a given element, precipitation methods described in analytical chemistry have been adapted to picoliter liquid droplets (Bonventre and Lechene, 1974). Liquid droplets of the samples are deposited under oil on the surface of a beryllium block or a vitreous carbon disk and droplets of precipitating reagent are added to the sample droplets. The precipitations are sedimented by centrifugation of the block supporting the samples under oil. After centrifugation, aliquots of the supernatant can be prepared for electron probe analysis on a separate beryllium block. To analyze the precipitate, the following procedure has been devised for washing the reagent. After centrifugation, the preparation is shock frozen and then dipped in absolute alcohol cooled to −70°C. In a short time there is sublimation of the reagent and a clean precipitate remains on the support. This precipitate can then be analyzed by electron probe analysis.

The presence of protein in picoliter fluid samples (plasma) analyzed by electron probe microanalysis can interfere with quantitative elemental analysis of these samples. In general, an organic matrix in the sample can provide several sources of artifacts. First, the protein makes the accurate delivery of picoliter aliquots with a picoliter pipet more difficult because the fluid sticks to the siliconized glass and lipoproteins will tend to emulsify with the oil in the pipet. This difficulty can be largely overcome by delivering only single droplets of the fluid onto the beryllium support and washing and resiliconizing the pipet between each droplet. Second, high concentrations of protein can cause absorption of weak X-ray emissions within the sample and thereby artificially lower the intensity of X-ray emissions from protein-containing solutions compared with emissions from standard solutions that are protein free. Finally, the presence of any amount of organic matrix may alter the crystallization pattern in these samples compared with the pattern in standard solutions. Samples can be ultrafiltered by microultrafiltration methods using a cuprophane membrane (Morel *et al.*, 1969) or one hollow fiber (Lechene, unpublished methods).

While quantitative electron probe analysis of deproteinated solutions is preferable to the analysis of protein-containing solutions, recent work has indicated that the latter solutions can be quantitatively analyzed. Originally, increasing amounts of crystalline bovine serum albumin (0.010–0.070 g/ml) were added to a stock solution of known elemental composition. Bovine serum albumin contains low concentrations of most of the elements but relatively high levels of Cl and S. The results of these experiments indicate that relatively accurate electron probe microanalyses of Na, Cl, K, Ca, Mg, S, and P can be obtained in the presence of concentrations of bovine serum albumin less than 0.050 g/ml. These results are consistent with analyses of mouse serum that have shown that ½ and ⅓ dilutions of the nondeproteinated samples are easier to pipet and give more accurate and reproducible results that are comparable to macroanalysis of the same samples (Borland *et al.*, unpublished data).

B. Minimum Detectable Levels and Precision of Electron Probe Analysis

The standard deviation (S.D.) of the total number of X-rays (T) counted during a given time is

$$S.D. = (T)^{1/2}$$

For example, 95% of the measurements of a given X-ray emission will fall within

2 S.D. of the mean value of the measurements, provided that the analytical conditions do not vary. The precision of measurement (S.D.%) is the value of S.D. expressed per 100 counts

$$\text{S.D.\%} = \frac{\text{S.D.}}{T} \times 100 = \frac{100}{(T)^{1/2}} \tag{1}$$

The concentration of polyvalent ions in tubular fluid is often low and therefore T is close to the background (B). The net number of counts (P) is $P = T - B$. The error or standard deviation of P is

$$\text{S.D.}_P = [(\text{S.D.}_T)^2 + (\text{S.D.}_B)^2]^{1/2} = (T + B)^{1/2}$$

The precision of the measurement is, similar to Eq. (1),

$$\text{S.D.}_P\% = \frac{(T + B)^{1/2}}{T - B} \times 100 \tag{2}$$

The minimum detectable concentration (MC) is defined in terms of 3 S.D. of the mean background value $(\bar{B})$ at the wavelength of the characteristic X-ray line. Indeed, 99.7% of all background counts will fall within ± 3 S.D. of $\bar{B}$. Therefore, any counts above

$$B + 3(\bar{B})^{1/2}$$

will represent true characteristic X-ray intensity counts. It follows that if C_s is a standard concentration of a characteristic X-ray line giving N_s counts, the concentration per counts will be C_s/N_s and the minimum detectable:

$$\text{MC} = 3(\bar{B})^{1/2} \times (C_s/N_s)$$

The precision is given by Eq. (2), where $T = B + 3(\bar{B})^{1/2}$.

Example: (1) In a given analytical condition, a 50-pl droplet of a solution containing 50 mM/liter of Mg gives Mg = 3500 counts/10 sec and $\bar{B}$ = 37 counts/10 sec.

Minimum detectable concentration = $3 \times (37)^{1/2} \times (50/3500)$ = 0.26 mM. Precision of the measurement of the minimum detectable concentration = $(37 + 55)^{1/2}/18$ = 53%. The minimum detectable will be 0.26 ± 0.14. (2) Increasing the counting time from 10 to 300 sec, Mg = 105,000 counts/300 sec and Bg = 1100 counts/300 sec. Minimum detectable concentration = $3 \times (1100)^{1/2} \times (50/10,500)$ = 0.05 mM/liter.

Precision of the measurement of the minimum detectable concentration = $(110 + 1210)^{1/2}/100$ = 48%. (3) Increasing the counting time to 20 min, Mg = 420,000 counts, Bg = 4440, and minimum detectable concentration = 0.02 mM/liter.

Precision of the measurement of the minimum detectable concentration = 47.7%. The minimum detectable concentration is decreased when the number of counts measured is increased (by increasing either the counting time or the beam current).

REFERENCES

Abramson, R. G., and Levitt, M. F. 1975. Micropuncture study of uric acid transport in rat kidney. *Am. J. Physiol., 228:*1597.

Adachi, S. 1964. Use of dimedon for the detection of keto sugars by paper chromatography. *Anal. Biochem., 9:*224.

Armsen, R., Schad, H., and Reinhardt, H. W. 1969. Die Harnkonzentrierung in der Niere. *Pflügers Arch., 313:*222.

Baeyer, H. von, Conta, C. von, Haeberle, D., and Deetjen, P. 1973. Determination of transport constants for glucose in proximal tubules of the rat kidney. *Pflügers Arch., 343:*273.

Barthelmai, W., and Czok, R. 1962. Enzymatische Bestimmungen der Glucose in Blut, Liquor und Harn. *Klin. Wschr., 40:*585.

Bastiaanse, A. J., and Meijers, C. A. M. 1968. A micromethod for the routine estimation of inorganic phosphate in serum and urine. *Z. Klin. Chem. Klin. Biochem., 6:*48.

Baumann, K., and Huang, K. C. 1969. Micropuncture and microperfusion study of L-glucose secretion in rat kidney. *Pflügers Arch., 305:*167.

Beale, R. N., and Croft, D. 1961. A sensitive method for the colorimetric determination of urea. *J. Clin. Pathol., 14:*418.

Beaman, D. R., Isasi, J. A. 1971. *Mater. Res. Stand., 11:*8.

Benson, J. R., and Hare, P. E. 1975. *o*-Phthalaldehyde: Fluorogenic detection of primary amines in the picomole range. Comparison with fluorescamine and ninhydrine. *Proc. Nat. Acad. Sci., 72:*619.

Birks, J. B. The theory and practice of scintillation counting. Packard Instrument Co., Inc., 2200 Warrenville Rd., Downers Grove, Illinois, 60515.

Birks, L. S. 1963. *Electron Probe Microanalysis*, p. 253. Interscience, New York.

Bloch, P. L., and Lata, G. F. 1970. Fluorescence assay for picomole quantities of uric acid: A new enzyme-coupled approach. *Anal. Biochem., 38:*1.

Bonventre, J. V., and Lechene, C. 1974. A method for electron probe microanalysis of organic components in picoliter samples. *Proc. Microbeam Analysis Soc. Ninth Ann. Conf.* (Ottawa) 8A-8D.

Bott, P. A. 1960. The determination of sodium and potassium in biological fluids with the dual channel ultramicroflame photometer. *Anal. Biochem., 1:*17.

Boudry, J. F., Troehler, U., Touabi, M., Fleisch, H., and Bonjour, J. P. 1975. Secretion of inorganic phosphate in the rat nephron. *Clin. Sci. Mol. Med., 48:*475.

Bransome, E. D. 1970. *The Current Status of Liquid Scintillation Counting.* Grune & Stratton, New York.

Bratton, C., and Marshall, E. K. 1939. A new coupling component for sulfanilamide determination. *J. Biol. Chem., 128:*537.

Bray, G. A. 1960. A simple efficient liquid scintillator for counting aqueous solutions in a liquid scintillation counter. *Anal. Biochem., 1:*279.

Brenner, B. M., Falchuk, K. H., Keimowitz, R. I., and Berliner, R. W. 1969. The relationship between peritubular capillary protein concentration and fluid reabsorption by the renal proximal tubule. *J. Clin. Invest., 48:*1519.

Briel, G., and Neuhoff, V. 1973. Microanalysis of amino acids and their determination in biological material using dansyl chloride. *Hoppe-Seyler's Z. Physiol. Chem., 353:*540.

Brown, M. N., and Boston, M. S. 1961. Ultramicro sugar determinations using 2,9-dimethyl 1,10-phenanthroline HCl (neocuproine). *Diabetes, 10:*60.

Brunette, M., Wen, S. F., Evanson, R. L., and Dirks, J. H. 1969. Micropuncture study of magnesium reabsorption in the proximal tubule of the dog. *Am. J. Physiol., 216:*1510.

Burg, M., and Green, M. 1973. Effect of ethacrynic acid on the thick ascending limb of Henle's loop. *Kidney Int., 4:*301.

Caflisch, C. R., and Carter, N. W. 1974. A micro pCO_2 electrode. *Anal. Biochem., 60:*252.

Capek, K., Fuchs, G., Rumrich, G., and Ullrich, K. J. 1966. Harnstoffpermeabilitaet der corticalen Tubulusabschnitte von Ratten in Antidiurese und Wasserdiurese. *Pflügers Arch., 290:*237.

Caraway, W. T. 1955. Determination of uric acid in serum by a carbonate method. *Am. J. Clin. Path.*, *25:*840.

Castaing, R. 1951. Application des sondes electroniques une methode d'analyse ponctuelle chimique et cristallographique. Ph.D. thesis, University of Paris. Onera, Publication 55, 92 pp.

Chandler, J. A. 1975. In: *Techniques of Biomedical and Biological Morphology,* Vol. 2, pp. 307–437. Ed. by Gluck, D. and Rosenbaum, R. M. Wiley-Interscience, New York.

Chen, P. S., Toribara, T. Y., and Warner, H. 1956. Microdetermination of phosphorus. *Anal. Chem., 28:*1756.

Chou, S. C., and Goldstein, A. 1969. Chromogenic groupings in the Lowry protein determination. *Biochem. J., 75:*109.

Clapp, J. R. 1966. Renal tubular reabsorption of urea in normal and protein-depleted rats. *Am. J. Physiol., 210:*1304.

Coleman, J. R., and Terepka, A. R. 1974. In: *Principles and Techniques of Electron Microscopy,* Vol. 4, pp. 159–207. Ed. by Hayat, M. A. Van Nostrand-Rheinhold, New York.

Conger, J. D., Rhoads, H. N., Christie, S. N., and Bruke, T. J. 1975. A modification of the fluorescence method for micro-inulin determinations. *Kidney Int., 8:*334.

Cortney, M. A., Mylle, M., Lassiter, W. E., and Gottschalk, C. W. 1965. Renal tubular transport of water, solute, and PAH in rats loaded with isotonic saline. *Am. J. Physiol., 209:*1199.

Deetjen, P., and Sonnenberg, H. 1965. Der tubulare Transport von *p*-Aminohippursaeure. Mikroperfusionsversuche am Einzelnephron der Rattenniere *in Situ. Pflügers Arch., 285:*35.

Dirks, J. H., Clapp, J. R., and Berliner, R. W. 1964. The protein concentration in the proximal tubule of the dog. *J. Clin. Invest., 43:*916.

Edwards, B. R., Baer, P. G., Sutton, R. A. L., and Dirks, J. H. 1973. Micropuncture study of diuretic effects on sodium and calcium reabsorption in the dog nephron. *J. Clin. Invest., 52:*2418.

Eisenbach, G. M., Weise, M., and Stolte, H. 1975. Amino acid reabsorption in the rat nephron. Free flow micropuncture study. *Pflügers Arch., 357:*63.

Fiske, G. H., and SubbaRow, Y. 1925. The colorimetric determination of phosphorus. *J. Biol. Chem., 66:*375.

Folin, O., and Denis, W. 1912–13. A new (colorimetric) method for the determination of uric acid in blood. *J. Biol. Chem., 13:*469.

Friedman, T. B., and Merril, C. R. 1973. A microradiochemical assay for urate oxidase. *Anal. Biochem., 55:*292.

Frohnert, P. P., Hoehmann, B., Zwiebel, R., and Baumann, K. 1970. Free flow micropuncture studies of glucose transport in the rat nephron. *Pflügers Arch., 315:*66.

Fuehr, J., Kaczmarczyk, J., and Krüttgen, C. D. 1955. Eine einfache colorimetrische Methode zur Inulinbestimmung fuer Nieren-Clearance-Untersuchungen bei Stoffwechselgesunden und Diabetikern. *Klin. Wschr., 33:*729.

Goldstein, J. I., and Yakowitz, H. 1975. *Practical Scanning Electron Microscopy,* p. 582. Plenum Press, New York.

Gomori, G. 1941–42. A modification of the colorimetric phosphorus determination for use with the photoelectric colorimeter. *J. Lab. Clin. Med., 27:*955.

Greger, R. 1976. Purine excretion by the rat kidney. In *Intern. Symp. Amino Acid and Uric Acid Transport,* pp. 192–201. Ed. by Silbernagl, S., Lang, F., and Greger, R. Thieme Verlag, Stuttgart.

Greger, R., Lang, F., and Deetjen, P. 1971. Handling of uric acid by the rat kidney. I. Microanalysis of uric acid in proximal tubular fluid. *Pflügers Arch., 324:*279.

Greger, R., Lang, F., Marchand, G., and Knox, F. 1976a. Re-examination of renal phosphate handling in acutely thyroparathyroidectomized and normal rats with an ultramodification of a chemical phosphate method. *Clin. Res., 24:*468.

Greger, R., Lang, F., Marchand, G., and Knox, F. 1976b. The postproximal site of phosphate (P)reabsorption in presence and absence of parathyroid hormone (PTH). In: *Phosphate Metabolism,* pp. 149–151. Ed. by Massry, S. G. and Ritz, E. Plenum Press, New York.

Greger, R., Lang, F., Deetjen, P., and Knox, F. G. 1977a. Sites of urate transport in the rat nephron.

In: *Purine Metabolism in Man. II. Physiology, Pharmacology and Clinical Aspects,* pp. 90–99. Ed. by Müller, M. M., Kaiser, E., and Seegmiller, J. E., Plenum Press, New York.

Greger, R., Lang, F., Marchand, G., and Knox, F. G. 1977b. Site of renal phosphate reabsorption. *Pflügers Arch., 369:*111.

Haeberle, D. 1975. Influence of glomerular filtration rate on the rate of para-aminohippurate secretion by the rat kidneys: Micropuncture and clearance studies. *Kidney Int., 7:*385.

Hagedorn, H. C., and Jensen, B. N. 1923. Zur Mikrobestimmung des Blutzuckers mittels Ferricyanid. *Biochem. Z., 135:*46.

Hendee, W. R. 1973. *Radioactive Isotopes in Biological Research.* Wiley, New York.

Hevert, F. 1973. Microdetermination of carbonate using a strain-gauge pressure transducer. *Pflügers Arch., 344:*271.

Hilger, H. H., Kluemper, J. D., and Ullrich, K. J. 1958. Wasserrueckresorption und Ionentransport durch Sammelrohrzellen der Saeugetierniere. *Pflügers Arch., 267:*218.

Holzer, F., and Hohenegger, M. 1974. Determination of sodium and potassium concentrations in nanoliter samples. Evaluation of commercially available helium glow photometer. *Microchim. Acta., 1974:*711.

Holzer, F., Hohenegger, M., and Kink, H. 1973. A simple method for measurement of inulin in nanoliter samples using glass capillaries. *Pflügers Arch., 343:*179.

Horrocks, D. L., and Peng, C. T. Organic scintillators and liquid scintillation counting. Packard Instrument Co., Inc., 2200 Warrenville Rd., Downers Grove, Il. 60515.

Ingram, M. J., and Hogben, C. A. 1967. Electrolyte analysis of biological fluid with the electron microprobe. *Anal. Biochem., 18:*54.

Itaya, K., and Ui, M. 1966. A new micromethod for the colorimetric determination of inorganic phosphate. *Clin. Chim. Acta. 14:*361.

Joppich, R., and Deetjen, P. 1971. The relation between the reabsorption of urea and of water in the distal tubule of the rat kidney. *Pflügers Arch., 329:*172.

Karlmark, B., and Sohtell, M. 1973. The determination of bicarbonate in nanoliter samples. *Anal. Biochem., 53:*1.

Knox, F. G., Willis, L. R., Strandhoy, J. W., Schneider, E. G., Navar, L. G., and Ott, C. E. 1972. Role of peritubular Starling forces in proximal reabsorption following albumin infusion. *Am. J. Physiol., 223:*741.

Lang, F., Greger, R., and Deetjen, P. 1974. *In vivo* studies on uricase activity in the rat. *Pflügers Arch., 351:*323.

Lechene, C. 1970. The use of the electron microprobe to analyze very minute amounts of liquid samples. In: *Proc. Fifth Nat. Conf. on Electron Probe Analysis,* p. 32. New York.

Lechene, C. 1974. Electron probe microanalysis of picoliter liquid samples. In: *Microprobe Analysis as Applied to Cells and Tissues,* p. 351. Ed. by Hall, T., Echlin, P., and Kaufmann, R. Academic Press, London.

Lechene, C., and Warner, R. 1977. Ultramicroanalysis X-ray spectrometry by electron beam excitation. *Am. Rev. Biophys. Bioeng. 6:*57.

Lechene, C. R., Morel, F., Guinnebault, M., and DeRouffignac, C. 1969. Etude par micropunction de l'élaboration de l'urine. I. Chez le rat dans differents états de diurese. *Nephron, 6:*457.

Liew, J. B., van, Buentig, W., Stolte, H., and Boylan, J. W. 1970. Protein excretion: Micropuncture study of rat capsular and proximal tubule fluid. *Am. J. Physiol., 219:*299.

Loeschke, K., and Baumann, K. 1969. Kinetische Studien der D-Glucoseresorption im proximalen Konvolute der Rattenniere. *Pflügers Arch., 305:*139.

Loeschke, K., Baumann, K., Renschler, H., and Ullrich, K. J. 1969. Differenzierung zwischen aktiver und passiver Komponente des D-Glucosetransportes am proximalen Konvolut der Rattenniere. *Pflügers Arch., 305:*118.

Lowry, O. H., Rosebrough, N. J., Farr, A. L., and Randall, R. J. 1951. Protein measurement with the Folin phenol reagent. *J. Biol. Chem., 193:*265.

Lowry, O. H., Rosebrough, N. J., Farr, A. L., and Randall, R. J. 1951. The measurement of pyridine nucleotides by enzymatic cycling. *J. Biol. Chem., 236:*2746.

Maffly, R. H. 1968. A conductometric method for measuring micromolar quantities of carbon dioxide. *Anal. Biochem., 23:*252.

Malnic, G., Klose, R. M., and Giebisch, G. 1964. Micropuncture study of renal potassium excretion in the rat. *Am. J. Physiol., 206:*674.

Marchand, G., Ott, C., Cuche, J., and Knox, F. 1976. A comparison of proximal tubule fluid-to-plasma ultrafiltrate chloride ratio in rats and dogs. *J. Appl. Physiol., 40:*1009.

Marsh, D. J., Frasier, C., and Decter, J. 1965. Measurement of urea concentrations in nanoliter specimens of renal tubular fluid and capillary blood. *Anal. Biochem., 11:*73.

Morel, F., Roinel, N., and LeGrimellec, C. 1969. Electron probe analysis of tubular fluid composition. *Nephron, 6:*350.

Mueller, P. 1958. Experiments on current flow and ionic movements in single myelinated nerve fibers. *Exptl. Cell Res., 5:*118.

Nagel, W., Wolff, G., Gigon, J. P., and Enderlin, F. 1967. Zur Bestimmung der Inulinclearance in Gegenwart von Dextran. *Klin. Wschr., 45:*137.

Neuhoff, V., Haar, F. von der, Schlimme, E., and Weise, M. 1969. Zweidimensionale Chromatographie von Dansyl-Aminosaeuren im pico-Mol Bereich, angewandt zur direkten Charakterisierung von Transfer-Ribonukleinsaeuren. *Hoppe Seyler's Z. Physiol. Chem., 350:*121.

Quinton, P. M. 1976. Construction of picoliter-nanoliter self-filling volumetric pipettes. *J. Appl. Physiol., 40:*260.

Ramsay, J. A. 1949. A new method of freezing-point determination for small quantities. *J. Exptl. Biol., 26:*57.

Ramsay, J. A., Brown, R. H. J., and Falloon, S. W. H. W. 1953. Simultaneous determination of sodium and potassium in small volumes of fluid by flame photometry. *J. Exptl. Biol., 30:*1.

Ramsay, J. A., Brown, R. H. J., and Croghan, P. C. 1955. Electrometric titration of chloride in small volumes. *J. Exptl. Biol., 32:*822.

Rapkin, E., Guide to preparation of samples for liquid scintillation counting. New England Nuclear, 575 Albany Street, Boston, Ma. 02118.

Roch-Ramel, F. 1967. An enzymic and fluorophotometric method for estimating urea concentrations in nanoliter specimens. *Anal. Biochem., 21:*372.

Roch-Ramel, F., and Weiner, I. M. 1973. Excretion of urate by the kidneys of cebus monkeys: A micropuncture study. *Am. J. Physiol., 224:*1369.

Roch-Ramel, F., and Weiner, I. M. 1975. Inhibition of urate excretion by pyrazinoate: A micropuncture study. *Am. J. Physiol., 229:*1604.

Roch-Ramel, F., Chomety, F., and Peters, G. 1968. Urea concentrations in tubular fluid and in renal tissue of nondiuretic rats. *Am. J. Physiol., 215:*429.

Roch-Ramel, F., Diezi, J., Chomety, F., Michoud, P., and Peters, G. 1970. Disposal of large urea overloads by the rat kidney: A micropuncture study. *Am. J. Physiol., 218:*1524.

Roch-Ramel, F., Rougemont, D.de, Peters, G., and Weiner, I. M. 1976a. Micropuncture study of urate excretion by the kidney of the rat, the cebus monkey and the rabbit. In: *Intern. Symp. Amino Acid and Uric Acid Transport*, pp. 188–192. Ed. by Silbernagl, S., Lang, F., Greger, R., Thieme Verlag, Stuttgart.

Roch-Ramel, F., Diezi, J., Chomety, F., Rougemont, D.de, Tellier, M., Widmer, J., and Peters, G. 1976b. Renal excretion of uric acid in the rat: A micropuncture and microperfusion study. *Am. J. Physiol., 230:*768.

Roch-Ramel, F., Wong, N. L. M., and Dirks, J. H. 1976c. Micropuncture study of urate transport in the mongrel and dalmation dog. *Fed. Proc., 35:*849.

Roth, M. 1971. Fluorescence reaction for amino acids. *Anal. Chem., 43:*880.

Roth, M., and Hampai, A. 1973. Column chromatography of amino acids with fluorescence detection. *J. Chromat., 83:*353.

Rohde, R., and Deetjen, P. 1968. Die Glukoseresorption in der Rattenniere. Mikropunktionsanalysen der tubulaeren Glukosekonzentration bei freiem Fluss. *Pflügers Arch., 302:*219.

Schachter, D. 1959. The fluorometric estimation of magnesium in serum and urine. *J. Lab. Clin. Med., 54:*763.

Schmidt, F. H. 1961. Die enzymatische Bestimmung von Glukose und Fructose nebeneinander. *Klin. Wschr., 39:*1244.

Schneider, W., and Greger, R. 1969. An improved microcuvette for photometric measurements. *Pflügers Arch., 311:*268.

Schnermann, J., and Thurau, K. 1965. Mikropunktionsversuche zum Verhalten der PAH-Konzentration im Vasa recta—Blut der Goldhamsterniere. *Pflügers Arch., 283:*171.

Schram, E. Organic scintillation detectors. Packard Instruments Co., Inc., 2200 Warrenville Rd., Downers Grove, Illinois 60515.

Silbernagl, S., and Bayliss, E. Personal communication. Column chromatography of amino acids in the picomole range.

Truniger, B., and Schmidt-Nielsen, B. 1964. Intrarenal distribution of urea and related compounds: Effects of nitrogen intake. *Am. J. Physiol., 207:*971.

Ullrich, K. J., and Hampel, A. 1958. Eine einfache Mikrokuvette fuer Monochromator Zeiss und Beckmann Modell DU. *Pflügers Arch., 268:*177.

Ullrich, K. J., Pehling, G., and Espinar-Lafuente, M. 1961. Wasser-und Elektrolytfluss im vaskulaeren Gegenstromsystem des Neiren-markes. *Pflügers Arch., 273:*562.

Ullrich, K. J., Rumrich, G., and Schmidt-Nielsen, B. 1967. Urea transport in the collecting duct of rats on normal and low protein diet. *Pflügers Arch., 295:*147.

Ullrich, K. J., Froemter, E., and Baumann, K. 1969. Micropuncture and microanalysis in kidney physiology. In: *Laboratory Techniques in Membrane Biophysics,* pp. 106–129. Ed. by Passow, H. and Staempfli, R. Springer Verlag, Berlin.

Vurek, G. G., and Bowman, R. L. 1965. Helium-glow photometer for picomole analysis of alkali metals. *Science, 149:*448.

Vurek, G. G., and Bowman, R. L. 1969. Fiber-optic colorimeter for submicroliter samples. *Anal. Biochem., 29:*238.

Vurek, G. G., and Pegram, S. 1966. Fluorometric method for the determination of nanogram quantities of inulin. *Anal. Biochem., 16:*409.

Vurek, G. G., Warnock, D. G., and Corsey, R. 1975. Measurement of picomole amounts of carbon dioxide by calorimetry. *Anal. Chem. 47:*765.

Walker, A. M., Bott, P. A., Oliver, J., and MacDowell, Mn C. 1941. The collection and analysis of fluid from single nephrons of the mammalian kidney. *Am. J. Physiol., 134:*580.

Warnock, D. G., and Burg, M. B. 1975. Heterogeneity of CO_2 transport in proximal straight tubules. *Am. Soc. Neph. Abstr.,* 96.

Zwiebel, R., Hoehmann, B., Frohnert, P., and Baumann, K. 1968. Fluorometrisch-enzymatische Mikro- und Ultra-mikrobestimmung von Inulin und Glukose. *Pflügers Arch., 307:*127.

Chapter **6**

Measurements of Glomerular Dynamics

Roland C. Blantz and Bryan J. Tucker

Department of Medicine
School of Medicine and Nephrology Division
University of California, San Diego
and Veterans Administration Hospital
San Diego, California

The rate of glomerular ultrafiltration is high in mammals and defines the filtered load to each nephron unit. The major focus in renal physiology has been upon the varied mechanisms involved in the process of tubular reabsorption of solute and water. However, it has long been apparent that equally exacting mechanisms are required in maintaining the load of solute and water to the tubule for volume homeostasis to be maintained (Smith, 1951). Analysis of the specific factors determining and controlling glomerular filtration has awaited the development of micro methods capable of providing the necessary measurements of all the pertinent pressures, flows, and permeabilities. During the past few years such systems of measurement have been developed (Brenner *et al.*, 1971; Blantz *et al.*, 1972) and knowledge of the specific factors contributing to glomerular ultrafiltration has advanced rapidly during this recent period (Brenner *et al.*, 1972; Deen *et al.*, 1972; Blantz, 1974; Maddox *et al.*, 1975; Blantz *et al.*, 1976). In this section, we will summarize the specifics of current methods used in the analysis of glomerular dynamics.

I. HISTORICAL BACKGROUND

A. N. Richards (1939) first utilized micropuncture techniques to provide meaningful information on the mechanism of glomerular filtration. Richards obtained fluid from Bowman's space and compared this fluid to that of plasma entering the kidney via the renal artery. Several pieces of information were derived from this analysis. First, macromolecules such as albumin and globulin were effectively excluded from Bowman's space and proximal tubule. Second, the volume of filtration was large. Third, the constituents of Bowman's space fluid were essentially identical to that in the aqueous phase of plasma and existed in similar concentrations. The findings of Richards provided evidence in support of the initial theories of Ludwig (1843, 1861) some years before, who proposed that fluid entered the reabsorbing tubule by a process of ultrafiltration across a capillary which, at the same time, excluded the major proteins. A secretory process was also effectively excluded by the data of Richards (1939).

Smith *et al.* (1940) also demonstrated a major interest in the process of glomerular filtration. The discovery of inulin provided an accurate method of assessing the rate of glomerular filtration in clearance studies, and, with the clearance of PAH as an estimate of renal plasma flow, Smith and Clarke (1938) were able to evaluate the effect of a variety of physiologic conditions and drugs upon the rate of glomerular filtration. Although Smith observed that the rate of glomerular filtration was regulated within certain narrow limits in a single animal, spontaneous changes in renal plasma flow, protein feeding, the administration of pyrogens and glucocorticoids were all examined and found to have an effect upon the GFR (Smith, 1937, 1951). Smith (1937, 1951) also concluded that glomerular filtration was not an intermittent process among nephrons, but continuous in all nephrons in the normal kidney.

During the past three decades there has been a decrease in research activity in the field of glomerular filtration, but this trend has reversed in the past few years. The issue of the distribution of the rate of glomerular filtration among nephron populations was one of the few areas of active interest over the past 10–12 years (Barger, 1966; Herrera-Acosta *et al.*, 1972). There have been a variety of stimuli which may have produced the renewed interest in the specific mechanisms for the control of filtration during the past 5–6 years. The continued interest in the tubulo-glomerular feedback hypothesis certainly has been a major reason (Thurau, 1964). The hypothesis states that variations in the rate of tubular reabsorption, possibly at the macula densa cell in the distal nephron, lead to a reciprocal alteration in the rate of glomerular filtration in the same nephron unit (Schnermann *et al.*, 1971a). Interest has been generated regarding the specific mechanisms mediating the efferent limb leading to changes in nephron filtration rate (Schnermann *et al.*, 1973; Blantz *et al.*, 1972; Hierholzer *et al.*, 1972). The specific contributions of hydrostatic pressure, the rate of plasma flow, and glomerular permeability to the efferent limb controlling nephron filtration rate remain unproven.

An interest in the potential technical artifacts involved in collection of nephron filtration rates also focused attention upon the role of hydrostatic pressures in contributing to errors during the collection of proximal tubular fluid (Schnermann *et al.*, 1971b; Andreucci *et al.*, 1971; Davidman *et al.*, 1971). Alterations in tubular pressure during collections may alter the filtration rate, but the exact degree of influence is markedly dependent upon whether the filtration forces (hydrostatic and oncotic pressures) come to equilibrium within the length of the glomerular capillary. In order to provide answers to these questions, techniques had to be developed which could provide accurate data on all the factors affecting the process of glomerular ultrafiltration.

The major interest in the role of peritubular capillary "physical factors" in determining the rate of proximal tubular reabsorption has also contributed to a renewed interest in the filtration process (Lewy and Windhager, 1968; Brenner et al., 1969; Blantz and Tucker, 1975). The major determinants of both the efferent peritubular oncotic and hydrostatic pressures are the changes in glomerular flows, resistances, and permeabilities. For these reasons, the control of the potentially important peritubular capillary "physical factors" is intimately related to the factors which affect glomerular ultrafiltration.

The specific data required for a complete analysis of factors affecting filtration rate consist of the hydrostatic pressures acting across the glomerular capillary, the profile of changing oncotic pressure along this capillary, and the rate of nephron plasma flow (Deen et al., 1972; Blantz, 1974). With these data the permeability coefficient and net driving pressure can be defined, and with quite different methods, the glomerular permeability coefficient is the initially defined factor (Lambert et al., 1972). We will now provide a description of the more recently developed, direct methods of measurement of these factors.

II. MEASUREMENT OF HYDROSTATIC PRESSURES

Critical to the evaluation of the determinants of glomerular ultrafiltration is an accurate method for the assessment of all relevant hydrostatic pressures. Gottschalk and Mylle (1957) first applied the method of Landis (1926) to the measurement of pressures in tubules and peritubular capillaries. The Landis technique is a manometric method which involves the equilibration of a colored isotonic fluid at the tip of a micropipet (usually 7–12 μm) at zero pressure on the kidney surface. After entering the structure to be measured, the colored dye is again reequilibrated and the resulting pressure in the open system is monitored with a manometer by observing the height of a column of saline continuous with the saline in the pipet. The Landis method is based upon simple principles and can provide accurate values for tubular pressure if properly performed. However, capillary pressures provide special problems with this method. First, the method is based upon a significant volume displacement through the pipet tip, such that fibrin deposition and cellular debris can cause either complete obstruction or significant alterations in tip resistance. In order to minimize this problem, larger pipet tips are required, which then limits the accurate measurement of pressure in smaller (<8 μm inner diameter) capillaries.

A modest advance in the measurement of intrarenal pressures was provided in the 1960s by development of the Kulite micropressure transducer (Wunderlich and Schnermann, 1969). The major advantage provided, when compared to the Landis method, is the continuous recording of pressures. The microtransducer is calibrated against known hydrostatic pressures through the pipet tip. Although this transducer eliminated some of the subjectivity inherent in the Landis equilibration method, major problems of partial tip obstruction by blood products prevented the accurate assessment of pressures in capillaries. In addition, the larger tips (5–9 μm) prevented the use of the Kulite micrometer in small diameter capillaries because of the increased risk of capillary rupture and bleeding.

In summary, both the Landis equilibration method and the Kulite micropressure transducer provide accurate measurements of hydrostatic pressure in tubules but present considerable technical difficulties when applied to the measurement of hydrostatic pressure in renal capillaries.

Accurate measurement of hydrostatic pressures within capillaries then requires a system which permits both the use of smaller (<3 μm tip) micropipets and does not require significant volume displacement into the tip of the pipet. The second criterion prevents changes in tip diameter due to deposition of fibrin and other debris. The development of servonulling systems by Wiederhielm *et al.* (1964) and improvements by Intaglietta *et al.* (1970) have provided a method which fulfills the criteria delineated. Falchuk *et al.* (1971) first applied a version of the servonulling system to the measurement of pressures in renal tubules and peritubular capillaries.

The Munich–Wistar rat, a strain in which glomeruli are present on the surface of the kidney, directly under the capsule, has permitted direct access to accurate measurement of glomerular capillary and Bowman's space hydrostatic pressures (Brenner *et al.*, 1971; Blantz *et al.*, 1972). We will describe the techniques involved in the direct measurement of glomerular capillary hydrostatic pressure in the Munich–Wistar rat in the following sections.

A. Direct Measurement of Glomerular Capillary Hydrostatic Pressure

1. The Animal Model—Preparation for Micropuncture

A critical element in the measurement of glomerular capillary pressure is the stability of the kidney, which permits the recording of stable pressure tracings. Movement of the kidney, vigorous transmission of arterial pressures and respiratory movement can all present considerable problems in obtaining stable and recognizable pressure tracings. Stability, however, must be accomplished without compromising renal blood flow or altering intrarenal pressures.

In Figure 1, the micropuncture surgical preparation that we have utilized is demonstrated graphically. The kidney is approached via a left subcostal incision. Perirenal fat is then carefully dissected from the dorsal-lateral, micropuncture surface. This aspect of the kidney is superior for pressure measurements because the capsule is thinner on this surface, an important factor when smaller tip pipets are utilized (A). Following dissection, the kidney is carefully placed into a Lucite cup (B), and care is taken to prevent stretch of the pedicle. The kidney is also not touched during this maneuver except by the Lucite cup. The cup is then lined with a thin padded material to the height of the cup (C). The space between the cup and kidney is then carefully filled with cotton soaked in saline in order to produce an elevated structure surrounding the micropuncture surface (D). One-to-two percent agar solution is heated to liquefy the solution

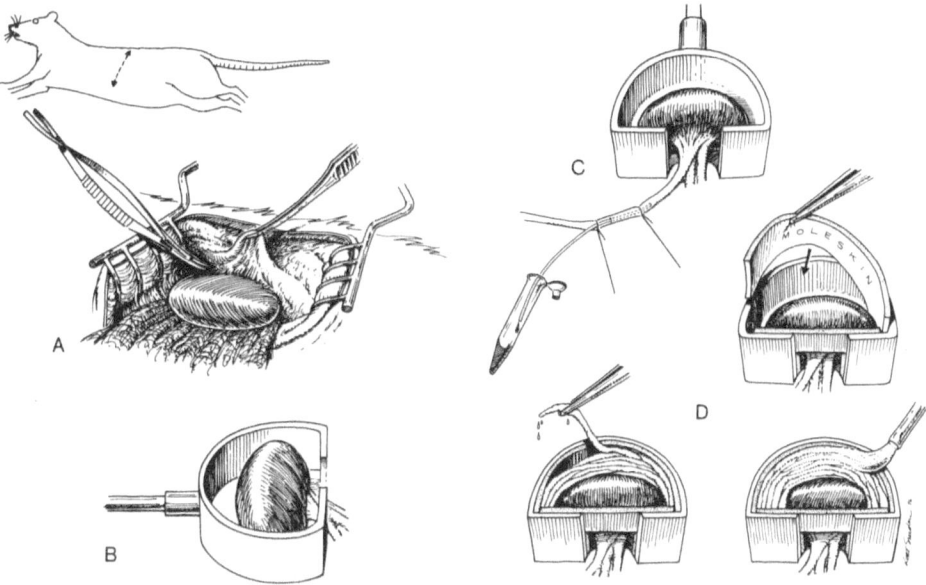

Figure 1. Preparation of the rat kidney for micropuncture measurements. (A) After a flank incision is made, the perirenal fat and adrenal are carefully separated from the kidney, allowing placement into the Lucite cup (B). The ureter is catheterized (C) for collection of urine, and care is taken to avoid stretch of the pedicle. The cup is then lined with moleskin (D) and cotton soaked in saline is placed around the kidney to create an amphitheater around the micropuncture surface. The cotton is then sealed with 1–2% agar to allow a warmed saline level to be maintained over the surface.

and dripped onto the cotton after cooling to ~40;°C to provide a saline-tight area around the kidney. (E). Care must be taken to exclude agar from the micropuncture surface. Heated NaCl–NaHCO$_3$ solution (37°C) is then delivered onto the micropuncture surface. In the Munich–Wistar rat usually 2–6 accessible glomeruli are present.

The Munich–Wistar rat has been reported to be growth hormone deficient (Martin *et al.*, 1974). However, we have reexamined this issue and found quite normal values for stimulated (PGE$_2$) and unstimulated growth hormone levels when compared to Sprague–Dawley rats (unpublished observations). The total kidney GFR and single nephron filtration rate (SNGFR) during hydropenia has also been observed to be quite normal and comparable to other strains at 1.0–1.1 ml/min/g kidney weight and 30–35 nl/min/g kidney weight respectively (Blantz, 1974; Blantz *et al.*, 1975, 1976).

2. The Servonulling Pressure System

The basic system is an electrical Wheatstone bridge. The high resistance point of one arm is at the tip of a 1–2 μm glass micropipet filled with hypertonic saline and mounted upon a Leitz micromanipulator (Figure 2). The pressure pipet is connected to a pressure drive motor by a hypertonic saline-filled

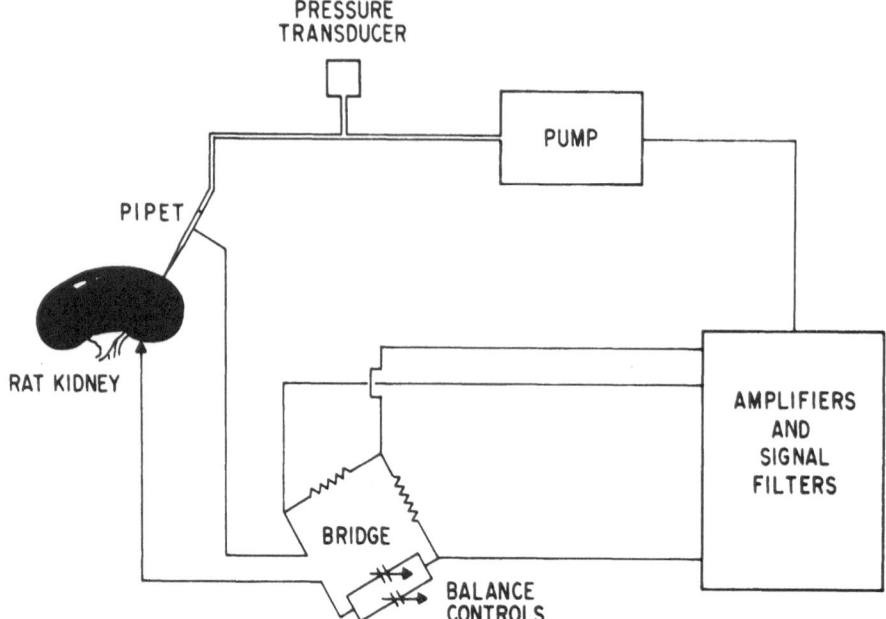

Figure 2. A basic schematic of the operation of the servonull pressure measuring system. A fluid interface is maintained at the tip of the pipet by a linear drive pump. The pump is activated by the change in tip resistance caused by movement of the interface due to alterations in pressure. The bridge becomes unbalanced, which in turn activates an amplifier to drive the pump until pressure within the pipet is equivalent to the external pressure measured, thereby balancing the bridge. The pressure can then be recorded from the pressure transducer.

nondistensible Teflon tubing. The pressure drive system is in turn filled with a 20-centistoke fluid (Dow-Corning 200) which interfaces with the hypertonic saline at a three-way stopcock in the line. Pressure generated within the pressure drive system is continuously monitored with a p23Db Statham pressure transducer. The pressure complexes are shown on a direct writing chart recorder and displayed on one channel of a two-channel oscilloscope (long phosphor) along with the femoral artery pressure complex.

The electrical control box is metered and is connected to the pressure drive system and a capacitance box located upon the Leitz manipulator (Figure 2). The circuit box is in turn grounded and attached to the pipet holder, completing the circuit of the Wheatstone bridge (Figure 2).

With the pressure pipet filled with hypertonic saline placed in isotonic saline over the surface of the kidney, the high resistance point of that arm of the bridge is at the pipet tip. The resistance increases as smaller tip pipets are utilized but can be decreased by increases in the concentration of saline filling the pipet. After the bridge is balanced at zero pressure in isotonic saline, movement of the pipet into renal structures of higher hydrostatic pressure will tend to displace hypertonic saline at the tip with the lower conductivity physiologic fluid. The net effect of entry into a higher pressure compartment is (1) to increase electrical resistance at the pipet tip, (2) unbalance the Wheatstone bridge, and (3) cause a net current flow across the bridge. This current flow is then sensed by the servo control box and the pressure drive system is activated instantaneously. The drive system continues until the interface between hypertonic and isotonic saline is "pushed" back to the tip, balancing the bridge. When the bridge is again balanced and there is no flow of current, the pressure drive system is stabilized. The pressure transducer records the pressure within the drive system that is required to displace the isotonic fluid at the tip and return the bridge to a balanced condition; it displays this pressure profile upon the chart recorder and oscilloscope. This process requires milliseconds.

The mechanics of measuring pressures involve (1) balancing the bridge on a test resistance to determine if the Wheatstone bridge is operative, and (2) balancing the bridge with the pipet in saline on the kidney surface at zero pressure. After the pipet is inserted into renal structures with hydrostatic pressures greater than zero, the tip must be free in the lumen or fluid space. If the pipet tip is against solid structures, the drive system generates maximum pressures and no pressure is recorded.

3. Measurement of Glomerular Capillary and Bowman's Space Pressures

The two major requirements for the accurate measurement of glomerular capillary hydrostatic pressure are properly manufactured pipets and a stable, yet finely controlled micromanipulator. We have found that sharpened glass micropipets of less than 2 μm size are the most suitable, preferably with a short taper if possible. In order to keep the breakage rate low, pipets are best sharpened to this size with an electrically driven, fine-surface grinding stone. The stone is frequently resurfaced on the grinding shaft utilizing a diamond bit. Before filling the pipet with hypertonic saline (0.5–1.2 M NaCl), this solution should be passed through a small pore filter to remove debris that could potentially plug the pipet tip.

A finely controlled micromanipulator is also needed because movement accuracy of 2–3 μm is required for stable pressure measurements. Although one can usually visualize capillary loops in the glomerulus, the exact position of the pipet tip within the capillary lumen cannot always be defined under direct vision (160–250×). Although the pipet tip may be within the capillary lumen, the pressure system often records an off-scale pressure until the tip is completely free in the lumen, accomplished by moving the tip a few microns within the capillary.

The long phosphor oscilloscope, upon which the servonulling pressure tracing and femoral artery pulse contour is displayed, is of considerable value in determining the exact location of the tip of the pressure pipet. The glomerular capillary pressure pattern should be in close synchrony with the femoral artery pulse. Also, the pressure tracing should be stable over at least 25–30 sec, with a rapid upstroke and a slower notched descent from a sharp peak. Occasionally pressure forms are obtained that are the same rate as systemic pulse rate but rounded and slightly delayed in time from the femoral artery pulse. We have concluded that these tracings are probably obtained from interstitial "space" immediately outside of a capillary loop. This conclusion was derived from the fact that when the pipet is further advanced, an acceptable glomerular capillary pressure is usually obtained, several millimeters Hg higher than the previous recording.

As long as the criteria designated are fulfilled (stable pressure tracings, a systemic pulse contour, and synchrony with the displayed femoral artery pulse contour), the pressure is most certainly derived from the glomerular capillary, since there are no other stable pressures of similar magnitude which meet these criteria within the glomerulus. In addition, there must be no evidence of disruption of the glomerular capillaries by the pressure pipet. In order for the pressure obtained to be considered a proper reflection of glomerular capillary pressure, there must be no evidence of bleeding either into Bowman's space, the proximal tubule, or onto the surface of the kidney.

The accurate measurement of Bowman's space pressure would seem a much simpler task than the measurement of glomerular capillary hydrostatic pressure. However, the micropuncturist must take care to measure and record Bowman's space pressure upon first entry into the glomerulus with the pressure pipet. Since the pipet is tapered, the Bowman's space pressure usually decreases if the pipet enters the capillary first and Bowman's space pressure is measured second in sequence, since there is increasing risk of dissipating the actual pressure onto the surface fluid through the larger aperture.

B. Indirect Estimation of Glomerular Capillary Hydrostatic Pressure

Direct assessment of glomerular capillary and Bowman's space hydrostatic pressures has not been technically possible in other species or in strains of rat other than the Munich–Wistar. An exception is the recent report of Maddox and co-workers (1974) in which capillary pressure was measured in the surface glomeruli of the squirrel monkey. Methods have been derived which utilize indirect evaluations of P_G to overcome the limitations in animals lacking surface glomeruli. We will describe the theoretical basis, assumptions involved, and the techniques utilized in these indirect approaches to the measurement of P_G.

1. Stop-Flow Method of Gertz

The basic principle of this method is that if proximal tubular flow is obstructed by an oil block, the pressure will rise to an equilibrium value at which no further filtration takes place. This value of tubular pressure is designated as the stop-flow pressure (SFP) (Gertz *et al.*, 1966). Consequently, systemic protein concentration (C) and oncotic pressure (π_A) will no longer rise along the length of the glomerular capillary, since ultrafiltration has been prevented. Therefore at equilibrium during tubular obstruction

$$P_G = \pi_A + \text{SFP}$$

This estimate of P_G will be in error to the extent that reabsorption continues in the segment between Bowman's space and the oil block, since some filtration would continue at stable values of SFP. The π_A would then be a small underestimate of mean glomerular capillary ($\overline{\pi_G}$), which will result in a small error in P_G (lower than the actual pressure). For this reason it is important to measure SFP very early in the proximal tubule in order to minimize this error by decreasing the length of the reabsorbing proximal segment. The oil block placed should also be of sufficient length or viscosity to remain stable during the measurement of SFP.

There have been several practical and theoretical objections raised as to the accuracy of stop-flow estimates of P_G. The original data on the tubulo-glomerular feedback hypothesis, provided by Schnermann *et al.* (1971a), was interpreted as effectively invalidating the stop-flow method. The authors initially concluded that acute reductions in delivery of fluid out of the proximal tubule should result in an increase in actual P_G through a feedback system triggered by reductions in reabsorption of NaCl at the macula densa cells of the distal nephron. Further examinations of this issue in studies by the same author (Schnermann *et al.*, 1973), using stop-flow techniques, and by Blantz *et al.* (1972) and Israelit *et al.* (1973), utilizing direct measurements of P_G in the Munich–Wistar rat, demonstrated that acute decreases in distal NaCl delivery from normal to essentially zero did not affect P_G estimates either by the stop-flow method or directly measured P_G. Therefore, the objections to the stop-flow method based on activation of a tubulo-glomerular feedback system have not been substantiated by examinations in the rat. However, Navar and co-workers (1975) have provided suggestive evidence that the stop-flow method in the dog may not provide accurate assessments of P_G, possibly through activation of the same feedback system.

The cessation of glomerular filtration which results from tubular obstruction during the stop-flow technique should result in an increase in glomerular capillary plasma flow of 10–20%. If vascular resistance does not change, P_G should rise above the value present prior to tubular obstruction. In the studies of Blantz *et al.* (1972), it was observed that P_G did rise transiently in hydropenic rats following tubular obstruction but fell again to the original value within 20–30 sec, suggesting compensating decreases in efferent vascular resistance. Aspiration of tubular fluid proximal to the oil block resulted in prompt reductions in P_G to the control level indicating that the initial rise in P_G was due to cessation of glomerular filtration and not due to activation of other factors. These data suggest that although the P_G determined by the SFP method may reflect true P_G, it does so through significant compensating alterations in efferent arteriolar resistance.

Specific comparisons in the same animal of direct and indirect estimates (SFP) of P_G in a variety of conditions are not abundantly available. Studies have shown (Blantz *et al.*, 1972) that when P_G and SFP estimates were performed in the same nephron in hydropenic and saline expanded rats, the values were indistinguishable. Data from the same study demonstrated that estimates of P_G by the SFP method in other surface nephrons were higher than P_G measured directly in surface glomeruli, but only in the hydropenic condition and not during saline expansion. A more complete comparison summarizing our experiences during hydropenia, mannitol infusion, hyperoncotic albumin expansion, and after the administration of the nephrotoxin, uranyl nitrate, is shown in Table I (contains unpublished observations). The pattern was rather inconsistent in that during hydropenia there was a significantly higher value for both ΔP and P_G when SFP estimates were utilized. This difference was less consistent in expanded states and after uranyl nitrate in which pressures were diffusely increased for reasons other than prior volume expansion. It seems fair to state that stop-flow estimates of P_G in the hydropenic rat are consistently higher than the directly measured values and are therefore in some doubt. The pattern is not consistent in other physiologic conditions. Therefore in experimental maneuvers utilizing hydropenia as a control, stop-flow estimates will not provide valid comparisons of P_G in the rat. No such data are available for the dog, but one would presume that similar problems exist.

Table I. Comparison of Direct and Indirect (Stop-Flow Method) Measurements of Glomerular Capillary Hydrostatic Pressure (P_G) and the Hydrostatic Pressure Gradient (ΔP) in a Variety of Physiologic and Pathophysiologic Conditions in the Rat

Condition	P_G (mm Hg)[a]		ΔP (mm Hg)	
	Direct	Indirect	Direct	Indirect
Hydropenia	46.1	50.0	30.3	36.5
	±0.8	±0.8	±0.8	1.0[b]
	($n = 39$)	($n = 54$)	($n = 39$)	($n = 54$)
	mean diff. = 3.9 mm Hg		mean diff. = 6.2 mm Hg	
	$p < 0.0005$[c]		$p < 0.0005$	
Mannitol infusion	48.5	50.0	29.8	32.7
	±1.9	±1.3	±1.7	±1.0
	($n = 13$)	($n = 28$)	($n = 13$)	($n = 28$)
			mean diff. = 3.0 mm Hg	
	$p > 0.5$		$p < 0.05$	
Hyperoncotic albumin expansion	62.7	62.2	36.4	36.4
	±1.2	±1.7	±1.2	±1.5
	($n = 19$)	($n = 25$)	($n = 19$)	($n = 25$)
	$p > 0.8$		$p > 0.9$	
Uranyl nitrate administration (acute renal failure)	60.5	53.1	24.2	27.0
	±1.9	±2.1	±2.6	±1.7
	($n = 11$)	($n = 19$)	($n = 11$)	($n = 19$)
	mean diff. = 7.4 mm Hg			
	$p < 0.005$		$p > 0.4$	

[a] Measurements obtained in the same rats, but P_G (direct) in surface glomeruli and P_G (indirect) in other proximal tubules on the kidney surface.
[b] ±S.E.M.
[c] Statistical difference defined by analysis of variance.

2. *Ureteral Occlusive Techniques*

Both Jaenicke (1970) and Navar (1970) have utilized ureteral occlusion techniques with measurement of the stop-flow pressure to estimate P_G and minimal afferent resistance. Recent studies by Blantz *et al.* (1975) have examined the glomerular hemodynamics before and during increases in ureteral pressure in both hydropenic and plasma expanded rats. Directly measured P_G rises with this maneuver in hydropenic rats but not in rats previously plasma expanded (2.5% body weight isoncotic plasma delivered over 60 min). Also, changes in vascular resistance were not limited to the afferent arteriole. It is clear that this method introduces greater compensating hemodynamic adjustments than are inherent to the single nephron stop-flow pressure estimates of P_G, and therefore should not provide accurate assessments of true glomerular capillary hydrostatic pressure (P_G).

Recent developments of micropressure systems capable of accurate assessment of glomerular capillary and Bowman's space hydrostatic pressures in the surface glomeruli of the Munich–Wistar rat have provided evidence that the hydrostatic driving forces for glomerular filtration are lower than previously proposed. At least in this strain of rat, the oncotic pressure rises to a value essentially equal to the hydrostatic pressure within the length of the filtering capillary (Brenner *et al.*, 1971; Blantz, 1974). This condition of filtration pressure equilibrium dictates considerable plasma flow dependence of filtration rate in the normally hydrated rat (Brenner *et al.*, 1972). The development of newer accurate methods for measurement of specific pressures has therefore considerably altered our previous concepts (Renkin and Gilmore, 1973) of the process of glomerular ultrafiltration.

II. EVALUATION OF ONCOTIC PRESSURES

An accurate analysis of protein concentration and the corresponding oncotic pressure (π) along the glomerular capillary is a critical requirement for the complete evaluation of glomerular dynamics. The afferent (C_A) and efferent protein concentrations (C_E) and the glomerular filtration rate define the nephron plasma flow. The corresponding blood flow can be further defined if the hematocrit is known. The oncotic pressure can be readily determined from the concentration, and is a necessary requirement (with ΔP) to calculate the effective filtration pressure acting across the glomerular capillary wall.

Mathematical models of glomerular filtration have been utilized by several investigators to obtain a profile of the forces producing ultrafiltration (Deen *et al.*, 1972; Blantz, 1974). From these mathematical models the oncotic pressure profile can be generated as shown in Figure 3. Graph A in Figure 3 is indicative of the oncotic pressure profile typical for hydropenic Munich–Wistar rats, the strain in which direct pressure measurements have been obtained. Nephron plasma flow (RPF) is ~80 nl/min and L_pA is sufficiently large to permit a condition of filtration pressure equilibrium ($\Delta P \approx \pi_E$). Graph B depicts the

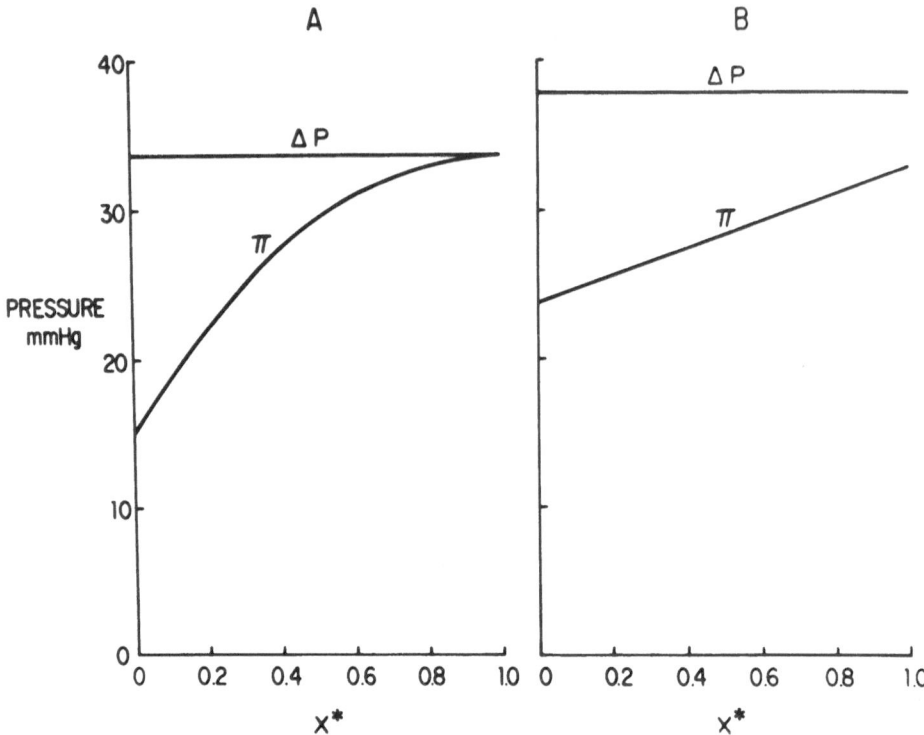

Figure 3. Profiles of oncotic pressure (π) along the glomerular capillary in hydropenia (A) and plasma volume expansion (B). (A) In hydropenia (RPF $\approx$ 8p nl/min), π increases rapidly along the length of the capillary (x^*) until $\pi = \Delta P (\Delta P = P_G - P_t)$, the point of filtration pressure equilibrium. (B) In the plasma volume expanded rat, π increases along the length of the capillary but usually does not achieve filtration pressure equilibrium ($\Delta P > \pi_E$).

pressure profile in rats in which nephron plasma flow (RPF) is increased to 200 nl/min. At higher RPF a positive effective filtration pressure persists at the end of the glomerular capillary ($\Delta P \gg \pi_E$). Such an increase in RPF can be produced by intravenous expansion with isoncotic plasma (2.5% body weight) (Deen et al., 1974; Blantz et al., 1975, 1976; Tucker and Blantz, 1977a).

Generation of such a π profile requires the following minimum data: (1) An arterial or systemic blood sample for the afferent protein concentration (C_A) and (2) a blood sample from the efferent peritubular capillaries nearest to the efferent arteriole, located directly on the surface of the kidney (C_E). Systemic protein concentration is assumed equivalent to that at the afferent arteriole and efferent peritubular protein concentrations are assumed equivalent to that which exists at the efferent arteriole.

Sampling of systemic protein concentration is fairly straightforward, requiring only a blood sample from a major artery. Considerable technical difficulty attends the sampling of efferent peritubular blood. The vessel is approximately 16–20 μm in diameter in the rat, which provides the major technical difficulties in obtaining blood samples.

A. Collection of Blood in Efferent Vessel

Collection of the efferent protein sample is accomplished by insertion of a sharpened glass pipet that has been tapered to a beveled point, 13–16 μm outside diameter. The pipet has been previously coated with a silicone fluid (Dow Corning 1107) (Blantz, 1974). The DC 1107 is diluted to a 3% solution with trichloroethylene and aspirated into the pipet and expelled out the tip. The pipets are then placed upright (beveled points upward) and heated to 200°C for 2–4 hr within 24 hr of their use. Prior to use the pipets are filled with mineral oil, stained with Sudan black.

Considerable care is required in the insertion of the pipet into "star" vessels in order to avoid (1) puncture of an adjacent tubule and dilution of blood with tubular fluid, (2) bleeding around the pipet, and (3) contamination with fluid from the surface of the kidney. After insertion of the pipet, initially and periodically, vigorous aspiration is required both to initiate and to maintain blood flow into the pipet. Aspiration is required because fibrin deposits within the tapered section of the pipet during the collection. Blood collections must be sufficiently large to pipet three 7–10 nl aliquots of plasma for the protein assay. The pipets are then sealed after collection with several applications of Eastman 910 (Eastman Chemicals, Inc.) (Figure 4). The sealed pipets are placed in a hematocrit centrifuge, tip outward, to separate the red blood cells from the plasma. These samples are then stored tip downward at 4°C until analysis of protein concentration is performed.

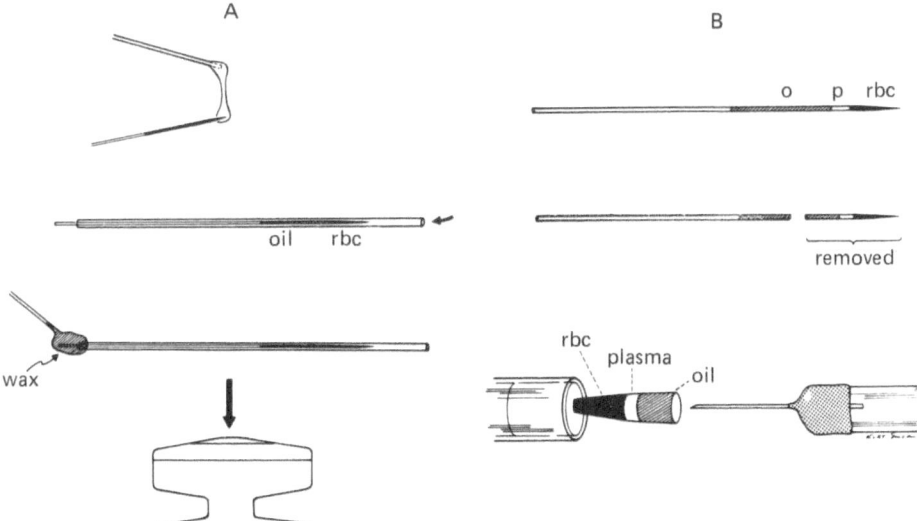

Figure 4. The sampling processing of efferent vessel blood for determination of plasma protein concentration. After collection of blood from the efferent arteriole, the tip is sealed with adhesive (A) and inserted into a capillary tube. The collection pipet is then held in the capillary tube with wax and centrifuged tip outward. After centrifugation, the tip of the pipet is separated (B) and inserted into a gum material in the end of a capillary tube. A constant volume pipet is then utilized to obtain aliquots of plasma for the determination of protein concentration by the microadaptation of the Lowry protein method.

B. Determination of Protein Concentration

The protein assay most commonly utilized for the determination of protein concentration in nanoliter quantities of plasma has been the microadaptation (Brenner *et al.*, 1969; Blantz, 1974) of the Lowry protein assay (Lowry *et al.*, 1951). Blood samples from the efferent vessels are small and evaporation through the mineral oil can produce an erroneously high protein concentration in the sample. Therefore the samples should not be stored for long periods prior to protein assay.

The collections are prepared for the assay by removing the tip from the shaft of the pipet and placing the tip in the end of a capillary tube filled with gum as shown in Figure 4. A constant volume 7–9-nl pipet is then inserted through the oil and the plasma aliquot aspirated into the pipet.

The constant volume (7–9 nl) Pyrex pipet is drawn from 90 μm o.d. tubing and sealed with wax into larger bore glass tubing (Figure 4). The aliquot of plasma is transferred into 20 μl of reagent A (a mixture of 2% Na_2CO_3 in 0.1 N NaOH and 0.02% Na tartrate–0.01% $CuSO_4$). The sample is set aside for 7–10 min to allow for diffusional mixing. Two microliters of reagent B (50% aqueous solution of 2 N phenol reagent) are added to the solution of reagent A and the solutions are mixed thoroughly. The reactants are then sealed to prevent evaporation and placed vertically for at least 1 hr for the development of color.

The development of color in each sample is compared to a standard curve pipetted and mixed in the same fashion and derived from protein concentrations from 2 to 10 g/100 ml at 2 g/100 ml intervals. Reaction solutions are read at 710 nm on a fiber-optic colorimeter designed for microliter quantities of fluid (American Instrument Co.). Three aliquots of each plasma sample and standard are evaluated. The resultant volume (22 μl) of the reaction mixture permits each sample to be read in triplicate since the volume of the cuvettes is 5–7 μl. Each of nine readings of the standards is applied to linear regression analysis and the mean of the readings from the blood collections is then applied to the resulting equation to obtain the protein concentration. The standard curves in the range of protein concentrations utilized are linear with a regression coefficient value of 0.98 or higher.

Either human serum albumin or concentrated rat plasma can be used for protein standards. The curves which result are identical, suggesting that both forms of albumin and rat globulin have the same number of reactive sites per gram protein in the Lowry assay.

C. Determination of Oncotic Pressure

The oncotic pressure generated by protein concentrations has been defined by Landis and Pappenheimer (1964) using an empirically derived mathematical relationship based upon measurements of pressure produced across a semipermeable membrane. If the albumin:globulin ratio (A/G) is 1:1, then the following relationship applies (reflection coefficient of proteins ≈ 1.0) (Landis and Pappenheimer, 1964):

$$\pi = 2.1C + 0.16C^2 + 0.009C^3$$

where π is the oncotic pressure in mm Hg and C is the protein concentration in grams/100 ml. This equation conforms closely to the oncotic pressures measured in rats with an albumin:globulin ratio of 1, utilizing a servonull pressure measuring instrument monitoring pressure changes across a semipermeable membrane. The A/G ratio of systemic plasma should be determined by protein electrophoresis in each experimental condition. It can be assumed that this ratio is not significantly different in efferent blood samples.

D. Potential Errors in the Determination of Oncotic Pressure

There are several potential errors in the method of analysis. Dealing with small sample sizes can lead to large errors if there are pipetting errors. A small change in the volume of the aliquot, caused by small air bubbles, will markedly alter the reading of the sample. Errors in pipetting of the reagents are not as critical but can contribute to variations in the final concentration of the mixture. Adequacy and uniformity of mixing of the sample and reagent A among assayed samples are critical, and partial mixing will lead to an erroneously low value for protein concentration. The potential error due to differing optical properties of the glass cuvettes is negligible since the fiber optic is in direct contact with the fluid. The formation of bubbles in the cuvette will, however, affect the reading in an unpredictable manner.

Errors can be introduced during the collection of blood from the efferent vessel. Contamination can occur for a variety of reasons: (1) Surface fluid entering the pipet, (2) formation of a fistula between tubule and blood vessel, allowing tubular fluid to gain access to the blood collection, and (3) dilution of the blood if water is mixed with the mineral oil contained in the pipet.

A theoretical problem relates to whether the "star" vessel blood is truly representative of the protein concentration of the blood at the efferent arteriole. Reabsorption of tubular fluid into the capillary between the efferent arteriole and the collection site could produce erroneously low values for C_E. Although there is no definite evidence for vascular shunts between the afferent and efferent arteriole (O'Dorisio et al., 1973), this remains a potential physiologic circumstance in which protein concentrations derived from "star" vessel blood collections may not reflect the protein concentrations at the end of the glomerular capillary. Baylis and co-workers (1976) have speculated that the apparent reductions in K_f (or L_pA) observed following the infusions of a variety of vasodilators may be the result of opening of potential afferent to efferent arteriolar shunts. Specific data on afferent and efferent vascular resistances, RPF and single nephron filtration rate (SNGFR) during blood collections from efferent vessels have not been available for obvious technical reasons. However, data from our experience and from the literature suggest that total filtration fraction and superficial filtration fraction are identical during hydropenia when evaluated by microprotein methods (Brenner *et al.*, 1971). Utilizing another method, Barratt *et al.* (1973) found the same results, suggesting that the filtration fractions derived from microprotein samples are accurate determinations.

IV. DETERMINATION OF NEPHRON PLASMA AND BLOOD FLOW

A. Calculations

Nephron plasma flow is calculated from single nephron filtration rate, systemic protein concentration (C_A), and the efferent arteriolar protein concentration (C_E) which can be determined as previously described. The specific equation is as follows:

$$RPF = SNGFR/(1 - C_A/C_E)$$

The term, $(1 - C_A/C_E)$, is the single nephron filtration fraction (SNFF) and the equation can be simplified to the following:

$$RPF = SNGFR/SNFF$$

Nephron blood flow is determined by the following relationship:

$$RBF = RPF/(1 - Hct)$$

where Hct is the hematocrit expressed as a fraction of one.

B. Potential Errors in Determination of RPF and RBF

There are well-defined sources of error in the measurements of SNGFR and plasma protein concentration, both of which are utilized in the calculation of RPF. Errors in the measurement of SNGFR have been defined in detail by previous studies on this issue (Schnermann *et al.*, 1971b; Andreucci *et al.*, 1971; Davidman *et al.*, 1971) and in Chapter 3 of Volume 4A in this series (Knox and Marchand). As previously described, the potential error in SNFF has been examined by several investigators (Brenner and Galla, 1971; Barratt *et al.*, 1973) by comparing SNFF by microprotein methods to the total kidney filtration fraction as defined by the extraction of inulin. In the hydropenic animal there were no significant differences between the two measured filtration fractions. Results from this laboratory also indicate that there is no difference in the two values by paired analysis in nine hydropenic animals [SNFF = 0.36 ($\pm$0.02) and total kidney filtration fraction 0.36 ($\pm$0.03) ($p > 0.40$)] (unpublished observations).

Other investigators have used changes in hematocrit across the glomerulus to determine SNFF (Brenner and Galla, 1971; Stein *et al.*, 1971). This method compares the systemic hematocrit to that in blood collected from the efferent arteriole, and this method provides similar results to the microprotein method.

Axial streaming of red blood cells in the kidney in certain physiologic conditions may increase the hematocrit entering the glomerulus to values higher than the systemic hematocrit, which would introduce errors into the calculation of RPF. The potential error involved in determination of nephron blood flow (RBF), other than that discussed for RPF previously, relates only to accuracy in determining hematocrit.

V. MATHEMATICAL MODELS OF GLOMERULAR ULTRAFILTRATION

A. Data Requirements and Definitions for Mathematical Models of Glomerular Ultrafiltration

Any method of data analysis which is applied to the process of glomerular ultrafiltration requires a delicate balance between the requirements for physiologic accuracy in accounting for all of the factors which could potentially influence the filtration process, and an awareness of the limitations upon the data which can be accurately determined with confidence. For purposes of both realism and simplicity, the mathematical models of glomerular ultrafiltration have utilized an idealized single conduit capillary of normalized length (x^*) across which the forces producing glomerular ultrafiltration act (Deen *et al.*, 1972; Blantz, 1974). The specific mathematical models are derived from a simple relationship where

$$\text{SNGFR} = L_p A \times \overline{\text{EFP}}$$

where the nephron filtration rate is the product of the glomerular ultrafiltration coefficient or permeability–surface area product ($L_p A$) and the mean effective filtration pressure ($\overline{\text{EFP}}$). The effective filtration pressure is defined as follows:

$$\text{EFP} = \Delta P - \pi$$

where $\Delta P = P_G - P_t$ and P_t equals proximal tubular or Bowman's space pressure. The mean EFP ($\overline{\text{EFP}}$) is defined as follows:

$$\overline{\text{EFP}} = \int_0^1 (\Delta P - \pi)_x^* \, dx^*$$

Changes in the rate of nephron plasma flow modify the $\overline{\text{EFP}}$ by influencing the rate of change of π along the capillary length (Brenner *et al.*, 1972; Blantz, 1974). Increases in RPF increase $\overline{\text{EFP}}$ and decreases in RPF will reduce $\overline{\text{EFP}}$. The EFP decreases along x^* as π rises, usually as a nonlinear function (ΔP is relatively constant along x^*). The specific profile of EFP is therefore influenced by variations in four factors: (1) RPF, (2) π_A, (3) ΔP, and (4) $L_p A$. A set of differential equations which describe the π_x^* and EFP_x^* functions have been derived from the basic relations (Deen *et al.*, 1972; Blantz, 1974). The specific profile of EFP and a value for $L_p A$ can be determined with the following input data: (1) RPF, (2) ΔP, (3) systemic protein concentration (C_A), and (4) efferent arteriolar protein concentration (C_E). Several publications have described the exact equations in more specific detail (Deen *et al.*, 1972). Protein concentration

(C) relates to oncotic pressure (π) as follows (Blantz *et al.*, 1974):

$$\pi = 1.76C + 0.28C^2$$

which is a simplification of the empirically derived relationship described by Landis and Pappenheimer (1964) which assumes that approximately 50% of total plasma proteins are albumin. Significant variations from this 50% value requires derivation of a different relationship between C and π (Blantz *et al.*, 1974).

    The existing mathematical models do not differ importantly in the basic differential equations utilized, but only in the methods utilized to integrate equations. The method of Deen *et al.* (1972) used a computer-based integration method and we have chosen a block iterative method (Blantz, 1974). The former is slightly more accurate, but the iterative method allows more diversity in data handling and has allowed us to carry through estimates of variance for all input variables in order to define a final estimate of variance for $\overline{\text{EFP}}$ and L_pA for each rat.

B. Assumptions of Existing Models of Ultrafiltration

    The present models utilized to determine $\overline{\text{EFP}}$ and L_pA (or K_f) reduce the parallel channels of the normal glomerular capillary to a single conduit of constant diameter and unit length, x^* (Deen *et al.*, 1972; Blantz, 1974). Based upon mathematical models, increases in RPF are applied to an increase in linear flow in a single conduit. However, in reality, RPF could also increase if flow was augmented by recruitment in capillaries with low or negligible flow. If the efferent effective filtration pressure was positive in the control condition, and remained constant after an increase in RPF, the model would conclude that SNGFR increased due to an increase in L_pA. However, these findings would also obtain if parallel conduits were recruited; a somewhat different biologic interpretation.

    The mathematical models assume also that L_p, hydraulic permeability, remains relatively constant along x^* and that L_p and L_pA are not functions of the other variables (π_A, ΔP, and RPF). It remains possible that within certain limits, L_pA may be a function of either ΔP or RPF, through variations in capillary surface area (A) (Blantz *et al.*, 1974; Tucker and Blantz, 1977b). Baylis and co-workers (1976) have recently provided objective data that L_pA (or K_f) is a function of π_A. Such a relationship between π_A and L_pA was also suggested by the studies of Blantz *et al.* (1974) and Blantz (1974) where increases in protein concentration with hyperoncotic albumin infusion were associated with increased L_pA (Blantz *et al.*, 1974) and acute reductions in protein concentration following mannitol infusion resulting in reductions in L_pA (Blantz, 1974). The fact that L_pA may be a function of π_A does not invalidate the application of mathematical models of filtration. However, if L_pA is a function of π, then L_p should increase along x^* due to the normal rise in π with ultrafiltration. Within certain limits, this should introduce some inaccuracy into the quantitative assessment of L_pA and the specific profile of the EFP curve along x^*. If the specific function describing the relationship of π and L_pA were known, this problem would again be circumvented and the profile could be defined with an acceptable, quantitative accuracy.

It is possible for the EFP profiles and L_pA determination to be affected by factors other than specific changes in A and the hydraulic permeability (L_p) of the capillary membrane. Concentration polarization occurs when there are significant differences between protein concentration (C) at the capillary membrane (C_m) and the axial flow at the center of the capillary lumen (C_1) at any value x^* (Deen *et al.*, 1974). These differences are due to the fact that ultrafiltration proceeds only at the capillary membrane and that albumin and globulin have finite diffusivities. The RPF, π_A, ΔP, and L_pA all can influence the magnitude of concentration polarization. The efferent arteriolar collections of blood are therefore admixtures of plasma at the capillary membrane (C_m) and at the central core flow (C_1). The greater the tendency for concentration polarization $(C_m \gg C_1)$ (decreased RPF, increased ΔP, and reduced π_A), the lower the calculated value for L_pA and the lower the absolute filtration at the capillary membrane. These effects are not artifacts, but real physiologic influences upon the filtration process, which affect measured and effective L_pA independent of real changes in either the structural characteristics of the capillary membrane or the total filtering surface area.

The last major limitation inherent to present techniques and methods of data analysis is the evaluation of the respective variables, hydraulic permeability (L_p), and effective surface area (A). Although the product of these two factors can be often defined with accuracy (L_pA), the respective contribution of L_p and A to change in L_pA cannot be readily assessed with available methods. Defining the meaning of A becomes difficult, since the area outside the capillary, on the epithelial surface, which is in contact with an aqueous phase cannot be determined, and changes in this potential variable are beyond the scope of the present quantitative methods. At present, it is rather pointless to make judgments as to whether changes in total hydraulic permeability result from variations in either L_p or A, since quantitative separation of these variables has not been accomplished.

VI. METHODS BASED UPON THE SIEVING OF MACROMOLECULES

During the past several years, there has been interest in the patterns of sieving of macromolecules by the kidney, as determined from the measurement of fractional clearances of macromolecules of a broad range of Stokes–Einstein radii (Robson *et al.*, 1974; Verniory *et al.*, 1973). Based upon the mathematical relationships proposed by Renkin and Collimore (1973) and Pappenheimer (1953), evaluation of sieving curves for macromolecules from 18 to 42 Å in size should permit an estimate of "pore size" which in turn can be utilized to determine a permeability coefficient for the kidney. Since the total glomerular filtration rate can be readily measured, a mean effective filtration pressure could also be determined (Lambert *et al.*, 1975). However, the specific profile of effective filtration pressure cannot be determined without a specific value for ΔP and π_A.

The specific fractional clearances of molecules between 18 and 42 Å radius are determined by both diffusional and convective forces (the larger the radius, the more important the diffusional component) (Chang *et al.*, 1975a). Recent studies have also shown that the charge of the macromolecule also markedly influences the fractional clearance (negatively charged macromolecules having reduced clearances when compared to neutral macromolecules) (Chang *et al.*, 1975b). The recent studies of Chang and co-workers have demonstrated that when evaluating changes in sieving profiles, the specific hemodynamic parameters, which define the effective filtration pressure (RPF, ΔP, and π_A) must be considered (Chang *et al.*, 1975c). These factors directly and significantly affect the fractional clearance of macromolecules independent of changes in radius of "pores," length of "pore" channel, and total filtering surface area. Therefore, interpretation of sieving profiles and changes in fractional clearances of macromolecules cannot be interpreted accurately in the absence of specific data on RPF, ΔP, and π_A.

VII. SUMMARY

Recent developments of microsystems for the evaluation of flows, hydrostatic and oncotic pressures within the surface glomeruli of the Munich–Wistar rat have produced rapid, recent advances in our understanding of the physiology of glomerular ultrafiltration. We have outlined some of the potential errors and limitations of the techniques. Application of such micromethods in renal physiologic laboratories will hopefully broaden the available techniques which can be applied to the analysis in both basic glomerular physiology and clinical models of disorders of glomerular ultrafiltration.

REFERENCES

Andreucci, V. E., Herrera-Acosta, J., Rector, F. C., Jr., and Seldin, D. W. 1971. Measurement of single nephron filtration rate by micropuncture: Analysis of error. *Am. J. Physiol., 222:*1551.
Barratt, L. J., Wallin, J. D., Rector, F. C., Jr., and Seldin, D. W. 1973. Influence of volume expansion on single nephron filtration rate and plasma flow in the rat. *Am. J. Physiol., 224:*643.
Baylis, C., Deen, W. M., Myers, B. D., and Brenner, B. M. 1976. Effects of some vasodilator drugs on transcapillary fluid exchange in the renal cortex. *Am. J. Physiol., 230:*1148.
Barger, A. C. 1966. Renal hemodynamic factors in congestive heart failure. *Ann. N.Y. Acad. Sci., 139:*279.
Blantz, R. C. 1974. Effect of mannitol on glomerular ultrafiltration in the hydropenic rat. *J. Clin. Invest., 54:*1135.
Blantz, R. C. 1975. The mechanism of acute renal failure after uranyl nitrate. *J. Clin. Invest., 55:*621.
Blantz, R. C., and Tucker, B. J. 1975. Determinants of peritubular capillary fluid uptake in hydropenia and saline and plasma expansion. *Am. J. Physiol., 228:*1927.
Blantz, R. C., Israelit, A. H., Rector, F. C., Jr., and Seldin, D. W. 1972. The relation of distal tubular NaCl delivery and glomerular hydrostatic pressure. *Kidney Int., 2:*22.
Blantz, R. C., Rector, F. C., Jr., and Seldin, D. W. 1974. The effect of hyperoncotic albumin expansion upon glomerular ultrafiltration in the rat. *Kidney Int., 6:*209.

Blantz, R. C., Konnen, K. S., and Tucker, B. J. 1975. Glomerular filtration response to elevated ureteral pressure in both the hydropenic and plasma expanded rat. *Circ. Res.*, 37:819.

Blantz, R. C., Konnen, K. S., and Tucker, B. J. 1976. Angiotensin II effects upon the glomerular microcirculation and ultrafiltration coefficient of the rat. *J. Clin. Invest.*, 57:419.

Brenner, B. M., and Galla, J. H. 1971. Influence of postglomerular hematocrit and protein concentration on rat nephron fluid transfer. *Am. J. Physiol.*, 220:148.

Brenner, B. M., Falchuk, K. H., Keimowitz, R. I., and Berliner, R. W. 1969. Relationship between peritubular capillary protein concentration and fluid reabsorption by the renal proximal tubule. *J. Clin. Invest.*, 48:1519.

Brenner, B. M., Troy, J. L., and Daugharty, T. M. 1971. The dynamics of glomerular ultrafiltration in the rat. *J. Clin. Invest.*, 50:1776.

Brenner, B. M., Troy, J. L., Daugharty, T. M., Deen, W. M., and Robertson, C. R. 1972. Dynamics of glomerular ultrafiltration in the rat. II. Plasma flow dependence of GFR. *Am. J. Physiol.*, 223:1184.

Chang, R. L. S., Robertson, C. R., Deen, W. M., and Brenner, B. M. 1975a. Permselectivity of the glomerular capillary wall to macromolecules. I. Theoretical considerations. *Biophys. J.*, 15:861.

Chang, R. L. S., Deen, W. M., Robertson, C. R., and Brenner, B. M. 1975b. Permselectivity of the glomerular capillary wall. III. Restricted transport of polyanions. *Kidney Int.*, 8:212.

Chang, R. L. S., Ueki, I. F., Troy, J. L., Deen, W. M., Robertson, C. R., and Brenner, B. M. 1975c. Permselectivity of the glomerular capillary wall to macromolecules. II. Experimental studies in rats using neutral dextrans. *Biophys. J.*, 15:887.

Davidman, M., Lalone, R. C., Alexander, E. A., and Levinsky, N. G. 1971. Some micropuncture techniques in the rat. *Am. J. Physiol.*, 221:1110.

Deen, W. M., Robertson, C. R., and Brenner, B. M. 1972. A model of glomerular ultrafiltration in the rat. *Am. J. Physiol.*, 223:1178.

Deen, W. M., Troy, J. L., Robertson, C. R., and Brenner, B. M. 1974. Dynamics of glomerular ultrafiltration in the rat. IV. Determination of the ultrafiltration coefficient. *J. Clin. Invest.*, 52:1500.

Deen, W. M., Robertson, C. R., and Brenner, B. M. 1974. Concentration polarization in an ultrafiltering capillary. *Biophys. J.*, 14:412.

Falchuk, K. H., Brenner, B. M., Tadokoro, M., and Berliner, R. W. 1971. Oncotic and hydrostatic pressures in peritubular capillaries and fluid reabsorption by proximal tubules. *Am. J. Physiol.*, 220:1427.

Gertz, K. H., Mangos, J. A., Braun, G., and Pagel, H. D. 1966. Pressure in the glomerular capillaries of the rat kidney in relation to arterial blood pressure. *Arch. Ges. Phys.*, 228:369.

Gottschalk, C. W., and Mylle, M. 1957. Micropuncture study of pressures in proximal and distal tubules and peritubular capillaries of the rat kidney during osmotic diuresis. *Am. J. Physiol.*, 189:323.

Herrera-Acosta, J., Andreucci, V. E., Rector, F. C., Jr., and Seldin, D. W. 1972. Effect of expansion of extracellular volume on single nephron filtration rates in the rat. *Am. J. Physiol.*, 222:938.

Hierholzer, K., Butz, M., Müller-Suur, R., and Lichtenstein, I. 1972. Pressure measurements in proximal surface tubules of the rat, single nephron filtration rate and tubulo-glomerular feedback. *Yale J. Biol. Med.*, 45:224.

Horster, M., and Thurau, K. 1968. Micropuncture studies on the filtration rate of single superficial and juxtamedullary glomeruli in the rat kidney. *Pflügers Arch.*, 301:162.

Intaglietta, M., Pavola, R. F., and Tompkins, W. R. 1970. Pressure measurements in the mammalian vasculature. *Microvasc. Res.*, 2:212.

Israelit, A. H., Rector, F. C., Jr., and Seldin, D. W. 1973. The influence of perfusate composition and perfusion rate on glomerular capillary hydrostatic pressure. *Am. Soc. Nephrol.*, 6:53.

Jaenicke, J. R. 1970. The renal response to ureteral obstruction. A model for the study of factors which influence glomerular filtration pressure. *J. Lab. Clin. Med.*, 76:373.

Lambert, P. P., Verniory, A., Gassée, J. P., and Ficheroulle, A. 1972. Sieving equations and effective glomerular filtration pressure. *Kidney Int.*, 2:131.

Lambert, P. P., DuBois, R., DeCoodt, P., Gassé, J. P., and Vernior, A. 1975. Determination of glomerular intracapillary and transcapillary pressure gradients from sieving data. II. A physiological study in the normal dog. *Pflügers Arch., 359:*1.

Landis, E. M. 1926. The capillary pressure in the frog mesentery as determined by micro-injection. *Am. J. Physiol., 75:*548.

Landis, E. M., and Pappenheimer, J. R. 1964. Exchange of substances through the capillary walls. In: *Handbook of Physiology,* Section 2, Circulation, pp. 961–1034. Ed. by Orloff, J., and Berliner, R., American Physiological Society, Washington, D.C.

Lewy, J. E., and Windhager, E. E. 1968. Peritubular control of proximal tubular fluid reabsorption in the rat kidney. *Am. J. Physiol., 214:*943.

Lowry, O. H., Rosebrough, N. J., Farr, A. L., and Randall, R. J. 1951. Protein measurement with the Folin phenol reagent. *J. Biol. Chem., 193:*265.

Ludwig, C. 1843. *Beiträge zur Lehre von Mechanisms der Harnsecretion.* N. G. Elwert, Marburg.

Ludwig, C. 1861. *Lehrbuch der Physiologie des Menschen.* C. F. Wintersche, Verlagshandlung, Heidelberg.

Maddox, D. A., Deen, W. M., and Brenner, B. M. 1974. Dynamics of glomerular ultrafiltration: VI. Studies in the primate. *Kidney Int., 5:*271.

Maddox, D. A., Bennett, C. M., Deen, W. M., Glassock, R. J., Knutson, D., Daugharty, T. M., and Brenner, B. M. 1975. Determinants of glomerular filtration in experimental glomerulonephritis in the rat. *J. Clin. Invest., 55:*305.

Martin, J. B., Harris, C. A., and Dirks, J. H. 1974. Evidence of GH deficiency in the Munich–Wistar rat. *Endocrin., 94:*1359.

Navar, L. G. 1970. Minimal preglomerular resistance and calculation of normal glomerular pressure. *Am. J. Physiol., 219:*1658.

Navar, L. G., Bungorn, C., and Bell, P. D. 1975. Absence of estimated glomerular pressure autoregulation during interrupted distal delivery. *Am. J. Physiol., 229:*1596.

O'Dorisio, T. M., Stein, J. H., Osgood, R. W., and Ferris, T. F. 1973. Absence of aglomerular blood flow during renal vasodilation and hemorrhage in the dog. *Proc. Soc. Exp. Biol. Med., 143:*612.

Pappenheimer, J. R. 1953. Passage of molecules through capillary walls. *Physiol. Rev., 33:*387.

Renkin, E. M., and Gilmore, J. P. 1973. Glomerular filtration. In: *Handbook of Physiology,* Section 8, Renal Physiology, pp. 185–248. Ed. by Orloff, J. and Berliner, R. American Physiological Society, Washington, D.C.

Richards, A. N. 1939. Process of urine formation: Croonian lecture, *Proc. Roy. Soc. London (Biol.), 126:*398.

Robson, A. M., Giangiacomo, J., Kienstra, K. A., Naqvi, S. T., and Ingelfinger, J. R. 1974. Normal glomerular permeability and its modification by minimal change nephrotic syndrome, *J. Clin. Invest., 54:*1190.

Schnermann, J., Wright, F. S., Davis, J. M., Stackelberg, W. v., and Grill, G. 1971a. Regulation of superficial nephron filtration rate by tubulo-glomerular feedback. *Pflügers Arch., 346:*263.

Schnermann, J., Davis, J. M., Wunderlich, P., Levine, D. Z., and Horster, M. 1971b. Technical problems in the micropuncture determination of nephron filtration rate and their functional implications. *Pflügers Arch., 329:*307.

Schnermann, J., Persson, A. E. G., and Agerup, B. 1973. Tubuloglomerular feedback. Nonlinear relation between glomerular hydrostatic pressure and loop of Henle perfusion rate. *J. Clin. Invest., 52:*862.

Smith, H. W. 1937. *The Physiology of the Kidney.* Oxford University Press, Oxford.

Smith, H. W. 1951. *The Kidney: Structure and Function in Health and Disease.* Oxford University Press, New York.

Smith, H. W., and Clarke, R. W. 1938. The excretion of inulin and creatinine by the anthropoid apes and other infrahuman primates. *Am. J. Physiol., 122:*132.

Smith, H. W., Chasis, H., Goldring, W., and Ranges, H. A. 1940. Glomerular dynamics in the normal human kidney. *J. Clin. Invest., 19:*751.

Stein, J. H., Rieneck, J. H., Osgood, R. W., and Ferris, T. F. 1971. Effect of acetylcholine on proximal tubular reabsorption in the dog. *Am. J. Physiol., 220:*227.

Thurau, K. 1964. Renal hemodynamics. *Am. J. Med., 36:*698.

Tucker, B. J., and Blantz, R. C. 1977a. Factors determining superficial nephron filtration in the mature growing rat. *Am. J. Physiol. 232:*F97.

Tucker, B. J. and Blantz, R. C. 1977b. An analysis of the determinants of nephron filtration rate (sngfr). *Am. J. Physiol. 232:*F477.

Verniory, A., DuBois, R., DeCoodt, P., Gassée, J. P., and Lambert, P. P. 1973. Measurement of the permeability of biological membranes: Application to the glomerular wall. *J. Gen. Physiol., 62:*489.

Wiederhielm, C. A., Woodbury, J. W., Kirk, S., and Rushmer, R. F. 1964. Pulsatile pressures in the microcirculation of frog's mesentery. *Am. J. Physiol., 207:*173.

Wunderlich, P., and Schnermann, J. 1969. Continuous recording of hydrostatic pressure in renal tubules and blood capillaries by use of a new pressure transducer, *Pflügers Arch., 313:*89.

Chapter **7**

Electrophysiological Measurements on the Renal Tubule

Emile L. Boulpaep and G. Giebisch

Department of Physiology
Yale University School of Medicine
New Haven, Connecticut

I. INTRODUCTION

The topic of electrical phenomena in the nephron has been surveyed in several recent reviews (Boulpaep, 1972b, 1976a,b; Frömter, 1972a, 1974; Giebisch and Windhager, 1973). These reviews are concerned, in general, with a discussion of electrical potential difference and conductance measurements across the epithelium of single renal tubules and their physiological interpretation. This chapter will emphasize technical aspects of electrophysiological measurements as they apply to the particular circumstances of renal tubule epithelium. In contrast to other epithelia where both cell boundaries are easily accessible to voltage-measuring or current-carrying electrodes, the geometry of renal tubules leads to a number of special problems. These have to do with the small size of the luminal fluid compartment, with the inaccessibility of certain nephron segments from the kidney surface *in vivo*, and with the frequent lack of mechanical and electrical stability of the tubular epithelium. Attempts to overcome these difficulties have centered on the use of luminal and peritubular microperfusion methods *in vivo*, the isolation of single tubular segments *in vitro*, and the use of tissue slices.

II. MICROELECTRODE TECHNIQUES

A. Electrolyte-Filled Micropipets

The Ling and Gerard (1949) microelectrode of less than 1 μm tip diameter, first introduced for the determination of transmembrane potential differences in single muscle fibers, has been the main tool for both transepithelial and single cell membrane electrical recordings in kidney tubules. The manufacture, the electrochemical properties, and the application of these microelectrodes have been extensively reviewed (Frank and Becker, 1964; Curtis, 1964; Geddes, 1972; Agin, 1969; Snell, 1969; Ferris, 1974; Bures *et al.*, 1976; Kuriyama and Ito, 1975). Two modifications of the Ling–Gerard electrode are potentially useful. (1) In view of the small cell size, particularly of mammalian tubular cells, very fine-tipped microelectrodes are advisable for intracellular impalements. Since such electrodes frequently have exceptionally high resistance and large tip potentials, attempts should be made to reduce partially the tip resistance by mechanical beveling (Brown and Flaming, 1974). (2) Using a different approach, recent attempts have also been made to overcome the problems related to the condition of a nonflowing liquid junction at the tip of the microelectrodes. Therefore, relatively large (2–11 μm outside diameter, o.d.), sharpened micropipets have been employed for transepithelial potential measurements (Barratt *et al.*, 1974, 1975; Frömter and Hegel, 1966; Hayslett *et al.*, 1976; Hegel *et al.*, 1967; Laurence and Marsh, 1971; Rau and Frömter, 1974a; Wilbrandt, 1938). These electrodes offer the advantage that they can be filled with solutions of lower electrolyte concentration, even with solutions approaching the composition of the relevant biological compartment which they are impaling.

A large number of filling techniques are available (Ling and Gerard, 1949; Nastuk, 1953; Tasaki *et al.*, 1954; Caldwell and Downing, 1955; Kennard, 1958; Curtis and Eccles, 1958; Kao, 1954; Duling and Berne, 1969; Zettler, 1970; Tasaki *et al.*, 1968; Cerf and Cerf, 1974; Biagi and Garcia-Filho, 1977). In order to avoid large tip potentials, preference should be given to those methods that do not involve a heating step. Appropriate and specific filling solutions will be discussed below. Multibarreled electrodes are useful for simultaneous voltage and current recordings and for cellular ion injection (Coombs *et al.*, 1955; del Castillo and Katz, 1957; Kennard, 1958; Vis, 1954). Recently, some useful special glass types have become available commercially, such as double-barreled theta-glass (R.D. Optical Systems, Inc., Spencerville, Md.) and "μ fiber" (omega dot) microcapillaries (Frederick Haer and Co., Ann Arbor, Mich.). A schematic description of cellular electrode impalement using Ling–Gerard microelectrodes is given in Figure 1.

B. Metal Microelectrodes

Axial insertion of metal wires for potential recording and current application was first made on nerve axons (Marmont, 1949; Cole, 1949; Hodgkin *et al.*, 1952). If metal electrodes are to be used, nonpolarizable reversible half cells should be employed to avoid electrolysis and gas formation within the prepara-

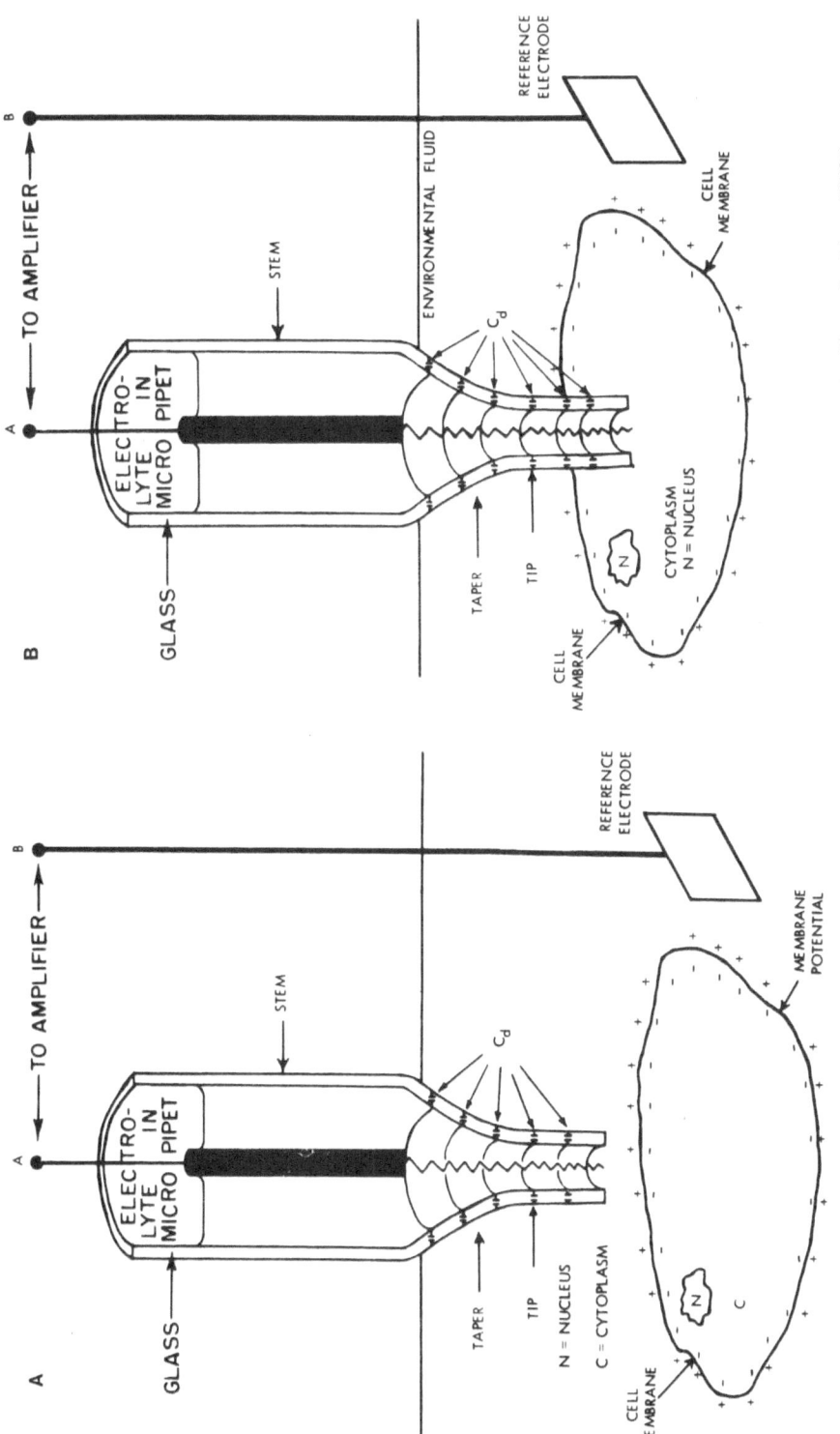

Figure 1. (A) Micropipet tip located outside a cell. (B) Micropipet tip located inside a cell. (From Geddes, 1972.)

tion during current passage. For potential recording, half cells are used in contact with solutions containing a soluble salt of the anion combining with the metal, e.g., silver–silver chloride electrodes in the presence of a chloride-containing solution. Spring and Paganelli (1972) and Spring (1972) developed an axial electrode made of 5–10 μm o.d. tungsten wire which was platinized and inserted into long straight segments of *Necturus* proximal tubule (Figure 2). The method permits current to pass across the epithelia although a platinum electrode can only be considered nonpolarizable for small current strengths. Electrical insulation is obtained by insulating columns of oil as shown in Figure 2. Current flow is restricted to the area of the split drop containing Ringer's solution. Transepithelial potential differences cannot be determined by means of a platinum electrode in view of the variable electrode potential at the metal–liquid interface. Hegel and Boulpaep (1975) used a hybrid Ag–AgCl filament electrode (15 μm o.d.) for both a-c current application and d-c transepithelial potential recording.

Electrical recordings on isolated perfused tubules are usually performed by means of large metal electrodes where the metal–liquid contact is made in the perfusion or collection pipet system. Insertion of an electrode into the lumen of the tubule segment itself may be appropriate for two-electrode applications of resistance measurements. Lutz *et al.* (1973) coated the outer surface of a

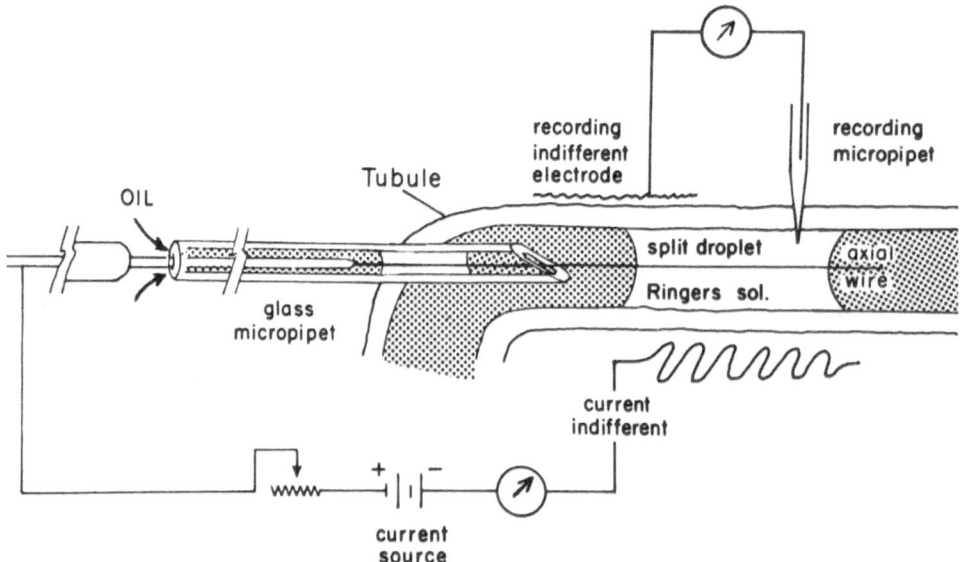

Figure 2. Electrode arrangement for voltage clamping of an injected droplet. The variable resistor in the circuit enables control of the current so that the potential difference is held at the desired value. The current-indifferent electrode is a large platinum wire lying under the kidney; the current record is displayed on an ammeter. The axial wire is moved hydraulically across the droplet, and additional droplets may be injected from the micropipet after reabsorption occurs. The voltage-recording micropipet is a 3 M KCl-filled glass microelectrode, the recording indifferent is a calomel wick electrode. Voltage is recorded by an electrometer–voltmeter–oscilloscope combination. (From Spring, 1972.)

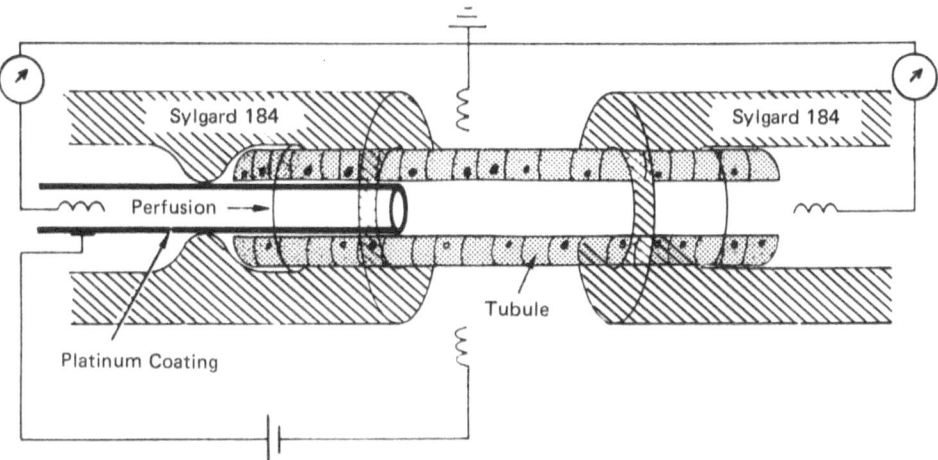

Figure 3. Arrangement for measuring transepithelial potential difference and resistance in isolated tubules using a single pipet coated with platinum black. (From Lutz *et al.*, 1973.)

perfusion pipet with platinum black for passing current and employed the core of the electrolyte-filled pipet for voltage recording (Figure 3).

C. Ion-Selective Microelectrodes

Ion-selective microelectrodes have been of three general types: metal, glass, and liquid ion-exchanger electrodes.

1. Metal Microelectrodes

pH-sensitive antimony microelectrodes have been arranged within single-barreled pipets (Malnic and Vieira, 1972; Malnic *et al.*, 1974) and within double-barreled pipets (Green and Giebisch, 1974). The properties and potential artifacts have been carefully defined (Malnic and Vieira, 1972; Malnic *et al.*, 1974; Green and Giebisch, 1974; Karlmark, 1973; Puschett and Zurbach, 1974; Caflish *et al.*, in press; Giebisch *et al.*, 1977; Quehenberger *et al.*, in press). These electrodes have been used (1) for the measurement of intratubular pH *in situ* in either free-flow or split-drop condition; (2) for the determination of pH of small collected fluid samples; and (3) for titration of small fluid samples to estimate titratable acid (Karlmark, 1973; Green and Giebisch, 1974). Chloride ion-selective metal microelectrodes have been developed for intracellular chloride activity determination in snail neurons (Neild and Thomas, 1973), but have not yet been used in renal tubules. Hegel and Boulpaep (unpublished) used an Ag-AgCl axial wire in the lumen of *Necturus* proximal tubule for intratubular chloride activity determination.

2. Glass Ion-Selective Microelectrodes

Glass ion-selective microelectrodes have been developed for the measurement of H^+, Na^+, and K^+ activities. The application of pH-sensitive glass electrodes to the measurement of tubular pH is discussed in Chapter 8 of this volume (Carter and Pucacco), and was reviewed by Khuri (1976). Carter and Pucacco, Hinke (1959), and Thomas (1974, 1976) have developed spear-type and recessed-tip glass electrodes for intracellular pH determinations. Cellular pH measurements on renal tubular cells have not yet been carried out. With respect to the measurement of Na activities, spear-type glass electrodes with sodium selectivity have also become available. Khuri *et al.* (1963) measured sodium activity *in situ* in small renal blood vessels, Bowman's capsule, and the lumen of proximal tubules. Miniaturization of sodium selective microelectrodes has been successfully accomplished by Thomas (1970, 1972, 1976) for measurement of intracellular sodium activity, but has not yet been applied to the kidney. Potassium-selective electrodes of the spear type were described (Hinke, 1959; Khuri *et al.*, 1963) and applied to the measurement of K activity of glomerular and tubular fluid *in vitro* (Khuri *et al.*, 1963). Khuri *et al.* (1968) have also described a flowthrough internal capillary glass microelectrode with potassium selectivity to measure tubular fluid activity.

3. Liquid Ion-Exchanger Microelectrodes

Liquid ion-exchanger microelectrodes are presently available for the determination of sodium, lithium, potassium, chloride, and bicarbonate. They consist of an organic electrolyte, dissolved in an organic solvent, and selective for a given ion species. Essentially, the liquid ion exchanger is introduced in the tip of a conventional Ling–Gerard-type microelectrode before impalements, and voltage measurements are carried out. Electrodes of this type are easier to manufacture than either glass recessed-tip or spear-type microelectrodes. The design of both single-barrel and double-barrel liquid ion-exchanger microelectrodes has been described (Khuri, 1976). The advantage of using double-barreled microelectrodes is the possibility of measuring intracellular electrical potentials at the same site as the intracellular ionic potential and thus to correct accurately for the electrical potential difference across the cell membrane.

Liquid ion-exchanger microelectrodes have been developed for measurements of lithium and sodium activities (Thomas *et al.*, 1975) but have not yet been applied to the study of electrolyte activity in the renal tubule. On the other hand, microelectrodes filled with a potassium-selective liquid ion exchanger (Walker, 1971; Khuri, 1972; Khuri *et al.*, 1971, 1972b) have been successfully applied to the measurement of cellular activities of single tubule cells both in the mammalian (Khuri, 1972; Khuri *et al.*, 1971, 1972a, 1974a) and amphibian tubule (Khuri, 1972c; Fujimoto *et al.*, 1977). It is important to note that the intracellular potassium activities have uniformly been found to be significantly less than the chemically measured concentration of cell potassium.

Cellular activities of chloride have been similarly measured by making use of chloride-sensitive liquid ion exchangers (Khuri *et al.*, 1975; Sohtell, in press; Fujimoto *et al.*, 1976; Spring and Kimura, 1977). These chloride measurements have accurately described the electrochemical potential difference of chloride across both the peritubular and luminal cell membrane of proximal and distal tubules. Finally, Khuri *et al.* (1974b) have measured intracellular bicarbonate activity in single cells of *Necturus* proximal tubules. The key observation is the finding of a relatively high bicarbonate concentration, necessitating an active cellular hydrogen-ion extrusion mechanism.

A different approach for manufacturing a sodium-selective liquid ion-exchange microelectrode was taken by Kraig and Nicholson (1976). A biologically synthesized compound, monensin, was introduced into presiliconized micropipets. These electrodes exhibit adequate sodium selectivity.

In view of the very high resistance of both glass and liquid exchanger ion-selective microelectrodes, it is necessary to record the potential differences by means of electrometers with higher input impedance than that necessary for electrolyte-filled Ling–Gerard electrodes. Garcia *et al.* (1976) have recently utilized a special electrometer (W.P. Instrument F-23B) which fulfills these requirements.

III. KIDNEY PREPARATIONS

A variety of renal preparations have been found useful for electrical measurements. Many of the problems are similar to those met in *in vivo* micropuncture (Greger *et al.*, Chapter 5, this volume), isolated perfused kidneys (Kaloyanides *et al.*, Chapter 13, this volume), isolated perfused tubules (Chonko *et al.*, Chapter 9, this volume), and renal cortical slices (Whittembury, 1965). Each approach offers specific advantages and limitations. It is often desirable to be able to control the composition of both luminal and peritubular fluid compartments. This can be achieved *in vivo* by simultaneous vascular and tubular microperfusion (Ullrich *et al.*, 1969; Spitzer and Windhager, 1970), or more conveniently by the use of isolated perfused tubules (Chonko *et al.*, Chapter 9). An alternative approach uses perfused kidneys (Seely and Boulpaep, 1971) and particularly amphibian preparations with dual blood supply (Giebisch, 1961) (see Figure 4).

With respect to the electrical study of specific nephron segments *in vivo*, mammalian preparations are only adequate for measurements on cortical and some selected papillary tubular structures. Concerning amphibian tubules, *Necturus* has been extensively used for measurements on proximal tubules (Giebisch, 1961) and *Amphiuma* for distal tubules (Sullivan, 1968). Other nephron segments can be studied by isolation of single tubules from subcortical areas (Chonko *et al.*, Chapter 9). Cortical slices offer appreciable stability but are limited to studies on average transmembrane potentials of single tubule cells (Whittembury, 1965).

In order to measure *transepithelial* potential differences over long time periods, methods applied to isolated tubules using an axial perfusion pipet as

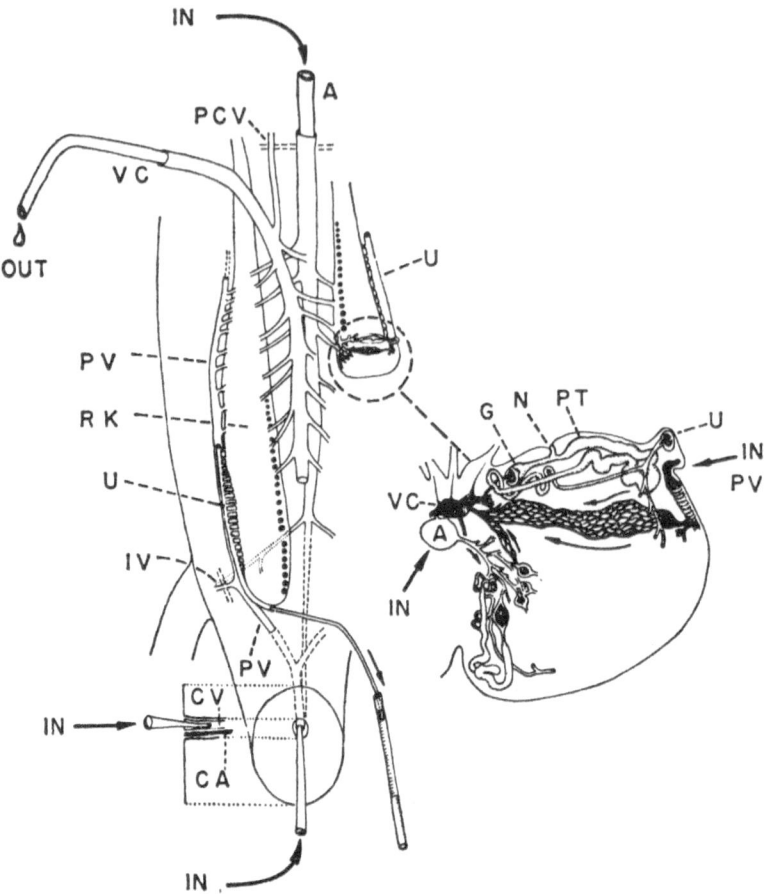

Figure 4. Schematic representation of the kidney perfusion in a male *Necturus*. The right kidney (RK) is shown. Catheters are placed in the aorta (A) and caudal vein (CV) for inflow (IN) of perfusion fluids. The inset (bottom left) shows how the caudal vein catheter occludes the caudal artery (CA). The caudal vein drains into the portal veins (PV) that flow along the lateral aspect of the kidneys dorsal to the ureter (U). The cephalic portion of the right ureter has been removed to show the portal vein (PV) more clearly. A small cannula inserted in the caudal portion of the ureter is used to collect urine in a glass capillary. The catheter in the vena cava (VC) for outflow of perfusion fluid is shown. Ligatures around the iliac vessels (IV) and around the cephalic end of the pelvic portion of the kidneys to obstruct the posterior cardinal veins (PCV) are indicated by two parallel lines. Part of the left kidney has been removed. The inset (right) illustrates how in the *Necturus* the fluid perfused via the portal vein circulates along the peritubular capillaries and bathes the peritubular spaces before draining into the VC. The fluid perfused via the aorta goes into the glomerulus (G) and drains into the VC after flowing through very short capillaries. N, nephrostome; PT, proximal tubule. (From Whittembury, 1972.)

recording electrode obviate the need for transepithelial impalement, which might introduce damage and leaks. Stable *cellular* potential recordings require a reasonable large cell size and stability, both of which are more easily attained in amphibian preparation such as *Necturus* (Giebisch, 1961), *Amphiuma* (Sullivan, 1968), *Triturus* (Hoshi and Sakai, 1967; Maruyama and Hoshi, 1972) and

Ambystoma (Sackin and Boulpaep, 1976). Some special aspects of accessibility, visualization, and mechanical stability of renal preparation for electrophysiological study have been reviewed (Boulpaep, 1972b; Ullrich *et al.*, 1969).

IV. MEASUREMENT OF POTENTIAL DIFFERENCES

A. Technical Problems

Despite the great variety of electrode arrangements used for different preparations, a problem common to all systems is the possible existence of electrical asymmetries, giving rise to an overall potential difference unrelated to the epithelium under study. Whichever recording or reference electrodes are used, a number of electrode potentials and diffusion potentials appear in series with the biological potential difference to be determined. The principle most commonly used is to arrange similar junctions on both sides of the epithelium, i.e., on the recording and the reference end, such that equal junctions of opposite sign cancel. Alternatively, the actual magnitude of dissimilar junctions should be determined separately.

Figure 5(A) illustrates the sequence of junctions typical for the use of electrolyte-filled microelectrodes and Figure 5(B) for the use of isolated tubule preparations. The interphases are numbered to indicate transitions between metal and liquid or between two liquids. Note three types of transitions.

1. At levels 1 and 2, and 10 and 11, a pair of half cells exist at the transition from solid to liquid phase. As long as identical metal electrodes on both ends are bathed with identical solutions as in Figure 5(A and B), the asymmetry cancels.

2. Since usually metal electrodes are bathed in high concentration electrolytes as, e.g., a calomel electrode in saturated KCl, the next transition will invariably involve a liquid interphase between a concentrated electrolyte solution and a solution of electrolyte strength similar to biological fluids. This would happen at junctions 3 or 4, depending on whether high concentration KCl or Ringer–agar bridges are used. Similarly, at the recording site, this type of junction would happen at interphase 8 for microelectrodes filled with KCl or K citrate (Rosenberg, 1973) [(see Figure 5(A)] or at interphase 8a or 9 for isolated tubule preparations, depending on the use of a KCl or Ringer bridge, respectively, within compartment 8a–9. Note that when macroelectrodes are used in *in vivo* preparations and are filled with Ringer's solution, junctions similar to Figure 5(B) apply, whereas macroelectrodes filled with KCl would essentially represent an arrangement similar to that in Figure 5(A). If the liquid–liquid junction potentials at each of these barriers 3 or 4 and 8, 8a, or 9 behave as truly flowing junctions, it is easily seen that (a) in Figure 5(A), junction 3 cancels 9, and 4 cancels 8 if lumen and bath have identical composition (or, if a Ringer–agar bridge was used in compartment 3–4, junction 3 cancels 8, assuming Ringer = bath = lumen or cytoplasm composition). (b) In Figure 5(B) junction 3 cancels 9, and 4 cancels 8a.

A special problem arises when one of the junctions between a concentrated

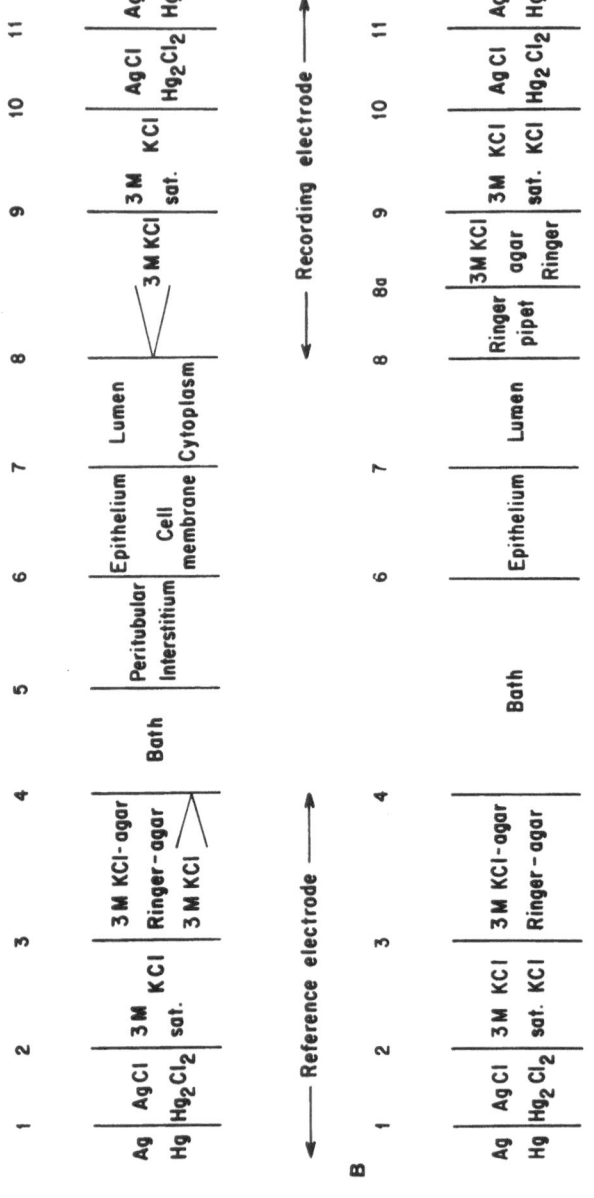

Figure 5. Schematic representation of the sequence of electrode, diffusion, and membrane potentials during measurement of transepithelial or transmembrane potential differences. (A) Arrangement frequently encountered during potential measurements using glass micropipets *in vivo*. (B) Arrangement frequently encountered during potential measurements using Ringer-filled micropipet to measure potential differences in isolated perfused tubules. (Modified from Boulpaep, 1972b.)

KCl and dilute solution does not balance as predicted by free solution ion mobilities. This is particularly the case for small Ling–Gerard microelectrodes where junction 8 of Figure 5(A) does not behave as a concentrated KCl bridge, but generates a unique asymmetry called "tip potential" of the microelectrode. Contrary to a KCl bridge, which is reasonably insensitive to the composition of the dilute compartment it is facing because of similar potassium and chloride ion mobilities, a microelectrode tip potential depends critically on the composition of compartment 7–8 (Adrian, 1956). Therefore it is essential to determine the tip potential, i.e., the potential difference of step 8 of Figure 5(A) for the various solutions which are experimentally perfusing the lumen. For free-flow conditions, tip potentials should be checked in solutions which mimic as closely as possible the tubular fluid. The problem of tip artifacts during intracellular impalements cannot be entirely overcome since cytoplasmic ionic activities are not known or cannot be artificially controlled. Errors of this type are thought to be minimized by the use of low-resistance microelectrodes with tip potentials in control Ringer's solution of less than 5 mV.

3. In the sequence of liquid–liquid junctions, additional biological compartments in series with the epithelium may differ in composition from the imposed perfusion media. A relevant example is the superfusion or peritubular perfusion of structures which are still surrounded by unstirred layers at a peritubular interstitium of different composition, for instance, as is likely in the renal papilla (Boulpaep, 1972b; Laurence and Marsh, 1971). These problems cannot be entirely avoided unless the composition of such an interstitial compartment is known or direct access to that compartment is made possible by means of a reference electrode at that site.

Changes in composition of the luminal (7–8) or bath (4–5) compartment are frequently carried out during potential or resistance measurements. The most favorable situation is probably that in which the transition at interphase 4 and 8 occurs between 3 M KCl and the modified bath or perfusion fluid. Nevertheless, time-dependent changes of these junctions may occur and salt dilutions or biionic junctions have been proposed instead because they are more independent of the actual concentration profile and time (Barry and Diamond, 1970).

Substitutions can be made in either peritubular bath or tubular lumen. (a) An alteration in composition of the *bath* or *peritubular perfusion* introduces a different potential difference at interphase 4. If the junction 4 is a truly flowing 3 M KCl junction, a change in bath composition will only slightly affect the asymmetry, and no correction would be required. If compartment 3–4 is not a flowing KCl junction but KCl-agar or Ringer-agar the change in junction potential should be determined. Calculation of ideal liquid junction potentials are often inadequate because free diffusion ion mobilities may not prevail. Experimental determination of junction potential 4 always requires another series arrangement of junctions and electrodes whose response to ion substitution is assumed to be known. In the absence of the epithelium, both reference and recording electrodes are placed in the bath. If the recording electrode side is an indifferent flowing KCl junction or a "known" liquid junction or a known metal-liquid junction, it is then possible to determine the response of junction 4 or the standard liquid potential expected between Ringer and the modified Ringer solution. An additional test may consist in using identical recording and reference electrodes, dipping them in the bath, and performing a bath composition switch. Symmetrical behavior is expected and no asymmetry should appear.

(b)An alteration in *luminal composition* when the sensitive electrode is a Ling-Gerard microelectrode requires the determination of the change in tip potential [junction 8 of Figure 5(A)] during luminal microperfusion. The microelectrode cannot be tested for tip potentials while inserted in the lumen. An *in vitro* test of possible tip potential changes should be performed, preferably before and after impalements. For example, the microelectrode is tested in a bath against a known reference system (flowing KCl junction, known liquid-liquid junction or liquid-metal junction), i.e., behavior of interphase 4 is now assumed to be known. Again, junctions are best minimized by the choice of an indifferent flowing KCl macroelectrode at interphase 4. The changes in overall asymmetry that result from specific ionic substitution in the *in vitro* system may be taken as the change in tip potential of the microelectrode. It is then assumed that the microelectrode, when located in the tubular lumen and exposed to similar perfusion fluid changes, would exhibit the same tip potential alterations. These tip potential changes are then subtracted from the total transepithelial potential reading.

(c) In isolated tubule preparations, luminal composition changes occur with a sensing electrode which is essentially large. However, corrections are also required. If tubular perfusion is fast enough so that the lumen remains identical in composition to the perfusion pipet, barrier 8 in Figure 5(B) may be neglected. The critical junction is now shifted back toward 8a. A composition change in compartment 8-8a when performed against 3 *M* KCl agar in compartment 8a-9 may approach that of the flowing KCl junction. However, this should be tested against a known reference, e.g., a 3 *M* KCl flowing electrode. More often, compartment 8a-9 contains control Ringer and a modified Ringer solution is applied to the perfusion pipet 8-8a; the change in junction 8a can be evaluated either in a bath which is also switched to contain modified Ringer, or directly against a 3 *M* KCl bath. Again, a final verification consists of an alteration in compartment 8-8a from control Ringer to modified Ringer, while both the bath and 8a-9 are filled with control Ringer. The latter situation should be symmetrical and cancel the asymmetry.

A problem particularly troublesome for all *in vivo* preparations, although in principle trivial, is the presence of spurious voltage effects caused by ground loops. These are frequently the result of electrical contacts of the kidney, abdominal cavity, or entire animal with grounded metal surfaces. A liquid-metal interphase develops which is different from the reference electrode and may result in unpredicted voltage changes. It is helpful to isolate electrically the preparation and to keep the resistance of the reference electrode assembly as low as possible.

Precise localization of the microelectrode tip within the renal epithelium is crucial. Several direct and indirect methods can be employed (Boulpaep, 1972b; Frömter, 1972a). The most convenient method for intraluminal localization relies on the observation of changes in transepithelial potential induced by luminal microperfusion with Ringer solutions modified in sodium and/or chloride concentrations (Boulpaep and Seely, 1971; Frömter *et al.*, 1971).

B. Transepithelial Potential Measurement

Figure 6 illustrates the methods for recording overall transepithelial potential differences. Such measurements can be carried out in free flow in cortical

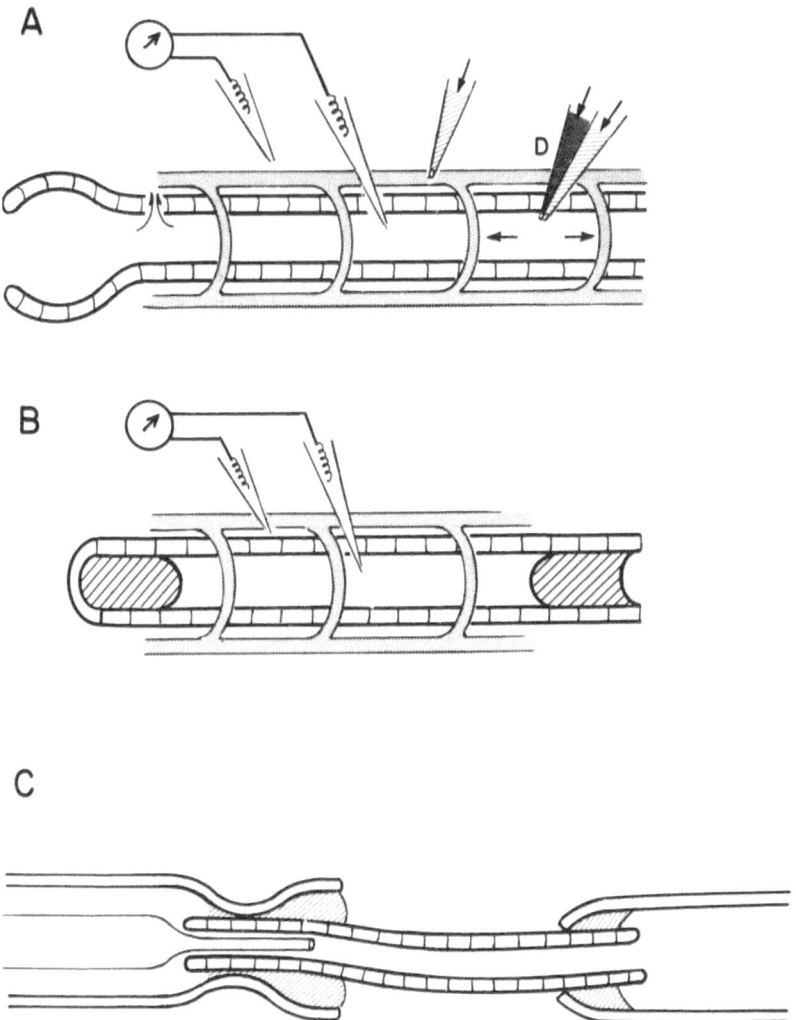

Figure 6. Methods for the measurement of transepithelial potential differences. (A) Potential measurement *in situ* during free flow. Recording and ground electrode on left. Double-barreled microperfusion pipet D (on right) can be used to perfuse a tubular segment with artificial solutions. In addition, it is possible to change the peritubular ionic environment by perfusion of peritubular capillaries surrounding the tubule. (B) Potential measurement as in (A) but during stationary microperfusion (split drop). (C) Potential measurement across isolated perfused tubular segment *in vitro*.

and medullary tubules between a single microelectrode impaling the lumen, and a reference electrode in an extratubular compartment in communication with the peritubular interstitium [Figure 6(A)]. By continuously microperfusing the lumen and/or the adjacent capillary network, one can either impose known ionic or osmotic gradients across the epithelium, or expose the given nephron segment to symmetrical solution changes (Windhager and Giebisch, 1965; Fromter, 1974; Boulpaep, 1976a,b).

Transepithelial potential differences can also be measured under stop-flow microperfusion conditions as shown in Figure 6(B) (Whittembury and Windhager, 1961; Maude, 1970; Spring and Paganelli, 1972; Malnic and Mello-Aires,

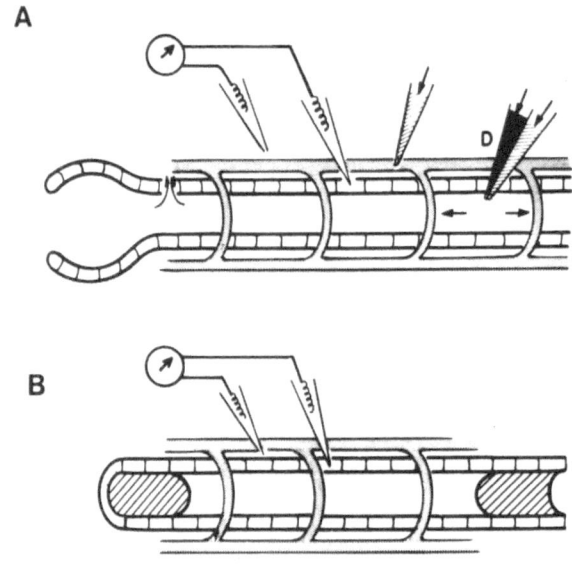

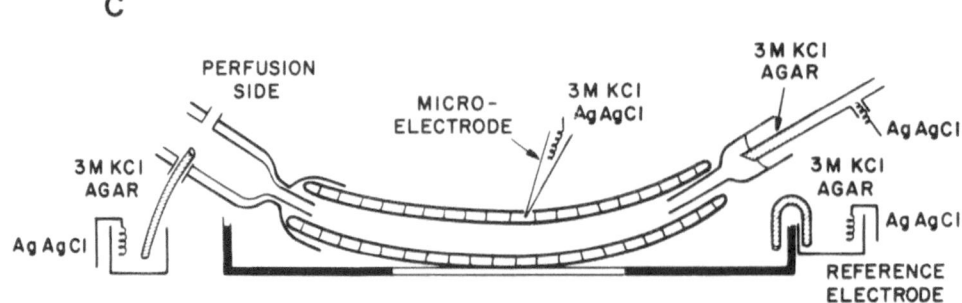

Figure 7. Methods for the measurement of transmembrane potential differences. (A) Cellular potential measurements *in situ* during free flow. Arrangement of recording and perfusion pipets similar to that in Figure 6. Note the intracellular position of the recording electrode tip. (B) Cellular potential measurement as in (A) but during stationary microperfusion (split drop). (C) Cellular potential measurement in perfused isolated tubule *in vitro*.

1971; Bentzel, 1974). It is noteworthy that with a limited small volume of the luminal compartment, it may be difficult to control its composition and hence to correct properly for junction potentials at the microelectrode tip, particularly when the luminal ionic contents change during the experimental procedure.

Finally, the method of measuring transepithelial potential differences has also been used in isolated perfused tubules as shown in Figure 6(C) (Burg and Orloff, 1970; Kokko and Rector, 1971; Lutz et al., 1973; Grantham et al., 1970; Helman et al., 1971; Schafer et al., 1974). The method has been greatly improved by the use of an insulating oil, Sylgard 184, at both the perfusion and collection end of the tubule. Special advantages of the perfused tubule preparation for transepithelial electrophysiological measurement are: (1) long-term stability due to the absence of leaks induced by the probing electrode itself, (2) the use of a relatively large recording electrode and hence the use of a low-resistance recording system, (3) the use of physiological solutions in the recording electrode [see Figure 5(B)] with avoidance of tip potential artifacts, (4) the ease with which luminal and extraluminal media can be rapidly altered.

The measurement of electrical potential differences across the total epithelial cell layer is useful to determine the driving force acting on individual ions under the simplifying assumption that only a single barrier represents the rate-limiting site. Knowledge of the chemical and electrical potential difference for a given ion, together with its partial conductance (see below), allows an estimate to be made of the passive flux of that particular ion. Furthermore, changes in the ion composition of the luminal or peritubular compartment, imposing either salt gradients or single ion gradients across the epithelium, allow the determination of artificially induced changes in transepithelial potential difference. From these changes in potential either transference numbers or relative permeability coefficients may be derived for specific ions. Imposition of osmotic gradients may result in the generation of apparent streaming potential differences which allow insight into the nature of electrical charges residing in the fluid pathway. In addition, diuretics, modifications of the metabolic rate, the presence or absence of cotransported organic solutes, changes in the diet or hormonal balance have been shown to influence the magnitude of the transepithelial potential differences. For reviews see Frömter (1974), Giebisch (1974), Boulpaep (1976a), Jacobson and Kokko (1976), and Burg (1976).

C. Transmembrane Potential Difference Measurement of Single Tubule Cells

Figure 7 illustrates the techniques for recording cell membrane potential differences in single tubule cells. Measurements of peritubular or basolateral cell membrane potential are obtained between a single microelectrode positioned in the cellular cytoplasm and a reference electrode in the bath (Figure 7). Luminal or apical cell membrane potentials can be measured directly, i.e., differentially between two microelectrodes, one impaling the cell and another positioned in the lumen. Alternatively and more conveniently, the potential difference of the luminal cell membrane can be calculated as the difference between the transepi-

thelial potential measurement [Figures 6(A and B)] and the peritubular cell
membrane potential recording [Figures 7(A and B)]. Instead of such sequential
impalements, a simultaneous measurement of transepithelial potential difference
and cell potential is obtained in the isolated tubule by a combination of an axial
electrode and an intracellular microelectrode [Figure 7(C)]. Immobilization of
the isolated tubule is a major problem and cell impalements have only been
performed on isolated cortical collecting tubules (Helman, 1973) and amphibian
isolated proximal tubules (Sackin and Boulpaep, 1976).

In principle, the same experimental manipulations can be applied for cell
potential measurements (Figure 7) as outlined in Figure 6(A–C) for transepithelial potential measurements. Of particular importance are the effects of changes
in either luminal, peritubular, or bilateral ion activities imposed by microperfusion or superfusion techniques. These studies have been recently expanded to
include the measurements of the electrical effects of the presence of organic
solutes, of metabolic inhibitors, of temperature changes, of different diets, and
hormones. For review see Boulpaep (1976a,b) and Frömter et al. (1971).

Cell potential measurements have been important for the assessment of net
driving forces responsible for passive movement of ions across single cell
membrane barriers. In principle, ion permeability properties of single cell
membranes can be calculated from the observed changes in potential difference
subsequent to alterations in external ion composition in the peritubular compartment directly facing the cell membrane. However, in order to compute either
cell membrane ion transference number or ion permeability coefficients, the
voltage displacement observed across a particular cell barrier should truly reflect
a response of an ionic electromotive force (emf) within that barrier. Actually, in
the presence of a low resistance paracellular shunt bypassing the cells, current
flow across the cell membranes leads to additional potential changes which may
obscure the true magnitude of the dependence of membrane emf on ion activity
changes (Boulpaep, 1976b).

Peritubular cell membrane potential measurements have also been useful in
assessing active transport properties of the cell membrane. In particular, the
observation of changes in peritubular potential differences stimulated by artificially induced alterations in transport rate and not directly related to changes in
diffusional emf's has been central to the demonstration of electrogenic or
rheogenic active transport. Sodium extrusion from the cell can be enhanced
either by rewarming sodium-enriched renal slices (Whittembury, 1971; Proverbio
and Whittembury, 1975), by imposition of quick temperature steps to isolated
tubules (Sackin and Boulpaep, 1976), by intracellular injection of sodium
electrophoretically (Tadakoro and Boulpaep, 1972), and more indirectly by step
changes in intraluminal sodium concentration (Wiederholt and Giebisch, 1974).
Consistent with the view of rheogenic sodium extrusion at the peritubular
membrane were the findings in the above experiments of a hyperpolarization of
the peritubular membrane associated with measured or presumed increments of
active sodium transport.

Finally, cell potential measurements are also important for the interpretation
of the electrode reading obtained with ion-selective electrodes. In order to obtain

the true half-cell potential of the ion-selective electrode and thus the ion activity within the cell, the overall transmembrane recording has to be corrected by the simultaneously determined cell membrane potential. Three approaches have been used experimentally: (1) true simultaneous measurement with double-barreled microelectrodes, (2) independent impalement of neighboring cells of the same tubule with an ion-selective *and* an indifferent microelectrode, and (3) the comparison of two populations of cell potential differences, one obtained with an ion-selective and the other determined with an nonselective microelectrode.

V. MEASUREMENT OF ELECTRICAL RESISTANCES AND CURRENT FLOW

A. Technical Problems

A resistance or conductance measurement involves application of current steps to tubular structures and the recording of the resulting voltage differences. Since this is most often done by using microelectrodes with relatively high resistance, some special problems arise.

First, the high resistance of the current-injecting barrel of a double-barreled microelectrode may place upper limits to the linear current-carrying capacity of the system. Microelectrodes may be either filled with special electrolyte solutions such as K-citrate, or, alternatively, at comparable external tip size, the tip may be beveled so as to carry higher currents (Brown and Flaming, 1974). For transepithelial applications in such leaky structures as the proximal tubule, large currents may be needed for resistance measurements. Special constant current sources are available (W.P. Instruments, New Haven, Ct.; Grass Instruments, Quincey, Mass.; Keithley Instruments, Cleveland, Ohio).

Second, the voltage-recording electrode should be properly separated from the current barrel such that no spurious coupling resistance exists which is common to the path of both the current and the voltage circuit. This is particularly critical when double-barreled microelectrodes are used. Corrections should be applied for any voltage deflection observed when the resistance to be measured is not in the circuit, e.g., when the double-barreled microelectrode is positioned in the reference bath.

B. Transepithelial Current Distribution and Resistance

Resistance determinations rely on two different approaches dictated by the unique cylindrical geometry of renal tubules. The first and most extensively used one depends on a point source for current application and nonuniform current density along the length of the tubule. Hence, a variety of cable analyses have been necessary (Taylor, 1964). The other method, so far only used in large amphibian proximal tubules, employs an axial current electrode extending along the entire length of the segment under study. In this case uniform transepithelial current density is achieved.

1. Inhomogeneous Current Distribution and Cable Analysis

Figure 8(A) illustrates the treatment of the renal tubule as a double-sided infinite cable extending from $-\infty$ to $+\infty$. A current electrode is placed in a properly located cortical segment which permits accurate length measurements between several electrodes. This current electrode may be a double-barreled

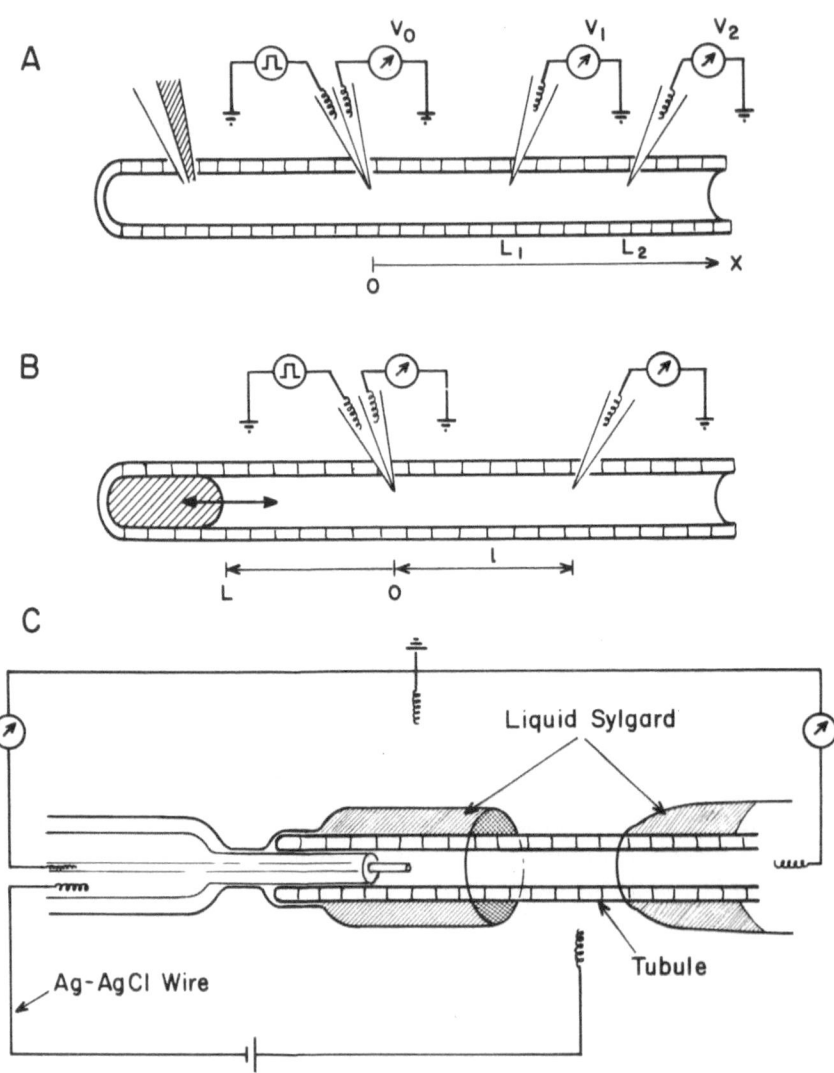

Figure 8. Methods for the measurement of transepithelial resistance. (A) Intratubular application current via double-barreled microelectrode during free flow, and measurement of voltage attenuation downstream by recording electrodes V_1 and V_2 at L_1 and L_2, respectively. (B) Transepithelial resistance measurement by recording the voltage change for a constant current pulse between two electrodes, separated by a constant interval l, during variations in position L of an occluding oil droplet on left. For details, see text. (From Hegel et al., 1967.) (C) Arrangement for measuring potential difference and resistance across isolated perfused tubule using separate pipets for passing current and recording voltage. (From Lutz et al., 1973.)

type to ascertain the intratubular localization by (a) recording the spontaneous transepithelial potential difference and (b) by its response to changes of intraluminal composition. At appropriate and known distances from the current electrode, voltage-sensing microelectrodes are placed into the tubular lumen and used to obtain information of the voltage attenuation along the tubule.

It is possible to either measure the voltage drop along the tubule by inserting a single electrode sequentially, or, although technically more demanding, by the simultaneous positioning of two voltage electrodes at different sites, as shown in Figure 8(A).[1] Assuming that the tubular segment under study extends infinitely in both directions without branching or change in diameter, the following relationships hold. Experimentally one may determine four parameters: (1) R_i, the resistivity of the solution in the core of the cable (ohm·cm). This value can be obtained for any particular solution *in vitro* from conductivity measurements. (2) a, the optical inner tubular radius. (3) λ, the length constant obtained from the inverse of the slope of the plot of ln $\Delta V_x/\Delta V_o$ against tubular length where ΔV_x and ΔV_o are the voltage deflections observed at distance x and o from the current electrode since $\Delta V_x = \Delta V_o e^{-x/\lambda}$. (4) R_{input}, input resistance or the ratio of $\Delta V_o/I_o$, where I is the amplitude of the applied current. For the purpose of determining the specific transepithelial resistance R_m (in ohm·cm^2) only three of the above parameters have to be known, hence R_m may be calculated in four different ways as follows:

$$R_m = \frac{2 R_i \lambda^2}{a} \tag{1}$$

$$R_m = \frac{8\pi^2 a^3 R_{input}^2}{R_i} \tag{2}$$

$$R_m = \sqrt{8\pi R_i \lambda^3 R_{input}} \tag{3}$$

$$R_m = 4\pi a \lambda R_{input} \tag{4}$$

As was pointed out by experimental application of each of these approaches to a set of data, Eq. (1) appears to give the most reliable result since it does not depend on the use of R_{input} (Boulpaep, 1972a; Grandchamp and Boulpaep, 1974). Estimates of R_{input} as $\Delta V_o/I$ do not agree with the value obtained by extrapolation of the voltage attenuation plot to distance $x = 0$ (Boulpaep, 1972a). Therefore, estimates of R_{input} by graphical extrapolation should be employed. Otherwise, the use of R_{input} may lead to errors in the estimates of R_m by means of Eqs. (2) to (4). Note that occasionally transepithelial resistance is not

---

[1] When a single recording electrode is used and sequential impalements are made at distances x_1 and x_2 from the current electrode, intervening damage to the epithelium between the two impalements or incomplete sealing of the first impalement site may lead to an error in the estimate of the length constant. Assuming that following damage the magnitude of the voltage deflections declines, sampling x_1 first yields an "untouched" high ΔV_1 whereas subsequent sampling of ΔV_2 with the same electrode would yield a value below the initial "untouched" value of ΔV_2. The slope of the plot of $\Delta V_x/\Delta V_o$ would thus be steeper and λ smaller than the correct value. An opposite sequence of events ΔV_2 sampled first, followed by ΔV_1 would tend to give an underestimated ΔV_1, value and thus a lesser slope of the plot $\Delta V_x/\Delta V_o$ and a λ larger than the correct value (Grandchamp and Boulpaep, 1974).

expressed per unit effective area (R_m) but per unit tubular length (r_m). The relationship between R_m and r_m is defined as

$$R_m = 2\pi a r_m \tag{5}$$

A special case shown in Figure 8(A) would be the tubule filled with oil, e.g., on the left side of $x = 0$, up to the point of current injection $x = 0$ (Rau and Frömter, 1974b). The cable then extends from $x = 0$ to $x = +\infty$. The same equations would apply except that the R_{input} for a one-sided infinite cable is twice the R_{input} of a double-sided infinite cable. Thus R_m can be calculated as in Eqs. (1) to (4) using a differently determined R_{input} value. The following equations hold for a single-sided infinite cable:

$$R_m = \frac{2R_i\lambda^2}{a} \tag{1a}$$

$$R_m = \frac{2\pi^2 a^3 R_{input}^2}{R_i} \tag{2a}$$

$$R_m = 2\sqrt{\pi R_i \lambda^3 R_{input}} \tag{3a}$$

$$R_m = 2\pi a\lambda R_{input} \tag{4a}$$

Figure 8(B) illustrates a special application of a tubular resistance measurement which does not rely upon multiple determinations of the voltage alteration along the tubule but instead depends on the measurement of the voltage deflection at a fixed distance (l) from the current-applying electrode ($x = 0$) (Hegel et al., 1967). Note that an oil block is moved on the left side of the current electrode at distances L ranging from 0 to $-\infty$. The voltage deflection at $x = 0$ is calculated from that recorded at $x = l$, assuming an exponential voltage decay since the right-hand side of the tubule is infinite. The relationship of ΔV_o at $x = 0$ against L, where L is the distance of the oil meniscus from the current electrode, is given by

$$\Delta V_{o(X=L)} = 2\,I_o R_{input} \frac{1}{1 + \tanh(L/\lambda)} \tag{6}$$

R_{input} in this equation is measured as the input resistance obtained when the oil meniscus is placed at $x = -\infty$, i.e., defined as in Eqs. (1) to (4). In addition, λ relates also to R_i, R_m, and a as in Eq. (1). Therefore, this approach allows the determination of (1) R_i as above, (2) a, as above, (3) λ from the plot of $\Delta V_{o(X=L)}$ against L, and (4) R_{input} as $\Delta V_{o(X=\infty)}/I_o$. Since R_{input} is here defined as for an infinite cable, application of one of the Eqs. (1) to (4) allows one to calculate R_m. Note that actually $\Delta V_{l(X=L)}$ is measured by the voltage electrode but since

$$\Delta V_{l(X=L)} = \Delta V_{o(X=L)} e^{-l/\lambda} \tag{7}$$

Eq. (6) would become

$$\Delta V_{l(X=L)} = 2\,I_o R_{input} \frac{e^{-l/\lambda}}{1 + \tanh(L/\lambda)} \tag{8}$$

A third case of a useful cable analysis appropriate for renal tubular resistance measurements is that of a terminated cable [see Figure 8(C) and Figure 3]. For practical purposes, a terminated tubular segment can be prepared by placing two oil blocks in tubules *in vivo* as was performed in medullary collecting duct segments (Rau and Frömter, 1974a,b).

This approach has been more extensively used on isolated perfused tubules where at either end of the excised segment a resistance $= \infty$ is imposed by Sylgard 184 seals placed on the outside of the tubule. The length of the finite cable is thus known as the tubular length exposed between the two Sylgard menisci as in Figure 8(C) and Figure 3. Current is injected at the perfusion end either via the perfusion pipet (Helman *et al.*, 1971) or through the coated outer surface on the perfusion pipet (Figure 3) (Lutz *et al.*, 1973), or via an additional pipet inserted in the perfusion pipet [Figure 8(C)]. Voltage deflections ΔV_o are recorded by the perfusion pipet in all three cases. In the first case where the perfusion pipet is used both to inject current as well as to measure the voltage displacement, a bridge circuit is employed to null the voltage deflection caused by the resistance of the pipet (Helman *et al.*, 1971). In addition, the voltage deflection at the collection pipet ΔV_L at distance $X = L$ is recorded.

Experimentally one may determine five parameters: (1) R_i (ohm·cm) defined as above, (2) a, the optical inner tubular radius, (3) λ, the length constant, (4) L, the total length of the perfused segment, (5) R_{input}, input resistance or the ratio of $\Delta V_o/I_o$. In this case λ is not obtained directly. Instead, the ratio L/λ is the characteristic parameter for the voltage attenuation according to

$$L/\lambda = \cosh^{-1} (\Delta V_o/\Delta V_L) \qquad (9)$$

For the purpose of determining specific transepithelial resistance, only four of the above parameters have to be known. R_m may be calculated in at least four different ways:

$$R_m = \frac{2R_i\lambda^2}{a} \qquad (10)$$

$$R_m = \frac{2\pi^2 a^3 R_{\text{input}} 2[\tanh(L/\lambda)]^2}{R_i} \qquad (11)$$

$$R_m = 2\sqrt{\pi R_i \lambda^3 R_{\text{input}}} \, \sqrt{\tanh (L/\lambda)} \qquad (12)$$

$$R_m = 2\pi a\lambda R_{\text{input}} \tanh L/\lambda \qquad (13)$$

Equation (12) is preferable since it does not employ an optical estimate of tubular radius. Electrical radii may also be calculated, and the comparison of electrical and optical radii provides an inherent check of the validity of the approach (Lutz *et al.*, 1973). Equation (13) was used on isolated cortical collecting ducts (Helman *et al.*, 1971), where the core resistivity is treated as an unknown. Note that for the infinite cable, preference was given to an equation of the type as in (10) because R_{input} directly measured was based on a problematic measurement. In contrast, in the isolated tubule, application of R_{input} is more reliable in view of the use of a rather large current-applying pipet.

Finally, a special treatment is available for the branched case of a one-sided infinite tubule applied to the medullary collecting duct tree (Rau and Frömter, 1974b).

2. Homogeneous Current Distribution

Figure 9(A) depicts an axial electrode system extending over the whole length (L) of an intraluminal split drop (Spring and Paganelli, 1972; Spring, 1972). Transepithelial resistance may be directly calculated from the input resistance $\Delta V/I$, where ΔV is recorded by means of a microelectrode and is assumed to be uniform over the entire exposed segment, and I is the constant current applied through the axial metal electrode:

$$R_m = R_{input}2\pi aL \qquad (14)$$

The method has been applied to straight segments of proximal tubules of *Necturus*. In principle, experiments involving long-term and uniform current applications may be performed such that the epithelium is effectively voltage clamped. A problem may arise during long-term current flows related to the release of ions from the metal electrode into the volume-restricted luminal compartment. Axial metal electrodes have been used in *Necturus* proximal tubule for transepithelial impedance measurement using a-c current (Hegel and Boulpaep, 1975).

Figure 9(B) shows an approach to achieve quasi-homogeneous current distribution. The method may be resorted to in small mammalian tubules in which an axial electrode impalement is not yet feasible. If the distances l_1, l_2, and l_3 and the length constant λ are known, the extent of inhomogeneity of voltage changes can be estimated from the ratio between the voltage deflection ΔV

A

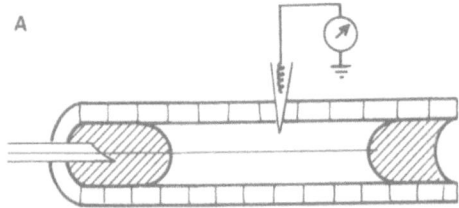

B

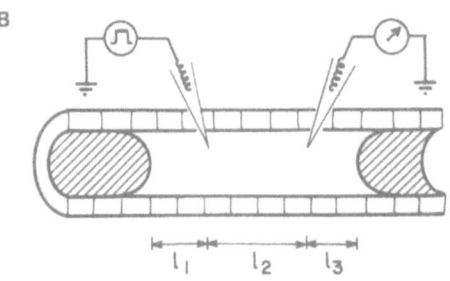

Figure 9. (A) Transepithelial resistance measurement with axial electrode. Current density is maintained constant by axial electrode and isolating oil droplets. The transepithelial potential difference is measured by conventional microelectrode. (From Spring, 1972.) (B) Restriction of current spread by insulating oil droplets. Point source of current application (left) and recording microelectrode (right). For details, see text. (From Garcia et al., 1976.)

measured by the voltage recording electrode, and the voltage deflection ΔV_o, expected at the site of the current application. As first approximation (Garcia *et al.*, 1976),

$$\frac{\Delta V}{\Delta V_o} = e^{-l_2/\lambda} + e^{-(l_2 + 2l_3)/\lambda} + e^{-(2l_1 + l_2)/\lambda} \tag{15}$$

Homogeneity of the voltage clamp is maximal when $\Delta V/\Delta V_o$ approaches unity.

C. Cellular Transmembrane Current Distribution and Resistance

The problem of measuring single-cell membrane resistance is usually met by injecting current into a cell and recording voltage deflection from the same. The R_{input} value multiplied by total plasma membrane area would theoretically yield specific resistance R_m. However, such methods are only satisfactory for mono-cellular preparations, separated cells, or certain cells in culture. In fact most cells, in particularly all epithelial cells studied thus far, are electrically coupled through specialized junctions (Loewenstein, 1966). This property, if the coupling is sufficiently uniform along two dimensions, may actually be used for assessing cell membrane resistance of unicellular epithelial layers. Providing the cytoplasmic resistivity together with the lateral junctions may be treated as a single bulk phase, current injected in one cell of an epithelial sheath will spread in two dimensions and effect a monotonic voltage alteration with distance. The apical or luminal membrane and the peritubular or basal membrane may be considered two uniform continuous limiting barriers which sandwich a cytoplasmatic fluid layer.

Figure 10(A) illustrates the method used in *Necturus* proximal tubules. Current is injected into a cell by a double-barreled microelectrode. Cells were found to be electrically coupled as additional recording electrodes detected significant voltage deflections in adjacent cells. From cable analysis it is possible to obtain the combined specific conductance $g_1 + g_2$ of both the outer and inner limiting membrane. The two-dimensional problem has been solved for an infinite flat sheet as may be appropriate in thin cardiac atrial muscle layers (Woodbury and Crill, 1961) and in planar epithelia (Frömter, 1972b; Reuss and Finn, 1975). In renal tubules, the geometry is that of a double core where the inner core is the tubular lumen and the outer core a cytoplasmatic ring.

As an extreme simplification, Hoshi and Sakai (1967) have treated the tubular wall as a plate conductor with cross-sectional dimensions determined by the height of the cell wall, and the inner and outer tubular perimeter. Current spread was treated only along a single dimension parallel to the axis of the tubule, thus neglecting any voltage decay in radial directions. In contrast, a two-dimensional approach was taken both by Windhager *et al.* (1966) and Anagnostopoulos and Velu (1974). This permits one to calculate the sum of the two cell membrane conductances $(1/R_1) + (1/R_2)$ in parallel.

In order to compute the specific resistance of one cell membrane separately, i.e., the peritubular membrane resistance R_1 or the luminal cell membrane resistance R_2, two different approaches may be taken. First, the lumen may be

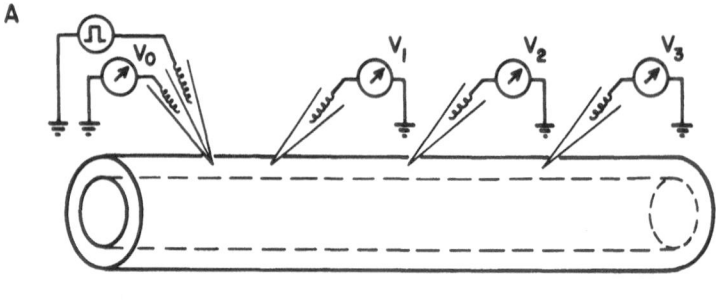

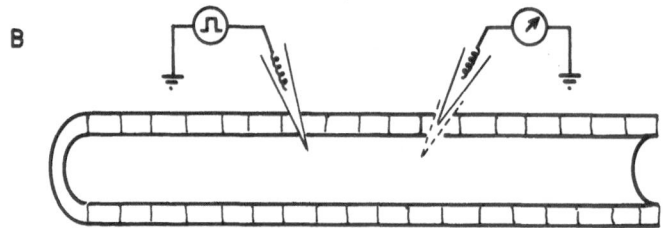

Figure 10. (A) Experimental arrangement to measure voltage attenuation along column of epithelial cells in the wall of a single renal tubule. Left: Double-barreled microelectrode for injection of current and for measurement of cellular transmembrane potential (to assure appropriate intracellular localization). Right: Recording electrodes V_1, V_2, and V_3 to measure changes in membrane potential as a function of distance from current-injecting electrode. (From Giebisch and Windhager, 1973.) (B) Experimental arrangement for measurement of relative resistance of luminal and peritubular cell membrane. Current is applied and the resulting voltage measured with the recording electrode pipet in a tubular cell and across the whole epithelium. For details, see text.

filled with a nonconducting medium and the experiment shown in Figure 10(A) repeated. Current passage is thus limited to the outer peritubular membrane. From this measurement, peritubular conductance $1/R_1$ is obtained. Alternatively, the ratio of the luminal cell membrane resistance to peritubular membrane resistance R_2/R_1 is obtained directly from the method illustrated in Figure 10(B). It is based on luminal current application at some distance and the sequential recording of the resulting voltage deflection ΔV_1 across the peritubular membrane first and subsequently the measurement of ΔV_3 across the entire epithelium at identical sites. Since current density for a cell at a given distance from the current electrode is the same across both peritubular and luminal cell membrane

$$R_2/R_1 = \frac{\Delta V_3 - \Delta V_1}{\Delta V_1} \tag{16}$$

This latter measurement, often called the "voltage divider" ratio, has been measured in a variety of circumstances and may provide a coarse estimate of the relative change in resistance of one of the two cell membranes (Whittembury *et al.*, 1973).

A special case of intracellular current application is that of microelectrophoresis of single ions into tubular cells. Double-barreled electrodes are used with one barrel filled with a salt of the ion to be injected and connected to a constant current source, and the other barrel serving to monitor the resulting voltage transient (Tadokoro and Boulpaep, 1972).

REFERENCES

Adrian, R. H. 1956. The effect of internal and external potassium concentration on the membrane potential of frog muscle. *J. Physiol., 133:*631.

Agin, D. P. 1969. Electrochemical properties of glass microelectrodes. In: *Glass Microelectrodes,* pp. 62–75. Ed. by Lavallee, M., Schanne, O. F., and Hebert, N. C. Wiley, New York.

Anagnostopoulos, T., and Velu, E. 1974. Electrical resistance of cell membranes in *Necturus* kidney. *Pflügers Arch., 346:*327.

Barratt, L. J., Rector, F. C., Kokko, J. P., and Seldin, D. W. 1974. Factors governing the transepithelial potential difference across the proximal tubule of the rat kidney, *J. Clin. Invest., 53:*454.

Barratt, L. J., Rector, F. C., Kokko, J. P., Tisher, C. C., and Seldin, D. W. 1975. Transepithelial potential difference profile of the distal tubule of the rat. *Kid. Internat., 8:*368.

Barry, P. H., and Diamond, J. M. 1970. Junction potentials, electrode standard potentials, and other problems in interpreting electrical properties of membranes. *J. Membr. Biol., 3:*93.

Bentzel, C. J. 1974. Expanding drop analysis of Na and H_2O flux across *Necturus* proximal tubule. *Am. J. Physiol., 226:*118.

Biagi, B., and Garcia-Filho, E. In press. A simple method for filling microelectrodes using centrifugation. *Pflügers Arch.*

Boulpaep, E. L. 1972a. Permeability changes of the proximal tubule of *Necturus* during saline loading. *Am. J. Physiol., 222:*517.

Boulpaep, E. L. 1972b. Electrophysiological techniques in kidney micropuncture. *Yale J. Biol. Med., 45:*397.

Boulpaep, E. L. 1976a. Recent advances in electrophysiology of the nephron. *Ann. Rev. Physiol., 38:*20.

Boulpaep, E. L. 1976b. Electrical phenomena in the nephron. *Kid. Internat., 9:*88.

Boulpaep, E. L., and Seely, J. F. 1971. Electrophysiology of proximal and distal tubules in autoperfused dog kidney. *Am. J. Physiol., 221:*1084.

Brown, K. T., and Flaming, D. G. 1974. Beveling of fine micropipette electrodes by a rapid precision method. *Science, 185:*693.

Bureš, J., Petráň, M., and Zachar, J. 1976. *Electrophysiological Methods in Biological Research,* Academic Press, New York.

Burg, M. 1976. Tubular chloride transport and the mode of action of some diuretics. *Kid. Internat., 9:*189.

Burg, M. B., and Green, N. 1973. Function of the thick ascending limb of Henle's loop. *Am. J. Physiol., 224:*659.

Burg, M. B., and Orloff, J. 1970. Electrical potential difference across proximal convoluted tubules. *Am. J. Physiol., 219:*1714.

Caflish, C. R., Pucacco, L. R., and Carter, N. W. In press. The manufacture and utilization of antimony pH electrodes. *Kid. Internat.*

Caldwell, P. C., and Downing, A. C. 1955. The preparation of capillary microelectrodes. *J. Physiol., 128:*31.

Cerf, J. A., and Cerf, E. 1974. A holder for rapid filling of micropipette electrodes by centrifugal action. *Pflügers Arch., 349:*87.

Cole, K. S. 1949. Dynamic electrical characteristics of the squid axon membrane. *Arch. Sci. Physiol., 3:*253.

Coombs, J. S., Eccles, J. C., and Fatt, P. 1955. The electrical properties of the motoneurone membrane. *J. Physiol., 130:*291.

Curtis, D. R. 1964. Microelectrodes. In: *Physical Techniques in Biological Research*, Vol. V, *Electrophysiological Methods*, Part A, p. 144. Ed. by Nastuk, W. L. Academic Press, New York.

Curtis, D. R., and Eccles, R. 1958. The excitation of Renshaw cells by pharmacological agents applied electrophoretically. *J. Physiol., 141:435.*

del Castillo, J., and Katz, B. 1957. A study of curare action with an electrical micro-method. *Proc. Roy. Soc. Lond.*, Ser. B, *146:339.*

Duling, B. R., and Berne, R. M. 1969. A rapid, small-volume method for filling micropipettes. *J. Appl. Physiol., 26:837.*

Ferris, C. D. 1974. *Introduction to Bioelectrodes*, Plenum, New York.

Frank, K., and Becker, M. C. 1964. Microelectrodes for recording and stimulation. In: *Physical Techniques in Biological Research*, Vol. V, *Electrophysiological Methods*, Part A, p. 23. Ed. by Nastuk, W. L. Academic Press, New York.

Frömter, E. 1972a. Progress in microelectrode techniques for kidney tubules. *Yale J. Biol. Med., 45:414.*

Frömter, E. 1972b. The route of passive ion movement through the epithelium of *Necturus* gall bladder, *J. Memb. Biol., 8:259.*

Frömter, E. 1974. Electrophysiology and isotonic fluid absorption of proximal tubules of mammalian kidney. In: *MTP International Review of Science*, Physiology Series I, Vol. 6, pp. 1–38. *Renal and Urinary Tract Physiology*, Ed. by Thurau, K. Butterworths–University Park Press, Baltimore, Md.

Frömter, E., and Hegel, U. 1966. Transtubuläre Potentialdifferenzen an proximalen und distalen Tubuli der Rattenniere. *Pflügers Arch., 291:107.*

Frömter, E., Mueller, C. W., and Wick, T. 1971. Permeability properties of proximal tubular epithelium of the rat kidney studied with electrophysiological methods. In: *Electrophysiology of Epithelial Cells*, pp. 119–146. Ed. by Giebisch, G. Schattauer, Stuttgart.

Fujimoto, M., and Kubota, T. 1976. Physiochemical properties of liquid ion exchanger microelectrode and its application to biological studies. *Jap. J. Physiol., 26:631.*

Fujimoto, M., Kubota, T., and Kotera, K. 1977. Electrochemical profile of K and Cl across the proximal tubule of bull frog kidneys. (A study of double-barreled ion-sensitive microelectrodes.) In: *Contributions to Nephrology*, Vol. 6, p. 114. Karger, Basel.

Garcia, E., Malnic, G., and Giebisch, G. 1976. Effects of changes in electrical potential difference upon distal tubular potassium concentrations, Abstr., p. 98. *Proc. 9th Ann. Mtg. Am. Soc. Nephrol.*

Geddes, L. A. 1972. *Electrodes and the Measurement of Bioelectric Events*. Wiley-Interscience, New York.

Giebisch, G. 1961. Measurements of electrical potential differences in perfused single proximal tubules in *Necturus* kidney. *J. Gen. Physiol., 44:659.*

Giebisch, G. 1974. The effects of drugs on the electrophysiological properties of kidney tubules. In: *Drugs and Transport Processes*, pp. 1–22. Ed. by Callingham, E., University Park Press, Baltimore, Md.

Giebisch, G., and Windhager, E. E. 1973. Electrolyte transport across renal tubular membranes. In: *Handbook of Physiology*, Section 8, *Renal Physiology*, pp. 315–376. Ed. by Orloff, J. and Berliner, R. W. American Physiological Society, Washington, D.C.

Giebisch, G., Malnic, G., deMello, G. B., and deMello-Aires, M. 1977. Kinetics of luminal acidification in cortical tubules of the rat kidney. *J. Physiol. 267:571.*

Grandchamp, A., and Boulpaep, E. L. 1974. Pressure control of sodium reabsorption and intercellular backflux across proximal kidney tubule. *J. Clin. Invest., 54:69.*

Grantham, J. J., Burg, M. E., and Orloff, J. 1970. The nature of transtubular Na and K transport in isolated rabbit renal collecting tubules. *J. Clin. Invest., 49:1815.*

Green, R., and Giebisch, G. 1974. Some problems with the antimony microelectrodes. In: *Ion Selective Microelectrodes*, pp. 43–53. Ed. by Berman, H. J. and Hebert, N. C. Plenum Press, New York.

Hayslett, J. P., Giebisch, G., and Boulpaep, E. L. 1976. Electrical properties of distal tubule epithelium. *Kid. Intern., 10:585.*

Hegel, U., and Boulpaep, E. L. 1975. Studies of electrical impedance of kidney proximal tubular epithelium in *Necturus*. Abstr., p. 45, *6th Intern. Congr. Nephr.*

Hegel, U., Frömter, E., and Wick, T. 1967. Der elektrische Wandwiderstand des proximalen Konvolutes des Ratteniere. *Pflügers Arch., 294:*274.

Helman, S. I. 1973. Microelectrode studies of isolated cortical collecting tubules. Abstr., p. 49. *6th Ann. Meet. Am. Soc. Nephrol.*

Helman, S. I., Grantham, J. J., and Burg, M. B. 1971. Effect of vasopressin on electrical resistance of renal cortical collecting tubules. *Am. J. Physiol., 220:*1825.

Hinke, J. A. M. 1959. Glass micro-electrodes for measuring intracellular activities of sodium and potassium. *Nature, 184:*1259.

Hodgkin, A. L., Huxley, A. F., and Katz, B. 1952. Measurement of current-voltage relations in the membrane of the giant axon of *Loligo*. *J. Physiol., 116:*424.

Hoshi, T., and Sakai, F. 1967. A comparison of the electrical resistances of the surface cell membrane and cellular wall in the proximal tubule of the newt kidney. *Jap. J. Physiol., 17:* 627.

Jacobson, H. R., and Kokko, J. P. 1976. Diuretics: sites and mechanisms of action. *Ann. Rev. Pharmacol. and Toxicol., 16:*201.

Kao, C. Y. 1954. A method of making prefilled microelectrodes. *Science, 119:*846.

Karlmark, B. 1973. The determination of titratable acid and ammonium ions in picomole amounts. *Anal. Biochem., 52:*69.

Kennard, D. W. 1958. Glass microcapillary electrodes. In: *Electronic Apparatus for Biological Research,* p. 718. Ed. by Donaldson, D. E. K. Butterworths, London.

Khuri, R. N. 1972. Intracellular potassium in cells of the distal tubule. *Yale J. Biol. & Med., 45:*384.

Khuri, R. N. 1976. Microelectrodes utilizing glass and liquid ion-exchanger sensors. In: *Ion and Enzyme Electrodes in Biology and Medicine,* pp. 123–130. Ed. by Kessler, M., Clark, L. C., Jr., Lubbers, D. W., Silver, I. A., and Simon, W. University Park Press, Baltimore, Md.

Khuri, R. N., Goldstein, D. A., Maude, D., Edmonds, C., and Solomon, A. K. 1963. Single proximal tubules of *Necturus* kidney, VIII. Na and K determinations by glass electrodes. *Am. J. Physiol., 204:*743.

Khuri, R. N., Agulian, S. K., and Harik, R. I. 1968. Internal capillary glass microelectrodes with a glass seal for pH, sodium and potassium, *Pflügers Arch., 301:*182.

Khuri, R. N., Agulian, S. K., and Wise, W. M. 1971. Potassium in the rat kidney proximal tubules in situ: Determination by K$^+$ selective liquid ion-exchange microelectrodes. *Pflügers Arch., 322:*39.

Khuri, R. N., Agulian, S. K., and Kalloghian, A. 1972a. Intracellular potassium in cells of the distal tubule. *Pflügers Arch., 335:*297.

Khuri, R. N., Hajjar, J. J., Agulian, S. K. 1972b. Measurements of Intracellular potassium with liquid ion-exchange microelectrodes. *J. Appl. Physiol., 32:*419.

Khuri, R. N., Hajjar, J. J., Agulian, S., Bogharian, K., Kalloghlian, A., and Bizri, H. 1972c. Intracellular potassium in cells of the proximal tubule of *Necturus* maculosus. *Pflügers Arch., 338:*73.

Khuri, R. N., Agulian, S. K., and Bogharian, K. 1974a. Electrochemical potentials of potassium in proximal renal tubule of rat. *Pflügers Arch., 346:*319.

Khuri, R. N., Agulian, S. R., Bogharian, K., Nassar, R., and Wise, W. 1974b. Intracellular bicarbonate in single cells of *Necturus* kidney proximal tubule. *Pflügers Arch., 349:*295.

Khuri, R. N., Agulian, S. K., and Bogharian, K. 1975. Electrochemical potential of chloride in distal renal tubule of the rat. *Am. J. Physiol., 227:*1354.

Kokko, J. P., and Rector, F. C. 1971. Flow dependence of transtubular potential difference in isolated perfused segments of rabbit proximal convoluted tubule. *J. Clin. Invest., 50:*2745.

Kraig, R. P., and Nicholson, C. 1976. Sodium liquid ion exchanger microelectrode used to measure large extracellular sodium transients. *Science, 194:*725.

Kuriyama, H., and Ito, Y. 1974. Recording of intracellular activity with microelectrodes. In: *Methods in Pharmacology, Vol. III, Smooth Muscle,* pp. 201–230. Ed. by E. Daniel and D. Paton, Plenum Press, New York.

Laurence, R., and Marsh, D. J. 1971. Effect of diuretic states on hamster collecting duct electrical potential differences. *Am. J. Physiol., 225:*1610.

Ling, G., and Gerard, R. W. 1949. The normal membrane potential of frog sartorius fibers. *J. Cell Comp. Physiol., 34:*383.

Loewenstein, W. R. 1966. Permeability of membrane junctions. In: *Biological Membranes: Recent Progress, Ann. N.Y. Acad. Sci., 137:*441.

Lutz, M. D., Cardinal, J., and Burg, M. B. 1973. Electrical resistance of renal proximal tubule perfused *in vitro. Am. J. Physiol., 225:*729.

Malnic, G., and Mello-Aires, M. 1971. Kinetic study of bicarbonate reabsorption in proximal tubule of the rat. *Am. J. Physiol., 220:*1759.

Malnic, G., and Vieira, F. L. 1972. The antimony microelectrode in kidney micropuncture. *Yale J. Biol. Med., 45:*356.

Malnic, G., Mello-Aires, M., and Cassola, A. C. 1974. Kinetic analysis of renal tubular acidification by antimony microelectrodes. In: *Ion Selective Microelectrodes*, pp. 89–108. Ed. by Berman, H. J. and Hebert, N. C. Plenum Press, New York.

Marmont, G. 1949. Studies on the axon membrane. *J. Cell. Comp. Physiol., 34:*351.

Maruyama, T., and Hoshi, T. 1972. The effect of D-glucose on the proximal electrical potential profile across the proximal tubule of newt kidney. *Biochem. Biophys. Acta, 282:*214.

Maude, D. L. 1970. Mechanism of salt transport and some permeability properties of rat proximal tubule. *Am. J. Physiol., 218:*1590.

Nastuk, W. 1953. The electrical activity of the muscle cell membrane at the neuromuscular junction. *J. Cell. Comp. Physiol., 42:*249.

Neild, T. O., and Thomas, R. C. 1973. New design for a chloride-sensitive microelectrode. *J. Physiol., 231:*7.

Neild, T. O., and Thomas, R. C. 1974. Intracellular chloride activity and the effects of acetylcholine in snail neurones. *J. Physiol., 242:*453.

Proverbio, F., and Whittembury, G. 1975. Cell electrical potentials during enhanced sodium extrusion in guinea-pig cortex slices. *J. Physiol., 250:*559.

Puschett, J. B., and Zurbach, P. E. 1974. Re-evaluation of microelectrode methodology for the *in vitro* determination of pH and bicarbonate. *Kid. Intern., 6:*81.

Quehenberger, P. In press. The influence of carbon dioxide, bicarbonate and other buffers on the potential of antimony microelectrodes. *Pflügers Arch.*

Rau, W. S., and Frömter, E. 1974a. Electrical properties of the medullary collecting ducts of the golden hamster kidney. I. The transepithelial potential difference, *Pflügers Arch., 351:*99.

Rau, W. S., and Frömter, E. 1974b. Electrical properties of the medullary collecting ducts of the golden hamster kidney. II. The transepithelial resistance. *Pflügers Arch., 351:*113.

Reuss, L., and Finn, A. L. 1975. Electrical properties of the cellular transepithelial pathway in *Necturus* gall bladder. I. Circuit analysis and steady-state effects of mucosal solution ionic substitution. *J. Membr. Biol., 25:*115.

Rosenberg, M. E. 1973. A comparison of chloride and citrate-filled microelectrodes for A-C recording. *J. Appl. Physiol., 35:*166.

Sackin, H., and Boulpaep, E. L. 1976. Simultaneous intracellular and transepithelial potential measurements in isolated perfused amphibian proximal tubules. Abstr., p. 111. *Proc. 9th Ann. Mtg. Am. Nephrol. Soc.*

Schafer, J. A., Troutman, S. L., and Andreoli, T. E. 1974. Volume reabsorption, transepithelial potential differences and ionic permeability properties in mammalian proximal straight tubules. *J. Gen. Physiol., 64:*582.

Seely, J. F., and Boulpaep, E. L. 1971. Renal function studies on the isobaric autoperfused dog kidney. *Am. J. Physiol., 221:*1075.

Snell, F. M. 1969. Some electrical properties of fine-tipped pipette microelectrodes. In: *Glass Microelectrodes*, pp. 111–123. Ed. by Lavallée, M., Schanne, O. F., and Hébert, N. C. Wiley, New York.

Sohtell, M. In press. Electrochemical forces for chloride transport in the proximal tubules of the rat kidney. *Acta Physiol. Scand.*

Sohtell, M., and Karlmark, B. 1976. *In vivo* micropuncture pCO_2 measurements. *Pflügers Arch., 363:*179.

Spitzer, A., and Windhager, E. E. 1970. Effect of peritubular oncotic pressure changes on proximal tubular fluid reabsorption. *Am. J. Physiol., 218:*1188.

Spring, K. 1972. Insertion of an axial electrode into renal proximal tubule. *Yale J. Biol. Med., 45:*426.

Spring, K., and Kimura, G. 1977. Luminal Cl entry into *Necturus* tubule cells. Abstr. *Proc. Int. Union Physiol. Sci.*, *13:*2119.

Spring, K., and Paganelli, C. B. 1972. Sodium flux in *Necturus* proximal tubule under voltage clamp. *J. Gen. Physiol.*, *60:*181.

Sullivan, J. 1968. Electrical potential differences across distal renal tubules of *Amphiuma*. *Am. J. Physiol.*, *214:*1096.

Tadokoro, M., and Boulpaep, E. L. 1972. Electrophoretic method of ion injection in single kidney cells. *Yale J. Biol. Med.*, *45:*432.

Tasaki, I., Polley, M., and Orrego, F. 1954. Action potentials from individual elements in cat geniculate and striage cortex. *J. Neurophysiol.*, *17:*454.

Tasaki, K., Tsukahara, Y., Ito, S., Wayner, M. J., and Yu, S. 1968. A simple direct and rapid method for filling microelectrodes. *Physiol. Behav.*, *3:*1009.

Taylor, R. E. 1964. Cable theory. In: *Physical Techniques in Biological Research*, Vol. VI, *Electrophysiological Methods*, Part B, pp. 219-262. Ed. by Nastuk, W. L. Academic Press, New York.

Thomas, R. C. 1970. A new design for sodium-sensitive glass microelectrode. *J. Physiol.*, *210:*82.

Thomas, R. C. 1972. Intracellular sodium activity and the sodium pump in snail neurones. *J. Physiol.*, *220:*55.

Thomas, R. C. 1974. Intracellular pH of snail neurones measured with a new pH-sensitive glass microelectrode. *J. Physiol.*, *238:*159.

Thomas, R. C. 1976. Construction and properties of recessed-tip microelectrodes for sodium and chloride ions and pH. In: *Ion and Enzyme Electrodes in Biology and Medicine*, pp. 141-148. Ed. by Kessler, R., Clark, L. C., Jr., Lubbers, D. W., Silver, I. A., and Simon, W., University Park Press, Baltimore, Md.

Thomas, R. C., W. Simon, and Oehme, M. 1975. Lithium accumulation by snail neurons measured by a new Li$^+$ sensitive microelectrode. *Nature*, *258:*754.

Ullrich, K. J., Frömter, E., and Baumann, K. 1969. Micropuncture and microanalysis in kidney physiology. In: *Laboratory Techniques in Membrane Biophysics*, pp. 106-129. Ed. by Passow, H. and Stampfli, R. Springer, New York.

Vis, V. A. 1954. A technique for making multiple bore microelectrodes. *Science*, *120:*152.

Walker, J. L. 1971. Ion specific liquid ion exchanger microelectrodes. *Anal. Chem.*, *43:*89A.

Whittembury, G. 1965. Sodium extrusion and potassium uptake in guinea pig kidney cortex slice. *J. Gen. Physiol.*, *48:*699.

Whittembury, G. 1971. Relationship between sodium extrusion and electrical potentials in kidney cells. In: *Electrophysiology of Epithelial Cells*, pp. 153-178. Ed. by Giebisch, G. F. K. Schattauer Verlag, Stuttgart-New York.

Whittembury, G. 1972. Cellular and paracellular mechanism in sodium transport in the proximal tubule. *Proc. 5th Int. Congr. Nephrol.*, Vol. 2, p. 18.

Whittembury, G., and Windhager, E. 1961. Electrical potential difference measurements in perfused single proximal tubules of *Necturus* kidney. *J. Gen. Physiol.*, *44:*679.

Whittembury, G., Rawlins, F. A., and Boulpaep, E. L. 1973. Paracellular pathway in kidney tubules: electrophysiological and morphological evidence. In: *Transport Mechanisms in Epithelia*, pp. 577-588. Ed. by Ussing, H. H. and Thorn, N. A. Academic Press, New York.

Wiederholt, M., and Giebisch, G. 1974. Some electrophysiological properties of the distal tubule of *Amphiuma* kidney. *Fed. Proc.*, *33:*387.

Wilbrandt, W. 1938. Electrical potential differences across the wall of kidney tubules of *Necturus*. *J. Cell Comp. Physiol.*, *11:*425.

Windhager, E. E., and Giebisch, G. 1965. Electrophysiology of the nephron. *Physiol. Rev.*, *45:*214.

Windhager, E. E., Boulpaep, E. L., and Giebisch, G. 1966. Electrophysiological studies on single nephrons. *Third Internat. Cong. of Nephrol.*, *1:*35.

Woodbury, J. W., and Crill, W. E. 1961. On the problem of impulse conduction in the atrium. In: *International Symposium on Nervous Inhibition*, pp. 124-135. Ed. by E. Florey, Pergamon, New York.

Zettler, F. 1970. Kaltgefüllte Mikroglaskapillaren und ihre elektrophysiologisch relevanten Eigenschaften. *Zeit. Vergl. Physiol.*, *67:*423.

Chapter **8**

Measurements of pH by Glass Microelectrodes

Norman W. Carter and Leo R. Pucacco

Department of Internal Medicine
University of Texas Health Science Center at Dallas
Southwestern Medical School
Dallas, Texas

I. INTRODUCTION

Both electrodes (Rector *et al.*, 1965; Vieira and Malnic, 1968) and dye indicators (Rector and Carter, 1963) have been used for the measurement of *in vivo* intraluminal pH of the nephron. Electrodes used for the measurement of pH have been of the antimony (Vieira and Malnic, 1968) and hydrogen ion (H^+) sensitive glass types. In our laboratory, two different types of H^+ sensitive glass electrodes have been miniaturized to the extent that they can be used for direct *in vivo* measurement of intraluminal pH in the typical micropuncture preparation (Carter *et al.*, 1967a; Pucacco and Carter, 1976). The newest of these electrodes (Pucacco and Carter, 1976) has also been used in our laboratory to measure pH in the microenvironment of the isolated tubule preparation.

In this chapter we will describe the construction of both electrodes, but the older electrode will be covered in only minimal detail since its manufacture and use has been well described previously (Carter *et al.*, 1967a,b; Carter, 1972). Moreover, we now favor the glass membrane, pH microelectrode over the ultramicroelectrode for most applications in renal physiology. The glass membrane, pH microelectrode is described in Section III of this chapter.

II. THE pH ULTRA-MICRO GLASS ELECTRODE

The main attribute of the pH ultra-micro glass electrode is the smallness of its micro tip. In the double-barreled type, scanning electron microscopy has shown that the tip diameter of the electrode is only 0.1 to 0.2 μm. In the case of a properly made electrode, the pH-sensitive portion of the tip extends back from 5 to 30 μm.

A. Materials

For the ultra-micro electrode, pH glass of the Corning 0150 type is used. The glass is obtained in capillary form with an outside diameter (o.d.) of 0.8 mm and a wall thickness of about 0.25 mm. This glass must be insulated, and for this purpose a glass enamel or glaze is fused onto the pH capillary.

The pH glass capillaries are cut to 10-cm lengths, one end is sealed, and the capillary dipped into a thin suspension of the glaze (200–250 g of glaze in oil mixed with 450 ml turpentine. Glaze in oil from Pemco, Division of Glidden Co., Baltimore, Md. TR-514-A supplied in No. 34 oil). The capillaries are hung and allowed to air dry; the dipping is then repeated. After a final air dry, the green, glazed capillaries are baked in a furnace at 600°C for from 6 to 10 min.

The glazed capillaries are now ready to make single-barreled pH electrodes or to be joined with a reference capillary to make double-barreled pH electrodes.

The glass used to make the reference barrel of the double-barreled electrode must thermally match the 0150 pH glass. After considerable investigation, it was found that Corning 0129 glass was the best available match. Unfortunately, this glass is not commercially available in capillary form. Many funnels of color television tubes are made of this glass, however, and capillaries can be blown from old tube funnels by the usual methods for lead glass. The capillary should be 1.0 mm o.d. with a wall thickness of 0.25 mm. The dimensions are important in that it is necessary to match this size with the 0.8 mm o.d. pH glass so that when the micro tip is pulled, the reference tip remains open while the pH tip of the electrode closes.

The reference capillary is cut to about 4-cm lengths and a piece is placed alongside the glazed pH capillary so that one end of the reference capillary is at one end of the pH capillary. The two capillaries are fastened together with any epoxy-type cement that can stand up to boiling water.

Both single- and double-barreled pH electrodes can be pulled to a micro tip on any standard vertical or horizontal pipet puller. The principle of the electrode is that on pulling the micro tip, "active" pH glass is pulled out from under the glaze (see insert, Figure 1). After pulling, electrodes are filled with distilled water using the heat and vacuum method. Prior to use, the water in the reference side of the double-barreled electrode is displaced with an electrolyte solution (2.5 M KCl, 0.5 M KNO$_3$; Carter, 1972) by means of a fine needle. The water in the pH barrel is not changed. By leaching the pH glass, it becomes a good electrolyte solution and is buffered to about pH 9.0 by alkali oxides from the glass.

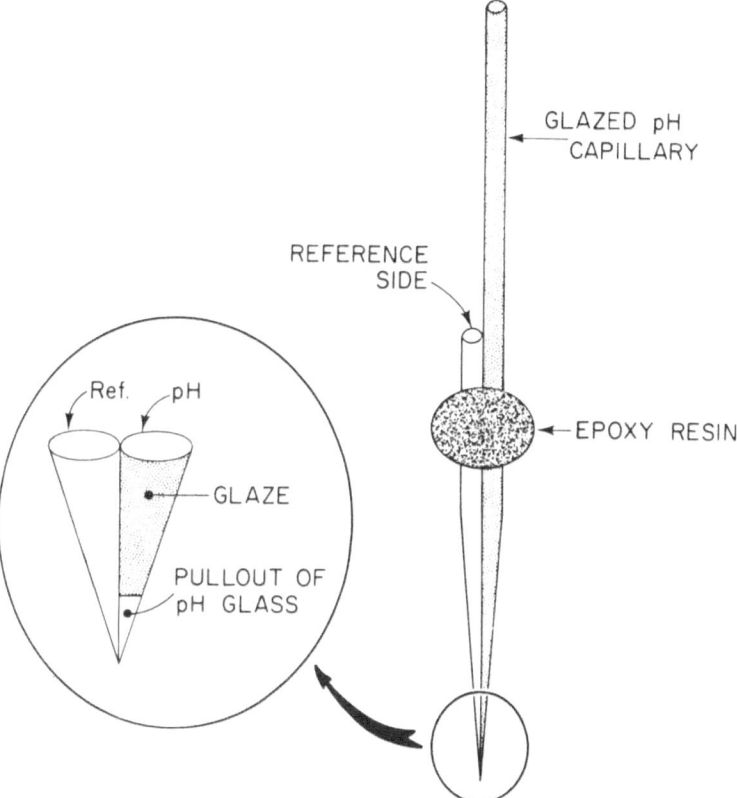

Figure 1. Double-barreled pH ultra-micro glass electrode.

The electrolyte solution in each barrel is connected to the appropriate reference electrodes and the pH electrodes are then ready for testing. Figure 1 shows a schematic representation of a double-barreled electrode.

B. Testing

The single-barreled pH electrodes or the pH side of the double-barreled electrodes are tested for pH sensitivity in standard buffers. The slope (millivolts per unit pH) of good electrodes varies from 45 to 55 mV. With these electrodes, theoretical slope is seldom achieved. The resistance of good electrodes can be measured by the method of Franks and Fuortes (1955) without damage to the electrode. It generally ranges from 5×10^8 to 8×10^9 ohms.

When an electrode reads pH with adequate slope, it should then be tested for the integrity of the tip, for even some electrodes that have a fairly high resistance and an adequate slope will be found to have the tip slightly open. This can be determined by measuring the pH of a known buffer of high ionic strength (an adequate buffer for this purpose can be made by adding 1 M KCl per liter to standard pH 7.0 buffer. Its ultimate pH must be determined by using a commercial pH electrode system). It has been found that when the tip of the pH barrel is closed, the micro pH electrode reads the pH of the high ionic strength buffer correctly. When the tip is slightly open, the micro pH electrode gives a falsely high or alkaline reading. Such electrodes should be discarded.

It must be carefully determined how far the sensitivity of the pH barrel extends from the electrode tip. This is required for both single- and double-barreled electrodes. Figure 2 is a schematic representation of the method used to test the insulation of the pH electrode (in this case a double-barreled pH electrode).

Buffer hardened with 3% agar is placed in a small cylindrical container. Over this is laid a piece of Parafilm® with a hole filled with latex or polyvinyl. The electrode, under microscopic observation, is put through the membrane a known number of microns. The pH of the hardened buffer is read. With a fine pipet, another buffer of different pH is placed above the Parafilm and around the electrode. The voltage reading should show only a transient deflection. Any permanent change in voltage suggests that uninsulated pH glass appears above the latex or polyvinyl membrane and therefore the electrode is not adequately insulated.

In addition, a known potential should be placed across the outer buffer drop and the solid buffer below. This should not unaccountably affect the voltage reading of the electrometer. If it does, the electrode should be discarded.

Electrodes passing the above tests are ready for use although it should be pointed out that the resistance and tip potential of the reference side of the double-barreled electrode should first be ascertained. Both high resistance and

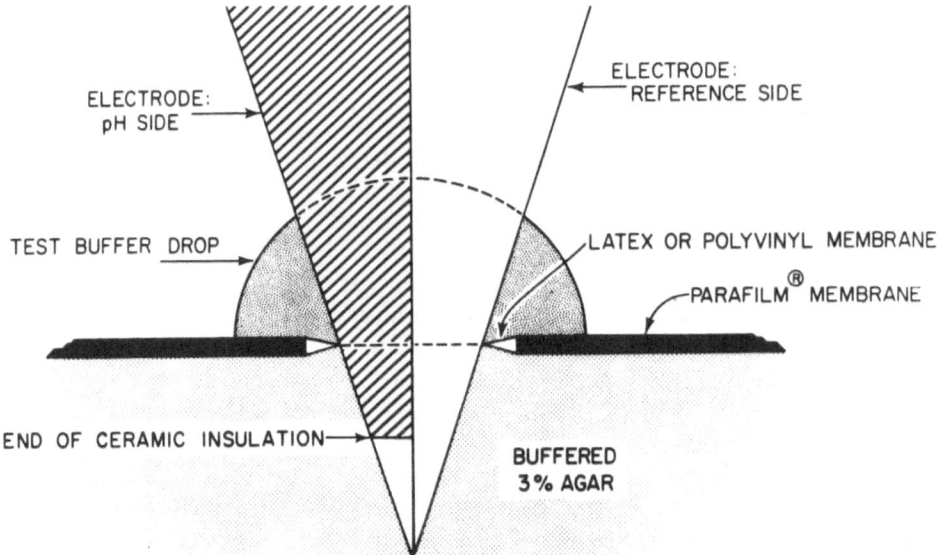

Figure 2. Technique employed to determine the length of the pH-sensitive portion of the pH ultra-micro glass electrode.

high tip potentials should be avoided. Applications of this electrode to pH measurements in renal physiology are similar to those for the glass membrane, pH microelectrode outlined in Section III-E.

III. THE GLASS MEMBRANE, pH MICROELECTRODE

The glass membrane, pH microelectrode is a miniature version of the original glass pH electrode developed by MacInnes and Dole (1929). Both of these electrodes make use of the fact that when glass is heated to its softening temperature it becomes sticky, and if it is touched by another piece of glass a glass-to-glass seal will be formed. MacInnes and Dole heated the opening of an indifferent glass tube to its softening temperature and then touched the softened orifice to a piece of thin (1 μm-thick) pH-sensitive glass. The result was an electrode which was pH insensitive everywhere except at the tip where the pH glass closed the orifice of the glass tube. The glass membrane, pH microelectrode described here was made by simply reversing this procedure, that is, the pH glass was heated to its softening point and then touched with the tip of an indifferent glass pipet. When the pH glass cooled, a glass-to-glass sealed was formed at the points of contact. The reason for reversing the procedure was that for making small electrodes (less than 200 μm) the tip of the pipet glass would close (fire-polishing) before it could be touched to the pH glass. By heating the pH glass instead of the pipet glass, this problem has been circumvented and thus small electrodes (1 μm) can be made.

The glass membrane, pH microelectrode senses pH ($-\log_{10}H^+$) as a potential difference (pd) which can be measured and recorded with the appropriate equipment. pH-Sensitive glass is a transducer in that it converts H^+ from millimoles/liter to millivolts. The parameters which determine the usability of a pH electrode are: size (tip diameter), sensitivity (slope; mV/unit pH), d-c resistance (ohms) and response time (time required for the electrode potential to reach its final value). There are two additional parameters which are particularly important with respect to pH microelectrodes: stability of intercept (how well does the electrode potential repeat at a specific pH) and lifetime (how long after manufacture will the electrode function).

The glass membrane, pH microelectrode can be made as small as 1 μm in tip diameter and as large as 100s of microns in tip diameter. The sensitivity or slope is always at or very near that which theory would dictate; 57–59 mV/pH at 22°C and 61–62 mV/pH at 37°C. The d-c resistance of the glass membrane, pH microelectrode varies from as low as 5×10^8 to as high as 5×10^{11} ohms. The resistance of this electrode is related to its size in that the smaller the electrode the higher the resistance. The resistance of the electrode limits its use in that the electrometer used to sense the potential developed by the electrode must have an input resistance at least 100 times that of the electrode. In addition, the resistance of the electrode is one of the component parts making up the response time (the other being capacitance), thus the larger the resistance the longer the response time. The response time of this electrode ranges from as fast as 15 sec to as long as 10 min. A response time of 3 min or less can be achieved for all size electrodes except that it is more difficult to achieve this goal with the smaller electrodes (less than 3 μm). The stability of this electrode is such that the potential developed for a specific pH, in most cases, will not vary more than 10% over a period of days and will not vary as a result of what types of solutions it comes in contact with (very strong acids and bases being a probable exception).

The glass membrane, pH microelectrode can also be made with an integral reference (double-barreled) so that the pH of a medium contained within a boundary having a potential difference (nephron distal tubule) can be accurately measured. These double-barreled electrodes have been made in the size range of 1–150 μm.

A. Materials

1. pH Glass

Two pH glasses were used in making the glass membrane, pH microelectrode. In our early work we used Corning 0150 pH glass and later changed to a uranium-containing pH glass made in our laboratory. The glass membrane, pH microelectrode has, by design, a small sensing surface area and therefore a high electrical resistance. The resistance is directly proportional to the thickness of the membrane and the specific resistance of the glass, but inversely proportional to the sensing surface area. As the size of the electrode was reduced, the surface area was reduced and thus the electrode resistance increased. Our design goal was the smallest possible electrode with a maximum resistance of 10^{12} ohms. This upper limit on the electrode resistance was dictated by the input resistance of the electrometer used to sense the potential developed by the pH membrane. We employed a Keithly Model 602 solid state electrometer which has a rated input resistance of 10^{14} ohms. In order to sense the total potential delivered to the input of an electrometer, the resistance of the source must be at least two orders of magnitude less than the resistance of the sensing instrument. If this is not the case, an attenuation of the input signal occurs as a result of voltage division between the source resistance and the input resistance. If the source resistance is $1/10$ the input resistance, a 10% error is incurred, while if the source resistance is $1/100$ the input resistance, the error incurred is only 1%. Since we minimized the thickness of the pH glass membrane by using the thinnest portion of a glass bubble blown from pH glass and we were attempting to reduce the surface area to its smallest possible value, we considered the possibility of reducing the specific resistance of the pH glass. There are pH glasses which have a specific resistance less than that of 0150 but these glasses cannot be reworked. That is to say, they cannot be reheated without devitrification and therefore could not be used since we must reheat our glass in the process of making the electrode. It has been reported (Schwabe, 1954) that if 5% to 6% of the SiO_2 of 0150 pH glass is replaced by UO_2, a pH glass with $1/10$ the specific resistance could be made. With this knowledge we made uranium-containing pH glass in our laboratory with various percentages of UO_2. The two UO_2-containing pH glasses we used to make pH electrodes are shown in Table I.

We varied the UO_2 from 0.129 mol % (0.52 wt. %) to 12 mol % (36 wt. %) in an attempt to determine the optimum percent of UO_2. The UO_2 quantity in each glass was exchanged for silica. The final glass, 2.1 wt. %, had the best characteristics, which were: least susceptible to heat damage (electrodes made from this glass rarely overheated to the point where they did not register pH), good chemical durability (electrodes made from this glass lasted longer than those made from the other compositions), and superior working characteristics (large working temperature range). All the UO_2 glasses had a characteristic which lent itself to the making of a glass membrane, pH microelectrode, that is, a larger working temperature range than the 0150 glass. Specifically, the UO_2-containing glass had working characteristics similar to a high lead glass. We found that the bubbles blown from UO_2-containing glass were thinner than those blown from 0150 glass and in the electrode-making procedure the UO_2 glass stretched more (changed colors) under the influence of heat and a penetrating pipet. Most of our developmental electrodes and all of our data-gathering electrodes were made with the UO_2-containing glass, therefore we were not able to confirm the reduction in the specific resistance of the pH glass. However, the thinnest of the UO_2 glass bubbles and its superior stretching characteristics during the electrode-making procedure were far better than with 0150 glass.

2. Pipet Glass

Four different glasses have been used for the body of the electrode, lead potash (Corning 0100), aluminosilicate (Corning 1720), borosilicate (Corning 7740), and 96% silica (Corning 7900). The lead potash glass was used in the early developmental stage because its temperature characteristics best matched those of the pH glass (Carter *et al.*, 1967a). It was felt that unless the two glasses were closely thermally matched, either the membrane glass or the pipet glass or possibly both would crack upon cooling (after being sealed or during filling). Actually, no cracking was apparent in the case of lead glass pipets and somewhat surprisingly, thermal cracks were not experienced with any of the

Table I. Composition of UO_2-Containing pH Glasses

	Original		Final	
	Mol. %	Wt. %	Mol. %	Wt. %
SiO_2	54.30	60	54.80	61.5
UO_2	1.03	4	0.52	2.1
MgO	13.74	8	13.74	8.1
NaO_2	30.90	28	30.90	28.3

above-mentioned pipet glasses, perhaps because of the small amounts of glass involved in the seal mismatch. The precise reasons for this fortuitous circumstance are not known. Although we did not encounter any problems with cracking using 0150 and 0100 glasses, we did experience difficulty with the electrode-making procedure as we attempted to reduce the size of the electrode below 15 μm. At this size we found that the lead glass was responding to the heat used to soften the pH glass by first fire-polishing at the tip and then bending. This occurred because the softening temperature of the lead glass and the pH glass were about the same, 660°C. We found that we could not make an electrode with lead glass below 15 μm because the lead pipet would bend instead of pushing through the pH glass membrane. To circumvent this problem, we tried another glass for the body of the electrode, aluminosilicate (Corning 1720), which has a higher softening temperature, 912°C. This meant that while the pH glass was soft at 660°C, during the electrode-making procedure, the pipet tip was 252°C below its softening temperature and so was unaffected. The problem incurred using 1720 as the pipet glass had to do with its thermal characteristics. Specifically, 0150 and 1720 are not good matches as far as thermal expansion and contraction are concerned. As a matter of fact, the coefficient of linear expansion for 0150 is about twice that of 1720. We tested the feasibility of using these two glasses by making glass membrane, pH microelectrodes and found that neither the pH nor the aluminosilicate glass cracked during cooling or filling. We were able to successfully make small electrodes (1 μm) with 1720 and observed no fire-polishing (tip stayed sharp and straight) or bending. In addition to 1720, two other high temperature glasses have been succcessfully used for the body of the electrode: borosilicate (Corning 7740) and 96% silica (Corning 7900). For most electrodes, the 1720 glass is the best choice for the pipet, however.

B. Equipment

1. Forge

In order to seal the tip of the glass pipet with pH-sensitive glass, a de Fonbrune microforge was used. The forge was modified and additions made so that the glass membrane, pH microelectrode could be manufactured. First the optical system was replaced. The de Fonbrune microforge is equipped with American Optical (A.O.) optics (4 or 8 × objectives and 10 or 15 × eyepieces). Although the magnification (120×) was sufficient, the acuity was not acceptable. In order to make a glass membrane, pH microelectrode, the tip of the pipet must be visible so that the pH glass and the heating filament can be precisely aligned. The A.O. optics were sufficient for making large electrodes (15 μm) but when making small electrodes (5 μm) we found it difficult if not impossible to complete the procedure successfully. We replaced the A.O. optical system with a Zeiss microscope having a 4× objective and 20× eyepieces. With this optical system we were able to properly align the pipet tip, pH glass, and heating element such that small electrodes could be made. Second, two tridirectional manipulators were added to the right-hand side of the forge in order to accommodate the

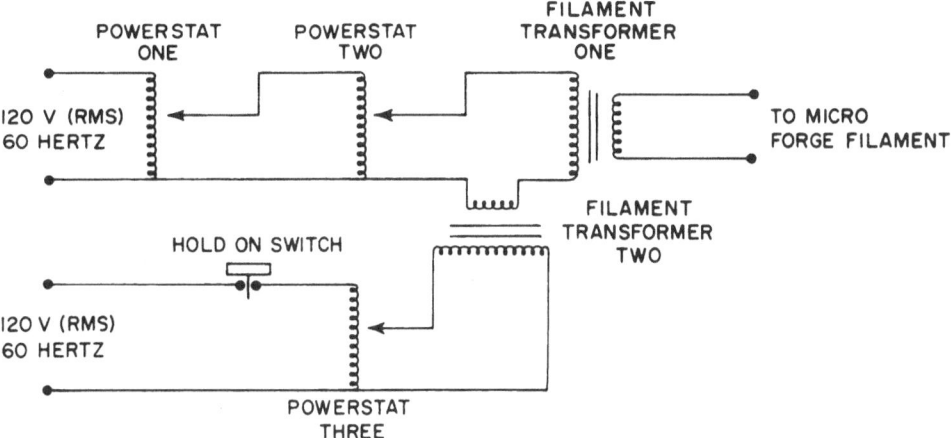

Figure 3. System providing fine control and bilevel operational capacity for the microforge heating element.

membrane mounting apparatus and a second heating filament. Third, the filament power supply and control system was disabled and replaced with the supply and control system shown in Figure 3. This power supply and control system allowed for bilevel heat capacity, which we found to be necessary when making small electrodes. Also, the dual Powerstat® arrangement and foot control activation allowed for fine temperature control and convenient operation. The fourth modification made to the forge was in the configuration of the filament. The reason for modifying the filament was that we found that the most critical parameter in the electrode-making procedure was the amount of heat used to seal the pH glass to the pipet. Insufficient heat resulted in a partially sealed electrode and too much heat resulted in dehydration (Isard, 1967) or loss of Na_2O (Hubbard and Rynders, 1948) from the pH glass. Both of these conditions resulted in nonfunctioning electrodes. In order to effectively control the amount of heat applied to the pH glass, a point source of heat was required. Platinum-iridium wire (40 gauge) was shaped into the desired form for use in the forge and then the tip of the filament was etched in a solution of saturated NaCN and 30% NaOH by an a-c electrical current (1–10 V, 60 Hz) (Frank and Becker, 1964). Only the tip of the filament was placed in the solution, therefore only the tip was etched. The result was a heating filament which was 75 μm in diameter everywhere but at the tip, where it was 10 μm in diameter. Figure 4 shows the configuration of the filament and the circuit used for etching the filament tip. This provided a localized source of heat, which minimized the possibility of overheating the pH glass. There is another factor concerning the source of heat which we found necessary for successful electrode making. We found it necessary to coat the tip of the filament (hot spot) with pH glass so as to block oxides of iridium and platinum from being liberated and coating the thin pH glass membrane. We found that with an uncoated filament an oxide layer is formed

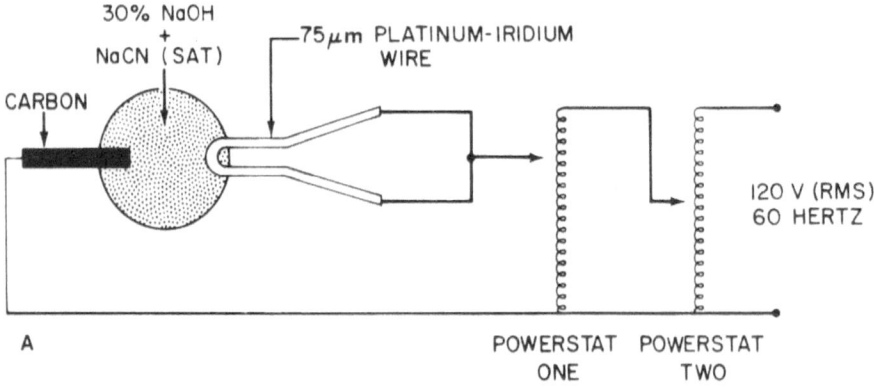

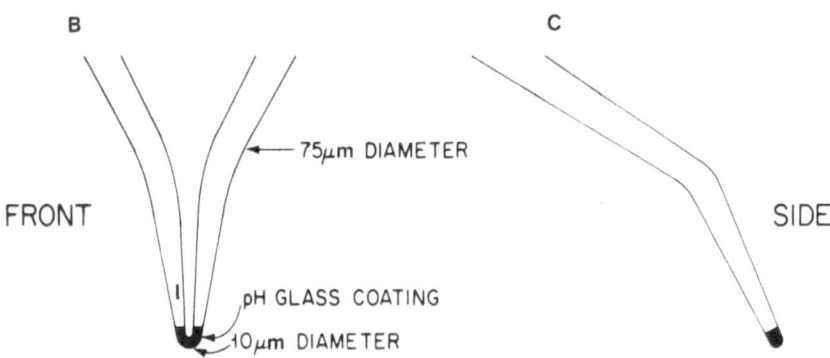

Figure 4. (A) System used to etch the tip of the heating filament used in the microforge. (B) Front view and (C) side view of the tapered platinum-iridum filament used to make glass membrane, pH microelectrodes.

over the pH glass which desensitizes it. This oxide layer can be dissolved in boiling aqua-regia, but the possibility of physically destroying the thin layer of pH glass made it an undesirable alternative. Coating the filament with a thin layer of pH glass solved the problem. It should be pointed out that the size of the filament is related to the size of the electrode being made. For small electrodes (1–5 μm), a filament made from 75 μm wire etched to 10 μm at the tip works well. If larger electrodes are desired, the filament size should be increased. For example, when making electrodes in the range of 5–50 μm, a filament made from 125 μm wire (36 gauge) etched to 25 μm at the tip works well, while a 240 μm wire (31 gauge) etched to 100 μm at the tip works well for electrodes in the range of 50–150 μm.

2. Grinder

The grinding of the body of the electrode to the desired tip diameter was accomplished with a silicon carbide 500 grit stone wheel. The grinding fluid used was acetone because it could more easily be blown out of the pipet after grinding. If the grinding fluid is not blown out of the pipet soon after grinding, small glass particles are left in and on the tip of the pipet and can interfere with the sealing of the pH glass to the pipet. If the ground tip is not scrupulously clean, the occurrence of partially sealed pH electrodes is high. The procedure we follow is to grind the pipet, blow out the acetone, place the tip in a ultrasonic cleaner (with acetone) and then place the tip of the electrode in a heat cone in order to evaporate the remaining acetone. With this procedure we can produce beveled pipets with perfectly clean tips. It should be pointed out that the pipet used as the body of the glass membrane, pH microelectrode can be ground at various angles in order to increase the sharpness and provide for an increased sensing surface area. It should also be pointed out that the grinding of the pipet is critical to the sealing procedure and therefore any chipping of, or dirt on, the ground surface must be avoided.

C. Manufacturing Procedure

1. Single-Barreled Electrodes

a. A 1-mm capillary (pipet glass: lead potash, aluminosilicate, borosilicate, 96% silica) is pulled to a submicrometer tip on a horizontal pipet puller.

b. Under microscopic observation the tip of the pipet is ground on a silicon carbide 500 grit stone wheel, with acetone as the grinding solution, to the desired size (1–500 μm).

c. The acetone in the pipet is blown out immediately after grinding by placing the tip in a heat funnel.

d. Thin, submicrometer pH glass membranes are made by blowing glass bubbles (Figure 5) from pH glass capillary (0150 or UO_2). The relative thickness of the glass can be determined by the color of the glass: red (0.107 μm), orange (0.1 μm), yellow (0.097 μm), green (0.087 μm), blue (0.08 μm), and violet (0.075 μm).

e. A small piece of thin pH glass is secured to the membrane mounting apparatus with Eastman 910® glue (Figure 6).

f. The membrane mounting apparatus is installed in a three-directional manipulator on the right side of the microforge.

g. The beveled glass pipet is installed in the pipet holder of the microforge with the tip up and the microscope focused on the tip.

h. The glass membrane is positioned into the middle of the field of view (above the electrode tip) with the edge of the desired color pH glass in focus.

i. The point source of heat (glass-covered, etched platinum-iridium wire) is positioned at the upper left corner of the field of view and in focus (Figure 7).

j. The electrode is brought up to a point just below the pH glass membrane [Figure 8(A)].

k. The heat source is brought down and over the pH membrane just to the left of the electrode tip [Figure 8(A)].

l. The heat source is turned on (or increased from baseline if bilevel

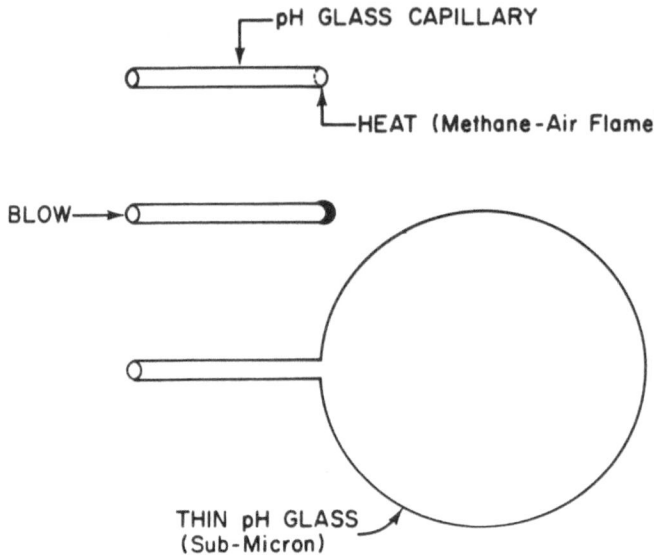

Figure 5. Method used to obtain submicron pH glass membranes from pH glass capillary.

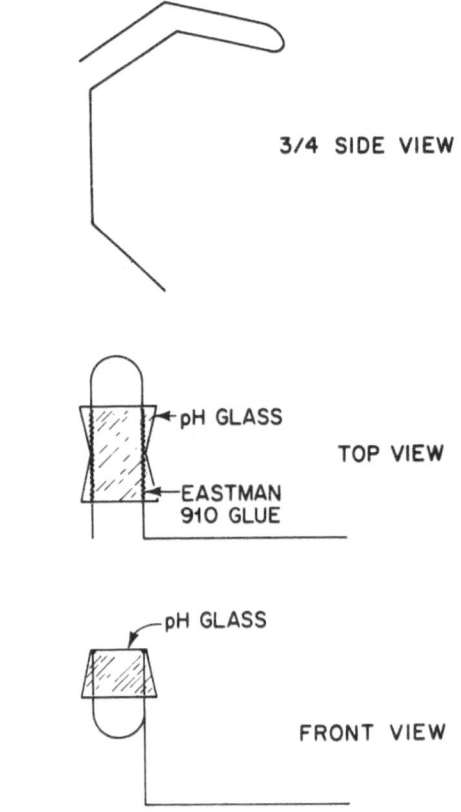

Figure 6. Apparatus used to mount pH glass membrane.

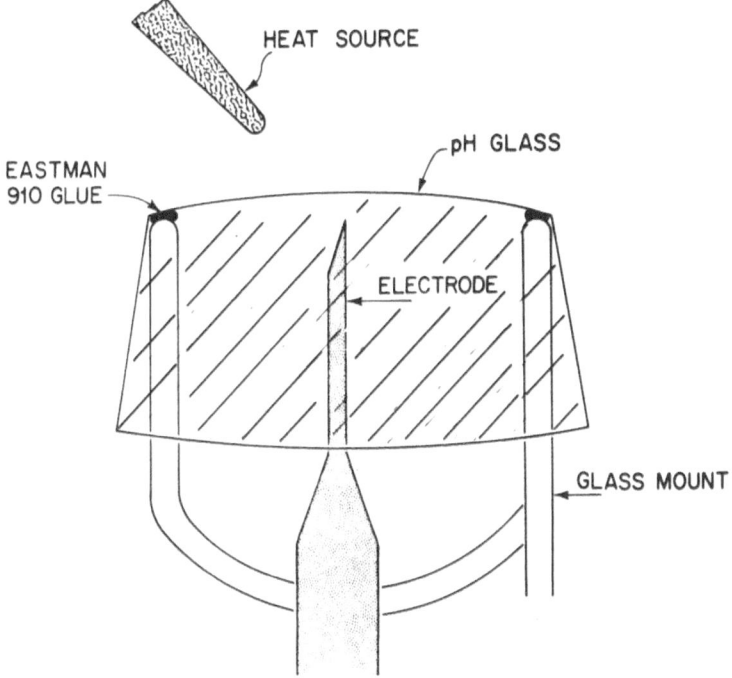

HEAT SOURCE

pH GLASS

EASTMAN
910 GLUE

ELECTRODE

GLASS MOUNT

Figure 7. Initial location of the three electrode-making components as viewed through the microscope at 20×.

temperature control is being used) and the electrode is advanced up to contact the pH glass membrane [Figure 8(A)].

m. The electrode is slowly advanced through the softened pH glass and simultaneously the heating filament is moved slightly to the left [Figure 8(B)].

n. As the electrode moves through the softened pH glass, the heat source is moved to the left so that the electrode can be advanced further [Figure 8(C)].

o. The electrode is advanced further until the thin pH glass overlaps a significant length of the pipet (50–1,000 μm, depending upon the tip diameter) [Figure 8(D)].

p. The heat source is removed and the electrode is gently advanced further until it breaks free from the pH glass membrane.

q. The pH glass control is moved down so as to break up the pH glass surrounding the electrode and then moved back to remove it from the electrode.

r. The glass membrane, pH microelectrode is removed from the holder and checked under the microscope for water uptake. This is accomplished by placing the tip of the electrode into a beaker of distilled water and then viewing the electrode under the microscope. If the electrode does not draw any water, the seal is usually sufficient. It should be pointed out that some electrodes that are water tight are found to be electrically open during the testing phase.

s. Electrodes to be filled are mounted on glass slides (using rubber bands) and the slides are mounted (using rubber bands) on a carousel-type holder with

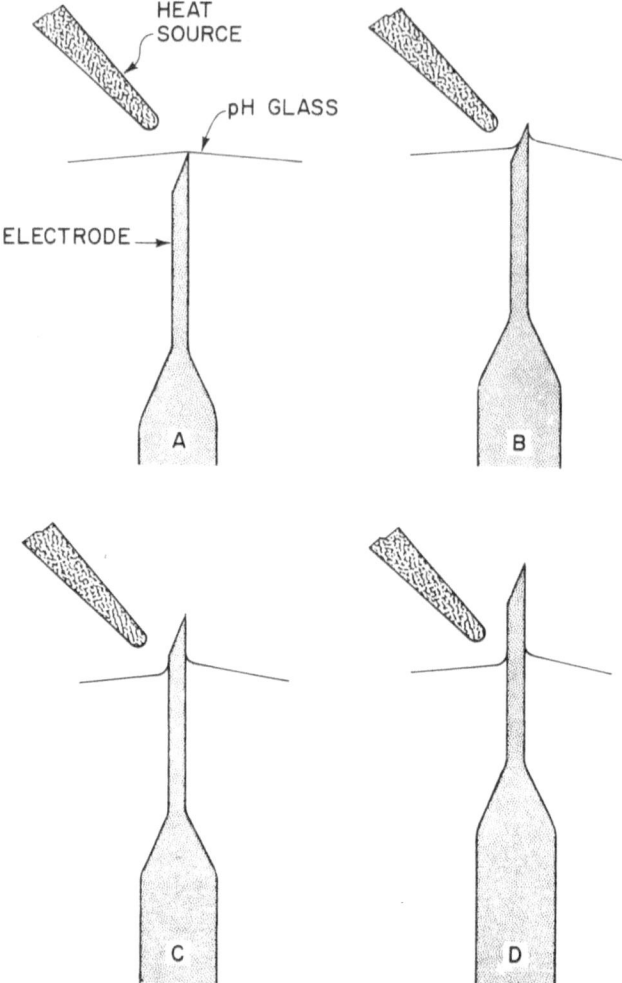

Figure 8. Method used to seal the opening of the indifferent glass pipet with pH glass.

the tips down. The carousel holder, with as many as 16 electrodes, is placed into a desiccator which is then filled with distilled water. The desiccator top is sealed with a water-soluble vacuum grease and placed into a steam pot (for heating) with a vacuum line attached to the desiccator.

t. The desiccator is exposed to steam (saturated at atmospheric pressure) for 30 min, which brings the temperature of the water inside the desiccator to 80–85°C. At this point, with the steam still on, 40 min of vacuum is applied by using a water aspirator. At the end of the 40 min the vacuum is gently broken and the steam turned off. An overnight cooldown follows in order to ensure a complete, bubbleless fill. This method of filling does not damage the thin pH glass membrane of the electrode.

u. The electrodes are then checked under the microscope for bubbles and if they do not appear, the water in the electrode is displaced (with a fine needle) with 1 *M* magnesium acetate saturated with AgCl. It was determined that this filling solution had minimal corrosive action on the pH glass membrane (Pucacco and Carter, 1976).

v. A silver, silver-chloride half cell is installed in the open end of the electrode and then sealed with molten dental wax. Figure 9 shows a completed single-barreled electrode.

2. Double-Barreled Electrodes (Side-by-Side Configuration)

a. Two glass capillaries (aluminosilicate or borosilicate) are glued together (at the end points) with Eastman 910 glue and then epoxy resin. The Eastman 910 is used as a preliminary seal because it is quick drying and holds the capillaries in position while the epoxy resin is applied. The epoxy resin is used because it is water-insoluble and can stand up to the pulling and filling procedures. The dimensions are: large capillary (for pH sensor) 7 cm long and 1.8 mm in diameter, and short capillary (reference barrel) 3 cm long and 0.9 mm in diameter.

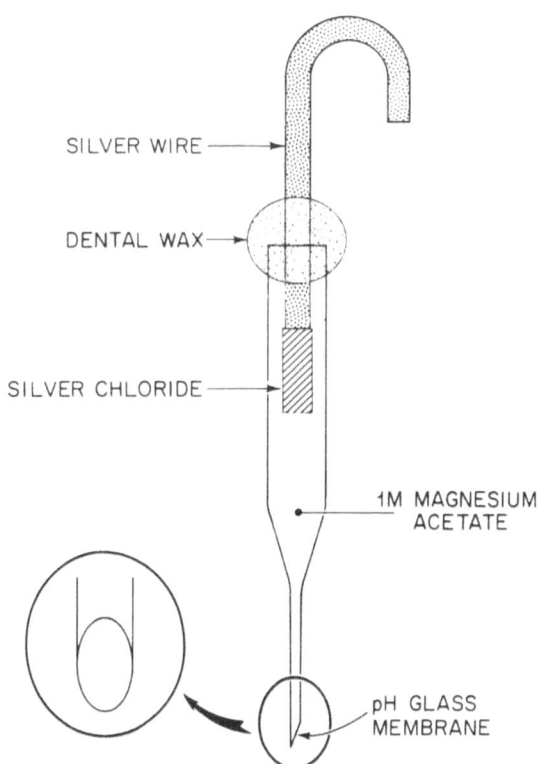

Figure 9. Single-barreled glass membrane, pH microelectrode.

b. The two capillaries are then pulled into a submicrometer pipet using a horizontal pipet puller and incorporating a 270° twist while the glass is in a softened state.

c. The electrode is ground to the desired tip diameter on a silicon carbide 500 grit stone wheel with acetone as the grinding fluid. The tip of the electrode is placed into an ultrasonic cleaner (filled with acetone) and then placed into a heat cone in order to evaporate the acetone.

d. When aluminosilicate glass is used the electrode is annealed (720°C for 10 min) in order to remove strain forces developed in the twisted portion during the pulling procedure. Failure to anneal these double-barreled pipets results in a large incidence of cracking occurring at the point of twist during the filling procedure.

e. The double-barreled electrode tip is sealed with pH glass in the same manner as the single-barreled electrode.

f. The double-barreled electrode is filled in the same manner as the single-barreled electrode.

g. The electrodes are checked under the microscope for bubbles and if they do not appear the water in the pH barrel is displaced with 1 M magnesium acetate (saturated with AgCl) and the water in the reference barrel is displaced with 2.5 M KCl, 0.5 M KNO$_3$ (Carter, 1972). A silver, silver-chloride half cell is installed in the open end of each barrel and sealed with molten dental wax.

h. The pH glass covering the orfice of the reference is removed by passing an a-c current through the tip of the reference barrel. The electrode tip is immersed in a saturated NaCl solution and the electrode terminals electrically connected as shown in Figure 10. The pH side of the electrode is electrically connected to the saturated NaCl solution in order to protect the thin pH glass membrane from a shunting current. The output of a 7500 V (secondary) transformer (controlled by a hold-on switch and regulated by a variable

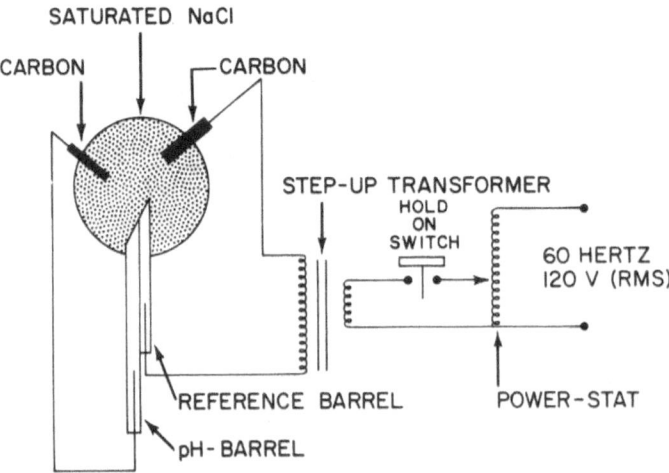

Figure 10. System used to remove glass membrane from the reference barrel of double-barreled electrodes.

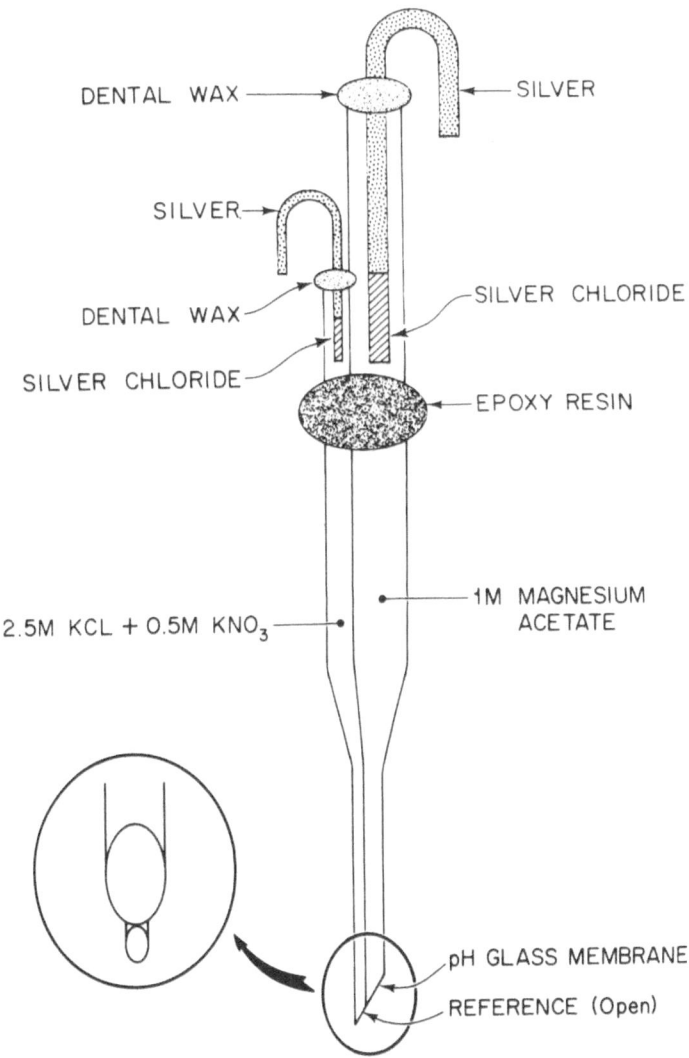

DENTAL WAX ──────► ◄──── SILVER

SILVER ──►

DENTAL WAX ─────► ◄── SILVER CHLORIDE

SILVER CHLORIDE ──

◄── EPOXY RESIN

2.5M KCL + 0.5M KNO_3 ──────►   ───── 1M MAGNESIUM ACETATE

pH GLASS MEMBRANE

REFERENCE (Open)

Figure 11. Double-barreled glass membrane, pH microelectrode (side-by-side configuration).

autotransformer) is placed across the reference membrane with connection to the NaCl solution made by means of a carbon rod. Depending upon the size of the electrode, from 100 to 600 V (RMS) is applied for 1 sec. In most cases one or two attempts are sufficient to open the reference side of the double-barreled electrode. Figure 11 shows a completed double-barreled electrode.

3. Double-Barreled Electrodes (Excentric Double-Lumen Configuration)

The reason for this second double-barreled electrode configuration is that this type of double-barreled pipet is easier to manufacture and is mechanically stronger. We found that in attempting to make double-barreled electrodes with tip diameters less than 4 μm, the side-by-side configuration was unusable because of its weakness. That is to say, the tips of the electrodes would frequently break either during the electrode-making procedure or while attempting to break the electrode free from the unused pH glass membrane [Figure 8(D)]. The excentric double-lumen configuration provided the mechanical strength which allowed us to make double-barreled electrodes as small as 1.5 μm. There is, however, a drawback to this configuration in that it is very difficult to get a good glass-to-glass seal between the pH glass and the back part (away from the tip) of the inner barrel. This is due to the fact that in most cases the inner barrel is undercut and as such does not always make good contact with the softened pH glass. When this condition occurs, it is impossible to open the reference barrel without damaging the pH barrel. Although the losses are high when making double-barreled electrodes in this configuration, the fact that smaller electrodes can be made justifies the difficulty.

a. Excentric double-lumen capillary (aluminosilicate or borosilicate) is made according to the procedure shown in Figure 12.

b. The excentric double-lumen capillary is pulled into a submicrometer pipet on a horizontal pipet puller.

c. The pipet is ground to the desired tip diameter in the same manner as the single-barreled electrode.

d. The electrode tip is sealed with pH glass in the same manner as the single-barreled electrode.

e. The electrode is filled in the same manner as the single-barreled electrode.

f. The electrodes are checked under the microscope for bubbles and if they do not appear, the water in the pH barrel is displaced with 1 M magnesium acetate and the water in the reference barrel is displaced with 2.5 M KCl, 0.5 M KNO$_3$.

g. The filling solutions are removed from about two-thirds of both barrels in order to isolate the two barrels (electrically).

h. A silver, silver-chloride half cell is installed in the open end of each barrel and positioned so that the silver-chloride portion is totally immersed in solution.

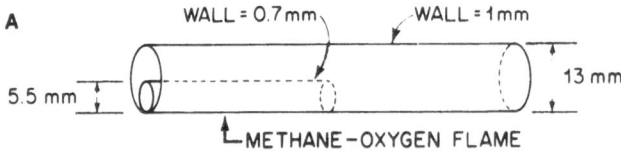

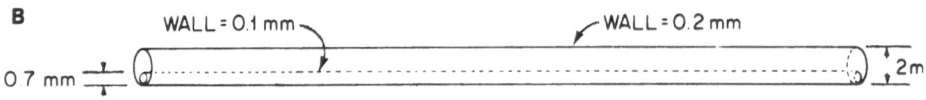

Figure 12. Method used to manufacture excentric double-lumen capillary.

i. Strands of dental wax (solid) are placed in each barrel so that they surround the silver wires.

j. The dental wax is then melted (employing a small-tiped soldering iron) in order to mechanically fix and electrically isolate the two silver, silver-chloride half cells.

k. The pH glass covering the orifice of the reference is removed in the same manner as the side-by-side configured double-barreled electrode. It should be pointed out that because of the marginal seal often incurred between the reference orfice and the pH glass, a large number of electrodes are lost while attempting to open the reference. By lost we mean that the pH membrane is also opened, thus causing the electrode to be unusable. We repeat, although the losses are high when employing this configuration, the ability to make a 1.5-μm electrode is sufficient justification. Figure 13 shows the completed excentric double-lumen double-barreled electrode.

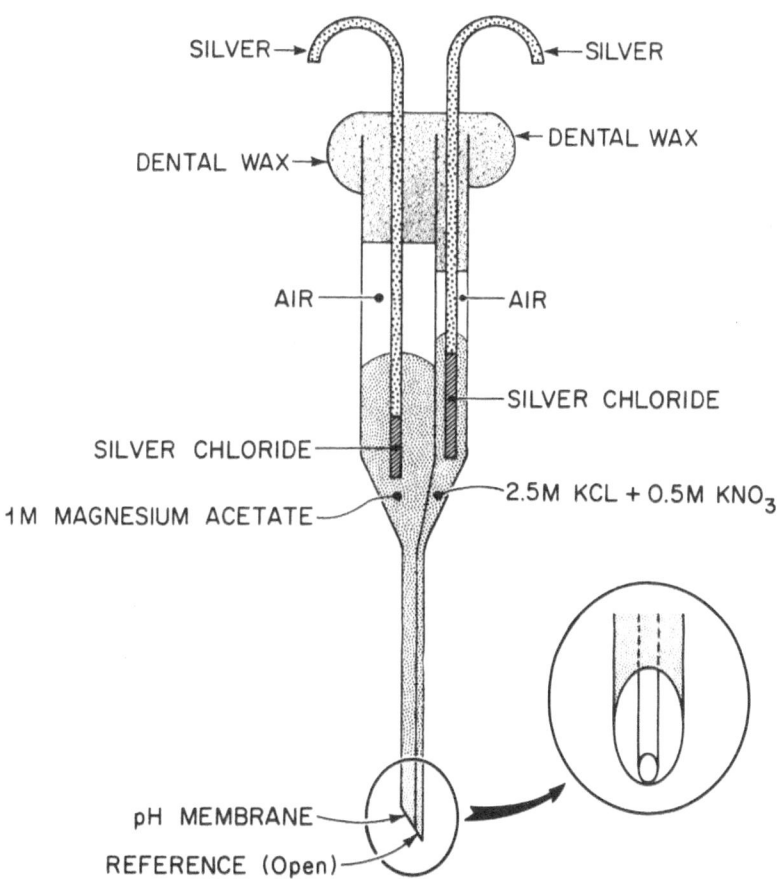

Figure 13. Double-barreled glass membrane, pH microelectrode (excentric double-lumen configuration).

4. Alternative Methods for Sealing the Orfice of the Pipet

When making small electrodes (less than 5 μm), a procedure we have called as "overhead" has proved to be superior to the procedure previously outlined (which we call "sidearm"). This new procedure minimizes the time that the pH glass is heated and thus produces electrodes with lower resistance and faster response times. The heat source is 31-gauge (240 μm) platinum-iridium wire which is formed into a "U" shape and ground flat on the bottom to about 100 μm in thickness. This thinned portion is covered with pH glass as the previous filament was and is similarly electrically excited by a bilevel current control system. Figure 14(A) shows the arrangement of the electrode, pH glass membrane, and the overhead heat source prior to current flow. When the baseline switch is closed (low heat), the pH glass tends to rise [Figure 14(B)] and at this point the high level switch is closed (high heat) and the pH glass is heated to its softening point and falls of its own weight [Figure 14(C)]. In the process of falling, it overlaps and seals to the electrode, thus closing the orfice of the electrode with pH-sensitive glass. The total time the heat is on is usually less

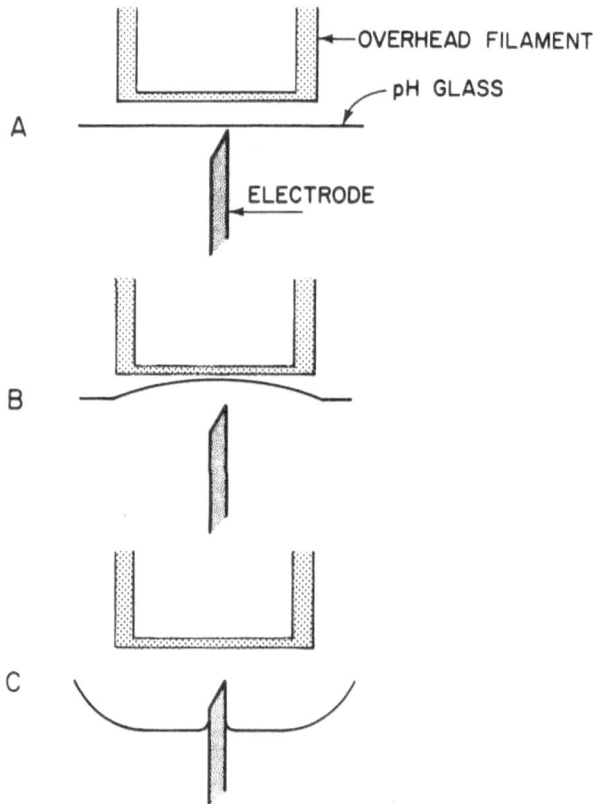

Figure 14. Method used to seal the opening of the indifferent glass pipet with pH glass employing the overhead heating filament.

than 3 sec and our results show that the electrical resistance of an electrode made with this procedure is lower than that of the same size made by the "side-arm" procedure. The only problem with this procedure is that it is rather difficult to get the electrode free from the pH glass membrane since the interface between the pH glass and the electrode is at a point where the electrode is very small in diameter and thus mechanically fragile. The only repeatable procedure which can be used to get the electrode free from the pH glass is to tap the microforge and cause the resulting vibration to break the pH glass–electrode connection. From the work thus far completed, three-fourths of the electrodes capped in this manner break rather than free themselves from the pH glass. The high rate of attrition is, however, acceptable since the electrical characteristics of these electrodes are superior. In addition, at 2 μm or less this is the only procedure which can make an acceptably responsive (time) electrode.

In our most recent work we have developed a third technique for making the glass membrane, pH microelectrode. This technique is a combination of the two previous techniques and has proved to be the best method for making small electrodes. First the electrode tip is sealed with pH glass by the overhead method as outlined. At this stage the electrode is in the state shown in Figure 14(C). A small (10–20 μm) sidearm point source of heat is used to advance the electrode through the pH glass to a point where the electrode is sufficiently strong to be freed from the pH glass without breaking. This second part of the new procedure is identical to that shown in Figure 8(D). Since the tip of the sidearm filament (hot spot) is below the tip of the electrode, little if any heat damage is incurred by the pH glass covering the orfice of the pipet. We have been able to make 2-mm single-barreled electrodes which respond in 1 min with this new technique. It should be pointed out that when making large electrodes (10 μm and greater), the original procedure (sidearm) can be used with no difficulty and the electrodes made will have acceptable resistances and response times.

D. Testing and Using

1. Single-Barreled Electrodes

The single-barreled, glass membrane, pH microelectrode is tested and used employing the circuit shown in Figure 15. The tip of the pH electrode and the reference calomel are placed in pH standard 4 and then in pH standard 7. It should be pointed out that during the testing procedure and unless absolutely necessary, buffers of extreme pH values (high and low) should be avoided. The potential developed across the pH membrane, along with the accompanying contact and liquid junction potentials, is sensed by the electrometer and recorded. The pH 4 intercept (final value) will be 171–177 mV more positive than the pH 7 intercept at 22°C and 180–186 mV more positive at 37°C. The pH of an unknown solution can then be determined by placing the pH electrode and the reference calomel into the solution, recording the resulting potential, and calculating the pH from the calibration intercepts (pH 4 and pH 7). A two-point calibration is sufficient because the potential vs. pH for the glass membrane, pH

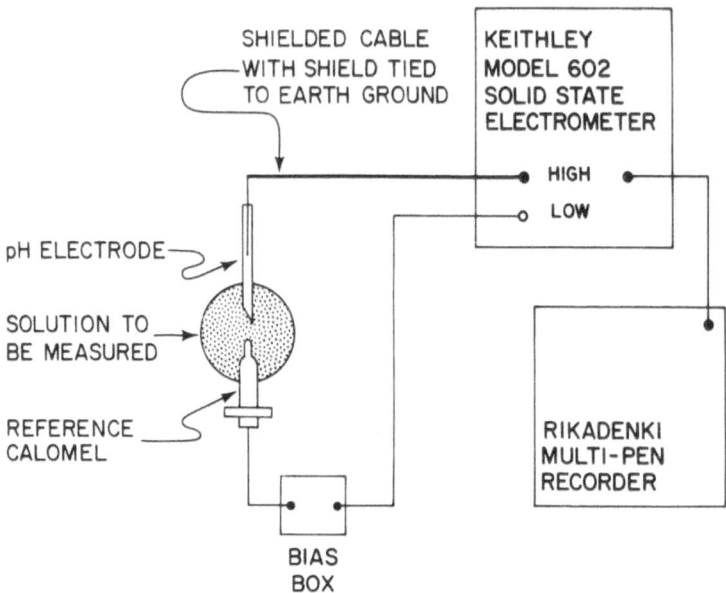

Figure 15. Circuit used to test the electrical characteristics of single-barreled electrodes.

microelectrode is linear from pH 1 to 10. If the pH of a medium which is enclosed by a semipermeable membrane (nephron tubule) across which a potential difference exists is to be measured, the procedure is slightly different. First the pH electrode is calibrated using pH standard 4 and pH standard 7 at the appropriate temperature. The pH electrode is inserted into the medium to be measured with the reference calomel in the solution (medium) on the outside of the membrane. The pH intercept recorded will be made up of both the pH millivolt equivalent of the medium being sensed plus the potential difference present across the membrane due to selective ionic permeabilities. A measurement of this potential must be made by means of another electrode system and the resulting millivolts subtracted or added to the pH intercept (depending on whether the potential difference across the membrane is positive or negative with respect to the reference calomel). Tubular punctures can be made with either the standard Ling-type electrode or a beveled pipet (1–4 μm) in the event a low resistance sensor is required.

2. Double-Barreled Electrodes

The double-barreled, glass membrane, pH microelectrode is tested and used employing the circuit shown in Figure 16. The tip of the electrode and the reference calomel are placed into pH standard 4 and then pH standard 7. The potential developed across the pH membrane, along with the accompanying contact and liquid junction potentials, is sensed by the electrometer and recorded. The pH 4 intercept will be 171–177 mV more positive than the pH 7

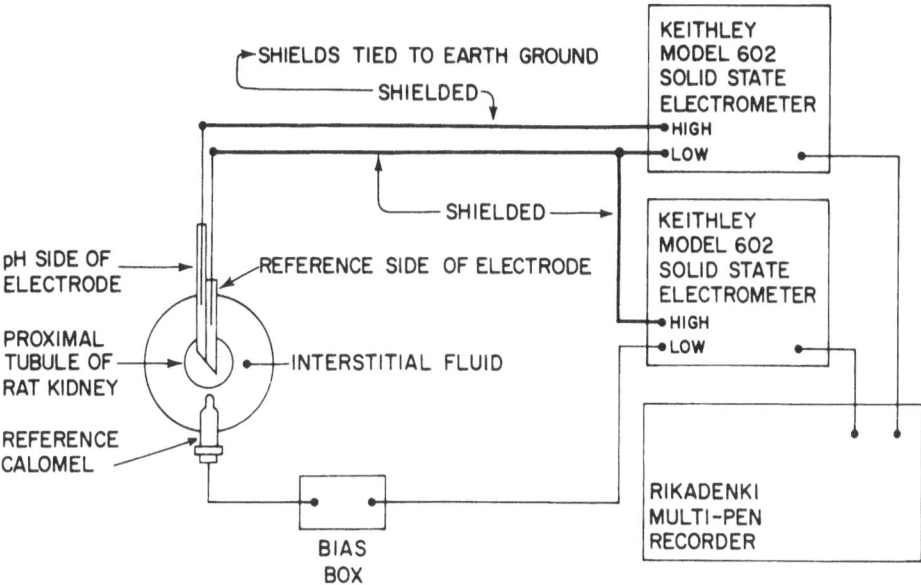

Figure 16. Circuit used to test the electrical characteristics of double-barreled electrodes.

intercept at 22°C and 180–186 mV more positive at 37°C. The potential sensed by the second electrometer represents the potential seen by the reference barrel of the pH electrode with respect to the reference calomel. This intercept should be the same in both pH standards and negative in polarity. If there is a difference in this intercept when the electrode is in pH standard 4 compared with pH standard 7, then the reference barrel of the pH electrode has a tip potential which must be taken into account when determining the slope of the electrode and the pH of the unknown solution. In most cases this tip potential will be less than 10 mV and if it is accounted for will not induce any error into the pH determination. An additional test is required for these double-barreled electrodes in order to ensure total isolation between the pH and reference loops. This test is important because if the isolation between the two loops is not adequate, an error can be induced into the pH intercept by the potential sensed by the reference loop. First, $+100$ mV and then -100 mV is applied to the reference loop using the bias control box (Figure 16) and if the two loops are totally isolated, the pH intercept will not be affected. This test can be performed in either pH 4 or pH 7. The double-barreled pH electrode was designed to measure the pH of a medium that is contained within a semipermeable membrane across which a potential difference exists (proximal and more appropriately the distal tubule of the kidney). First the electrode is calibrated using pH standard 4 and pH standard 7 at the appropriate temperature. The pH electrode is inserted into the medium to be measured with the reference calomel in the solution (medium) on the other side of the membrane. The pH electrometer will sense and record the H^+ activity of the medium being measured without sensing the potential difference across the membrane, i.e., no pH intercept correction is required. The reference loop simultaneously senses and records the potential difference across the membrane. If the potential difference across the medium-separating membrane is of no interest, then the second electrometer can be eliminated (along with the reference calomel and associated wiring) and the remaining electrometer will sense and record the pH without being affected by the transmembrane potential difference. A word of caution should be added here in that the electrical characteristics of the reference loop are of paramount importance and should be monitored closely. That is to say, the reference intercept should be negative in both standard buffers, the difference in the reference intercept between the two buffers should be small (10 mV or less), there should be no effect (except a short time duration transient) on the pH intercept when external potentials are applied (via bias control box) to the reference loop, and the d-c resistance of the reference loop should be at least two orders of magnitude less than the pH loop.

The glass membrane, pH microelectrode is a high resistance (10^8–10^{11} ohms) sensor and therefore certain precautions should be taken in order to prevent experimental artifacts from inducing error. First, since the electrical resistance of the electrode is so high, the experimental area should be inclosed in a Faraday cage. This cage should be connected to an earth ground. Second, all a-c powered equipment used in the experiment should be placed outside the cage if possible. Third, all equipment inside the cage should have cases connected to an earth ground. Fourth, all leads within the cage should be as short as possible and shielded, with the shields connected to an earth ground. Finally, the experimental setup should be so arranged that laboratory personnel do not pass by the open side of the cage.

3. Further Testing of Electrodes

It has been found that *good* electrodes made by the methods described have a slope (mV per unit pH) within 1 or 2 mV of that predicted by the Nernst equation for the particular temperature at which the electrode is being used. However, some electrodes do have a slope which is less than the Nernst value by more than 2 mV. It has been found that there are primarily two reasons for this:

a. The resistance of the electrode is greater than two orders of magnitude less than the input resistance of the electrometer being used. Generally this will be apparent because of the slow response time of the electrode. In addition, the resistance of the electrode can be measured. Rather than applying a current to the electrode, and observing the potential change, it is more satisfactory to parallel known resistances across the input of the electrometer and calculate the electrode resistance from the fall in potential (Frank and Fuortes, 1955).

b. We have found that the most common cause for a decreased slope is a hole in the pH glass membrane (most likely an inadequate seal between the pH glass membrane and the pipet). This can be objectively determined by attempting to measure the pH of a standard buffer which has a high ionic strength (described in Section II-B.). An electrode which has a small hole in the pH membrane tends to read the pH of this buffer lower than it should be. Note that this is the reverse of the error found with this test using open-tip ultramicroelectrodes. Likewise, we have observed that electrodes with a small hole in the pH membrane read Tris-buffered solutions incorrectly, whereas good electrodes read the pH of these solutions correctly.

Unusually fast-responding glass membrane, pH microelectrodes (too fast for their size) tend to have low slopes and generally will not pass the above tests. In some cases the electrode will totally open (have no pH-sensitivity at all) while pH measurements are being made with these inappropriately fast responding electrodes.

4. Aging and Longevity of Electrodes

Although most good electrodes have adequately fast response times immediately after being filled with electrolyte, some have been found to dramatically reduce their response time some time after being made and filled. For this reason we store all completed electrodes with inappropriately long response times in distilled water at 4°C. In most cases the response time of these electrodes will fall from 20 min to 2 min over several days. Thus an unusable electrode becomes a satisfactory electrode. Those electrodes which have a satisfactory response time when first tested we choose to store at 4°C in air. It seems that storing electrodes in distilled water tends to reduce the response time while storing in air tends to extend the lifetime.

One of the better points regarding the 2.1 wt.% UO_2-containing pH glass is the apparent good chemical durability. This characteristic is apparent in the ability to store electrodes for many days (and weeks) after manufacture without destruction of the small, thin pH glass membranes. Nevertheless, it is wise not to keep the electrode tips in either very acidic or very basic solutions for long periods.

E. Applications of the Glass Membrane, pH Microelectrode

Time has been insufficient to exploit to the fullest this electrode in renal research. However, preliminary experiments have been undertaken in our laboratory. Single-barreled, glass membrane pH microelectrodes have been used to estimate the pH of the effluent of the luminal perfusate of isolated portions of the rabbit nephron. Both single- and double-barreled electrodes have been used to measure the intraluminal pH of the superficial rat nephron in *situ*. In both cases, no technical artifacts have been seen and the ability to make the electrode tip diameters to suit the experimental situation of pH measurement has been an advantage.

The glass membrane, pH microelectrode is currently being adapted for use in the pCO_2 microelectrode previously described by this laboratory (Caflisch and Carter, 1974). Originally, the ultra micro ceramic insulated pH microelectrode was used in making the pCO_2 electrode. It has, however, been found that the ease of manufacture, stability, and full slope of the glass membrane, pH microelectrode offers advantages in constructing the pCO_2 microelectrode.

ACKNOWLEDGMENT

The authors wish to acknowledge the excellent technical services of Mr. Allen C. Nunn.

This research was supported in part by National Institutes of Health (NIH) Program Project Grant 1 PO1 HL 11662.

The second author performed these studies under the auspices of an NIH Special Research Fellowship, 1 FO3 GM 57750-01.

REFERENCES

Caflisch, C. R., and Carter, N. W. 1974. A micro pCO_2 electrode. *Anal. Biochem., 60:*252.

Carter, N. W. 1972. The production and testing of double-barreled pH glass microelectrodes for measurement of intratubular pH. *Yale J. Biol. Med., 45:*349.

Carter, N. W., Rector, F. C., Campion, D. S., and Seldin, D. W. 1967a. Measurement of intracellular pH of skeletal muscle with pH-sensitive glass microelectrodes. *J. Clin. Invest., 46:*920.

Carter, N. W., Rector, F. C., Campion, D. S., and Seldin, D. W. 1967b. Measurement of intracellular pH with glass microelectrodes. *Fed. Proc., 26:*1322.

Frank, K., and Becker, M. C. 1964. Microelectrodes for recording and stimulation. In: *Physical Techniques in Biological Research,* Vol. V, pp. 32–33. Ed. by Nastuk, W. L. Academic Press, New York.

Frank, K., and Fuortes, M. G. F. 1955. Potentials recorded from the spinal cord with microelectrodes. *J. Physiol. (Lond.), 130:*625.

Hubbard, D., and Rynders, G. F. 1948. Effect of annealing and other heat treatments on the pH response of the glass electrode. *J. Res. Nat. Bur. Stand., 40:*105.

Isard, J. O. 1967. The dependence of glass-electrode properties on composition. In: *Glass Electrodes for Hydrogen and Other Cations,* p. 88. Ed. by Eisenman, G. Dekker, New York.

MacInnes, D. A., and Dole, M. 1929. Tests of a new type of glass electrode. *Ind. Eng. Chem. (Anal. Ed.), 1:*57.

Pucacco, L. R., and Carter, N. W. 1976. A glass-membrane pH microelectrode. *Anal. Biochem., 73:*501.

Rector, F. C., and Carter, N. W. 1963. Evidence for a disequilibrium pH in the proximal tubule of rat kidney. *Proc. Soc. Exp. Biol. Med.* (New York), *112:*466.

Rector, F. C., Carter, N. W., and Seldin, D. W. 1965. The mechanism of bicarbonate reabsorption in the proximal and distal tubule of the kidney. *J. Clin. Invest., 44:*278.

Schwabe, K. 1954. Über neue hochleitfähige Gläser zur pH-Messung. *Chem. Tech.* (Berlin), *6:*301.

Vieira, F. L., and Malnic, G. 1968. Hydrogen ion secretion by rat renal cortical tubules as studied by an antimony microelectrode. *Am. J. Physiol., 214:*710.

Chapter **9**

Microperfusion of Isolated Tubules

Arnold M. Chonko, James M. Irish III,
and Dan J. Welling

Department of Medicine, Division of Nephrology
and Departments of Pathology and Physiology
University of Kansas Medical Center College
of Health Sciences and Hospital
Kansas City, Kansas

I. INTRODUCTION

"The responsibility for maintaining the composition of the blood in respect to other constituents devolves largely upon the kidneys. It is no exaggeration to say that the composition of the blood is determined not by what the mouth ingests but by what the kidneys keep; they are the master chemists of our internal environment, which, so to speak, they synthesize in reverse. . . . Bones can break, muscles can atrophy, glands can loaf, even the brain can go to sleep, without immediately endangering our survival, but when the kidneys fail to manufacture the proper kind of blood, neither bone, muscle, gland nor brain can carry on. Recognizing that we have the kind of blood that we have because we have the kind of kidney that we have, we must acknowledge that our kidneys constitute the major foundation of our physiological freedom. Superficially, it might be said that the function of the kidneys is to make urine; but in a more considered view one could say the kidneys make the stuff of philosophy itself" (Smith, 1939).

It has been almost four decades since Homer W. Smith expressed that opinion during the course of the Ninth Porter Lecture which he delivered at the University of Kansas. In the 38 years that have passed since his lectureship, significant advances have been made in our knowledge of the mechanisms of solute and water transport by which the kidney regulates our internal milieu. Smith and his colleagues developed in great measure the facts and theory underlying much of modern renal physiology through the use of clearance methods for reliably evaluating glomerular filtration rate, renal blood flow, and net tubular reabsorptive and secretory transport. With the renaissance of micropuncture that occurred in the 1950s, further characterization of the functional capacities of the individual segments of the mammalian nephron was undertaken. This process continues to the present day. However, clearance techniques cannot precisely localize function to specific nephron segments, cannot always clearly separate reabsorption or secretion of substances that undergo both processes, cannot accurately distinguish variation among nephrons, and cannot incisively define transport mechanisms. Although *in situ* micropuncture techniques can accomplish many of these goals, only those segments of the nephron that lie along either the cortical or papillary surfaces of the kidney are accessible to direct micropuncture (Figure 1). Significant portions of the nephron, such as the straight segment of the proximal tubule, the loop of Henle, and the cortical and medullary collecting tubules, lie beneath the renal surface and are therefore not accessible to direct puncture. Moreover, only one nephron population, the superficial cortical nephrons, can be conveniently studied with micropuncture techniques since the juxtamedullary nephron population is too deep for direct puncture, except in the region of the renal papilla.

Frustrated by these limitations and disenchanted with tissue slice and suspension methods for investigating tubular transport processes—techniques

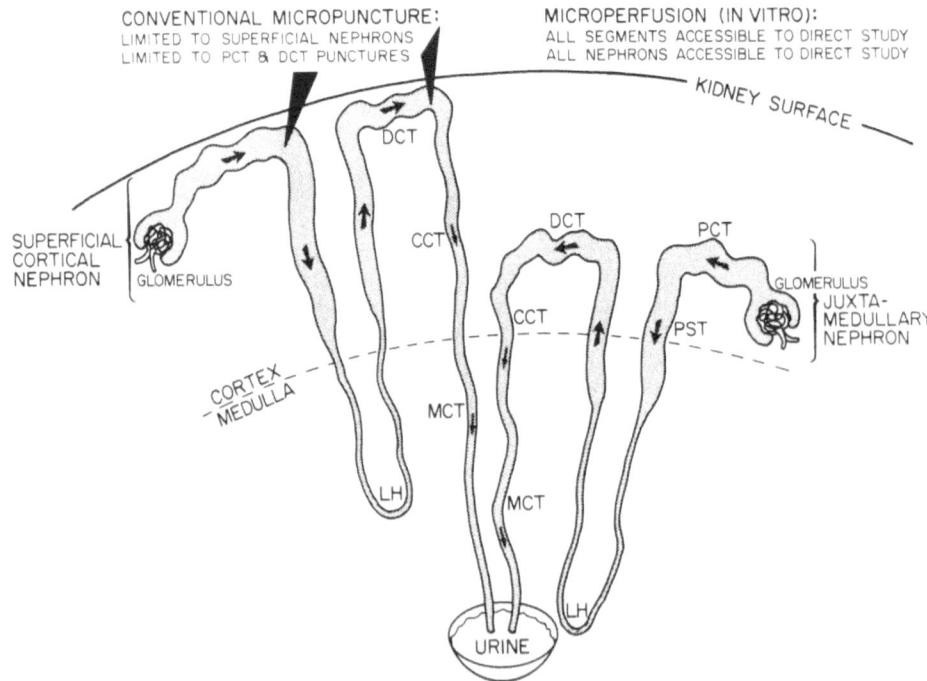

Figure 1. Diagram of the renal cortex. Two populations of nephron, superficial and juxtamedullary, are located within the cortex. All segments of the nephron can be dissected and microperfused *in vitro*. PCT, proximal convolution; PST, proximal straight; DCT, distal convolution; LH, loop of Henle; CCT, cortical collecting tubule; MCT, medullary collecting tubule.

which only allow examination of the peritubular cell membrane—Burg, Grantham, Abramow, and Orloff in 1966 introduced a technique for the perfusion of isolated segments of rabbit nephron *in vitro*. In brief, the main advantages of this method are: (1) essentially all segments of the nephron can be dissected, isolated, and studied directly, (2) the extratubular environment—oxygen content, temperature, pH, oncotic and hydrostatic forces and osmotic regulation—can be rigorously controlled, (3) the tissues can be observed directly at high magnification to facilitate correlation between changes in function and changes in tubular structure, (4) the constituents of the perfusate or bathing fluid can be varied in the midst of the experiment while tubular flow and the integrity of the tubular epithelium remain undisturbed, and (5) analogous segments of superficial, intermediate, and juxtamedullary cortical nephrons can be dissected and perfused so that a study of functional nephron heterogeneity can be carried out. Since the polarity of the tubule is maintained during microperfusion and the tubular fluid, bathing fluid, and tubular epithelium can be recovered for analysis, a three-compartment model of transport (lumen fluid, cell compartment, bath fluid) can be derived for any substance which can be isotopically or microanalytically quantified. The explicit analysis of "transport steps" is a powerful attribute of the *in vitro* microperfusion method.

Herbert Spencer (1863) once stated that evolution is "a change from an indefinite incoherent homogeneity to a definite coherent heterogeneity." If one surveys the structure of the "kidney" as an organ from the level of the teleost through the first bony fishes, the amphibians, the reptiles, the birds, to the mammals—and man—the increased complexity of vascular and tubular structures is clear. Although in its ontogenetic development the kidney of higher mammals recapitulates phylogenetic evolutionary change, the only feature common to all adult species from teleost to man is the monologous "brush border" segment of the renal tubule. Since the time of Smith and his contemporaries, investigators have turned to experimental approaches that remove "levels of heterogeneity" from the kidney as a whole and allow for direct examination of the transport capacities of the various portions of the renal tubular epithelium. The *in vitro* microperfusion technique provides an excellent tool for the creative investigator, to define mechanisms of transport located in the various segments of the individual nephron and to clarify differences in function among various types of nephron. In the remainder of this chapter we discuss many of the technical aspects of performing *in vitro* microperfusion experiments. We do not claim to be comprehensive; we offer this discussion as an empirical approach. In the concluding section of this chapter, a formulation of solute and fluid transport in isolated perfused tubules under various experimental conditions is presented.

II. TECHNICAL ASPECTS

A. Overview of the Microperfusion Technique

For those totally unfamiliar with the *in vitro* microperfusion method, a few introductory remarks are in order. The female New Zealand white rabbit has

been used most extensively for these studies, although *in vitro* microperfusion
has been successfully performed with tubules dissected from flounder, snake,
Necturus, frog, and human fetal tissue. Although it is not possible to dissect an
intact nephron from the kidney, 1–4 mm segments of each portion of the rabbit
nephron have been successfully dissected and perfused.

To conduct an experiment, the animals (2–3 kg) are sacrificed, the kidney
quickly removed, and a 2-mm sagittal section taken and immediately immersed
in rabbit serum at 4°C. The slice is teased apart with fine-tipped forceps under
direct visualization through a binocular microscope (10–90×). Once a suitable
tubule is isolated, it is transferred within a small volume of serum to a
thermostatically controlled perfusion chamber. The perfusion chamber consists
of a 2 × 0.5 cm slot cut through a 0.5-cm translucent acrylic plate. The bottom of
the chamber is formed by an ordinary 2-cm glass slide cover which is joined to
the acrylic plate from below with beeswax [Figure 2(C)]. High-magnification
(100–600×) inspection of tubular morphology is facilitated by an arrangement in
which the perfusion chamber is mounted above an inverted microscope and
illuminated from above (Figure 3). Any tubule with evidence of excessive trauma
due to dissection, such as cell swelling, breaks in the tubular basement
membrane, or areas of increased opacity, is discarded.

To perfuse a suitable tubule, a glass micropipet (holding pipet) is maneuvered so that one end of the tubule is engaged by gentle suction. A concentri-

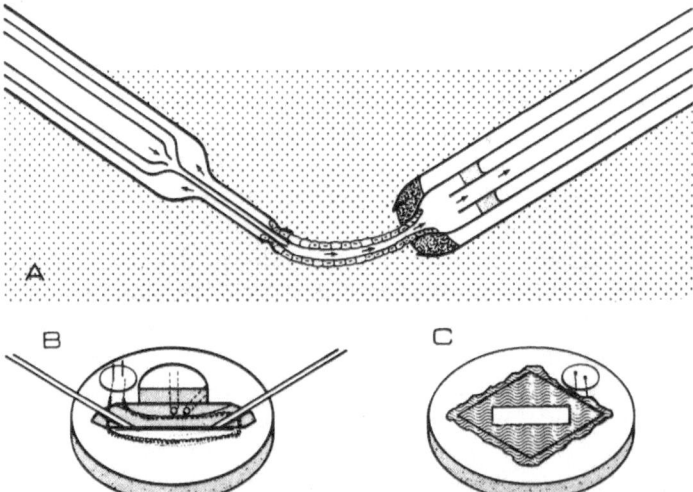

Figure 2. (A) Arrangement for perfusing kidney tubule segments. Pipets on the left of figure
from outside to inside: holding, perfusion, and fluid exchange pipet. Pipets on the right of
figure from outside to inside: Sylgard holding, collecting, and constant bore capillary
collecting pipet. Arrow in holding pipet indicates negative pressure that is applied to the
tubule. Arrows in fluid exchange pipet, tubular segment, and collecting pipet indicate direction
of perfusate flow. (B) Acrylic perfusion chamber with holding and collecting pipets in place.
Heating wire used to maintain 37°C temperature surrounds the perfusion chamber well. (C)
Acrylic perfusion chamber viewed from below. The glass cover slip that forms the bottom of
the perfusion chamber is held in place with beeswax.

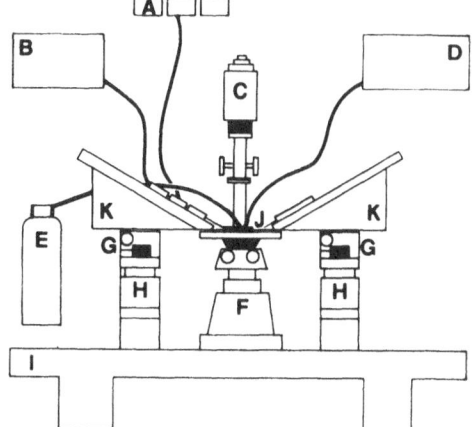

Figure 3. Block diagram of equipment used in microperfusion experiments. A, perfusate reservoir; B, pump; C, light source; D, temperature controller; E, O/CO₂ gas source; F, invested microscope; G, micromanipulator; H, elevation; I, stable base; J, chamber; K, V-track.

cally mounted pipet (perfusion pipet) is then inserted into the tubule lumen (Figure 2). The other end of the tubule is then gently aspirated into another micropipet (collecting pipet). Either a microsyringe pump or simple hydrostatic pressure is used to propel perfusion fluid through the tubule into the collecting pipet where it accumulates beneath a column of water-equilibrated oil. The oil prevents evaporation but provides no significant resistance to flow. A wide range of relatively stable rates of outflow can be obtained. All the accumulated fluid is collected at periodic intervals by inserting a calibrated collecting pipet through the oil column in the collecting pipet. The tubule length is measured with a micrometer in the microscope eyepiece. The absolute volume reabsorption is determined (nl/mm per min) from the change in concentration in the collected fluid of an impermeant marker such as [^{14}C]inulin or [^{125}I]iothalamate.

The glass micropipets are mounted in acrylic holding pieces which are fitted within specifically designed aluminum V-tracts (Jim White Instrument Co., Bradbury Park, Md.). Each V-track is mounted at a 30° angle to the horizontal plane and rests atop a rack-and-pinion micromanipulator (Stoelting Co., Chicago, Il.). The micromanipulator arrangement provides for movement along both axes of the horizontal plane (Figure 3). Vertical movement of the pipet arrangement is provided by elevating column supports (J. H. Emerson Co., Cambridge, Ma.) which are positioned below the micromanipulators (Figure 3). The exquisite stability, prerequisite for microperfusion, is accomplished by mounting the inverted microscope, with the perfusion chamber and the micromanipulators, on an aluminum base plate which is fastened to a stable laboratory bench (Figure 3).

The goal of *in vitro* microperfusion is to mimic to great degree the *in situ* condition in which an ultrafiltrate of plasma courses along the tubule from glomerulus to the papillary collecting tubule. Thus, in many experiments conducted on proximal tubules, an isotonic ultrafiltrate of rabbit serum is perfused while the tubule is immersed in a bath of rabbit serum. In the decade that has passed since the introduction of this technique, various investigators have employed certain changes in both perfusion and bath fluid composition in order to gain insight into the mechanism of salt and water transport in specific segments of the rabbit nephron.

The perfusion chamber holds approximately 1 ml of bathing medium which is exchanged throughout the course of an experiment without disturbing the tubule. Control of the bathing medium pH and PO_2 is accomplished via insufflation of various O_2/CO_2 gas mixtures over the surface of the chamber from above (Figure 3). A constant bath temperature within the perfusion chamber is maintained by adjusting the current flow through a platinum-iridium wire which is embedded within the acrylic plate surrounding the perfusion trough [Figure 2(A)]. Constant monitoring of the bath temperature is accomplished via a temperature probe which is immersed in the bath fluid through a slot in the perfusion chamber wall. A negative feedback servonulling arrangement (Yellow Springs Instrument Co., Yellow Springs, Ohio) regulates the current flow to the heating coil.

The basic equipment costs necessary to undertake microperfusion experiments are listed in Table I. Some investigators have performed *in vitro* microperfusion with a less expensive setup through the use of a "top-viewing" binocular microscope (Irish and Dantzler, 1976). However, the inverted microscope provides the high-power magnification necessary to verify the integrity of the tubule while it is perfused. A camera conveniently records structure–function correlations at high-power magnification.

Precise control of the tonicity and pH of the perfusate and bath fluid is a prerequisite for obtaining meaningful data. Therefore, access to an osmometer

Table I. Present Costs of Basic Equipment Necessary for *In Vitro* Microperfusion Experimentation

Item	Approximate cost ($)
Vertical pipet puller	650.00
Microforge	2,200.00
Dissecting microscope	800.00
Fiber light illuminator	120.00
Inverted microscope	2,200.00
Micromanipulators X 2	450.00
Elevating column supports	550.00
V-tracks × 2	1,200.00
Acrylic perfusion chamber	300.00
Acrylic holding pieces	2,000.00
Temperature probe	190.00
Temperature regulator	450.00
Variable voltage power supply	50.00
Base plate	500.00
Microsyringe pump	600.00
Osmometer	2,500.00
pH meter	2,000.00

and a pH meter is essential. Although hydrostatic pressure can be used to propel perfusate along the tubule, it is advisable to use a microsyringe pump for experiments that require a more nearly constant flow rate.

When isotopes are used, the investigator must have access to either a gamma or a liquid scintillation counter. In a modification of the perfusion arrangement, which eliminates the need for isotopes, the distal end of the tubule is occluded and the movement of an oil drop, contained within the shaft of the perfusion pipet, is used to calculate absolute volume reabsorption or volume secretion (Grantham *et al.*, 1973).

There are many potential "pitfalls" en route to a successful microperfusion experiment. Careful pipet manufacture, fluid preparation, and dissection technique are required for success with this method. A detailed discussion of these procedures follows since they are "rate limiting" to the success of any microperfusion experiment.

B. Pipet Preparation and Assembly

Prior to removing the kidney tissue, glass pipets to hold and perfuse the tubule must be manufactured and assembled. Properly prepared and aligned pipets are critically important to the success of the experiments.

In this laboratory, perfusion pipets and holding pipets are fashioned from flint glass which is ordered from Drummond Scientific (Broomwall, Pa.). Precision capillary tubing used to make calibrated collecting pipets can be purchased from Friedrich and Dimmock (Millville, N.J.) or Corning Glass (Corning, N.Y.). The various pipets used in the laboratory, together with their respective glass sizes, are listed in Table II.

The following pipet nomenclature will be used in this discussion of pipet design (Figure 4). The shaft is the unconstricted portion of the pipet. The segment of the pipet exhibiting the largest degree of taper is called the shoulder. The pipet shank is the long, constricted segment of the pipet. The tip refers to the end of the pipet which either perfuses the tubule or collects the perfused fluid.

The perfusion pipets and holding pipets are initially pulled to a taper on a vertical pipet puller (Stoelting, Chicago, Il.). The slope and wall thickness of the

Table II. Dimensions of Glass Used to Manufacture Pipets

Pipet	Outside diameter (inch)	Inside diameter (inch)
Holding, collecting	0.084	0.064
Perfusion	0.047	0.040
Volumetric collecting	0.047	0.027
Fluid exchange	0.018	0.008
Sylgard holding	0.157	0.126

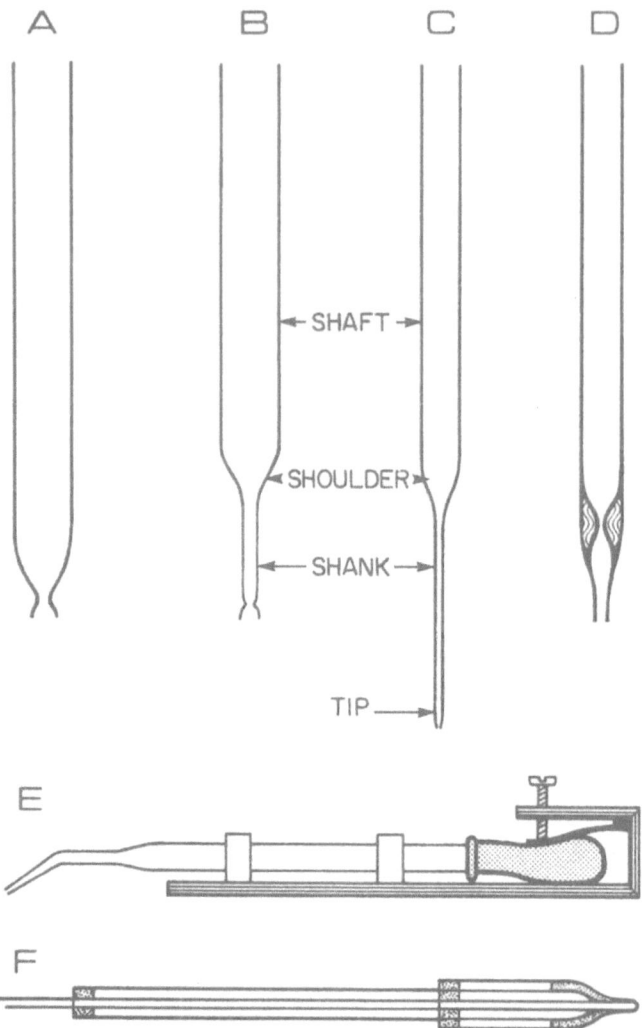

Figure 4. The various pipets used in microperfusion experiments: (A) Collecting pipet. (B) Holding pipet. (C) Perfusion pipet. (D) Volumetric collecting pipet. (E) Transfer pipet mounted in holder. (F) Constant bore capillary collecting pipet.

pipet can be varied by using different combinations of heat intensity and weights on the pipet. The weights, ranging from 1.25 to 2.5 g, consist of various lengths of plastic rod in which holes have been drilled to accommodate the glass. The weight is attached to the glass with plasticine [Figure 5(A)]. The shank is snapped off 2–3 cm from the shoulder of the pipet after the glass rod has been pulled to a taper.

A microforge (Stoelting, Chicago, Il.) is used to bring the various pipets to final form. A hook is fashioned at the tip of the pipet so that a weight may be hung to provide a pulling force (Figure 5). To form the hook, the pipet tip is touched to the activated heating wire. When the glass has adhered to the wire, the wire is moved to the side and upward while the heat is released (Figure 5). The pipet is then positioned with the heating wire surrounding the pipet shank just above the hook. After placing the appropriate weight on the hook, the glass is heated so that it bends slightly. The bend brings the weight directly under the pipet shank and further heating will not cause the shank to bend (Figure 5). To this point, all pipets are formed in the same manner. Various modifications are used to manufacture the specific pipets.

The holding and collecting pipets have a similar design at the pipet tip (Figure 4). However, these pipets differ in that the constriction in the collecting pipet is made at the junction of the shoulder and the shank at about 0.5 mm inside diameter (i.d.) [Figure 4(A)], while the constriction in the holding pipet is made in the pipet shank 1.5 cm beyond the shoulder [Figure 4(B)]. In both cases, the heating wire is positioned around the pipet and a 1-g weight is hung on the hook. The pipet is heated until the constriction diameter is about 60 μm as measured with an eyepiece reticle (Figure 5). The weight is then changed to a 5-mg weight and the pipet is again heated until the desired constriction is reached. The desired size of the constriction will be determined by the size of the tubule segment being perfused. Ideally, the pipet combination on the perfusion side should form a tight seal between the constriction of the holding pipet and the outside of the tubule, and another seal between the inside of the tubule and the perfusion pipet. A successful combination for most rabbit proximal tubules (2–3-kg rabbit) is a 34-μm i.d. holding pipet and a 15-μm o.d. perfusion pipet.

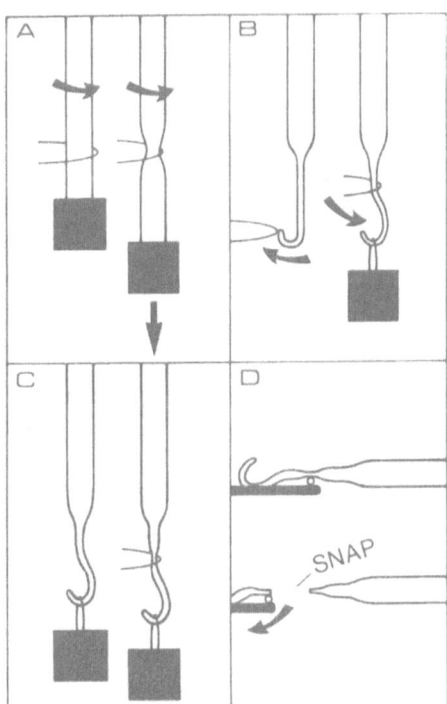

Figure 5. Steps in pipet preparation. (A) Rotating pipet being pulled to a tip on vertical pipet puller. The Lucite rod attached to the pipet provides enough weight to pull the pipet when heat is applied. (B) The pipet on the left shows formation of the hook. On the right, the pipet is heated gently to bring the weight directly in line with the central axis of the pipet. (C) Formation of the constriction. (D) Breaking of the pipet. Note the glass bead on the wire which bonds to the pipet on heating.

All pipets except the perfusion and constant-bore calibrated pipet are completed by breaking off the excess glass below the constriction. This is accomplished with the pipet in the horizontal position [Figure 5(D)]. The holding and collecting pipets are broken at the point where the inside diameter measures 50 μm. It is important to have a small bead of glass on the heating wire to which the pipet can adhere. The heating wire is brought to the surface of the pipet from below [Figure 5(D)]. The glass bead is then positioned on the pipet a short distance from where the pipet is to be broken since the wire migrates as heat is applied. As soon as the bead and the pipet fuse, the heat is released. The stress applied by the "cooling migration" of the heating wire causes the glass to break at the point of fusion. The broken end of the pipet is then fire polished by bringing the pipet in proximity to the heating wire. Care must be taken not to alter the pipet design during fire polishing.

The collecting pipets are made in a range of sizes (28–40 μm) to provide a tight seal between the tubule segment and the pipet. The quality of the seal can be improved by precoating the pipets with encapsulating resin, Sylgard 184 (Dow Corning Corp., Midland, Mi.). This is done by immersing the pipet briefly in the proper 10:1 mixture of encapsulating resin and curing agent so that the Sylgard 184 migrates up the lumen to the level of the constriction. With the pipet mounted vertically in the microforge, suction is applied to the back end of the pipet. The heating element is again positioned around the pipet at the constricted portion and gentle heat applied until the Sylgard 184 hardens on the glass. The pipet can be stored for use.

The perfusion pipet [Figure 4(C)] is made with 0.047 inch o.d., 0.040 inch i.d. glass. The flint glass used to make the perfusion pipet is thoroughly rinsed with distilled water and dried in an oven prior to forming the pipet. Failure to clean the glass may lead to an obstructed pipet during the experiment. The tip, formed 2 cm from the shoulder, should be pulled to a constant bore at 15 μm i.d. for about 1 mm before being pulled to a sealed tip (100 mg wt.). The sealed tip is snapped off with forceps after the perfusion pipet has been filled with perfusate and inserted in the holding pipet following final assembly of the pipets in their respective holding pieces.

There are two types of calibrated collecting pipets: a constant bore capillary tube [Figure 4(F)] which allows a sample of variable volume to be collected, and a volumetric pipet [Figure 4(D)] which provides for constant volume collection. The calibrated volumetric pipet allows for the collection of serial samples without emptying the pipet between collections.

The constant bore capillary collecting pipet is constructed by fusing the larger diameter support glass to the capillary glass. A hook is fashioned in tapered 0.047-inch o.d., 0.027-inch i.d. glass. The 0.018-inch o.d. glass and the capillary glass are advanced into the 0.047-inch o.d. glass until stopped by the constriction [Figure 4(F)]. With a 1-g weight on the hook, the glass is heated at the junction of the 0.047-inch o.d. and the 0.018-inch o.d. glass until fusion occurs. The process is repeated at the junction of the 0.047-inch o.d. glass and the capillary glass. The pipet tip is then snapped off with forceps. Finally, the junction of capillary and 0.018-inch o.d. glass, and the junction of 0.018-inch o.d. and 0.047-inch o.d. glass are sealed with beeswax.

The design of the volumetric collecting pipet [Figure 4(D)] requires some planning. The expected perfusion rate and the desired collection time will determine the necessary volume of the pipet. For any given volume, a balance must be struck between the diameter and the length of the volumetric pipet. Large diameter pipets may cause the collected fluid to migrate between the volumetric pipet and collecting pipet. Excessive length from pipet tip to constriction will place the constriction beyond the range of focus of the microscope, thus preventing observation of the collected volume. To form this type of calibrated collecting pipet, the 0.047-inch o.d. glass is mounted in the microforge and a 5-mg weight attached. The upper constriction, started at 390 μm i.d., is fashioned by heating the pipet until the lumen is constricted to 5–7 μm [Figure 4(D)]. The pipet is moved up 1 mm and is then pulled to a tip using the 0.5-g weight. The tip is broken back to about 10 μm i.d. diameter with forceps and fire polished with the microforge. A pipet with these dimensions will contain approximately 60 nl.

The fluid exchange pipet, made from 0.018 inch o.d. glass, is the only pipet which is not pulled to a taper before the hook is formed. With a 5-mg weight attached and slight positive pressure applied via syringe and polyethylene tubing, the pipet is heated just above the hook. Heating causes lumen expansion at the expense of the wall thickness. This process should continue until the lumen becomes oval shaped. This thin-walled portion is used to form the pipet tip. The 0.5-g weight is attached and the pipet pulled to a tip. The pipet is broken off at 0.01-inch o.d. and fire polished with the microforge.

The Sylgard holding pipet (Figure 2) is fashioned from 4 mm o.d. glass. The pipet is pulled to a taper, broken off at 500 μm i.d., fire polished and coated with polymerized Sylgard 184 as previously described.

Once the pipets have been formed, they must be assembled into a cohesive functional unit. All the pipets are held in place within cylinders of acrylic plastic which are machined to fit tightly within the V-track aluminum carriages (Figure 6). Each holding piece is constructed in two parts: a main body, approximately 2 cm in length, and a sealing portion, approximately 0.5 cm in length (Figure 6). The latter is threaded into either the front or rear of the main body of the holding piece. Each acrylic holding piece has been drilled at its center to specifically fit the outer diameter of the shaft of a holding pipet, collecting pipet, perfusion pipet, or fluid exchange pipet (Table II). Once properly inserted into their holding pieces, all the various pipets are held firmly in place. Sylastic seals are applied to the shaft of the pipets at the junction of the body and sealing portions of the holding pieces. Thus, negative or positive pressure can be applied to any pipet independently.

Assembly of the pipets on the V-track carriages is performed away from the perfusion chamber. We use a wooden block to hold the V-track carriages in the horizontal position while the holding pieces (with pipets) are inserted on the track. The holding pipet [Figure 4(B)] is placed on the track and advanced to the front edge of the carriage. The perfusion pipet is carefully inserted through the rear of the holding pipet and advanced until the tip approaches the narrow constriction at the tip of the holding pipet. Care is taken during insertion of the perfusion pipet into the rear of the holding pipet lest the perfusion pipet tip be

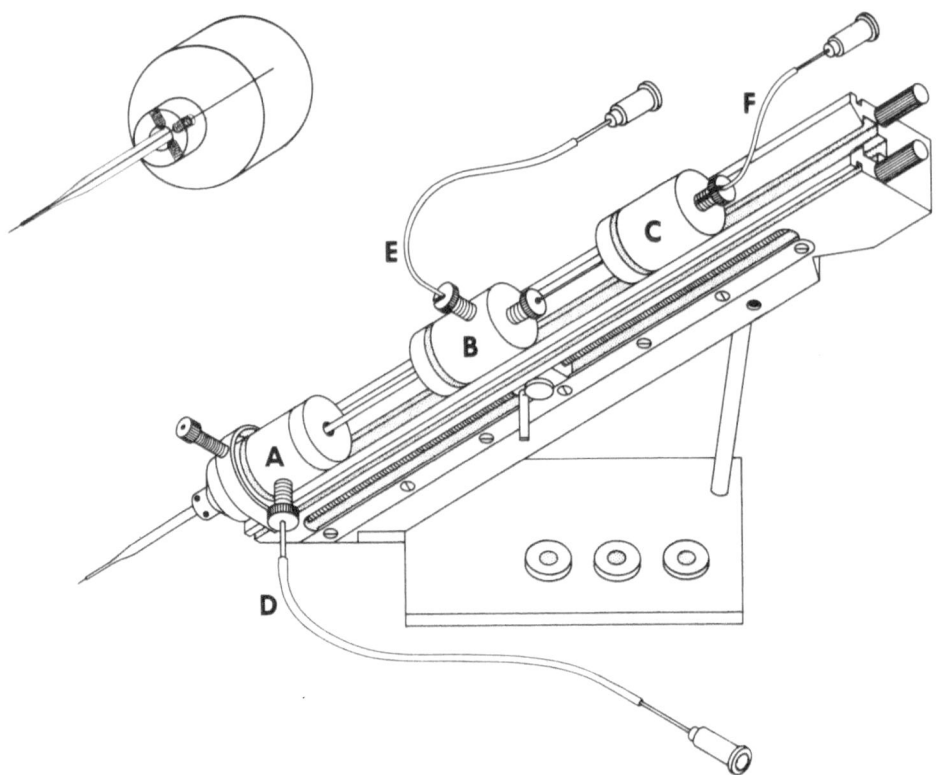

Figure 6. V-Track carriage and arrangement of perfusion pipets. A,B,C are the acrylic holding pieces for the holding pipet, perfusion pipet, and fluid exchange pipet respectively; D, connection for applying suction to draw the tubule into the holding pipet; E, outflow from discarded perfusion fluid; F, delivery point for perfusion fluid and pressure to drive the perfusate. Insert: Absolute concentricity of the perfusion pipet within the holding pipet can often be obtained by adjusting the screws contained within the front end of the acrylic holding piece for the holding pipet.

shattered. This procedure is performed with the visual aid of a binocular microscope. The holding piece for the perfusion pipet is connected to a threaded rod which when turned advances or retracts the perfusion pipet (within its holding piece) along the V-track (Figure 6).

Final advance of the perfusion pipet through the most constricted portion of the holding pipet is carried out under microscopic visualization (20–30×). Adherence of the perfusion pipet to the inner wall of the shank of the holding pipet occasionally occurs. Filling the holding pipet tip with distilled water for 1 cm obviates this problem.

Once the perfusion pipet tip emerges from the holding pipet, the relative concentricity of the pipet arrangement is examined under the microscope (30×). The relationship of the perfusion pipet and holding pipet is inspected in both the horizontal and vertical axes. Even with "straight" pipets, the perfusion pipet at times is centered in one plane but rests against the edge of the holding pipet in the second plane. Absolute concentricity of the pipet arrangement is obtained by adjusting set screws placed within the forward edge of the body of the holding piece (insert, Figure 6). The perfusion pipet is discarded if concentricity is not obtained since it is difficult to cannulate a tubule with pipets that are not perfectly aligned.

The first *in vitro* microperfusion experiments were performed with a single perfusion pipet and holding pipet at the proximal end of the tubule. The development of the fluid exchange pipet has broadened the scope of the microperfusion technique. With the fluid exchange pipet in place, perfusate can be exchanged in the midst of an experiment without disrupting tubule perfusion. Thus, a single tubule can serve as its own control while pertubations in luminal fluid or bath fluid are made. The fluid exchange pipet is also held in place with a holding piece (Figure 6). It is the last pipet to be placed in the V-track carriage and is advanced or retracted independently via a second threaded rod (Figure 6).

If pipet alignment proves satisfactory, perfusion fluid is added to the perfusion pipet. If the two-pipet system is used, a 30-gauge needle (Popper and Sons, Inc., New Hyde Park, N.Y.) is inserted through the rear of the perfusion pipet and advanced to the shoulder of the pipet. The perfusion fluid is introduced into the perfusion pipet under positive pressure and the needle is slowly withdrawn as the pipet fills with fluid. With a three-pipet system, the perfusion fluid is introduced at the rear of the fluid exchange pipet [Figure 6(F)] and advanced along the fluid exchange pipet to fill the perfusion pipet in retrograde fashion. Excess perfusion fluid is drained from the perfusion pipet via polyethylene tubing which is connected to the rear of the perfusion pipet [Figure 6(E)]. This drainage pathway is sealed during perfusion of a tubule.

The final assembly of the "perfusion complex" is carried out with the V-track attached to the micromanipulator (Figure 3). This maneuver is performed with the elevating column extended so that the holding and perfusion pipet tips are suspended 5 cm above the perfusion chamber. Thus, the pipets are less likely to be crushed against the walls of the perfusion chamber if unanticipated movements of the V-track occur. The connections to the microsyringe pump and the glass syringe used for applying suction to the holding pipets are threaded in place. The pipets are carefully lowered into the perfusion chamber.

Whatever perfusion system is used, the driving force for perfusion is applied to the last pipet in the system—either the perfusion pipet (two-pipet system) or the fluid exchange pipet (three-pipet system). A 27-gauge needle (Jim White Instrument Co., Bradbury Park, Md.) is inserted into the rear of the last holding piece in the system to serve as the connection between the series of glass pipets and the driving force for perfusion—either a 10-μl gas-tight syringe (Hamilton Co., Reno, Nv.) driven by a microsyringe pump (Sage Instruments, White Plains, N.Y.), or a hydrostatic pressure reservoir. The steel needle is inserted through a rubber gasket which prevents fluid leaks at the rear of the pipet system.

The collecting pipet "complex" is much simpler in design (outer Sylgard holding pipet and inner collecting pipet, Figure 2). It is assembled while the V-track carriage is attached to its micromanipulator at the general perfusion arrangement. The holding pieces for the collecting and outer Sylgard pipet are similar in construction to those previously described. Stability of the pipet system is maintained by inserting the holding pieces within the V-track and clamping them in place. The rear of the collecting pipet is open to the atmosphere. Thus, the smaller bore calibrated collecting pipet can be inserted within the collecting pipet to retrieve accumulated fluid. A rack-and-pinion device is attached to the top end of the V-track to guide the movement of the calibrated collecting pipet.

C. Bath and Perfusion Fluid Preparation

Early micropuncture experiments (Wearn and Richards, 1924) indicated that the fluid entering the early proximal convoluted tubule closely resembled an ultrafiltrate of plasma. Thus, in the initial *in vitro* experiments with proximal convoluted tubules, an ultrafiltrate of rabbit serum was perfused while the tubule was bathed in rabbit serum (Burg and Orloff, 1968). Subsequently, cortical collecting tubules were perfused with a hypotonic perfusion solution that more closely resembled the *in situ* condition of tubular fluid along this segment (Grantham and Orloff, 1968).

In our laboratory, rabbit serum (Microbiological Assoc., Bethesda, Md.) is decomplemented soon after its arrival. This is done by heating the serum to 55°C for 30 min. The serum is frozen and stored. Serum is thawed and used daily to minimize bacterial contamination. Prior to use, the serum is filtered through an 8-μm filter (Millipore Corp., Bedford, Ma.) and the serum adjusted to pH 7.3–7.4 by bubbling with 80% O_2/20% CO_2. The osmolality is determined (Fiske Assoc., Uxbridge, Ma.). The serum is placed in a 50-ml syringe and capped to prevent changes in pH or tonicity. Serum is delivered directly from syringe to the bathing chamber during the course of an experiment.

Ultrafiltrates of rabbit serum are prepared with a standard ultrafiltration apparatus (Amicon Corp., Lexington, Ma.). Nitrogen gas at 10–20 psi drives filtration of the serum through a "Diaflo" ultrafiltration membrane (PM 30, Amicon Corp., Lexington, Ma.). Low driving pressure minimizes the problem of forming a hyposmotic ultrafiltrate. We perform this procedure under hypothermic conditions (4°C) to suppress bacterial growth. The ultrafiltrate is bubbled with 80% O_2/20% CO_2 to adjust the pH to the physiologic range. It is also filtered through a 0.45-μm filter (Millipore Corp., Bedford, Ma.) to remove any particulate matter that can obstruct the perfusion pipet. Ultrafiltrate repeatedly thawed and frozen will become hypotonic over several weeks. It is essential that the osmolality of the perfusate be checked prior to use. Exposure of proximal tubules to markedly hypotonic perfusate (perfusate osmolality 15–20 mOsM/kg less than bath fluid osmolality) produces rapid cell swelling and sluffing of the tubular epithelium. The osmolality of 5 μl of perfusate is accurately measured with a vapor pressure osmometer (Wescor Corp., Logan, Ut.).

In most experiments, an isotopic impermeant solute is added to the perfusate as a marker for the determination of fluid absorption across the tubule.

[³H]inulin, and [¹²⁵I]iothalamate have sufficiently high specific activities so that very small volumes of isotope are required ($\geqq 1:100$ dilution). The isotope is added directly into the ultrafiltrate with an accurate micropipet.

In the past decade, numerous artificial perfusion fluids have been devised for all of the various segments of the rabbit nephron. Several of these artificial perfusates are listed in Table III. Standard gravimetric techniques are used to manufacture these fluids. The adjustments of pH and tonicity and filtration of these solutions are performed in the same fashion as described for rabbit serum.

Kokko (1973) developed an artificial perfusate (solution C, Table III) in an effort to duplicate an ultrafiltrate of rabbit serum. The potential difference generated by the proximal convoluted tubule was 13% lower in tubules perfused with artificial perfusate when compared with tubules perfused with an ultrafiltrate of rabbit serum (-5 mV vs. -6.1 mV). Volume absorption was also slightly less in tubules perfused with artificial perfusate. There is evidence that additional organic solutes in the perfusion fluid increase net fluid absorption (Burg *et al.*, 1976).

Proximal straight tubules perfused with an ultrafiltrate of rabbit serum and bathed in rabbit serum (Burg and Orloff, 1968) absorbed fluid at an average rate of 0.42 nl $\text{mm}^{-1}\text{min}^{-1}$. Proximal straight tubules perfused with a synthetic perfusate (solution C, Table III) had very similar average fluid absorption rates (0.47 nl $\text{mm}^{-1}\text{min}^{-1}$, Kawamura *et al.*, 1975). When another artificial perfusate was used to perfuse proximal straight tubules (solution D, Table III), net fluid absorption averaged only 0.31 nl $\text{mm}^{-1}\text{min}^{-1}$ (Kawamura *et al.*, 1975).

Microperfusion experiments with segments of Henle's loop have been performed with a combination of ultrafiltrate as the perfusate and rabbit serum in the bath (Kokko, 1972; Rocha and Kokko, 1973; Imai and Kokko, 1974). Burg and Green (1973a) utilized a synthetic perfusate (solution A, Table III) with thick ascending limbs of the medullary portion of the loop of Henle. The same

Table III. Synthetic Perfusate Solutions[a]

	A	B	C	D	E	F	G
NaCl	115	60	105	141	140	126	80
KCl	5		5	5	2.5	3	2.5
NaHCO₃	25		25	5	5	24	24
NaC₂H₃O₂	10		10	5			
NaH₂PO₄	1.2		4	4	0.5	0.72	1
MgSO₄	1.2	1.2	1	1		1.2	
CaCl₂	1.0	1.0	1.8	1.8	1.5	1.8	
K₂HPO₄		2.5					
MgCl₂					1		1
Dextrose	5.5		8.3		5		5.5
Alanine			5				

[a] Concentration in mmol/liter⁻¹.

solution, with the addition of 5% v/v rabbit serum was used as bathing media in those experiments (Burg and Green, 1973a).

Gross et al. (1975) perfused distal convoluted tubules and cortical collecting tubules with artificial perfusate (solution C, Table III). This solution, with the addition of 5% v/v fetal calf serum, was also used to bathe the tubules. Transtubule potential differences reported for the perfused cortical collecting tubules were similar to data reported by Helman et al. (1971).

Several aspects of renal function in nonmammalian vertebrates have been examined with *in vitro* microperfusion. The perfusion solutions for the proximal tubules differed somewhat from those used in similar studies in mammalian proximal tubules. Synthetic perfusion and bath fluids (solutions E, F, and G, respectively, Table III) were used in experiments with flounder (Burg and Weller, 1969), garter snake (Dantzler, 1974), and bullfrog (Irish and Dantzler, 1976).

Any of the perfusion solutions listed in Table III can be used as bathing solutions with the addition of protein or a large molecular weight substance. Some samples include: bovine serum albumin, 6 g dl^{-1} final conc. (Dellasega and Grantham, 1973); 5% v/v rabbit serum (Burg and Green, 1973a); and, in snakes, 4 g dl^{-1} 40,000 mol. wt. dextran (Dantzler and Bentley, 1976). However, perfused rabbit proximal tubules exposed to a bath in which dextran or polyvinylpyrrolidone was substituted for protein exhibited cell sloughing (Imai and Kokko, 1974).

D. Dissection Technique

Adequate dissection of the rabbit kidney tubule remains the most difficult part of preparing the tubule for *in vitro* microperfusion. We dissect in a glass petri dish (diameter 60 mm, height 15 mm) which is inserted into a circular slot in a wooden box (18.5 cm × 13 cm × 5.5 cm). The box fits over an ordinary pint can (Figure 7). A water–antifreeze mixture in the can cools the underside of the dissecting dish. The tissue is observed through a binocular microscope (10–40×, American Optical Corp., Buffalo, N.Y.). A fiber optic light source (Dolan-Jenner Ind., Melrose, Ma.) illuminates the tissue. A gas mixture of 80% O_2/20% CO_2 suffused over the dissecting solution maintains the pH of the serum in the physiologic range. The petri dish rests on a disk of black paper so that the tubules are contrasted against a dark background. Notches 2 mm apart scratched on the bottom of the petri dish provide a reference for determining tubule length during the course of dissection.

We have not found differences in the function of perfused tubules in relation to the method of sacrifice—decapitation vs. intravenous injection of pentobarbital. The animal is sacrificed, the abdomen opened with scissors, and the kidney removed. A microtome knife (Arthur H. Thomas Co., Philadelphia, Pa.) is used to remove a 2-mm sagittal section through the area of the papilla. The tissue is quickly transferred to the dissection dish which contains either chilled rabbit serum or isotonic Krebs–Ringer solution. Tubules adhere to the bottom of the dissection dish when Krebs–Ringer solution alone is used. However, adding a

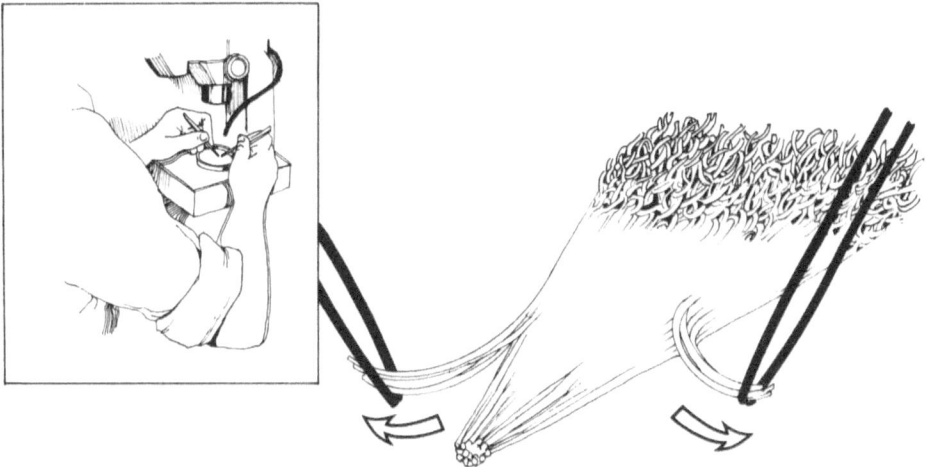

Figure 7. The method used to dissect tubules. Note that the tissue is held against the bottom of the dissection dish with one forcep while the other forcep is used to strip tissue from the medulla outward through the cortex.

small amount of bovine serum albumin to the Krebs–Ringer solution alleviates this problem. Adherence of the tubules to the dish does not occur when dissection is performed in rabbit serum.

We have found consistent results with tubules dissected at 4°C although cortical collecting tubules have been successfully dissected in a Krebs–Ringer solution at room temperature (Grantham and Orloff, 1968). A wedge of tissue, from papilla to cortex, is removed from the original section with fine-tipped forceps (A. Dumont and Sons, Switzerland). The wedge is reduced to finer strips of tissue by stripping the tissue through the cortex with the forceps (Figure 7). A smaller bundle of tissue, now with approximately 25–30 tubules, is gently teased apart. With practice, suitable lengths (1.4–4.0 mm) from any of the various segments of the rabbit nephron can be isolated within 15 min. However, the relative ease of dissection of the tissue varies from rabbit to rabbit. We use another rabbit if the dissection extends beyond 30 min, particularly if we are attempting to isolate segments from the proximal tubule. Segments of the loop of Henle or collecting tubule are more hardy and can be successfully perfused after an hour of dissection at 4°C.

Ideally, the tubule is touched at only one end of the segment. The basement membrane will seal the end of the tubule if pinched together during the course of dissection. This can prevent proper cannulation of the tubule. This is a problem with segments dissected from the proximal tubule. However, cannulation of cortical collecting tubules is often facilitated by repeatedly crushing one end of the tubule with the forceps during dissection.

Progressive removal of tissue from the papilla outward is a convenient way to obtain segments from the loop of Henle, collecting tubule, proximal straight tubule, and juxtamedullary proximal convoluted tubule. A different technique has been developed for dissecting segments of superficial proximal and distal convoluted tubules. A tangential slice of the superficial cortex under the capsule of the kidney is taken instead of the usual sagittal slice. The tips of the forceps are inserted into the thin layer of the superficial cortex and carefully spread apart. A patient dissector can free a 2-mm segment of convoluted tubule by redirecting the forcep tips and spreading the tissue in several directions. It is usually necessary to cut off one end of the tubule to free it from a bundle of tissue. This is done by pulling the forcep tips in opposite directions across the tubule.

There are some characteristic anatomic features of the various nephron segments that aid in their recognition during dissection. The proximal and distal convoluted tubules are coiled within the cortex and behave like tiny springs when dissection is attempted. Often glomeruli will remain attached to the early segments of the proximal convoluted tubules. Recognition of distal convoluted tubules is difficult, particularly when a glomerulus clings to this segment (Gross et al., 1975). However, distal convoluted tubules are thinner (30 μm average diameter) than proximal convoluted tubules (40 μm average diameter) when collapsed.

Proximal straight segments are approximately 30–35 μm in diameter and have a characteristic "ground glass" appearance. Their outer contours are smooth.

Cortical collecting tubules are approximately 20–25 μm in diameter, and are more nearly straight than are proximal straight tubules. Cortical collecting tubules also have a "fuzzy" appearance when viewed in the dissecting dish at high-power magnification (35×). This is due to the irregular outer contour of this segment.

Segments of the thin limb of the loop of Henle range from 10 to 15 μm in diameter. This segment is most easily recognized when it remains attached to the medullary end of a proximal straight tubule.

Segments of the thick ascending limb of the loop of Henle are intermediate in size between cortical collecting tubules and proximal straight tubules. Differentiating among these segments is at times difficult. However, the ascending thick limb of the loop of Henle lacks the characteristic "fuzzy" appearance of the cortical collecting tubules. They are also on the average somewhat thinner (25–30 μm diameter) than are the proximal straight tubules. Thick ascending limbs are also quite translucent; they lack the "ground glass" appearance that is characteristic of proximal straight tubules.

At times, final identification of a particular segment rests with inspection of the tubule at high power magnification in the perfusion chamber.

Tubules are transferred to the perfusion chamber with a small volume of serum once the dissection is complete. The transfer pipet is made from a Pasteur pipet [Figure 4(E)] which is bent at a 45° angle. The pipet is coated with silicone and the tip fire polished to prevent adherence of tubules to the pipet. A metal holder supports the pipet. An adjustable screw that presses on a rubber bulb at the rear of the pipet is used to propel fluid in and out of the pipet [Figure 4(E)].

The tubules are removed from the dissecting dish by placing the transfer pipet adjacent to the tubules and applying negative pressure to the pipet with the pressure adjustment screw. Reversing this process deposits the tubules in the perfusion chamber. A single tubule can be transferred in 10 μl of fluid using this technique.

Final inspection of the tubule at high magnification (100–600$\times$) is performed with the tubule in the perfusion chamber. We have established several criteria that must be met prior to using a tubule for study. If the basement membrane is ruptured at any point along the tubule, the dissection has been too rough. Narrowing or abrupt constriction in the diameter of the tubule implies overzealous stretching in the course of dissection. The presence of large vacuoles or opacified areas in the tubules suggests that the metabolic machinery of the cell has been damaged. Two additional observations can be made regarding the viability of the tubule. Normal tubules reabsorb fluid at 37°C. Consequently, any lumen present at the time of transfer to the bathing chamber should disappear within a few minutes after warming. With proximal straight tubules we use another helpful indicator. These tubules normally secrete p-aminohippurate (PAH) into the lumen to the extent that fluid is obligated as well (Grantham *et al.*, 1974). If lumen expansion does not occur within 5–10 min after the addition of $10^{-3}M$ PAH to the bath (37°C), the metabolism of the cell may have been compromised by the dissection.

E. Perfusion Technique

Gentle aspiration of the tubule onto the perfusion pipet is done with minimal difficulty if the perfusion pipet and holding pipet are properly aligned. The pipet tips are lowered to within several micrometers of the bottom of the chamber. The tubules, which are lying on the bottom of the perfusion chamber, serve as a reference point on which to focus, so that the pipets are not crushed against the bottom of the chamber. The tip of the perfusion pipet is withdrawn to a point just beyond the narrow constricted portion of the holding pipet. The holding pipet serves as a funnel to direct the tubule onto the tip of the perfusion pipet. During cannulation, perfusate must flow from the perfusion pipet. If there is no fluid flowing, bathing medium can be drawn into the perfusion pipet when aspiration of the tubule is attempted. This results in dilution of the volume marker contained in the perfusate. Errors in the determination of volume absorption across the tubule can result.

The tip of the perfusion pipet is advanced to the tip of the holding pipet once the tubule has been cannulated. Negative pressure within the holding pipet is maintained with closure of a stopcock that connects the tubing leading to the aspiration syringe [Figure 6(D)]. Extension of the perfusion pipet for several micrometers beyond the tip of the collecting pipet can cause puncture of the tubule when bath fluid is exchanged. However, if electric measurements are to be obtained, the perfusion tip is extended into the lumen for a distance of several micrometers in order to obtain the best results.

The perfusion pipet complex is raised off the bottom of the perfusion chamber once the proximal end of the tubule is wedged between the holding and perfusion pipets. Thus, the pipets will not be broken should the micromanipulators be bumped inadvertently during the experiment.

Perfusion fluid is propelled through the tubule by raising the perfusate reservoir above the tip of the perfusion pipet (or by increasing the microsyringe pump speed). The hydrostatic pressure within the tubule lumen is increased gradually. Too vigorous a rise in pressure can tear the tubule at its proximal end and allow infiltration of perfusate along the tubular basement membrane. If this occurs, the epithelium at the proximal end of the tubule develops a characteristic dark, granulated appearance, and in minutes obstructs the tubule. This is referred to fondly as "proximal rot" and has ended many an experiment for a neophyte microperfusionist. A markedly hypotonic perfusate can cause similar changes with perfused proximal tubules.

The tissue is once again inspected (37°C) with perfusate flowing freely along the tubule and into the bath. Strict criteria must be fulfilled before the tubule is accepted for study. Cells should uniformly line the basement membrane. Swelling or absence of individual cells implies rough handling in dissection. In proximal segments, brush borders are an excellent guide to the integrity of the preparation. The brush border is easily seen at 200–400× magnification. Absence of brush border on a large number of cells indicates the initial perfusion was too vigorous. Nuclei of most segments are oriented toward the base of the cells—the cortical ascending limb being an exception. When cells die, the nucleus is often extruded into the lumen. With perfused cortical collecting tubules, two cell types can be recognized. The predominant cell has a cobblestone shape and is "ground glass" in appearance. Interspaced among these cells are "dark cells" which are most easily recognized by focusing along the back wall of the tubule. These cells are more heavily granulated. There are, on the average, two to four dark cells visible per millimeter cortical collecting tubule. Finally, an easy test of viability in proximal segments involves lowering perfusion pressure to zero whereupon the lumen should collapse completely at 37°C.

If the tubule is intact, the distal end is gently aspirated into the collecting pipet (Figure 2). A large supply of collecting pipets with different internal diameters (20–40 μm at the inner constriction) should be available! A collecting pipet is selected that fits the distal end of the tubule tightly—much like a shoe is selected to fit a particular foot. The tubule should not slide within the collecting pipet when gentle, positive, or negative pressure is applied. Some investigators routinely use an external pipet filled with Sylgard to surround the collecting pipet to help seal the distal end of the perfused tubule within the collecting pipet (Figure 2).

The distal end of the tubule is pulled just beyond the constriction in the collecting pipet. If an excess of tissue is pulled beyond the constriction, this portion of the tubule can be aspirated into the calibrated collecting pipet when sampling is attempted. Disruption of the system can result when the calibrated collecting pipet is withdrawn.

Bath fluid is drawn into the collection pipet during aspiration of the tubule into the collecting pipet. This fluid is removed before samples of collected perfusate are obtained. This is accomplished with a tapered, unfinished perfusion pipet which is inserted within the collecting pipet and advanced within several micrometers of the distal end of the tubule. Gentle aspiration of the accumulated fluid does not cause a leak of bath fluid into the collecting pipet.

A layer of colored, water-equilibrated oil (10 μm) is placed over the accumulated perfusate once the bath fluid is removed from the collecting pipet. A meniscus, formed at the oil–fluid interface within the collecting pipet (Figure 2), is clearly visible through the microscope. An estimate of the perfusion rate is made by following the movement of the meniscus. A leak from the bath into the collecting pipet, around the outer walls of the tubule, is present if the meniscus continues to move after the perfusion pressure is reduced to zero.

Once the tubule is cannulated and perfusion established, sample collection becomes a primary concern. The rate at which the sample collects is a function of the perfusion rate and the absorptive and secretory forces regulating fluid movement. The sample is retrieved using either the constant bore capillary collecting pipet or the volumetric pipet.

The constant bore capillary collecting pipet is advanced down the collection holding pipet and the accumulated fluid is collected by suction at the end of a given time interval. The pipet is withdrawn and the length of the fluid sample is measured with an accurate ruler under a microscope. An oil column brackets the sample in the capillary glass and prevents evaporation during handling. The sample is ejected into a counting vial for determination of isotope concentraion with either standard gamma or liquid scintillation counting. Sodium and potassium concentration can be determined on the perfused and collected fluid with a helium glow photometer (American Instrument Co., Silver Springs, Md.); chloride concentration can be determined by electrometric means (Burg and Green, 1973a).

The volumetric pipet, placed in the collecting fluid, fills by capillary action. The collection period ends when the volumetric pipet is full. The volumetric pipet can be used to make serial sample collections without emptying the pipet between sample collections. The pipet tip is retracted into the oil column until a short column of oil is drawn into the tip of the volumetric collecting pipet. The pipet tip is again advanced into the collecting fluid to obtain the next sample. Care must be taken to ensure the separation of the samples when they are emptied to undergo analysis. This step is performed with the help of a microscope so that each sample is clearly recognized.

The pipets are calibrated with isotopic standards at the termination of each experiment to account for minimal changes in the glass. Reproducible results can be obtained only if the pipet is thoroughly flushed with water and chloroform and dried with acetone. This is done between experiments with the volumetric pipet; between individual sample collections with the constant bore capillary pipet. Loss of mental concentration during collection and cleaning will transform a functional pipet into a rubble of silica. However, gentle handling and attention to detail will prolong the life of the pipet indefinitely.

The introduction of the fluid exchange pipet broadened the scope of the microperfusion technique. Perfusate can be exchanged during an experiment without disrupting the hookup of the tubule under study. Thus, a single tubule can serve as its own control. The provocative discovery that chloride and not sodium is actively transported across the tubule along the length of the thick ascending limb of the loop of Henle was made with the use of the fluid exchange pipet (Rocha and Kokko, 1973; Burg and Green, 1973a). Furthermore, Burg and associates (1973) discovered that the diuretic action of furosemide was dependent on the inhibition of the "active chloride pump" located along the thick ascending limb of the loop of Henle. The drug was more effective from the luminal side of the membrane. Similar findings have been reported for other potent diuretics such as mersalyl (Burg and Green, 1973b) and ethacrynic acid (Burg and Green, 1973c).

The perfusion pipet arrangement shown in Figure 2 depicts the paths (arrows, Figure 2) of perfusion fluid flow during the course of an experiment. Hydrostatic pressure applied through the exchange pipet forces the perfusate out the perfusion pipet through the tubule during normal perfusion. Perfusion of the tubule is continued during the process of perfusate exchange by positioning the outflow valve below the tip of the perfusion pipet. To initiate exchange, the outflow valve to collection perfusate is opened, followed by the opening of the valve to the new perfusate. The exchange of 1 ml of perfusate requires about 2 min. Normal perfusion is resumed when the outflow valve leading to the waste perfusate [Figure 6(E)] is closed.

Perfusion fluid exchange eliminates the problem of dilution of the perfusion fluid during the tubule hookup. This problem was previously diminished by maintaining a positive pressure on the perfusion pipet during cannulation and perfusing for a 20 min period prior to beginning an experiment. The perfusion exchange allows cannulation and perfusion to be established with a nonradioactive perfusate. Once the system has stabilized, the nonisotopic perfusate is exchanged with isotopic perfusate and the experiment begun.

F. Control of the Extratubular Environment

Bath fluid exchange serves several purposes. First, regular bath replacement decreases the difficulty of maintaining a constant peritubular environment throughout the course of an experiment. Second, bath replacement allows for the periodic collection of the bathing solution which can be conveniently analyzed for isotopic content. Thus, major leaks of an impermeant marker (such as [125I]iothalamate) are detectable early in the course of an experiment. Therefore, the investigator will not invest valuable time with a tubule that is not properly cannulated. Finally, bath fluid exchange permits the introduction of a variable (physical factor or drug) into the peritubular environment and its effect on the transport properties of the tubule can be evaluated.

Complete fluid exchange requires thorough flushing of the bath chamber. The total volume exchanged with fresh bathing fluid should exceed the volume of the chamber severalfold. Exchange is best made by serially evacuating most of the fluid covering the tubule and filling the chamber with new bath fluid. Gentle suction through polyethylene tubing is applied to one end of the chamber while the fresh bath solution is added to the other end of the chamber with a small syringe. Flexible polyethylene tubing is attached to the syringe. This allows for a less turbulent entry of the fresh bathing medium into the chamber, particularly if the tubing is placed against the side wall of the chamber. Care must be taken during bath exchange not to damage the tubule segment or dislodge it from the holding pipets. If the perfusion pipet extends into the tubule lumen far beyond the holding pipet, excessive tubule movement may rupture the cells adjacent to the perfusion pipet. Bath fluid may be evacuated directly into a scintillation vial to allow for isotopic counting.

A number of physical factors in the peritubular environment influence net solute and water transport in both directions across microperfused tubules *in vitro*. The peritubular environment (oxygen content, temperature, pH, oncotic forces, and osmotic regulation) must be rigorously controlled if meaningful data are to be obtained with the microperfusion method.

Burg and Orloff (1968) observed that net fluid transport was exquisitely temperature sensitive. At 37°C the proximal convoluted tubule reabsorbed fluid at approximately 1.18 nl/mm/min, while the proximal straight segment did so at approximately 0.42 nl/mm/min. With the reduction in bath temperature to 13°C, the fluid transport ceased in the proximal convoluted segment. The reversibility of the hypothermic effect was interpreted to indicate that fluid transport was dependent on metabolism. Several investigators (Kokko *et al.*, 1971; Grantham *et al.*, 1972; Hamburger *et al.*, 1974) have since confirmed the presence of functional heterogeneity within the proximal tubules in regards to net fluid transport. Grantham (1973) also found that hypothermia elicited a proportional reduction of transport in the proximal straight segment as well as the convoluted segment (lowering bath temperature to 25°C resulted in a 50% reduction in net fluid transport in both segments). Moreover, this investigator found that net fluid secretion by the proximal straight tubule, as initiated by the addition of *p*-aminohippurate to the bath, was exquisitively sensitive to the effect of hypothermia (Grantham *et al.*, 1974). This phenomenon has recently been demonstrated for uric acid secretion by the proximal straight tubule (Chonko *et al.*, 1975). Therefore, investigations of transport parameters which utilize the *in vitro* microperfusion method should be conducted at a reasonably constant temperature. Indeed, an important advantage of the microperfusion technique, in contrast to the renal slice or suspension techniques, is that at 37°C the segment probably can transport solutes at rates closer to the *in vivo* condition.

Initial studies with microperfused cortical collecting tubules (Grantham and Burg, 1966) were performed at room temperature since the thermostatically controlled perfusion chamber had yet not been developed. Subsequent studies with this nephron segment were also performed at 25°C until Gross and his colleagues (1975) perfused cortical collecting tubules at 37°C and compared their functional characteristics to those of microperfused distal convoluted tubules. Recently Hall and Grantham (in press) discovered that the hydraulic water permeability of microperfused cortical collecting tubules, in the presence of vasopressin at 37°C, decreased over the course of 60–180 min. This phenomenon did not occur at 25°C. Thus, the experimentalist must be aware of the transient nature of the response to vasopressin with cortical collecting tubules that are perfused at 37°C.

Lewy and Windhager (1968) and Brenner and his associates (1969) on the basis of micropuncture studies *in situ* suggested that the balance of Starling forces across the renal peritubular capillary influenced the control of fluid absorption across the proximal tubule. Stated in a different way, so-called "glomerulotubular balance" was not an intrinsic functional characteristic of the tubular epithelium, but was related to factors extrinsic to the tubule. Microperfusion studies by Imai and Kokko (1972, 1974) and Grantham and colleagues (1972) have verified the importance of the peritubular protein concentration upon net fluid reabsorption in both segments of the proximal tubule. In these studies a reduction of protein content in the bath from 6.4 g/100 ml to less than 0.3 g/100 ml caused a 40% reduction in net volume flux. However, in contrast to *in vivo* micropuncture studies, the oncotic effects of protein were dissociated from changes in peritubular hydrostatic pressure, extratubular interstitial volume, and renal blood flow, since the normal capillary relationship to the tubules had been disrupted.

The passive movement of fluid across the isolated microperfused tubule in response to osmotic forces can be significant. The osmotic water permeability of the proximal tubule, in particular, is sufficiently high that small changes in the osmolality of the bath may cause a serious error in the estimation of "active" solute and volume absorption. This complicating factor is especially troublesome when perfusion rates greater than 10 nl/min are used (Kokko, 1972). As a practical point, it is emphasized that evaporation occurs from the bathing chamber at 37°C to a significant extent. Accordingly, the osmolality of the bathing medium should be monitored carefully in the course of *in vitro* microperfusion studies and distilled water added to the bath chamber to replace evaporative losses. A rapid estimate of evaporative losses can be obtained by measuring the changes in protein concentration in a few drops of aspirated bath fluid with a refractometer (American Optical Corp., Buffalo, N.Y.).

The pH of the bathing medium can be maintained in a narrow range if various O_2/CO_2 gas mixtures are bubbled through the bath fluid. However, the turbulence created can lead to dislodgement of the tubule from the holding pipets. Moreover, visualization of the tubule is obscured when small bubbles accumulate at the surface of the bathing solution. In our laboratory we do not bubble the O_2/CO_2 mixture directly into the bath chamber, but insufflate the gas mixture over the surface of the bathing solution from above. A clear plastic lid fits over the top of the perfusion chamber and reduces evaporative losses and blunts, but does not totally eliminate, changes in pH. If the CO_2 content of the bath solution is not regulated, the pH of the bath solution will rise to 7.6 over the course of 7 min. Insufflation of 80% O_2/20% CO_2 prevents any increase in bath pH if the bath fluid is exchanged at 10-min intervals. The pH of the bath fluid is monitored prior to each bath exchange (Radiometer Corp., Copenhagen, Denmark).

The importance of maintaining a physiologic pH in the bathing medium has recently been pointed out by Dennis and associates (1976). These investigators found that net fluid absorption across microperfused proximal convoluted tubules decreased when the bath pH exceeded 7.5. In the pH range 7.0–7.5, volume flux was maintained at approximately 1.0 nl/mm/min. In addition, Dellasega and Grantham (1973) found that isolated nonperfused segments of proximal straight tubule when treated with ouabain $10^{-5}M$ (in the bath) swelled to a greater extent in alkaline bathing media. Indeed, in our laboratory we recently have found that [^{14}C]uric acid uptake by nonperfused isolated proximal straight tubules is diminished when the bathing solution pH exceeds 7.50.

G. Electrical Measurements

The ability to measure the electrical potential difference (PD) and resistance across the epithelium of the perfused tubule provides an insight into electrical forces regulating ion movement and permeability properties of the epithelium. Electrical measurements in isolated microperfusion experiments have provided a partial segmental analysis of the electrical properties of the rabbit nephron (Burg *et al.*, 1968; Helman *et al.*, 1971; Burg and Orloff, 1970; Helman, 1972 Lutz *et al.*, 1973; Rocha and Kokko, 1973; Burg and Green, 1973a; Stoner *et al.*, 1974; Gross *et al.*, 1975). The description which follows is but one approach. Many modifications have been made in the various laboratories making electrical measurements on the isolated perfused tubule.

Agar bridges are used to connect the perfusion apparatus to the electronics used to measure the potential difference. These bridges are made by filling 240 polyethylene tubing with warm agar solution. This polyethylene tubing must be trimmed back to the agar, which shrinks during cooling, to provide electrical continuity. One end of the agar bridge is connected to the perfusion pipet and the other end is placed in a saturated KCl solution. A calomel half cell provides continuity between the saturated KCl solution and an electrometer (Keithley Instrument Inc., Cleveland, Ohio). An agar bridge connects the bath to another calomel electrode in saturated KCl solution, which in turn is connected to a voltage reference source (Heath Co., Benton Harbor, Mi.). The PD can be read directly from the electrometer or recorded on a strip chart.

Prior to cannulation of the tubule, the perfusion pipet is placed in a bath containing perfusion fluid and the electrometer is set to zero. Perfusion and bath solutions that differ in composition generate junction potentials which must be considered when a determination is made of actual PD generated by the tubule segment. Kokko (1973) has presented a discussion of the limitations and sources of error in calculations of the liquid junction potential.

Tubule perfusion does not differ from the procedures described previously in this paper. However, care must be exercised to ensure adequate seals at each end of the nephron segment to prevent short circuiting. This is accomplished by sealing the tubule in the holding pipet and collecting pipet with Sylgard 184 (Dow Corp., Midland, Mi.).

The other electrical measurement commonly obtained with isolated microperfused tubules is the electrical resistance (Helman *et al.*, 1971; Lutz *et al.*, 1973; Burg and Green, 1973a). The circuitry resembles the PD measurement arrangements but in this case it is necessary to insert a separate circuit to pass current into the tubule lumen.

H. Tissue Compartment Analysis

The tubular epithelium can be recovered for analysis at the completion of microperfusion. Thus, a three-compartment model (lumen fluid, cell compartment, bath fluid) can be derived for any substance that can be microanalytically or isotopically quantified. Models of transport have been proposed for p-aminohippurate secretion (active transport across the peritubular membrane into the cell with passive diffusion across the luminal membrane) and glucose reabsorption (active transport across the luminal membrane into the cell) in microperfused rabbit proximal tubules (Tune et al., 1969; Tune and Burg, 1971). Secretion of uric acid across isolated perfused proximal straight tubules occurs in a manner similar to that for p-aminohippurate (Chonko et al., 1976). Three-compartment models of transport also have been established for p-aminohippurate secretion across microperfused proximal tubules in the snake (Dantzler, 1974) and frog (Irish and Dantzler, 1976).

To recover the epithelium, the tubule is gently dislodged from the holding pipets. The pipets are retracted from the bath and the tubule is aspirated from the perfusion chamber and transferred to a dish of chilled isotonic saline. A thin glass needle (15–20 μm) is used to swirl the tubule vigorously through the saline in order to rinse off the extracellular fluid. The tubule is not allowed to sink to the bottom of the chamber lest it adhere to the glass and rupture. A 1-min rinse in the chilled saline is sufficient to remove the bulk of extracellular fluid. The tubule is lifted from the rinse solution on the tip of the glass needle. The needle is broken off into a counting vial with forceps if isotopes are to be measured. The cell volume of the tubule is calculated from measurements of photographs taken at high power magnification while the tubule is lying on the bottom of the perfusion chamber. Alternatively, the tubule can be extracted with trichloroacetic acid to remove the isotope and the tubule weighed on a quartz fiber ultramicrobalance (Bonting and Maynon, 1961).

Structural correlates of the cellular compartment can be conveniently obtained with the microperfusion method. The bath is exchanged for an isotonic glutaraldehyde solution which "fixes" the tubule almost instantaneously. The tissue is retrieved from the bottom of the chamber with the transfer pipet [modified Pasteur pipet, Figure 4(E)]. However, the tubule will stick to the glass pipets when exposed to glutaraldehyde. The perfusion pipet usually can be manipulated to free the proximal end of the tubule from the holding pipet. In most situations, the tip of the collecting pipet must be broken against the bottom of the perfusion chamber in order to free the distal end of the tubule. Standard dehydrating and embedding techniques are used to prepare the tubule for electron microscopy (Ganote et al., 1968). Grantham and his colleagues (1969) utilized these techniques to examine the paths of transtubular water flow in isolated perfused cortical collecting tubules. Welling and Welling (1976), likewise, investigated the shape of epithelial cells and the intercellular channels in microperfused rabbit proximal tubules.

A more detailed review of segmental function as derived from in vitro microperfusion experiments is beyond the scope of this presentation. Recently two extensive reviews of this material have been published (Chonko and Grantham, 1976; Grantham *et al.*, 1978).

Nowhere in the literature can one find a concise analysis of the formulas used to quantify solute and water transport across microperfused tubules. The next section of this presentation aims to fill this void.

III. FORMULATION

The following discussion of fluid flow in renal tubule segments is relevant to *in vitro* microperfusion experiments in which flow into the tubule lumen is determined principally by hydrostatic pressure applied by gravity to a perfusion pipet. A typical experimental situation is depicted in Figure 8. Volume flow, $F_x(0)$, into the tubule lumen in the steady state is equal to the sum of the radial absorbed volume flow, $F_{ABS}(l)$, and the longitudinal flow passing out of the distal end of the tubule, $F_x(l)$. P_a is the hydrostatic pressure applied by gravity (ρgh) to the perfusion pipet and is expressed in units of manometer height (h). P_B. is the hydrostatic pressure in the bath or peritubular medium and usually is equal to atmospheric pressure. $P(x)$ is luminal hydrostatic pressure averaged over a tubule cross section at a longitudinal distance x.

A. Steady-State Mass Balance

The radial volume flow (vol/time), $F_{ABS}(x)$, crossing outward (absorbed) through a length x of tubule wall is defined by the mass balance,

$$F_x(0) - F_x(x) = F_{ABS}(x) = 2\pi r \int_0^x V_r(x)\, dx \qquad (1)$$

where $V_r(x)$ is the outward radial velocity of the fluid at the internal radius r and tubule length x, and $F_x(x) = \pi r^2 V_x(x)$ is the longitudinal volume flow at x where $V_x(x)$ represents the longitudinal velocity averaged over the tubule cross section. The symbol $J_v(x)$ is often used in the literature to represent $V_x(x)$. Equation (1)

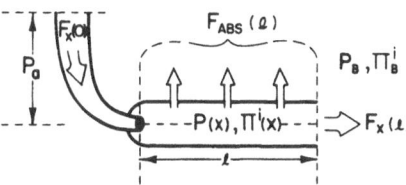

Figure 8. Depiction of the various parameters for tubule perfusion. P_a is the hydrostatic pressure applied by gravity (manometer height); $F_x(0)$ is the perfusion rate; $P(x)$ and $\Pi^i(x)$ are respectively the hydrostatic pressure, and the osmotic pressure exerted by solution i at tubule length x; $F_{ABS}(l)$ is the volume flow traversing the entire tubule wall of length l (total absorbed flow); P_B and $\Pi_B{}^i$ are respectively the hydrostatic pressure and osmotic pressure exerted by solution i in the bath; $F_x(l)$ is the volume flow exiting the tubule.

may also be expressed in the convenient differential form,

$$dF_{ABS}/dx = -dF_x/dx = 2\pi r V_r(x) \tag{2}$$

Similarly, the flow of any solute i, $F_{ABS}^i(x)$ (mol/time), crossing outward through a length x of tubule wall is defined by the solute balance equation,

$$\pi r^2[J_x^i(0) - J_x^i(x)] = F_{ABS}^i(x) = 2\pi r \int_0^x J_r^i(x)\,dx \tag{3}$$

where $\pi r^2 J_x^i(x)$ and $J_x^i(x) = C^i(x)V_x^i(x)$ are respectively the solute flow (mol/time) and the solute flux (mol/cm²/time) in the longitudinal direction. $C^i(x)$ is the concentration (mol/vol) of solute i at x and is understood to be averaged over a tubule cross section, and $J_r^i(x)$ is the solute flux in the radial direction. All of the solutes to be considered are dilute and usually their concentrations are independent of tubule radius. Large-molecular-weight solutes such as proteins are exceptions and appropriate modifications may be necessary (Deen *et al.*, 1974). In analogy to Eq. (2), the differential form of Eq. (3) is written

$$dF_{ABS}^i/dx = -\pi r^2\,dJ_x^i/dx = 2\pi r J_r^i(x) \tag{4}$$

B. Phenomenology

To obtain those relations applicable to the various experimental situations, it is necessary to introduce the functional dependence of the flows on those forces which can act across and within the tubule membrane. To this end we shall utilize those phenomenological equations deduced from irreversible thermodynamics for dilute solutions near thermodynamic equilibrium. These were first expressed in a convenient form for biology by Kedem and Katchalsky (1961) and subsequently in an excellent text by Katchalsky and Curran (1965).

In terms of the parameters appropriate to the perfused tubule, the phenomenological equation for the radial velocity of water is of the form

$$V_r(x) = L_p\left\{P(x) - P_B - \sum_i^n \sigma^i[\Pi^i(x) - \Pi_B^i]\right\} + V_r^E + V_r^A \tag{5}$$

where L_p is the hydraulic conductivity of the tubular membrane (length/time/pressure), $\Pi^i(x)$ and σ^i are respectively the osmotic pressure and reflection coefficient of the perfused solute i of the total number of solutes n, Π_B^i is the osmotic pressure exerted by solute i in the bath, and V_r^E and V_r^A are the radial water velocities due to electroosmosis and active transport respectively (House, 1974). The mode of water movement expressed by V_r^A is caused by those forces or "pumps" which are internal to the membrane. In what follows the osmotic pressure will be considered a linear function of the solute concentration, i.e., $\Pi^i(x) = RTC^i(x)$ where R is the molar gas constant and T is the absolute temperature. Osmotic pressure as a nonlinear function of concentration is important when considering sufficient concentrations of large molecular weight solutes such as serum albumin (Landis and Pappenheimer, 1963). The appropriate modifications of equations for such cases are usually very complicated and should be considered on an individual basis.

The phenomenological equation for solute movement (flux) across membranes can be written in several equivalent forms (Katchalsky and Curran, 1965; House, 1974). The most convenient and general equation for our purposes is of the form,

$$J_r^i(x) = (1 - \sigma^i)\bar{C}^i V_r + \omega^i(\Delta\Pi^i + z^i F\bar{C}^i \Delta\psi) + N^i \tag{6}$$

where ω^i is the permeability of solute i (mol/cm²/atm/sec), $\Delta\psi$ is the transepithelial potential difference from lumen to bath measured with saturated KCl bridges, $\Delta\Pi^i$ is the transtubular osmotic pressure difference from lumen to bath of solute i, z^i is the valence of the ith ionic species, and F is the Faraday constant. ($z^i F$ expresses the coulombs of charge per mole of ionic species i). $\bar{C}$ is the logarithmic average concentration and is given by $\bar{C}^i = (C^i + C_B^i i/h\ln C^i/C_B)$ where C^i and C_B^i are respectively the concentrations in the lumen and bath. N^i is the flux of solute i due to active transport. Finally, it is often convenient to express the solute permeability ω^i as a coefficient of concentration rather than osmotic pressure. For that case the symbol P^i (length/time) is used with the conversion $P^i \equiv RT\omega^i$. The hydraulic conductivity L_p is sometimes given in units of permeability and in that case $L_p RT/\bar{V}_w = P^w$ where $\bar{V}_w$ is the partial volume of water.

The experimental determinations of these various parameters by means of *in vitro* microperfusion have been discussed in numerous publications and various mathematical formulas here have been given supplementary to the particular experiments. We shall present below some of the most basic derivations together with the experimental conditions necessary for applicability.

C. Measurement of Hydraulic Conductivity, Using an Impermeant Solute

In general, the volume flow can be determined as a function of the driving forces by substituting Eq. (5) into Eq. (2). Since several unknown parameters are present, it is necessary to devise experimental maneuvers so that each parameter can be determined separately. From a theoretical standpoint, one of the simplest maneuvers is the use of an impermeant solute to determine the hydraulic conductivity of the tubular membrane. In this case then, if i represents the impermeant species, $\sigma^i = 1$ and $J_r^i(x) = 0$.

D. Impermeant Solute in the Bath

If the impermeant solute is placed only in the bath where it exerts an osmotic pressure Π_B, we find using Eq. (5) in (2) and integrating from $x = 0$ to $x = l$,

$$F_{ABS}(l) = F_x(0) - F_x(l) = (2\pi r l L_p)(\Pi_B + k) \tag{7}$$

where k represents the integration over the transtubular hydrostatic and other solute osmotic pressures plus possible contributions from V_r^E and V_r^A. Thus, if k remains constant while Π_B is changed, a plot of the experimentally determined flow $F_{ABS}(l)$ vs. Π_B will be a straight line of slope $(L_p 2\pi r l)$. The alteration of k by a change in Π_B could occur since the concentration differences of other solutes could be altered by the change in solvent drag. This is not observed to occur in the usual cases (Kokko *et al.*, 1971). This experimental technique provides an easy method for determining the hydraulic conductivity of the intact tubule membrane when flow occurs from lumen to bath. These results are of course subject to unstirred layers, which means L_p may be underestimated. Furthermore, any values obtained for the hydraulic conductivity of intact tubules are meaningful only in relation to other intact values similarly obtained. Since the composite membrane is composed of various single membranes and unknown water routes, any value obtained for the total conductivity cannot easily be compared with single tissue values without further modeling of the intra- and intercellular pathways.

E. Impermeant Solute in the Perfusate

In this case the impermeant solute is also added to the perfusion fluid and flow can be induced from lumen to bath or bath to lumen, depending on the relative transtubular concentrations. Since the tubular volume is small compared to the bath, the concentration of impermeant solute can change markedly as water moves across the tubular wall. While this case is more complicated than the previous one, a value for the hydraulic conductivity can be determined easily if further experimental conditions can be imposed.

Conditions will always be such that the tubule perfusion $F_x(0)$, and tubule length are large enough so that longitudinal solute diffusion is negligible compared to convective flow. Therefore, the longitudinal solute flux is given by

$$\pi r^2 J_x^i(x) = \Pi^i(x) F_x(x)/RT \tag{8}$$

where $\Pi^i(x)$ is the osmotic pressure at x of the impermeant solute i in the tubular lumen. Since $J_r^i = 0$, Eq. (4) together with (8) gives

$$d(\Pi^i F_x)/dx = 0 \tag{9}$$

so that

$$\Pi^i(x) F_x(x) = \Pi^i(0) F_x(0) = \Pi^i(l) F_x(l) \tag{10}$$

and

$$dF_x/dx = -[\Pi^i(0) F_x(0)/(\Pi^i)^2] \, d\Pi^i/dx \tag{11}$$

The simplest and most informative solution of Eq. (11) is obtained when the experimental conditions are such that the transtubular osmotic pressures exerted by the impermeant solutes dominate all other terms in Eq. (5). This situation may not always be satisfied, particularly in those cases where large changes in permeant solutes occur over short tubule segments and where large contributions to absorbed flow are made by the pumps V_r^A. Nevertheless, if the impermeant solute can be made to dominate Eq. (5), then substitution into Eq. (2) gives

$$dF_x/dx = -2\pi r L_p [\Pi_B^i - \Pi^i(x)] \tag{12}$$

Substituting Eq. (12) into (11) gives

$$[\Pi^i(0)F_x(0)/(\Pi^i)^2]\,d\Pi^i/dx = 2\pi r L_p[\Pi^i_B - \Pi^i(x)] \tag{13}$$

Equation (13) can be integrated directly and has the solution

$$2\pi r l L_p = \left\{\left[\frac{\Pi^i_B}{\Pi^i(0)} - \frac{\Pi^i_B}{\Pi^i(l)}\right] + \ln\left[\frac{\Pi^i_B}{\Pi^i(0)} - 1\right]\Big/\left[\frac{\Pi^i_B}{\Pi^i(l)} - 1\right]\right\}\Pi^i(0)F_x(0)/(\Pi^i_B)^2 \tag{14}$$

where Eq. (14) expresses the results in terms of the experimental values $F_x(0)$, $\Pi^i(l)$, $\Pi^i(0)$ and Π^i_B. In Eq. (14) it can be seen that $\Pi^i(l)$ approaches Π^i_B asymptotically. Those regions where $\Pi^i(l)$ is close to Π^i_B should be experimentally avoided since the effect of other solutes can become important there. For those tubules where Π^i_B is maintained large compared to $\Pi^i(x)$ (or vice versa), the flow is nearly linear and $\Pi^i(x)$ remains linear provided the absorbed flow is small compared to the perfusion flow. This condition can usually be maintained for the range of hydraulic conductivity measured. A typical curve of $\Pi^i(l)$ vs. l is given in Figure 9 for the case when $\Pi^i_B/RT = 290$ mOsM and $\Pi^i(0)/RT = 125$ mOsM for $F_x(0) = 5$, 15, and 30 nl/min and $L_p = 1.5 \times 10^{-5}$ cm/sec atm with $r = 10\ \mu$m.

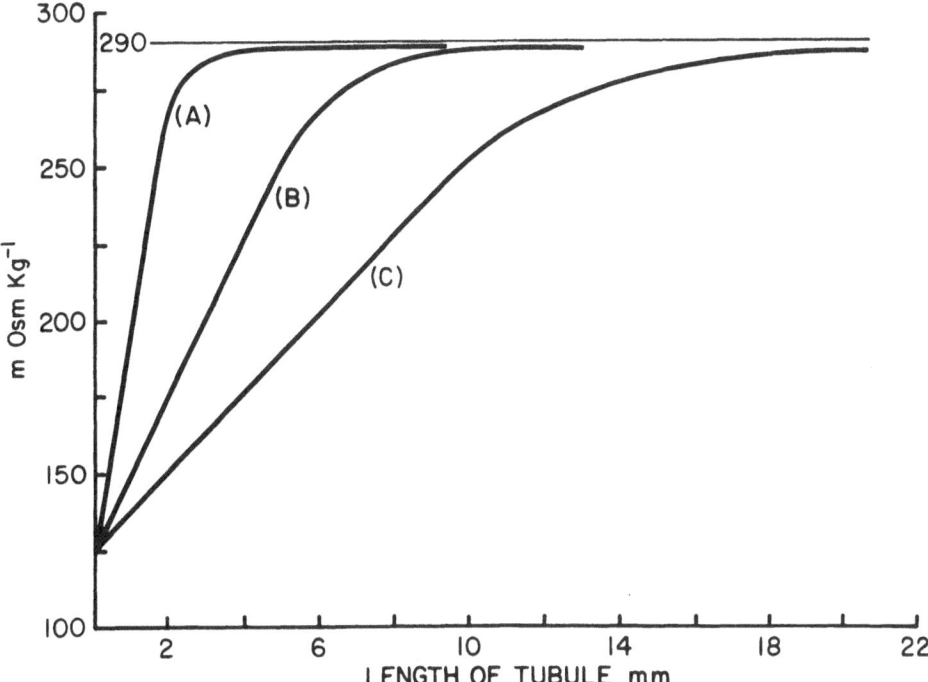

Figure 9. Osmotic pressure exerted by impermeant solutes at tubule end as a function of tubule length l. $\Pi^i(l)$ is plotted against l from Eq. (14) for the case when Π^i_B/RT equals 290 mOsM and $\Pi^i(0)/RT$ equals 125 mOsM for perfusion rates: (A), $F_x(0) = 5$nl min^{-1}; (B) $F_x(0) = 15$ nl min^{-1}; (C) $F_x(0) = 30$ nl min^{-1} and tubule hydraulic conductivity $L_p = 1.5 \times 10^{-5}$ cm sec^{-1} atm^{-1} with an internal radius $r = 10\ \mu$.

If flow response to active transport is a contributing factor to total reabsorption, and if impermeant solute can be added to the perfusion fluid so that no volume flow occurs when the perfusion fluid is Π', then the hydraulic conductivity is given by Eq. (14) with Π_B^i replaced by Π'.

F. Measurement of Solute Permeability

The simplest derivation of an equation for computing the solute permeability is obtained when the volume flow across the tubule wall is held to zero. When experimentally possible, this is usually accomplished by adding an impermeant solute such as raffinose to the perfusate, which provides a sufficient transtubular osmotic pressure to stop volume reabsorption. If no active transport exists and if the transtubular potential is zero, or small relative to the transtubular concentration of the solute in question, Eq. (6) is simplified and when substituted into Eq. 4 gives

$$dC^i/dx = -2\pi r\omega^i RT[C^i(x) - C_B^i]/F_x \tag{15}$$

where $C^i(x) = \Pi^i/RT$ is the concentration of the lumenal solute at x, C_B^i is the concentration of the measured solute in the bath, and F_x is the constant perfusion flow. The solution of Eq. (15) is of the form

$$P^i = RT\omega^i = (F_x/2\pi rl) \ln \{[C^i(o) - C_B^i]/[C^i(l) - C_B^i]\} \tag{16}$$

where $C^i(0)$ and $C^i(l)$ are the solute concentrations at $x = 0$ and $x = l$ respectively.

The derivation of equations for the solute permeability in the presence of transtubular electrical potentials and active transport is somewhat more difficult and is subject to further restrictions. It is beyond the scope and purpose of this article to consider in detail the theoretical problems associated with electrophysiology. Basic theoretical treatments related to tubule perfusion can be found in review articles by Fromter (1974) and by Ullrich and Sauer (1973).

In general, the nephron tubule cannot be easily short circuited and the derived permeability values must be considered in that framework. Several simple formulas can be derived for these "corrected" permeabilities when transtubular volume flow is zero ($V_r = 0$) but experimental measurements are required both when solute is moving radially ($J_r^i \neq 0$) and when it is not ($J_r^i = 0$). This requires the additional assumption that the permeability and active transport remain constant for these two conditions, i.e., that the solute flux is given by Eq. (6), where P^i and N^i are constants. This assumption may not be true, particularly if the active transport generates an electrical potential difference. The following derivation, therefore, is presented for the determination of solute permeability in a perfused tubule under the restriction of the assumption that N^i and P^i remain constant both when solute moves radially and when it does not.

The presence of active transport is usually determined when the radial movement of the solute together with the radial volume flow is stopped ($J_r^i = V_r = 0$) by adding enough of the permeable solute to the bath. Then according to

Eq. (6), the ratio of active transport to permeability, $\Delta = N^i/P^i$ for solute i is given by

$$\Delta = N^i/P^i = (\Delta C^i - z^i F \bar{C}^i \, \Delta\Phi/RT) \tag{17}$$

where ΔC is the transtubular concentration difference for the solute measured from bath to lumen, $\bar{C}$ is the average transtubular concentration, and $\Delta\Phi$ is the transtubular potential difference measured from lumen to bath, all for the situation when $J_r^i = V_r = 0$. It should be noted that $\Delta\Phi$ measured at zero solute and volume flow may be different than $\Delta\psi$ measured only at zero volume flow. If it is now assumed that Δ remains the same for the case when only solute is allowed to move across the tubular wall, Eq. (17) may be substituted into Eqs. (6) and (4) to give

$$dC^i/dx = 2\pi P^i[C^i(1 + z^i F \Delta\psi/2RT) - C_B^i(1 - z^i F \Delta\psi/2RT) + \Delta] \tag{18}$$

where it is also assumed that C^i and C_B^i differ by an amount small enough so that the average transtubular concentration can be given by the simple arithmetic average $\bar{C} = (C^i + C_B^i)/2$. (Further consideration of this assumption is given below.) Equation (18) can then be integrated to yield

$$P^i = [F_x/2\pi rl(1 + z^i F \Delta\psi/2RT)] \ln \{[C^i(0) - C_B^{i\prime} + \Delta']/[C^i(l) - C_B^{i\prime} + \Delta']\} \tag{19}$$

where $C_B^{i\prime} = C_B^i(1 - z^i F \Delta\psi/2RT)/(1 + z^i F \Delta\psi/2RT)$ and $\Delta' = \Delta/(1 + z^i F \Delta\psi/2RT)$. The "corrected" value of the permeability as given by Eq. (19) is smaller than that given by Eq. (16) because of the presence of the active transport term Δ'. With P^i computed from Eq. (19), the active transport can be determined using $N^i = P^i \Delta$. The values for the permeability and active transport are determined consistent with the several assumptions and only for the experimental situations stated. Determinations of these parameters under different experimental conditions may give different values.

G. Permeability Measurements in the Presence of Volume Reabsorption

In some cases it is either not possible or convenient to stop the volume reabsorption independent of solute movement and one is confronted with a situation in which volume flow and solute move across the tubule wall simultaneously but at different rates. In general, the substitution of Eq. (6) into Eq. (4) does not lead to analytic solutions without further simplifying assumptions. Other than the case of no volume reabsorption as discussed above, the simplest solution is obtained when the radial water velocity V_r is assumed constant over the tubule length. This assumption is probably reasonable due to the short lengths of the perfused tubule segments and the relative homogeneity of their function. This assumption has been made in several experimental investigations (Grantham and Burg, 1966; Kokko *et al.*, 1971; Schafer and Andreoli, 1972), and provides a single relation between concentration and permeability, thus allowing a determination of the latter if the former is known from experiment.

If V_r is assumed constant, then the longitudinal flow is a linear function of x and Eq. (1) gives

$$F_x(x) = F_x(0) - F_{ABS}(l)x/l \qquad (20)$$

Substituting Eqs. (20) and (6) into Eq. (4) gives

$$F_x(dC^i/dx) = C^i(1 + \sigma^i)F_{ABS}(l)/2l + 2\pi r P^i C^i \qquad (21)$$

where we have considered the case when $N^i = \Delta\psi = C_B^i = 0$ and $\bar{C}^i = C^i/2$. It is perhaps worthwhile to note at this point that the average transtubular concentration is usually taken as the arithmetic rather than the logarithmic average as derived from irreversible thermodynamics for dilute solutions which obey ideal gas laws (Katchalsky and Curran, 1965). If the ratio of concentrations on each side of the membrane is small compared to unity, the logarithmic average can be well approximated by the arithmetic average. However, when one concentration is zero, the logarithmic average equals zero, not the arithmetic average. This means simply that if we strictly set one concentration to zero we have not allowed a continuity through the membrane and solute does not move. Obviously this is not the case just at the membrane periphery and so it is assumed that in this case the arithmetic average remains a good approximation. For the logarithmic average to equal the arithmetic average, $C^i/2$, the ratio of concentrations C_B/C^i must be about $1:5$, which is not unreasonable. Then, integrating Eq. (21) making use of (20) gives

$$P^i = \{[F_x(0) - F_x(l)]/2\pi rl\} \left[\frac{\ln C^i(0)/C^i(l)}{\ln F^i(0)/F^i(l)} + \frac{(1 + \sigma^i)}{2} \right] \qquad (22)$$

This equation is somewhat different than Eq. (16) derived for the case when $V_r = 0$. Equation (22) necessarily involves the reflection coefficient σ^i of the solute in question and so more information is necessary to compute the solute permeability by this method than that given by Eq. (16). Furthermore, this method involves two added assumptions, namely, $V_r = $ constant and $\bar{C}^i = C^i/2$. If concentration is added to the bath so that $C_B^i \neq 0$ or $N^i \neq 0$ or $\Delta\psi \neq 0$, the derived equation becomes transcendental in P^i and the calculation is much more cumbersome.

H. Determination of the Reflection Coefficient

From the standpoint of derivation, the simplest method for determining the reflection coefficient of a given solute is to use a solute which is known to be impermeant ($\sigma = 1$) but which is otherwise similar to the desired permeant solute. Two separate experiments are then performed, one with the unknown solute, the other with the impermeant species such that in both cases the radial volume flow $F_x(0) - F_x(l)$, is made equal. Then, from Eq. (5), if the factors of hydrostatic pressure, V_r^E, V_r^A are known to be equal for the two species, it follows that

$$\sigma^i(\Pi^i - \Pi_B^i) = (\Pi^j - \Pi_B^j) \qquad (23)$$

where j represents the impermeant species. Since Π^i, Π_B^i, Π^j, and Π_B^j are known, σ^i can be computed. It is assumed that Π^i and Π^j do not vary significantly over the length of tubule considered.

Often, such a comparison experiment is impossible because the other factors in Eq. (5) are not equal or the solute in question is not easily separated from other solutes in the solution. A second method can be used, but it also involves special conditions. In this case the lumen and bath concentrations of the desired solute are not allowed to deviate very much from each other so that $\bar{C} \simeq C^i \simeq C_B^i$ and the lumen concentration C^i is maintained at a relatively constant value over the length of tubule segment. From Eqs. (2) and (4) it follows that if $C^i = $ constant, $J_r^i = C^i V_r$. Thus, Eq. (6) can be rearranged so that

$$J_r^i - \bar{C}^i V_r = \sigma^i \bar{C}^i V_r + P^i(\Delta C^i + z^i F \bar{C}^i \, \Delta\psi / RT) + N^i \qquad (24)$$

and since $\bar{C}^i \simeq C^i$, the left side of (24) is approximately zero so that

$$\bar{C}^i V_r \simeq C^i V_r = -(P^i/\sigma^i)(\Delta C^i + zFC^i \, \Delta\psi / RT) - N^i/\sigma^i \qquad (25)$$

If then an impermeant solute such as raffinose is added to the perfusate, V_r can be made to change consistent with observed changes $(\Delta C^i + z^i F C^i \, \Delta\psi / RT)$. By plotting $C^i V_r$ against $(\Delta C^i + z^i F C^i \, \Delta\psi / RT)$, a straight line will be obtained of slope P^i/σ^i and intercept N^i/σ^i. If P^i has been previously determined, then σ^i and N^i can be computed (Ullrich and Sauer, 1973).

I. Determination of Solute Flux from Bath to Lumen

It is sometimes desirable to determine the solute movement from the bath into the tubule lumen. If active transport and transepithelial potential are small and if the volume flow across the tubule wall is zero, then Eq. (6) defines the flux of solute i from bath to lumen as $J_{BL}^i = P^i C_B^i$. If other terms are present in Eq. (6), the bath-to-lumen flux is not so easily defined. If each parameter can be separately measured as described in the preceding sections, then in principle the unidirectional fluxes can be identified using Eq. (6). Since the individual components cannot always be easily measured, a less specific method for determining J_{BL}^i can be used (Burg et al., 1976). The experimental arrangement is such that volume reabsorption is present and the solute permeability can be determined by Eq. (22). The perfusion fluid is then cleared of the desired solute while the bath is changed from zero concentration to C_B^i. It is then assumed that the bath to lumen flux, J_{BL}^i, is relatively constant over the tubule length compared with the concentration of that solute which appears in the lumen $C^i(x)$. (The average transluminal concentration must not change significantly). Thus, the net radial solute flux, J_r^i, can be written in the form

$$J_r^i = P^i C^i(x) - J_{BL}^i \qquad (26)$$

so that using Eqs. (4) and (8) with (26) gives

$$dC^i(x) F_x / dx = -2\pi r[P^i C^i(x) - J_{BL}^i] \qquad (27)$$

Then if the volume reabsorption can be assumed constant along the tubule length, Eq. (20) can be substituted into (27) to give

$$F_x dC^i/dx = -2\pi r[P^i C^i(x) - J^i_{BL} - F_{ABS}(l)C^i/A] \tag{28}$$

where $A = 2\pi rl$ is the area of the tubule lumen. Integrating Eq. (28) from $x = 0$ to $x = l$ yields an expression for the bath to lumen solute flux,

$$J^i_{BL} = \frac{C^i(l)[P^i - F_{ABS}(l)/A]}{\{1 - [F_x(0)/F_x(l)]^{[1 - P^i A/F_{ABS}(l)]}\}} \tag{29}$$

where $C^i(0) = 0$. If J^i_{BL} is due only to diffusion from bath to lumen, then Eq. (29) must equal $P^i C^i_B$.

ACKNOWLEDGMENTS

We wish to thank Karen Robson, LaVerna Carrigan, Alice Dworzack, Judy Irish, and Dawn Varney for their excellent assistance in the preparation of this manuscript. We also thank Dr. Sandy Helman for helpful discussions concerning the formulation section and Dr. Jared Grantham for his advice and criticism concerning the overall manuscript.

REFERENCES

Bonting, S. L., and Mayron, B. R. 1961. Construction, calibration, and use of a modified quartz fiber "fishpole" ultramicrobalance. *Microchem. J., 5:*31.

Brenner, B. M., Falchuk, K. H., Deimowitz, R. I., and Berliner, R. W. 1969. The relationship between peritubular capillary protein concentration and fluid reabsorption by the renal proximal tubule. *J. Clin. Invest., 48:*1519.

Burg, M., and Green, N. 1973a. Function of the thick ascending limb of Henle's loop. *Am. J. Physiol., 224:*659.

Burg, M., and Green, N. 1973b. Effect of mersalyl on the thick ascending limb of Henle's loop, *Kidney Int., 4:*245.

Burg, M., and Green, N. 1973c. Effect of ethacrynic acid on the thick ascending limb of Henle's loop. *Kidney Int., 4:*301.

Burg, M., Grantham, J., Abramow, M., and Orloff, J. 1966. Preparation and study of fragments of single rabbit nephrons. *Am. J. Physiol., 210:*1293.

Burg, M., and Orloff, J. 1968. Control of fluid absorption in the renal proximal tubule. *J. Clin. Invest., 47:*2016.

Burg, M., and Orloff, J. 1970. Electrical potential difference across proximal convoluted tubules. *Am. J. Physiol., 219:*1714.

Burg, M., and Weller, P. F. 1969. Iodopyracet transport by isolated perfused flounder proximal renal tubules. *Am. J. Physiol., 217:*1053.

Burg, M., Isaacson, L., Grantham, J., and Orloff, J. (with appendix by Patlak, C.) 1968. Electrical properties of isolated perfused rabbit renal tubules. *Am. J. Physiol., 215:*788.

Burg, M., Stoner, L., Cardinal, J., and Green, N. 1973. Furosemide effect on isolated perfused tubules. *Am. J. Physiol., 225:*119.

Burg, M., Patlak, C., N., and Villey, D. 1976. Organic solutes in fluid adsorption by renal proximal convoluted tubules, *Am. J. Physiol., 231:*627.

Chonko, A. M., and Grantham, J. J. 1976. The use of the isolated tubule preparation for the investigation of diuretics. In: *Methods in Pharmacology,* Vol. 4A, pp. 47-71. Ed. by Martinez-Maldonado, M. Plenum Press, New York.

Chonko, A. M., Lowe, C. M., and Grantham, J. J. 1975. Uric acid secretion in isolated perfused rabbit kidney tubules. Comparison of proximal convoluted, proximal straight and cortical collecting tubules. *Clin. Res., 23:*358 (April).

Chonko, A. M., Dellasega, M., Varney, D., and Grantham, J. J. 1976. Mechanism of uric acid secretion by proximal straight tubules of rabbit nephron. *Clin. Res., 24:*553 (October).

Dantzler, W. H. 1974. PAH transport by snake proximal renal tubules, differences from urate transport. *Am. J. Physiol., 226:*634.

Dantzler, W. H., and Bentley, S. K. 1976. Low Na^+ effects on PAH transport and permeabilities in isolated snake renal tubules. *Am. J. Physiol., 230:*256.

Deen, W. M., Robertson, C. R., and Brenner, B. M. 1974. Concentration polarization in an ultrafiltering capillary. *Biophys. J., 14:*412.

Dellasega, M., and Grantham, J. J. 1973. Regulation of renal tubule cell volume in hypotonic media. *Am. J. Physiol., 224:*1288.

Dennis, V. W., Woodhall, P. B., and Robinson, R. R. 1976. Characteristics of phosphate transport in isolated proximal tubule. *Am. J. Physiol., 231:*979.

Fromter, E. 1974. Electrophysiology and isotopic fluid absorption of proximal tubules of mammalian kidney. In: *Kidney and Urinary Tract Physiology*, pp. 1–38. Ed. by Thurau, K. University Park Press, Baltimore, Md.

Ganote, C. E., Grantham, J. J., Moses, H. L., Burg, M. D., and Orloff, J. 1968. Ultrastructural studies of vasopressin effect on isolated perfused renal collecting tubules of the rabbit. *J. Cell Biol., 36:*355.

Grantham, J. 1973. Sodium transport in isolated renal isolated renal tubules. In: *Modern Diuretic Therapy in the Treatment of Cardiovascular and Renal Disease*, pp. 220–228. Ed. by Lant, E. F. and Wilson, G. M. Excerpta Medical Foundation, Amsterdam.

Grantham, J. J., and Burg, M. 1966. Effect of vasopressin and cyclic AMP on permeability of isolated collecting tubules. *Am. J. Physiol., 211:*255.

Grantham, J. J., and Orloff, J. 1968. Effect of prostaglandin E_1 on the permeability response of the isolated collecting tubule to vasopressin, adenosine 3′,5′-monophosphate, and theophylline. *J. Clin. Invest., 47:*1154.

Grantham, J. J., Ganote, C. E., Burg, M., and Orloff, J. 1969. Paths of transtubular water flow in isolated renal collecting tubules. *J. Cell Biol., 41:*562.

Grantham, J. J., Qualizza, P. B., and Welling, L. W. 1972. Influence of serum proteins on net fluid reabsorption of isolated proximal tubules. *Kidney Int., 2:*66.

Grantham, J. J., Irwin, R. L., Qualizza, P. B., Tucker, D. R., and Whittier, F. C. 1973. Fluid secretion in isolated proximal straight renal tubules. *J. Clin. Invest., 52:*2441.

Grantham, J. J., Irish, J. M. III, and Hall, D. A. 1978. Isolated perfused kidney tubules *in vitro*, *Annual Review of Physiology, 40:*223.

Grantham, J. J., Qualizza, P. B., and Irwin, R. I. 1974. Net fluid secretion in proximal straight renal tubules in vitro: role of PAH. *Am. J. Physiol. 226:*191–197.

Gross, J. B., Imai, M., and Kokko, J. P. 1975. A functional comparison of the cortical collecting tubule and the distal convoluted tubule. *J. Clin. Invest., 55:*1284.

Hall, D. A., and Grantham, J. J. In press. Transient response to vasopressin in isolated perfused cortical collecting tubules. *Fed. Proc.*

Hamburger, R. J., Lawson, N. L., and Dennis, V. W. 1974. Effects of cyclic adenosine and nucleotides on fluid absorption by different segments of the proximal tubule. *Am. J. Physiol., 227:*396.

Helman, S. I. 1972. Determination of electrical resistance of the isolated collecting tubule and its possible anatomic location. *Yale J. Biol. Med., 45:*339.

Helman, S. I., Grantham, J. J., and Burg, M. B. 1971. Effect of vasopressin on electrical resistance of renal cortical collecting tubules. *Am. J. Physiol., 220:*1825.

House, C. R. 1974. *Water Transport in Cells and Tissues*. Edward Arnold (Publishers), London.

Imai, M., and Kokko, J. P. 1972. Effect of peritubular protein concentration on reabsorption of sodium and water in isolated perfused proximal tubules. *J. Clin. Invest., 51:*314.

Imai, M., and Kokko, J. P. 1974. Transtubular oncotic pressure gradients and net fluid transport in isolated proximal tubules. *Kidney Int., 6:*138.

Irish, J. M. III, and Dantzler, W. H. 1976. PAH transport and fluid absorption by isolated perfused frog proximal renal tubules. *Am. J. Physiol., 230:*1509.

Katchalsky, A., and Curran, P. F. 1965. *Nonequilibrium Thermodynamics in Biophysics.* Harvard University Press, Cambridge, Ma.

Kawamura, S., Imai, M., Seldin, D. W., and Kokko, J. P. 1975. Characteristics of salt and water transport in superficial and juxtamedullary straight segments of proximal tubules. *J. Clin. Invest., 55:*1269.

Kedem, O., and Katchalsky, A. 1961. A physical interpretation of the phenomenological coefficients of membrane permeability. *J. Gen. Physiol., 45:*143.

Kokko, J. P. 1972. Qualitative and quantitative importance of the constituents used in microperfusion experiments. *Yale J. Biol. Med., 55:*1269.

Kokko, J. P. 1973. Proximal tubule potential differences. *J. Clin. Invest., 52:*1362.

Kokko, J. P., Burg, M., and Orloff, J. 1971. Characteristics of NaCl and water transport in the renal proximal tubule. *J. Clin. Invest., 50:*69.

Landis, E. M., and Pappenheimer, J. R. 1963. Exchange of substances through the capillary walls. In: *Handbook of Physiology,* Vol. 2. *Circulation,* pp. 961–1034. Ed. by Hamilton, W. F. Williams and Wilkins Co., Baltimore, Maryland.

Lewy, J. E., and Windhager, E. E. 1968. Peritubular control of proximal tubular fluid reabsorption in the rat kidney. *Am. J. Physiol., 214:*943.

Lutz, M. D., Cardinal, J., and Burg, M. B. 1973. Electrical resistance of renal proximal tubule perfused *in vitro. Am. J. Physiol., 225:*729.

Rocha, A. S., and Kokko, J. P. 1973. Sodium chloride and water transport in the medullary thick ascending limb of Henle. *J. Clin. Invest., 52:*612.

Schafer, J. A., and Andreoli, T. E. 1972. The effect of antidiuretic hormone on solute flows in mammalian collecting tubules. *J. Clin. Invest., 51:*1279.

Smith, H. W. 1939. *Newer Methods of Study of Renal Function in Man.* University of Kansas Press, Lawrence, Kan.

Spencer, H. 1863. *First Principles.* Chapter 16, p. 138. Williams and Norgate, London.

Stoner, L., Burg, M., and Orloff, J. 1974. Ion transport in cortical collecting tubule: Effect of amiloride. *Am. J. Physiol., 227:*453.

Tune, B. M., and Burg, M. B. 1971. Glucose transport by proximal renal tubules. *Am. J. Physiol., 221:*580.

Tune, B. M., Burg, M. B., and Patlak, C. S. 1969. Characteristics of *p*-aminohippurate transport in proximal renal tubules. *Am. J. Physiol., 217:*1057.

Ullrich, K. J., and Sauer, F. 1973. Permeability characteristics of the mammalian nephron. In: *Handbook of Renal Physiology,* Vol. II, pp. 377–414. Ed. by Orloff, J. and Berliner, R. W. American Physiological Society, Washington, D.C.

Wearn, J. T., and Richards, A. N. 1924. Observations on the composition of glomerular urine, with particular reference to the problem of reabsorption in the renal tubules. *Am. J. Physiol., 71:*209.

Welling, L. W., and Welling, D. J. 1976. Shape of epithelial cells and intercellular channels in the rabbit proximal nephron. *Kidney Int., 9:*385.

Chapter **10**

Sodium–Potassium-Activated Adenosine Triphosphatase: Methodology for Quantification in Microdissected Renal Tubule Segments from Freeze-Dried and Fresh Tissue

Udo Schmidt

Enzyme Laboratory, Medical Polyclinic
Department of Internal Medicine
University of Basel
Basel, Switzerland
and Institute of Pathology
University of Tübingen
Tübingen, Germany

and

Michael Horster

Institute of Physiology
University of Munich
Munich, Germany

I. INTRODUCTION

Since Na–K-ATPase, a part of the system responsible for the active transport of cations across the cell membrane, is firmly associated with the membrane structure, different procedures have been developed to separate the enzyme and quantify its specific activity. Purification of the enzyme has been attempted in a variety of tissues using surface-active agents such as deoxycho-

259

late (Skou, 1971), digitonin (Somogyi *et al.*, 1969), Triton-X-100, and Lubrol (Banerjee *et al.*, 1970) to solubilize the Na–K-ATPase.

The untreated homogenate of rabbit renal outer medulla, a tissue with a large capacity of Na–K-ATPase, reveals a specific activity of Na–K-ATPase under optimal conditions of 0.2 U (mg protein)$^{-1}$.[1] Demasking the latent enzyme activity of Na–K-ATPase by treatment with detergents elevates the specific activity of the enzyme in homogenates of this tissue to about 1 U (mg protein)$^{-1}$ (Jørgensen, 1974). In the microsomal fraction, a crude membrane preparation, the activity is 4–5 U (mg protein)$^{-1}$ (Jørgensen, 1974). Incubation of the microsomal fraction with deoxycholate followed by isopycnic-zonal (15 U) and rate-zonal centrifugations (25 U) results in a five-to-sixfold increase of enzyme activity.

Finally, treatment of the microsomal fraction with sodium dodecyl sulfate in the presence of ATP yields a specific activity of 36 U (mg protein)$^{-1}$ in a single isopycnic-zonal centrifugation, corresponding to a seven-to-ninefold purification of the Na–K-ATPase (Jørgensen, 1974).

The use of detergents for isolation and purification of a membrane-bound enzyme system raises some serious problems. All detergents increase the Na–K-ATPase activity up to a certain concentration, and higher detergent concentrations cause a marked loss of activity. Exposure to detergents could lead to an opening of vesicular structures, which would result in a greater accessibility of substrate and activators (Jørgensen and Skou, 1971). Furthermore, detergents such as deoxycholate, Triton, and Lubrol might increase the number of Na–K-ATPase molecules by partial replacement of lipids and proteins from the cell membrane.

The difficulty encountered in purifying Na–K-ATPase is apparent also from the fact that the activity of this enzyme depends on a certain integrity of the cell membrane, e.g., the Na–K-ATPase is known to require lipids for catalytic activity (Jørgensen, 1975). It is possible, therefore, that all procedures for purifying Na–K-ATPase change to some extent the matrix for the enzyme, resulting in a modulated conformation of Na–K-ATPase.

Optimal activation of a purified Na–K-ATPase preparation is achieved with sodium and potassium concentrations of 120 mM and 30 mM respectively, which are unbiologically high for a sodium activating site on the inside of the cell membrane, and a potassium activating site on the outside. *In vivo*, we expect an intracellular sodium concentration of 10 mM sodium (Dörge *et al.*, 1976) only, a concentration below the K_m value of most studies working with a purified enzyme preparation.

In our own laboratory we have been studying Na–K-ATPase activity within single segments of the nephron, microdissected from freeze-dried and from fresh renal tissue sections. The dissected samples are transferred without previous homogenization or treatment by detergents directly into the highly diluted assay reagent (5 ng dry tissue per 0.7 μl reagent).

Under these conditions we observed that an optimal stimulation of Na–K-

---

[1] The unit for enzyme activity (U) is μmol $P_i \times$ min^{-1}.

ATPase is achieved with sodium concentrations of 30–50 mM (K_m 10 mM), a potassium concentration of 5 mM (K_m 0.8 mM) and ATP concentration of 2 mM (K_m 0.6 mM). Thus, in untreated microdissected nephron segments, Na–K-ATPase works best with those concentrations of cations and substrate which we assume to be present *in vivo* inside and outside the cell (Schmidt *et al.*, 1974). The enzyme-enriched part of the distal nephron, i.e., the medullary thick ascending limb of Henle's loop, reveals an activity value of 0.8 U (mg protein)$^{-1}$. In addition, the first demonstration of a parallel change in Na–K-ATPase and renal sodium absorption came from our studies on single isolated nephron segments (Schmidt and Dubach, 1971a; Schmidt and Dubach, 1974; Schmidt *et al.*, 1975).

From these observations it might be concluded that the method of tissue preparation for assaying Na–K-ATPase will influence importantly the functional behavior of the enzyme.

The aim of the present survey is to provide a useful manual for preparing well-defined nephron segments and for assaying Na–K-ATPase with a sensitivity sufficient to calculate the activity within a single homogeneous segment of the nephron.

II. METHODS

A. Isolation of Nephron Segments from Freeze-Dried Renal Tissue Slices

The methodology described in the first part of this chapter is based on the fundamental techniques in quantitative histochemistry developed by Lowry and his collaborators in the Department of Pharmacology at the University of St. Louis. The details of the equipment used for quantitative histochemistry as well as the various assay conditions for microsamples and their application to different tissues have been described extensively (Lowry and Passoneau, 1972; Schmidt and Dubach, 1971b).

A scheme of the entire procedure is given in Figure 1. The main steps are: quick freezing of a small piece of renal tissue, slicing in a cryostat, lyophilization of the slices, identification and dissection of the desired nephron structure, weighing of the samples on a highly sensitive quartz fiber balance, and finally assaying the chemical constituents of the nephron segment with the oil-well technique combined with chemical amplification by enzymatic cycling.

1. Excision and Freezing

The animal is sacrificed by decapitation and the kidney removed as fast as possible, decapsulated on a petri dish, and cut in slices of 1 mm thickness with a razor blade. This thickness prevents fractures in the tissue when it is dropped into a medium of a temperature of more than $-80°C$. A cone containing cortex, outer medulla, and papilla is excised (Figure 2) from each slice.

One of these cones is mounted upright on a tissue holder using tragacanth or

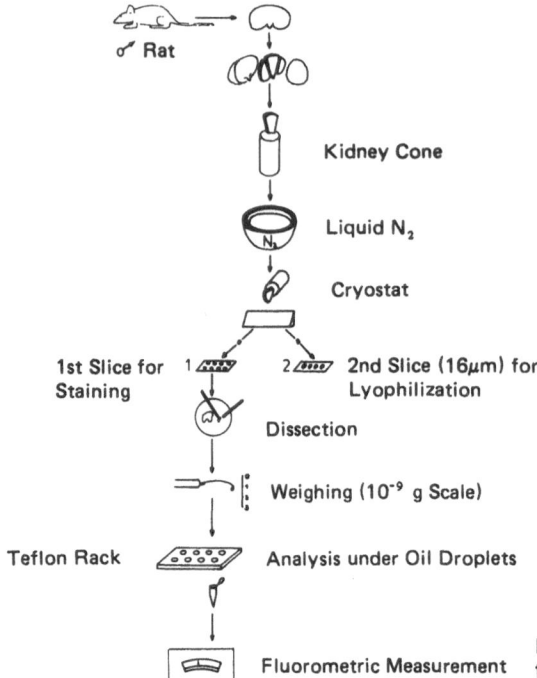

Figure 1. Survey of the procedure used for quantitative histochemistry of kidney tissue. For detailed explanation see text.

a paste of brain tissue prepared for this purpose. Tragacanth powder is mixed slowly under stirring at 60°C into a 4% sodium chloride solution to obtain a paste. The paste is stored in a freezer at −25°C and rewarmed before use. The other cone is mounted in such a way that each slice to be cut in the cryostat contains cortex, outer medulla, and papilla.

The tissue block in upright position yields sections from defined levels between subcapsular cortex and papilla (Figure 3). This sectioning technique ensures an exact classification of the nephron segments into those from the superficial and the juxtamedullary nephron type (see below) and into cortical and medullary nephron segments.

The loaded cryostat block (Figure 2) is plunged into liquid nitrogen. Chilled propane or isopentane is not used since these solutions affect the phospholipid content of the cell membrane.

The frozen block is removed and transferred to a petri dish which is kept in a cryostat at −25°C. The cap of the petri dish is sealed with silicone stopcock grease to avoid drying the tissue. At least 1 hr of temperature equilibration is allowed before slicing is begun. Usually, about 30 sec have elapsed from the sacrifice of the animal to the freezing of the tissue cone.

The frozen tissue samples which are not sectioned immediately can be stored at −80°C for several months without ice crystal growth, or loss of enzyme and of labile metabolites.

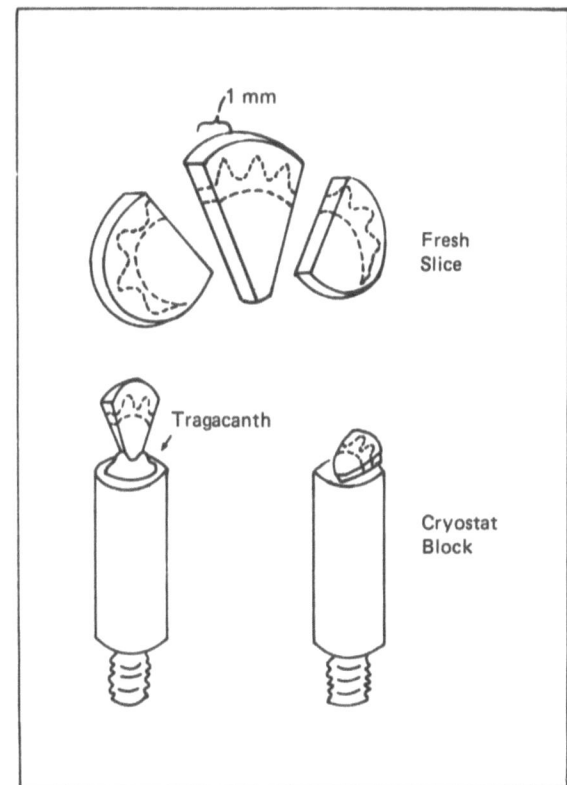

Figure 2. Procedure for slicing the removed kidney and mounting the slices on suitable tissue holders for the cryostat. The left holder carries the slice in an upright position whereas the right holder carries it flat.

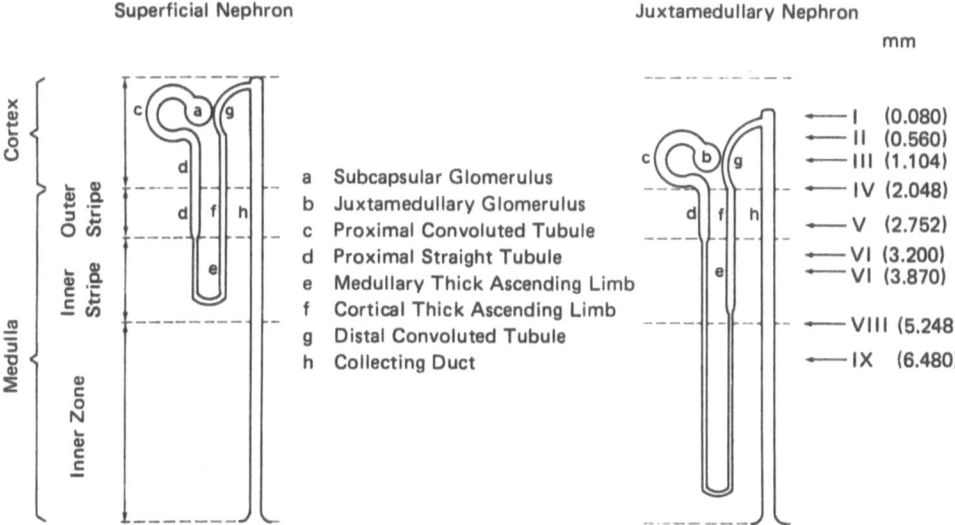

a Subcapsular Glomerulus
b Juxtamedullary Glomerulus
c Proximal Convoluted Tubule
d Proximal Straight Tubule
e Medullary Thick Ascending Limb
f Cortical Thick Ascending Limb
g Distal Convoluted Tubule
h Collecting Duct

Figure 3. Schematic drawing of the superficial (subcapsular) and the juxtamedullary nephron. The segments a–h can be isolated individually by microdissection from freeze-dried renal tissue sections. The arrows on the right side indicate the depth of the defined section level from the cortex toward the papilla.

2. Slicing

In general, the thicker the section, the higher the temperature required in the cryostat since the section otherwise will fracture as it comes off the knife. We prefer a thickness of 16 μm for sectioning kidney tissue; the nephron segments are easily distinguished after drying and their dry weight is adequate for enzyme analysis. A convenient temperature for cutting the renal tissue is $-25°C$.

The cutting is usually completed within 1 hr because the temperature in the cooling chamber will slowly rise by about 3°C. At higher temperatures (i.e., about $-15°C$), tissue deformation occurs during cutting.

Serial sections are cut from each tissue sample in the following way: Three consecutive sections are cut from each of the well-defined levels throughout the kidney zones (Figure 3); the first section is put into the hole of a special tissue holder (Figure 4) which consists of a drilled plastic block sandwiched between glass slides. The second section is mounted on a glass slide. The glass slide is treated with albumin-glycerin to prevent the section from coming off the slide during the staining procedure. The third section put into the same hole where the first one has been kept. This procedure is important for maintaining an exact sequence which ensures a correlation of the stained tubule segment in the middle section to the corresponding freeze-dried unstained tubule segments in the first and third sections.

When the plastic block is filled with sections, the cover is replaced to prevent drying at the temperature of the cryostat.

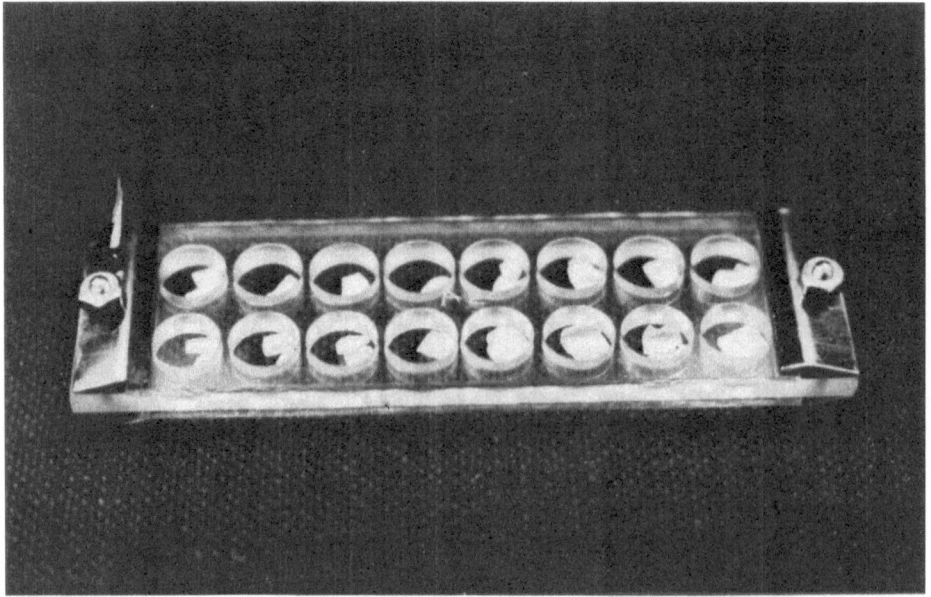

Figure 4. Tissue holder loaded with lyophilized sections of 16 μm thickness. The holder is 90 × 25 mm, the diameter of a hole is 7 mm.

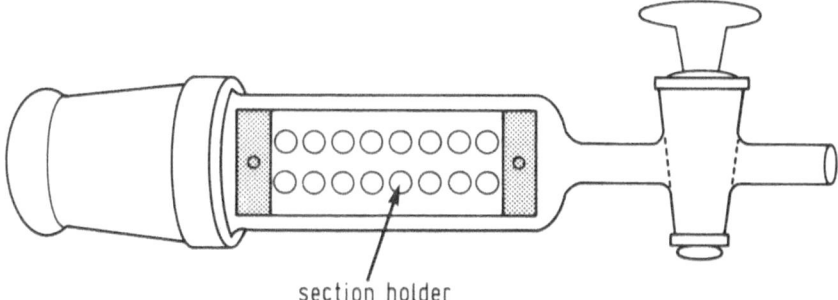

section holder

Figure 5. Schematic drawing of the glass vacuum tube containing the section holder used for freeze-drying renal tissue. The length of the tube (without the cap) is 220 mm; the inner diameter is 34 mm.

Two or four of the loaded plastic blocks are placed in a Pyrex glass tube (Figure 5) built with a stopcock at one end and a cap on the other end. The stopcock and the cap are greased with silicone and care should be taken to prevent grease from entering the airway. The tube is transferred without rewarming into a freezer at $-40°C$ where it is connected to a vacuum system.

3. Staining Procedures

The second of three consecutive sections is used for staining and serves as guiding map for identification of the desired nephron structures within the lyophilized first and third section. The periodic acid–Schiff (PAS) procedure is an intensive and adequate staining method for kidney tissue because of the carbohydrate-enriched coat of the tubule epithelial cells. In addition, the various nephron segments can also be distinguished by the thickness of their cell coat.

The two solvents used for periodic acid are water and ethyl alcohol.

Periodic Acid–Schiff Stain with an Aqueous Periodic Acid: Preparation of Schiff reagent.

1. One gram of basic fuchsin is dissolved in 200 ml boiling distilled water. The solution is cooled to room temperature.
2. 20 ml of 1 N hydrochloric acid, in which 1 g of sodium metabisulfite ($Na_2S_2O_5$) is dissolved, are added to (1).
3. The mixture is shaken for 3 min.
4. After storage for at least 12 hr in the dark, 2 g of activated charcoal are added and shaken for 1 min.
5. The charcoal is removed by filtration and the solution is stored in the dark at 4°C.
6. The solution should be clear; otherwise steps (4) and (5) should be repeated.

Staining procedure: Periodic acid (0.5%) must be freshly prepared before each staining procedure.

1. When the glass slides loaded with tissue sections are taken out of the cryostat chamber, they should be dried for 15 min at room temperature.

2. Sections must first be oxidized with periodic acid to get them to react with Schiff reagent. The time of exposure to periodic acid should be kept to a minimum and not exceed 10 min at room temperature. Longer exposure to periodic acid will cause proteins to become PAS positive. The sections are exposed to periodic acid for 5 min.
3. Sections are washed in running water for 5 min and rinsed in distilled water.
4. They are treated with Schiff reagent for 10–30 min, depending on the intensity of the staining.
5. The sections are washed in warm water (45°C) and
6. counterstained with hematoxylin for 1 min.
7. The slides are transferred into 20, 40, 70, 96, and 100% alcohol for 5 min each.
8. Transfer them into xylol for 5 min and
9. mount in Canada balsam.

Periodic Acid–Schiff Stain with Alcohol-Buffered Periodic Acid: Solutions

1. Schiff reagent (see p. 265)
2. Alcoholic periodic acid: 0.7 g of periodic acid is dissolved in 30 ml sulfuric acid (6%) and 70 ml of absolute alcohol are added.
3. Acid-reducing rinse: 1.5 g of sodium hydrogen sulfite are dissolved in 300 ml of distilled water and 15 ml of 1 N hydrochloric acid are added.

Solutions (2) and (3) are freshly prepared.
Staining procedure

1. The sections are put in alcoholic periodic acid for 20 min,
2. rinsed in distilled water,
3. treated with Schiff reagent for 45 min,
4. treated with acid-reducing rinse for 1 min,
5. washed in running water for 2 hr,
6. counterstained with hematoxylin, and
7. further prepared as described above.

For renal sections we prefer a simple aqueous solution of periodic acid which will give equally good, if not better, results compared to buffered alcoholic periodic acid.

4. Drying

Evacuation of the Pyrex glass vacuum tube is performed at a temperature of −40°C at a vacuum equivalent of 0.01 mm Hg. Two dry ice traps are interposed between pump and Pyrex glass vacuum tube to adsorp the moisture (Figure 6). Usually, evacuation is carried out overnight although most of the water will be removed within 1 hr. If ice crystals remain in the tube, evacuation is continued at room temperature since even a few crystals could ruin the sections. As soon as drying is completed, the stopcock outlet is plugged with a cork or covered with a rubber cap to prevent ice crystal formation at the stopcock. This precaution taken, the tube can be stored for long periods in a freezer at −40°C

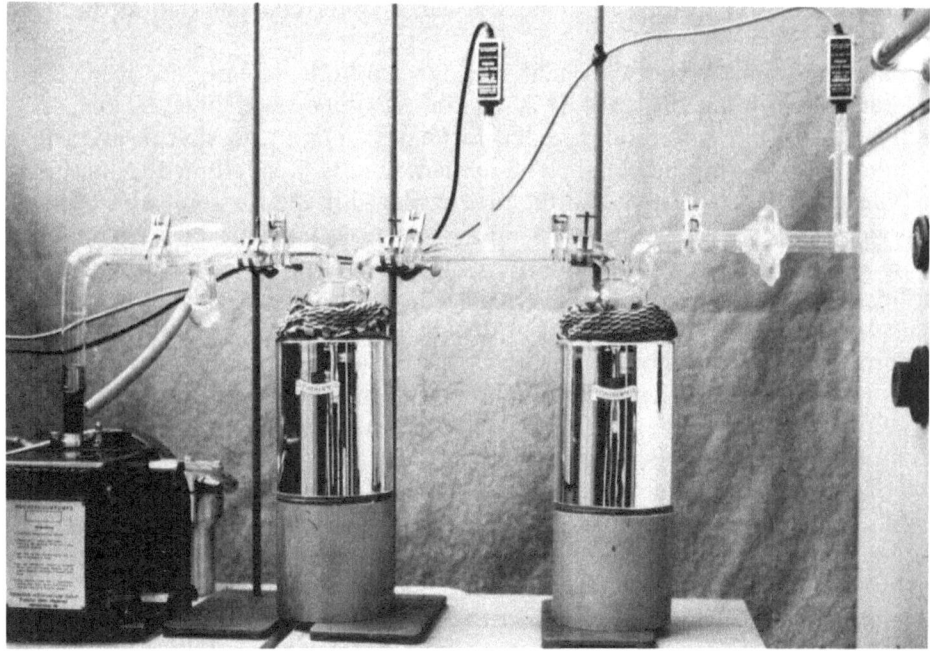

Figure 6. Vacuum system used for drying renal tissue. A pump is on the left side, a freezer with the glass vacuum tube inside is on the right side. Between pump and freezer are two traps filled with a dry ice–acetone mixture.

(for enzymes) or −80°C (for metabolites). Dried sections kept under vacuum can be stored in this way for many years without loss of enzyme activity or without breakdown of labile metabolites (Lowry and Passonneau, 1972).

5. Dissection of the Freeze-Dried Nephron Segments

The dissection of the nephron segments, the weighing of the isolated portions, and the transfer of the dried samples to the reagent are performed in a room where temperature and humidity are controlled. The temperature should not exceed 25°C and the humidity should not be above 50%. For example, labile pyridine nucleotides are stable for several hours at 25°C if the relative humidity is 50% or less (Lowry and Passonneau, 1972).

To raise the tissue temperature for dissection, the tube is taken out of the freezer and connected to the vacuum pump at room temperature. As soon as a vacuum of 0.01 mm Hg is reached, the stopcock is opened; this step allows one to check whether or not the tube vacuum was stable during storage in the freezer. If a change in vacuum is observed upon opening the stopcock, the rewarming is extended to at least 3 hr to ascertain complete drying. Usually, the warming process is accelerated by wrapping the tube in a warmed wet towel (45°C). Because heat transfer across the evacuated tube to the specimens is minimal, warming usually requires 1 hr. If the rewarming period is too short, the air entering the tube during opening will cause water condensation at the cool section holders.

The rewarmed tube is brought into the controlled room and opened. In general, although enzyme activity in the dry sections is relatively stable, it is preferable to keep the sections under vacuum as long as possible. Only a few sections are taken for dissection. The tissue holder is then returned to the tube, the vacuum is reestablished, and the tube is placed in the freezer.

The dry section is transferred on a solid plastic plate which is mounted under a stereomicroscope. The plastic plate is translucent to allow illumination of the section from below. In the freeze-dried and unstained renal tissue section, the various tubule segments cannot be distinguished. Therefore, the PAS-stained corresponding and neighboring section is essential as a guiding map for exact identification and dissection of the nephron segments within the dried section.

An exact knowledge of renal cytoarchitecture is needed to identify the nephron segments in the freeze-dried section and is the cornerstone of a successful application of the ultramicrochemical assay technique. Recent research on intrarenal topography has yielded important new information which facilitates the exact recovery of almost all of the nephron segments defined so far by functional and ultrastructural differences (Kriz, 1967; Kriz *et al.*, 1972; Kriz and Koepsell, 1974).

The kidney tissue can be separated into cortex and medulla. The cortex consists of the cortical labyrinth and the medullary rays which penetrate into the labyrinth, almost reaching the renal surface.

The medulla consists of an outer and inner zone. The outer zone contains an outer and inner stripe. The outer zone is the "red medulla" whereas the inner zone is the "white medulla" or "papilla." The thickness of the zones for a 200-g rat are 1.5 mm for the cortex, 0.65 mm for the outer stripe, 1.2 mm for the inner stripe, and 3.7 mm for the inner zone (Kriz, 1967).

The nephron populations consist of a superficial (subcapsular) and a juxtamedullary nephron type. The loop of Henle of the short-looped superficial nephron turns at the border of the outer to inner medullary zone, whereas the juxtamedullary nephron extends its long loop into the inner zone and a minor part into the papillary tip. In the rat kidney, 68% of all nephrons have been estimated to be short-looped, superficial type nephrons. The tubular part of the nephron consists of a proximal and a distal convoluted tubule connected by a loop of Henle. The straight portion (pars recta) of the proximal tubule is the first part of the loop of Henle followed by the thin limb, by the bend of the loop, by the thin ascending limb (only in long loops) and finally by the thick ascending limb.

Superficial or Subcapsular Nephron. The proximal and distal convoluted tubules are located peripheral from the corresponding glomerulus toward the renal surface. The straight portions of the proximal tubule and the thick ascending limb together with the initial part of the collecting duct constitute the apical part of the medullary ray. Descending and ascending parts from the same loop of Henle are adjacent throughout the length of the medullary ray.

Juxtamedullary Nephrons. The proximal convolutions appear as transversally arranged segments bordering the bases of the medullary rays. The proximal straight portions are not localized in the medullary rays, but penetrate directly into the outer stripe of the outer medullary zone and are tortuous when traversing the outer stripe. The thick ascending limbs of Henle's loop reach the convoluted portions without penetrating into the medullary rays. The inner stripe of the outer medulla is characterized by the vascular bundles. The ascending limbs of the long loops are situated next to vascular bundles whereas the same segment from the subcapsular nephron is located more distally next to the collecting duct.

Table I lists some of the properties helpful for dissecting defined segments of the rat nephron. The proximal and distal convolutions are dissected close to their glomerulus. In the PAS-stained section, the deep red color of the brush border permits easy differentiation between the proximal and distal convolutions. Special attention is given to the distinction between the proximal convoluted and the proximal straight portion by the localization of the latter within the medullary rays.

The distal convolution is distinguished from the cortical collecting duct by its localization near the glomerulus. The cross section of the distal convolution reveals nuclei arranged in a star-shaped configuration close to the luminal area. The cortical collecting duct displays dispersed nuclei in the cross section and is localized peripheral to the glomerulus. Within the medullary ray, the proximal straight portion is distinguishable from the thick ascending limb of Henle by the deep red color of its brush border. In the dried section, the collecting duct can be distinguished from the thick ascending limb by its open lumen and a remarkably thin wall.

The thick ascending limb of Henle can be best isolated from the inner stripe of the outer medulla. In the stained section, thick ascending limbs reveal cells with a brown-violet cytoplasm and longitudinally arranged nuclei. The collecting duct in this kidney zone demonstrates cells with a shiny, red cytoplasm and round nuclei which are localized at the cell base. In the dried section the thick ascending limb is recognizable by its relatively thick wall and a usually collapsed lumen. The collecting duct has a thin wall and the lumen is generally patent.

The two populations of nephrons of the mammalian kidney are distinguished by the location and depth of penetration into the medulla of their loops of Henle. Since it has been established that the two nephron populations differ also in glomerular filtration rate, and other functional properties (Horster and Thurau, 1968; Schmidt and Dubach, 1969; Jacobson and Kokko, 1976), it should be strongly emphasized that any microdissected tubular segment must be correctly identified as belonging to the superficial (subcapsular) or juxtamedullary nephron type.

From reconstruction studies, it is known that the proximal convolution is attached to the capsule of its own glomerulus. Therefore, proximal convolutions from the superficial nephron are dissected off the glomeruli just below the capsule and those from juxtamedullary nephrons off the glomeruli in the depth of the labyrinth between two medullary rays.

The tip of the medullary ray consists of proximal straight portions belonging

Table I. Characteristics during Dissection of Freeze-dried Rat Nephron Segments

Structure	Localization		PAS staining			Lyophilized section
	Cortex	Medulla outer	Brush border	Cytoplasm	Nuclei	
Proximal tubule						
Pars convoluta	Adjacent glomeruli		Deep red	Bright red	Basal, round	—[a]
Pars recta	Peripheral glomeruli		Deep red	Pale red	Basal, round	—[a]
Distal tubule						
Pars convoluta	Adjacent glomeruli		Absent	Bright red	Apical, oblong	—[a]
Thick ascending limb		Inner stripe	Absent	Brown–violet	Apical, oblong	Closed lumen
Collecting duct						
Cortical	Peripheral glomeruli		Absent	Deep red	Dispersed, round	—[a]
Medullary		Inner stripe	Absent	Deep red	Basal, round	Open lumen

[a] Not characteristic.

exclusively to the superficial nephron. In the deeper outer stripe of the medulla, a mixture of proximal straight portions belonging to the superficial and juxtamedullary nephron is found. The differentiation in the deeper outer stripe between the two nephron types is successful when the particular arrangement of the straight portions to vascular bundles and the characteristic course in this layer of the outer stripe is considered. The vascular bundles at their beginning in the outer stripe are surrounded by proximal straight portions belonging to the juxtamedullary nephrons. In addition, the cross section shows that the proximal straight portions of the juxtamedullary nephron have a tortuous course and are therefore cut longitudinally, while those segments from the superficial nephron are sectioned transversally. As mentioned before, the attribution of the different proximal tubule segments to the two major nephron populations is facilitated by defined kidney sections from the cortex toward the outer medulla.

It has so far not been possible to microdissect thin descending or thin ascending limbs from the freeze-dried section.

The dissection is performed freehand without a micromanipulator under a stereomicroscope (100× magnification). Structures of even 10 μm in diameter, e.g., a cross section of the distal tubule, may be dissected freehand. The identification of the desired nephron structure in the freeze-dried section is ascertained by the stained alternate section, which is examined under a second microscope next to the dissection stereomicroscope (Figure 7).

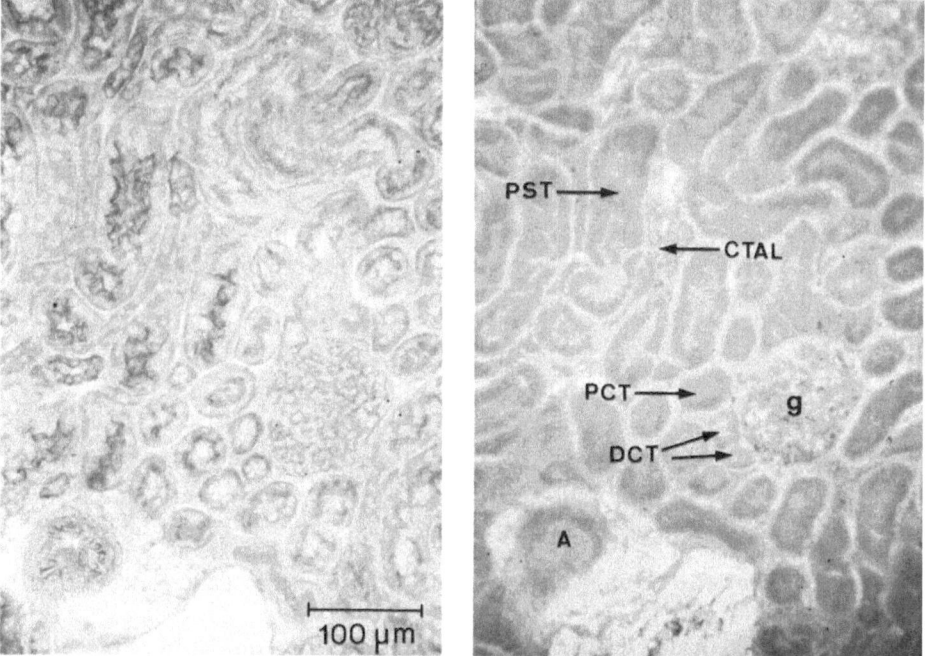

Figure 7. PAS stained (left) and corresponding freeze-dried (right) renal section from the midcortical level. A, artery; CTAL, cortical thick ascending loop; DCT, distal convoluted tubule; g, glomerulus; PCT, proximal convoluted tubule; PST, proximal straight tubule.

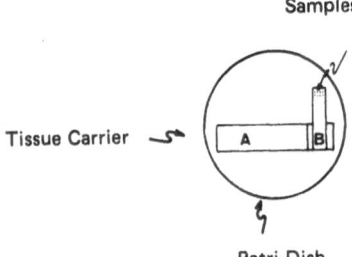

Figure 8. Schematic drawing of the sample carrier within a petri dish. The body of the carrier (A) is made of wood (40 × 10 mm), and the carrier (B) is made of glass cut from a microscope slide (30 × 5 mm).

Appropriate instruments for the dissection in freeze-dried sections are small knives which are splinters of a razor blade mounted on a piece of polyethylene tube. The tube is fixed on a pencil-shaped glass holder. The flexibility of the polyethylene reduces the tremor. In addition, short injection needles (1 cm in length) mounted on a tuberculin syringe are used.

During dissection, tissue specimens consisting of 6–10 tubules are separated with the knife from the freeze-dried section. The single desired structure is then dissected with needles from the separated specimen. Finally, the knife is used to cut off fragments of interstitium which almost always adhere to the isolated freeze-dried tubular structure.

The dissected nephron segments are placed on a special tissue carrier for transfer to the balance and for temporary storage (Figure 8). The loaded carrier is placed into a petri dish to prevent air currents from changing the sequence of the tubules. The loaded petri dish should be handled gently since the electrostatic charge on the cover glass may cause samples to jump off the carrier.

The microdissected samples are picked up and transferred with a hair glued to a pencil-shaped glass holder. The size of the hair tip and its stiffness are chosen to fit different sample sizes. Human eyebrow hair or a quartz fiber are suitable.

Electrostatic forces are sometimes a serious problem during handling of the sections or of isolated nephron segments. Low-dose radium radiation prevents samples from sticking to the plastic surface, to instruments for microdissection, or to the hair tip.

6. Weighing

The microdissected nephron segments from the 16-μm-thick freeze-dried renal section are 5 to 100 μm in length; the weight is in the range of 4 to 50 ng. Determination of the dry weight is made on a quartz fiber balance. The construction of balances with appropriate sensitivity has been carefully described by Lowry (Lowry and Passonneau, 1972) and the reader is referred to this work.

Briefly, the balance consists of a chamber in which a quartz fiber of defined length and diameter is attached to the end of a plunger (Figure 9). A syringe of 5 ml volume is used as chamber; the closed end of the syringe barrel is cut off, and the plunger is reserved. A piece of copper wire of suitable flexibility is glued to

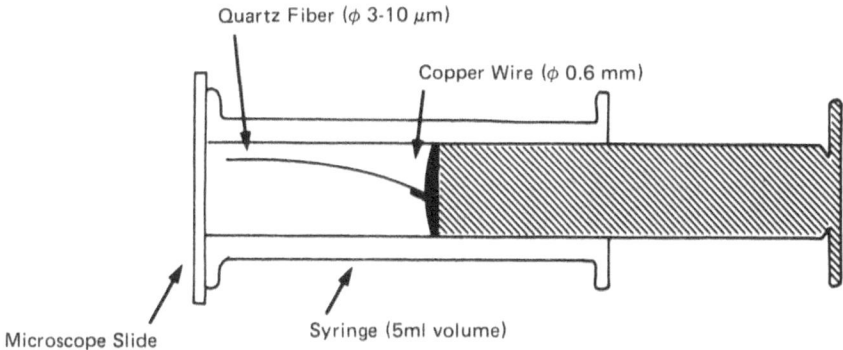

Figure 9. Schematic drawing of a quartz fiber balance. For detailed explanation see text.

the end of the plunger with epoxy resin so that 5 mm of the wire extend straight out of the center. The quartz fiber is sealed to the copper wire with epoxy resin. The sensitivity of the quartz fiber can be calculated from the equation (Lowry and Passonneau, 1972)

$$S = L^3/d^4 \ (\text{mm}/\mu\text{g})$$

where L is the length in millimeters and d is the diameter in microns. Commercially produced quartz fibers are now available in sizes down to 3 μm. A quartz fiber of 16 mm length and 3 μm diameter measures linearly up to 55 ng and has a sensitivity of 6×10^{-9} g/mm (Figure 10).

To avoid air currents and dust within the balance, the chamber is closed with a piece of flat glass. This glass consists of a microscope slide or part of it; wire hooks are sealed to the glass to attach nylon filaments with small wire springs which hold the glass plate in place. The wire springs permit removal of the plate without displacement of the balance and provide firm closure. The syringe plunger with the fiber is set to give a distance between the free end of the fiber and the glass plate of 1 mm.

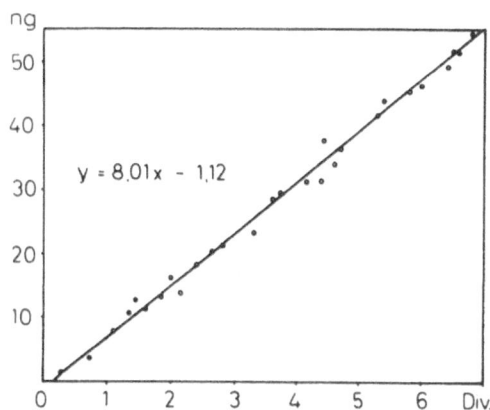

Figure 10. Calibration curve of a quartz fiber balance. The quartz fiber is 3 μm in diameter at a length of 16 mm. One division on the abscissa corresponds to 6.9 ng.

The balance is fixed to the table using a metal stand so that the open end of the syringe barrel faces the operator at approximately eye level when the operator sits at the table. A convenient hand support can be provided by a horizontal heavy wooden bar mounted separately on the table at a level approximately 1 cm below the barrel of the balance chamber. This bar should be large enough to provide room for the specimen carriers close to the balance, and it should be solid enough to firmly support the hand of the operator while his elbows rest on the table so that the loading process can be well controlled.

The displacement of the balance tip after loading is measured on an ocular micrometer scale in a stereomicroscope. The stereomicroscope is mounted in front of the balance. A 5-mm ocular scale divided into 0.1-mm divisions is convenient.

Next to the microscope, a simple manipulator serves to move the sample holder in and out of the balance. The magnification is selected so that both the balance and the tissue holder are in focus.

During weighing, the zero point is adjusted, the balance chamber opened, and the samples on the holder are moved into the balance chamber just under the tip of the fiber. A sample is loaded on the fiber tip with a hair tip and the holder is withdrawn. The glass cover is put back and the reading is made after fiber stabilization (about 5 sec). The chamber is opened, the sample holder is inserted, and the sample taken off the fiber tip with the hair tip, and returned to the sample holder. Usually, two to three samples can be measured this way within 1 min.

The dry weights of the different nephron segments dissected from a 16-μm-thick renal section are listed in Table II. It should be remembered that the tubule segments are dissected from thin sections (16 μm) and represent only part of the total circumference, particularly in the proximal convoluted tubule. This fact also influences the relation between weight and length. The dry-weight-to-length relation in the rat nephron segments are: proximal convoluted tubule, 26 ng/100

Table II. Dry Weight of Nephron Segments Dissected from a Rat Renal Slice (16 μm)

Structure	Dry weight (nanograms)	
	Superficial	Juxtamedullary
Glomerulus	25	35
Proximal convoluted tubule	20	25
Proximal straight tubule	23	27
Medullary thick ascending loop of Henle	10	10
Cortical thick ascending loop of Henle	8	8
Distal convoluted tubule	5	5
Cortical collecting duct	8	8
Medullary collecting duct	7	7
Papillary collecting duct	15	15

μm; medullary thick ascending limb of Henle's loop, 16 ng/100 μm; distal convoluted tubule, 11 ng/100 μm.

The freeze-dried tissue adsorbs O_2, N_2, and moisture (Lowry and Passonneau, 1972). This adsorptive process is completed within a few seconds after opening the tube in the controlled room. The adsorbed O_2 and N_2 add 2% to the weight, the amount of moisture adsorbed is proportional to the humidity and is 1% of weight increase for each 10% of humidity. In a controlled room with 50% humidity, therefore, a sample weight is 7% above the true weight.

The balance in the nanogram range is calibrated fluorometrically with crystals of quinine hydrobromide. Crystals of different size are put on the tip of the fiber and the fiber deflection is read. The single crystals are dissolved in 1 ml of 0.1 N H_2SO_4 and read against two standards (0.005 μg/ml and 0.05 μg/ml).

A diagram of crystal weight versus scale divisions is shown in Figure 10, demonstrating that one division corresponds to 6.9 ng.

The sensitivity of the balance has been found to be constant for years. When the unloaded fiber moves below the zero point, dirt may have covered the fiber. Suitable cleaning fluids are ethanol or fuming HNO_3. A droplet of the cleaning fluid is placed with a micropipet on the fiber near the origin at the copper wire and moved with the pipet along the fiber.

B. Microdissection of Nephron Segments from Fresh Renal Tissue Slices

The principles of some of the techniques described in this section have been developed by Burg and his collaborators at the National Institutes of Health for *in vitro* studies on isolated perfused nephron segments (Burg *et al.*, 1966; Kokko *et al.*, 1971; Horster *et al.*, 1973). In mammalian species, nephron segments from rabbit kidneys only have been systematically studied during *in vitro* perfusion. Therefore, new aspects of the technique for rabbit nephron segments will be emphasized.

A schematic outline of the entire procedure for analysis of Na–K-ATPase in single tubule segments dissected from fresh tissue is presented in Figure 11. Briefly, the procedure consists of transfer of a fresh slice into the dissection medium, dissection of defined segments, freezing, and lyophilization. Subsequent steps are identical to those described for the freeze-dried tissue analysis.

1. Preparation and Transfer of the Slice for Microdissection

The animals used are white New Zealand rabbits kept on a defined salt intake. The body weight of the animals is 1.0–1.5 kg, corresponding to 3–4 months of postnatal age. Neonatal animals (2–8 days of postnatal age) can also be studied by nephron microdissection and analysis. Technical details and results of these studies have been reported elsewhere (Schmidt and Horster, 1977).

The animals are sacrificed by a blow to the neck, the left kidney is immediately removed and cut into slices of 1 mm thickness. The slices are plunged directly from the knife into a cooled (4°C) special artificial solution (see

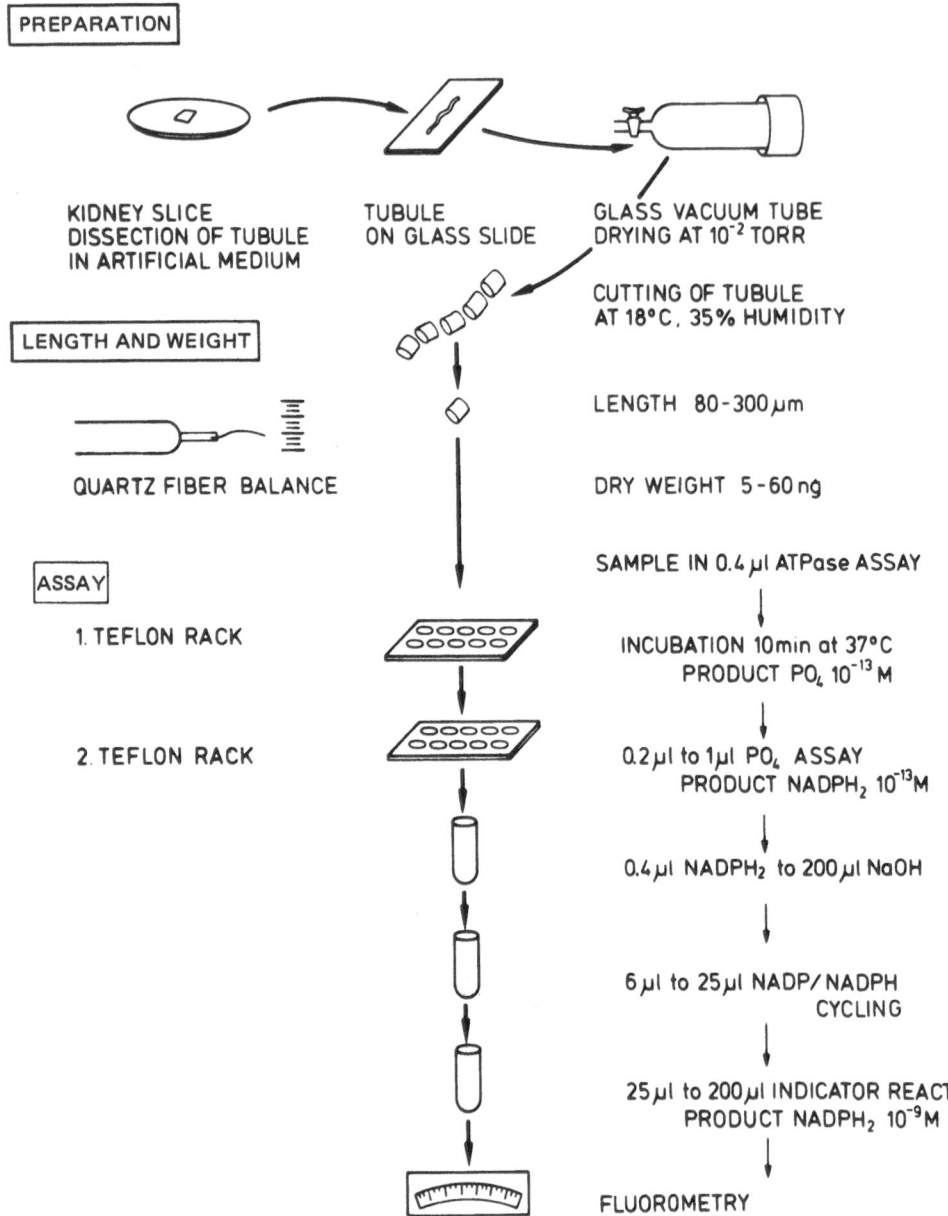

PREPARATION

KIDNEY SLICE
DISSECTION OF TUBULE
IN ARTIFICIAL MEDIUM

TUBULE
ON GLASS SLIDE

GLASS VACUUM TUBE
DRYING AT 10^{-2} TORR

CUTTING OF TUBULE
AT 18°C, 35% HUMIDITY

LENGTH AND WEIGHT

QUARTZ FIBER BALANCE

LENGTH 80-300 μm

DRY WEIGHT 5-60 ng

ASSAY

1. TEFLON RACK

2. TEFLON RACK

SAMPLE IN 0.4 μl ATPase ASSAY

INCUBATION 10 min at 37°C
PRODUCT PO_4 10^{-13} M

0.2 μl to 1 μl PO_4 ASSAY
PRODUCT $NADPH_2$ 10^{-13} M

0.4 μl $NADPH_2$ to 200 μl NaOH

6 μl to 25 μl NADP/ NADPH
CYCLING

25 μl to 200 μl INDICATOR REACT.
PRODUCT $NADPH_2$ 10^{-9} M

FLUOROMETRY

Figure 11. Scheme of the complete procedure for Na–K-ATPase ultramicroanalysis in single rabbit tubules microdissected *in vitro* from fresh renal slices.

below). This step clears the tissue from blood. Thereafter the slices are transferred to the dissection chamber containing the identical solution. From sacrifice, 1–2 min have passed.

The artificial medium, which is used in our laboratory besides other solutions such as rabbit ultrafiltrate for *in vitro* nephron perfusion, contains:

NaCl, 115 mM; NaHCO$_3$, 25 mM; Na-acetate, 10 mM; KCl, 5 mM; CaCl$_2$, 1.0 mM; MgSO$_4$, 1.2 mM; NaH$_2$PO$_4$ 1.0 mM; glucose, 5.5 mM. The solutions used in the tissue-wash-step and in the dissection chamber are gassed with 95%/5% CO$_2$ before and during the experiment to assure a constant pH of 7.4. The osmolality of this medium is 290 mosmol/liter, the sodium and potassium concentrations are 153 and 5.5 mEq/liter, respectively. In the rabbit, addition of collagenase or any other tissue-digesting enzyme is not only unnecessary but also harmful, since it may cause disruption of cells from the tubule basement membrane (Burg *et al.*, 1966).

A scheme of the dissection chamber is shown in Figure 12. The chamber is mounted below the surface into the top of a heavy table. This position facilitates the dissection because arms and hands rest comfortably on the table. A light source (Wild-Heerbrugg) is attached below the table directly to the bottom of the chamber for transmission and dark field illumination. Zoom microscopes (Wild; Zeiss) are used for dissection at 20 to 100× magnification. The dissection chamber is built from Lucite material as a flowthrough system. From a cryothermostat (Colora WK 5), a cooling fluid (Antifrogen) is perfused continuously through the bottom and side walls of the chamber to yield a constant temperature of 4°C in the dissection medium.

Dissection is carried out in a glass petri dish partially covered with a Lucite top and positioned into the chamber. An oil layer may be placed between petri dish and chamber for better cooling.

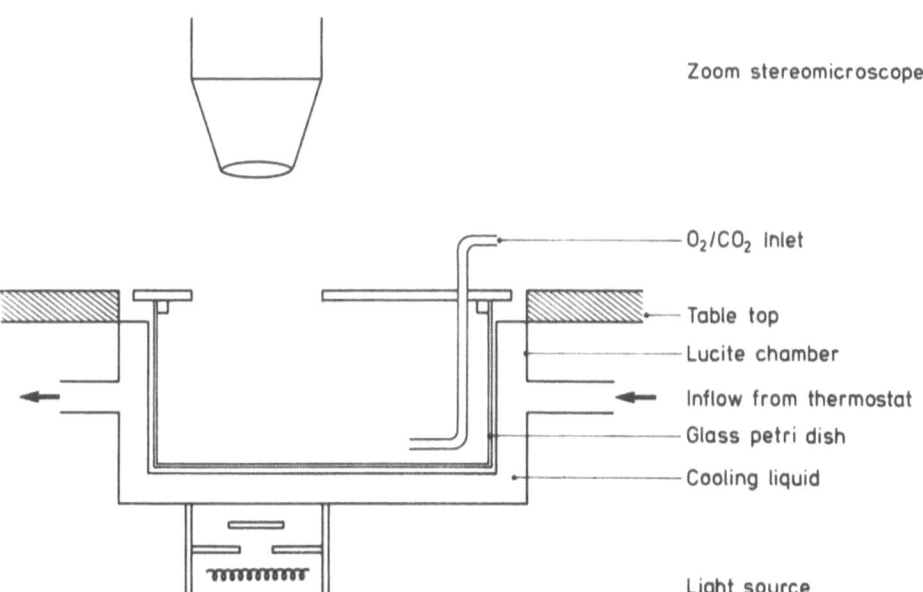

Figure 12. Arrangement used for *in vitro* dissection of single nephron segments from fresh rabbit renal slices.

2. Dissection

Routinely, only two steel forceps (Dumont) are used for dissection. These have been specially sharpened on a grindstone (Degussa) to a branch tip size of 30 μm. One edge of each branch has been prepared to be used like a knife. Dissection is begun by removing the renal capsule from the slice and separating cortical from medullary tissue along the corticomedullary boundary. The difference in color between these two parts and the rigidity of the large vessels along the border allow an easy orientation.

It has been advantageous for dissection of functionally and ultrastructurally intact segments (Larsson and Horster, 1976; Horster and Larsson, 1976) to develop specific techniques for each nephron segment. In the following section, identification by localization and appearance for a variety of segments will be described together with specific isolation techniques. For guidance, the characteristics of different nephron segments during *in vitro* dissection from fresh renal tissue are illustrated in Figure 13.

Proximal Convoluted Tubule. The two forceps are inserted with open branches into the cortical tissue block, about 0.5 cm apart, and the tissue is gently torn sidewise. Numerous proximal convoluted segments and some collecting ducts spread between the two tissue blocks. Among those, a particularly long proximal segment is chosen for further isolation. One or two slices are screened for proximal tubules in this way. This approach is thought to cause minimal tension to long segments since shorter segments will absorb most of the traction before it reaches the long tubules. For further isolation of the desired segment, the proximal and distal end are followed into the tissue blocks as far as possible and the tubule ends are cut sharply using a specially prepared branch of the forceps. During the entire procedure the tubule need not be touched except for transfer. Proximal convoluted tubules from the superficial nephron type differ greatly from the juxtamedullary type. Apart from their localization within the cortex, juxtamedullary convolutions can easily be detected by their tortuous structure, their milky, dense appearance, and by their larger diameter.

Pars Recta of the Proximal Tubule and Cortical Collecting Duct. Both structures are readily detected in the medullary rays of the cortex. The appearance (diameter, transparency, granularity) of the pars recta closely resembles that of the superficial proximal convoluted tubule. The cortical collecting duct, in contrast, is much smaller in diameter and somewhat more translucent, with a distinctly granular surface. Both segments can easily be separated from adjacent tissue.

Juxtaglomerular Apparatus. These can readily be dissected from an interlobular artery in the midcortex. Tubule tissue is removed to isolate a group of glomeruli branching from the same artery. Some of these are connected intact to the arterial tree and may contain the macula densa segment with parts of the ascending loop of Henle and distal convoluted tubule, as well as the beginning of the proximal convoluted tubule. Final separation begins with cutting by a microknife of an interlobular artery segment carrying one afferent arteriole with juxtaglomerular apparatus.

Cortical Thick Ascending Limb of Henle's Loop. This segment, to which an

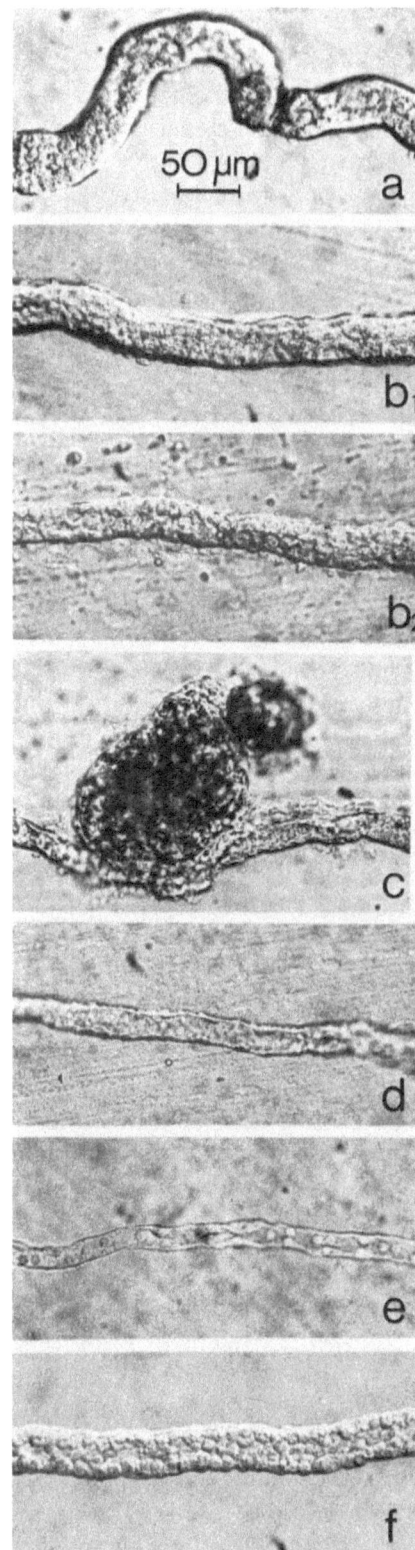

Figure 13. Characteristic microscopic appearance of rabbit nephron segments during *in vitro* dissection using transmission illumination. All segments are from the same kidney at identical magnification. For detailed description of the appearance see text. The segments are: (a) superficial proximal convoluted tubule; (b_1) pars recta; (b_2) cortical collecting duct; (c) glomerulus with macula densa segment; (d) cortical thick ascending loop of Henle; (e) medullary thick ascending loop of Henle; (f) medullary collecting duct.

active chloride transport has been attributed (Burg and Green, 1973), traverses the cortex along with the pars recta and the collecting duct in the medullary rays from the corticomedullary border to its glomerulus. The cortical ascending loop is characterized by its close association to the cortical collecting duct, by a diameter smaller than that of the collecting duct, and specifically by a transparent inner (luminal) line bordered by dense outer (basal) lines in the collapsed state. The cortical thick ascending loop is usually difficult to separate from the cortical collecting duct and attempts to do so may result in injuries although the continuity of the loop in the dissection chamber appears to be maintained. Therefore, small fragments of collecting duct or tissue from other loops are often left attached to the basement membrane of the thick ascending loop if the segment is perfused subsequently; these fragments, however, are meticulously cut off with a branch of the forceps before the segment is transferred for quantitative histochemistry.

Medullary Thick Ascending Limb of Henle's Loop. Dissection of medullary structures is begun by pulling strips of tissue longitudinally from the medulla. This simple step usually produces some loops and collecting ducts to spread between the tissue strips. Separation into outer and inner medullary segments, of course, is facilitated by the intense red color of the vascular bundles in the outer medulla during fresh dissection. The medullary thick ascending loop in the outer medulla is similar in appearance to the cortical thick ascending loop in that two dense outer lines border a transparent inner line when the tubule is collapsed. The diameter is somewhat larger than that of the cortical thick ascending loop, but it is still much smaller than that of the medullary collecting duct. In general, separation of the medullary thick ascending loop from adjacent tubule structures is easier than in the cortical thick ascending loop. However, medullary loops adjacent to vascular structures appear to come off more readily than those next to collecting ducts.

Medullary Collecting Duct. Extensive branching of this segment occurs in the inner medulla; dissection, therefore, of long segments is easier in the outer parts of the medulla. The granularity and the large diameter distinguish the collecting duct from other medullary tubule segments.

Thin Segments of the Loop of Henle. These segments have been successfully dissected from fresh rabbit renal slices and perfused *in vitro* (Kokko, 1970). For determination of Na–K-ATPase, these segments, similar to the pars recta, are not particularly promising in view of their low enzyme activities.

Several observations, not specific to any tubule segment, during renal tubule microdissection may be useful to report. At times, most of the proximal convoluted tubules appear to be milky-dense in the dissection chamber, and soon after the onset of dissection a layer of small cellular fragments covers the bottom of the petri dish. From such a kidney long and intact portions of any tubule segment have rarely been harvested, and the decision to discard the preparation should be made early in the course of the dissection. A good preparation, on the other hand, is defined by the ease of segment separation from adjacent tissue and by a certain transparency of all superficial-type proximal tubules. These optimal conditions are found more often in neonatal and young than in mature animals. Occasionally, loop of Henle segments and collecting ducts, in particular, will stick to the dissection forceps. Although addition of protein (5 g/100 ml) to the medium may solve this problem, a careful cleaning of small tubule fragments from the forceps during dissection also prevents this complication.

The time required for complete isolation of a segment long enough for enzymatic and perfusion analysis, of course, varies with experience and duration of training. In a good preparation it takes no more than 5 min to dissect a complete segment, except for the juxtaglomerular apparatus which requires about 15 min for complete isolation.

3. Transfer of Single Dissected Segments for Lyophilization

Before transfer, the length of each dissected segment is measured in a calibrated ocular micrometer. Obviously, this measurement is somewhat arbitrary for extensively convoluted proximal tubules. The segment to be transferred for enzyme analysis is put aside in the cooled and oxygenized dissection chamber until a reasonable number of similar segments has been collected. Glass slides (2.5 × 1.0 cm) have been prepared from a large slide, numbered with a glazier's diamond, and cleaned in acid, water, and acetone solutions. Immediately before transfer, a drop of 1 μl volume of bidistilled water is pipetted onto the flat glass slide. The slide is moved under the dissection microscope and a defined tubule segment is transferred directly into the water drop without intermediate washing. For transfer, only a forceps is used to hold a tubule end. Some fluid as well is transported between the branches of the forceps into the drop. This fluid, however, facilitates the release of the tubule into the water drop. The tubule drifts for some seconds through the water drop and usually settles firmly on the glass slide surface. Most segments, except for proximal convoluted tubules, settle in a straight configuration. Some need to be stretched out using a second forceps. In all tubules, the appearance after settling on the surface of the glass slide is identical to that in the dissection chamber. One segment only is transferred into a drop of water; two samples are put on a glass slide.

The loaded glass slide is set on an aluminum block kept on dry ice in a styrofoam box. The tubule freezes instantaneously upon contact of the slide with the block. In this way, several glass slides are kept on dry ice while collecting enough slides to fill the lyophilization Pyrex vacuum tube. Before lyophilization is begun, the glass slides are inserted into an aluminum rack carrier holding about 20 to 30 slides. The carrier is placed into the Pyrex vacuum tube. Lyophilization as well as subsequent analytical steps are identical to those already described for freeze-dried tubule segments.

4. Processing Microdissected Rabbit Nephron Segments

After rewarming the glass vacuum containing the aluminum block in vacuum, the sample carrier is taken out and a glass slide containing two samples is brought under the stereomicroscope. The dried nephron segment is recogniz-

Table III. Dry Weight (ng) of Nephron Segments
Microdissected from Rabbit Kidney (1.5 kg body weight)
in Relation to Segment Length (100 μm)

Nephron segment	Nanograms per 100 μm of length
Subcapsular proximal convoluted tubule	30.4 ± 2.1
Juxtamedullary proximal convoluted tubule	36.7 ± 3.1
Medullary thick ascending loop of Henle	11.8 ± 1.2
Cortical thick ascending loop of Henle	10.4 ± 1.3
Cortical collecting duct	13.8 ± 1.8
Medullary collecting duct	30.2 ± 2.6

able within the salt. When the salt has been carefully removed from the surface of the nephron segment, the segment is picked up from the glass slide and transferred to the microdissection dish where the segment length is measured under the stereomicroscope. If the drying process was adequate, it is easy to remove the nephron segment from its carrier with a hair tip. The length of the lyophilized structure is smaller by about 35% in all structures when compared to the length of the freshly dissected structure.

Since Na–K-ATPase activity changes with the segment along the nephron, structures are cut into smaller pieces of 80–300 μm with a hand-made knife. Each of these pieces is transferred to the sample holder and weighed. Table III lists the dry weight of nephron segments from the rabbit kidney in relation to segment length.

C. Microchemical Analysis of Na–K-ATPase

When the inorganic phosphate (P_i) split from ATP during the ATPase reaction is measured directly with the molybdate reaction in a microcuvette of 40 μl final volume, a sensitivity in the range of nanomoles of P_i is achieved (Schmidt and Dubach, 1971a; Bonting et al., 1961). With this sensitivity, a dry weight of 1.8×10^{-7} g for glomeruli, 1.2×10^{-7} g for proximal, and 0.7×10^{-7} g for distal tubules is necessary for each analysis when the tissue mass is diluted in 5 μl reagent volume. As can be calculated from Table II, the direct P_i measurement requires that single microdissected nephron segments be pooled.

The pooled tissue is placed on the bottom of a dry microtest tube (40 mm in length and 3 mm inner diameter) using a manipulator under microscopic control. The microtest tube is held horizontally on a manipulator to which a needle of quartz glass is attached. After the tip of the needle is loaded with single nephron segments, the tube is moved so that the needle enters the tube. When the tip of the needle is just at the bottom of the tube, a slight push to the back of the needle will cause the tissue to jump onto the bottom of the tube.

During this transfer the stereomicroscope is used to check that the sample has not been lost. The loading procedure is performed under the same controlled temperature and humidity as the microdissection.

To each tube 5 μl of reagent are added and the tube is carefully covered with Parafilm before it is placed on a rack in an ice bath. During pipetting, the tip should be kept off the samples to prevent the sample from sticking to the pipet. The reagent delivery from the pipet should be gentle to avoid bubbles and blowing the samples. After this dilution step, the micro test tube should not be shaken.

The reagent for the total ATPase consists of:

Tris–HCl, pH 7.4	100 mM
ATP	2 mM
MgCl$_2$	2 mM
KCl	5 mM
NaCl	55 mM
EDTA	0.1 mM
Bovine serum albumin[2]	0.05 %

and for the ouabain-insensitive ATPase:

Tris–HCl, pH 7.4	100 mM
ATP	2 mM
MgCl$_2$	2 mM
NaCl	60 mM
EDTA	0.1 mM
Bovine serum albumin	0.05 %
Ouabain	2 mM

At zero time the rack is placed in a water bath at 37°C. After 15 min the rack is returned into ice water and to each tube 25 μl of 10% trichloric acid are added. After centrifugation at 12,000 rev/min for 10 min at 4°C, 25 μl of the supernatant fluid are transferred to a tube containing 25 μl color reagent. The color reagent is prepared just before use by dissolving 200 mg FeSO$_4$ in 2.5 ml of a 1% NH$_4$-molybdate solution in 1.15 N H$_2$SO$_4$. The color reagent is stable for only 2 hr.

Ten minutes after dilution, the resulting color is read at 700 nm in a microcuvette (containing a final volume of 45 μl) within a spectrophotometer.

Reagent blanks, tissue blanks, and standards (the standards are equivalent to 5, 25, and 75 $\times$ 10^{-9} mol of inorganic phosphate) are used in each experiment to express the optical density of the samples in moles of inorganic phosphate liberated per kilogram dry weight per hour (MKH units).

Generally, the range of the samples is from 4 to 30 $\times$ 10^{-9} mol of inorganic phosphate. Under these assay conditions, less than 12% (0.2 $\times$ 10^{-3} M, determined chromatographically) of the substrate (ATP) is split by *total* ATPase

---

[2] To maintain enzyme stability at high dilution, total protein content should not be below 0.02% in volumes down to 5 μl. Therefore, bovine serum albumin is added to all reagents used for microtests. A 1-μg dry tissue sample in a 10-μl volume constitutes a 0.005–0.01% protein solution (Lowry and Passonneau, 1972). In volumes smaller than 5 μl, the protein content should not be below 0.05 to 0.1%.

and 5% ($0.1 \times 10^{-3} M$) by ouabain-insensitive ATPase using a dry weight of 5.0 $\times 10^{-7}$ g in 10 min at 37°C.

The activity of Na–K-ATPase is calculated from the difference between total ATPase and ouabain-insensitive ATPase.

D. Ultramicrochemical Analysis of Na–K-ATPase

The sensitivity of the molybdate reaction is limited to the range of 10^{-9} mol P_i. For quantifying Na–K-ATPase in single microdissected tubules, this technique is not sensitive enough. One microdissected piece of the proximal tubule of 30 ng dry weight yields only 10 ng for total ATPase and 10 ng for ouabain-insensitive ATPase; distal tubule dry tissue yields even less for each ATPase. However, the sensitivity of the assay for inorganic phosphate quantification can be increased by introducing a technical and a chemical refinement, i.e., the oil-well technique (Lowry and Passonneau, 1972) and the enzymatic measurement of inorganic phosphate (Schulz *et al.*, 1967b) in combination with a chemical amplification system, the enzymatic cycling reaction (Schulz *et al.*, 1967a).

1. Enzymatic P_i Analysis

Three reactions are carried out in a single analytical step [see reaction sequence (2) in Figure 14]: (1) The liberated P_i from the ATPase reaction phosphorylizes glucose, which is separated from glycogen by phosphorylase a. (2) Glucose-1-phosphate formed is converted to glucose-6-phosphate by phosphoglucomutase. (3) Glucose-6-phosphate is thereafter oxidized to 6-phosphogluconate by glucose-6-phosphate dehydrogenase.

This reaction sequence yields NADPH. Since NADPH can be measured by enzymatic cycling (Schulz *et al.*, 1967a), the sensitivity is virtually unlimited.

The advantages of the enzymatic P_i analysis are (a) the high specificity, (b) the enzymatic reactions at neutral pH, and (c) an unlimited sensitivity which can easily be carried to a 10^{-13} mol P_i level with the cycling step.

2. Enzymatic Cycling

The pyridine nucleotides NADP/NADPH and NAD/NADH have become essential components of nearly every micromethod because of their unique properties (Lowry and Passonneau, 1972). (1) They serve as oxidizing and reducing agents in a wide variety of specific enzyme reactions. Therefore, innumerable compounds can be selectively oxidized or reduced with the appropriate enzyme as catalyst. (2) The reduced forms of the pyridine nucleotide are fluorescent, whereas the oxidized forms are not measurable directly but can be converted to a highly fluorescent form in strong alkali. The oxidized and reduced forms of the pyridine nucleotide can be measured at concentrations down to $10^{-8} M$. (3) The reduced forms can be completely destroyed in acid without any effect on the oxidized forms; conversely, the oxidized forms are destroyed in alkali with no effect on the reduced forms. Thus, at the end of a

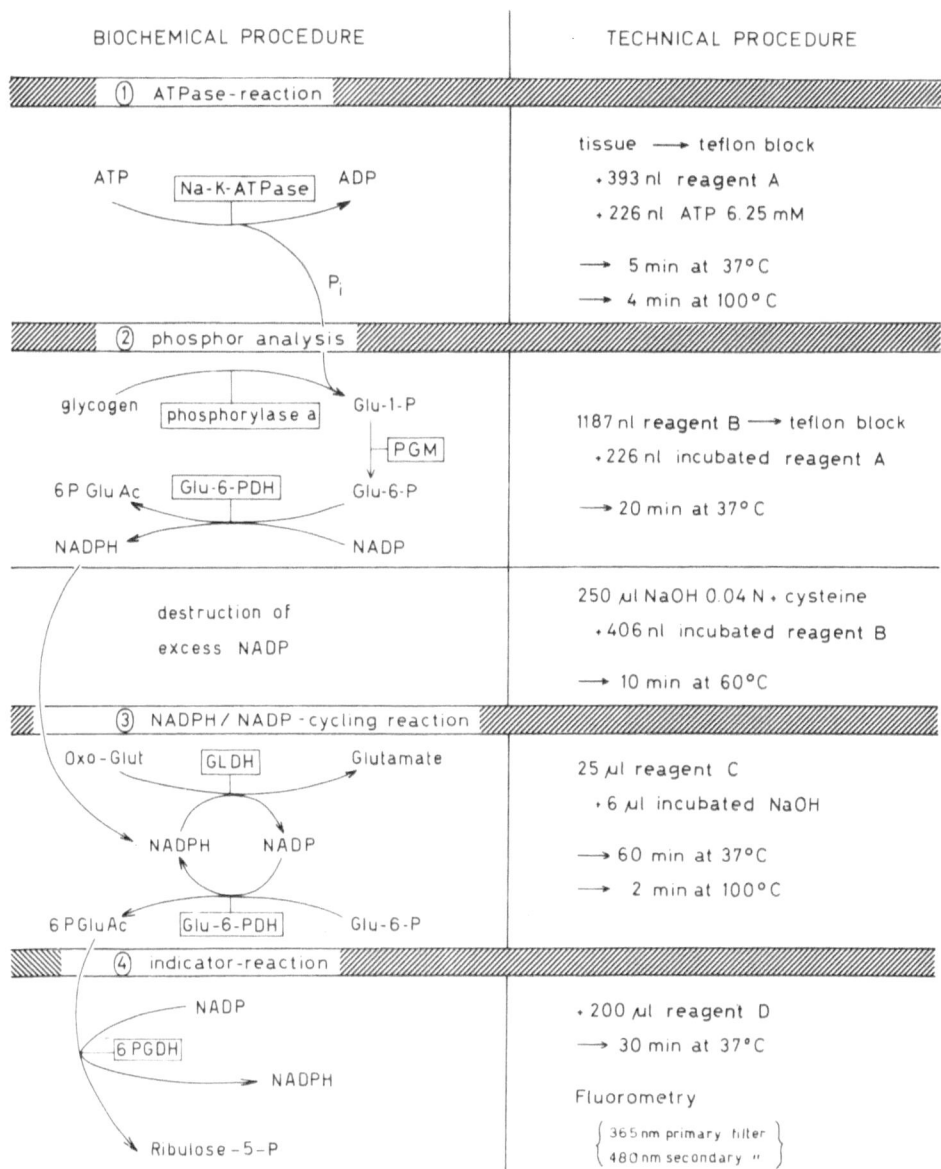

Figure 14. Survey of the ATPase analysis on the ultramicrochemical scale. For detailed explanations see text.

reaction the excess pyridine nucleotide of the reagent can be eliminated, leaving that fraction intact which has to be measured. (4) To further increase the sensitivity up to 10^{-12} M, the pyridine nucleotides in low concentrations, e.g., 10^{-15} mol of NADPH, are used as catalysts in an enzymatic cycling reaction between two enzyme systems [see step (3) in Figure 14]. In a first step, oxoglutarate is converted to glutamate by glutamate dehydrogenase whereby NADPH is oxidized to NADP; in a second step, glucose-6-phosphate is oxidized to 6-phosphogluconate by glucose-6-phosphate dehydrogenase whereby the oxidized form NADP serves as coenzyme and is reduced to NADPH. The NADPH from the second step is the catalyst for the first step.

With excess of glutamate dehydrogenase, glucose-6-phosphate dehydrogenase, and the substrates oxoglutarate and glucose-6-phosphate, for one molecule of pyridine nucleotide present there are 20,000 molecules of 6-phosphogluconate and glutamate formed in 1 hr at 37°C. Glutamate or 6-phosphogluconate is then measured as indicator in a final reaction [see step (4) in Figure 14].

3. Oil-Well Technique

In order to further increase the sensitivity of the enzymatic P_i analysis, the first two steps in Figure 14 are carried out in very small volumes of less than 1 μl which are kept under a droplet of oil to prevent evaporation. The pipetting of volumes in the nanoliter range is done in holes which are drilled in a block of Teflon. Teflon is a hydrophobic and chemically inert material which can be heated up to 100°C and cooled to 4°C easily; in each case the ambient temperature is reached within 10 min. The cleaning of the Teflon block is done the following way: the oil is removed with chloroform and the Teflon is boiled for 10 min in 1 N NaOH. After the Teflon is rinsed with tapwater and deionized water, it is dried in an oven at 100°C. The cleaned rack is wrapped in aluminum foil and stored.

The size of the rack and of the wells can be varied as required. Volumes from 100 nl to 1 μl can be pipetted in a Teflon rack of 80 × 50 × 5 mm, containing 40 holes of 8 mm surface diameter; the walls of the holes are tapered off to the bottom. Volumes less than 100 nl are put into Teflon racks of 60 × 25 mm with 30 holes of 3 mm surface diameter.

The Teflon rack can be heated either in an oven or on a copper bench covered with aluminum foil which is placed in a closed water bath. (The foil protects the rack from any condensation of water.) For cooling, it is put on a copper box filled with crushed ice positioned in an ice bath.

It is also possible to heat the rack up to 100°C; this should be done for 3 min only since otherwise the convection currents bring the droplets to the surface, where they will evaporate. To stop an enzymatic reaction, it is convenient to heat the rack to 80°C, which can be done for at least 20 min without loss of sample volume.

The oil for this special technique must have an appropriate viscosity to prevent any CO_2 adsorption from the air and to permit the droplet to fall on the bottom of the well when delivered from the pipet. Commercial paraffin oil

(Merck) has been found to be satisfactory; in can be used without further cleaning or dilution with hexadecane (Lowry and Passonneau, 1972).

The pipets for the oil-well technique are simple tubes of Pyrex glass with an inner diameter of a few micrometers and a corresponding length of one or two centimeters. They are built the following way: a 10-cm piece is cut from a Pyrex glass tube of 3 mm inner diameter and held with slow rotation into the flame of an oxygen burner. As soon as the glass turns red, it is removed from the flame and quickly pulled out with moderate force. When the glass tube has been cooled, the ends are separated. The inner diameter of the tube is measured under a stereomicroscope and the tube is cut to an appropriate length determined by

$$L = V/r^2$$

where L is the length, V is the desired volume, and r is the inner diameter. The pipet is mounted in a pencil-shaped glass tube, centered carefully, and its opening is slightly reduced in the flame. This last step prevents a rapid delivery, which produces bubbles that destroy the sample. The pipet is filled by adhesive forces only, which ensures reproducible volumes. After every pipetting procedure, the pipet is cleaned with chloroform, 1 N NaOH, bidistilled water (3 times) and finally with acetone.

The pipet is calibrated fluorometrically with a quinine hydrobromide solution. The oil-well technique is performed under a stereomicroscope with a

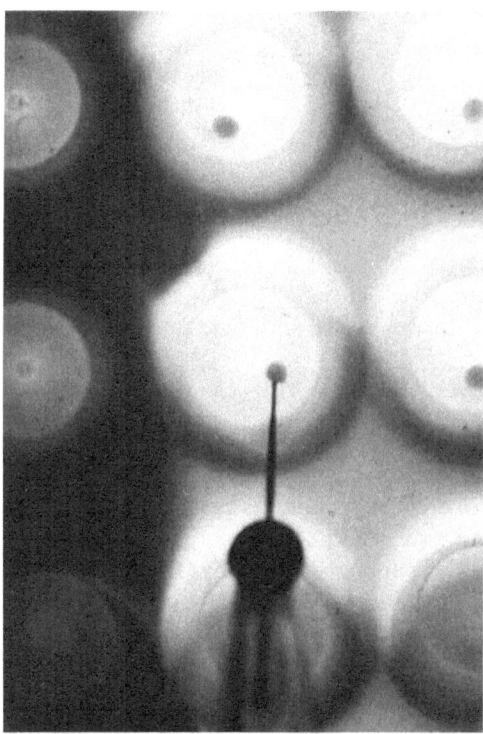

Figure 15. Illustration of the oil-well technique carried out under a stereomicroscope (25×).

magnification of 25×. A long focal distance is achieved when the microscope is mounted on a stand extending over the Teflon surface.

The rack is illuminated from above (Figure 15). Using an initial volume of more than 100 nl, the mixing of the samples with the reagent is performed the following way: The rack is placed under the stereomicroscope; the sample holder is brought close to the rack so that the well and the samples can be controlled simultaneously with the microscope. First, the volume of the initial step is placed on the wall of the well. Second, a freeze-dried sample is picked up from the sample holder with a hair tip and brought into the liquid. Third, the loaded reagent is covered with two droplets of paraffin oil.

4. Special Procedure for Na–K-ATPase (Schmidt and Dubach, 1971c)

As cited above, Na–K-ATPase is calculated by subtracting the activity of the ouabain-insensitive ATPase from the total ATPase. For measuring Na–K-ATPase in one dissected tubule segment, it is useful to divide the sample into two halves: one for the total ATPase and the other one for ouabain-insensitive ATPase.

The initial step whereby the samples and reagent are brought together occurs in the same room where the dissection and weighing was performed.

In each well 400 nl of reagent A (Figure 14) are pipetted, containing for total ATPase:

Tris–HCl, pH 7.4	100 mM
NaCl	55 mM
KCl	5 mM
MgCl$_2$	2 mM
EDTA	0.1 mM
Bovine serum albumin	0.1 %

and for ouabain-insensitive ATPase:

Tris–HCl, pH 7.4	100 mM
NaCl	60 mM
MgCl$_2$	2 mM
EDTA	0.1 mM
Ouabain	2 mM
Bovine serum albumin	0.1 %

Thereafter, a sample is picked up from the sample holder, put into the fluid, and covered as quickly as possible with two droplets of oil. The next well is loaded the same way.

As soon as the rack is filled, it is placed on a copper box filled with crushed ice, positioned in an ice bath, and cooled. Ten minutes later, 200 nl of ATP disodium salt (6.25 mM) are added: the filled 200-nl pipet is pushed through the oil and the contents delivered slowly into reagent A. Before delivery, the pipet has been checked outside the reagent to see whether it contains the total 200-nl volume.

In the next step, the rack is put in a covered water bath at 37°C for 12 min of incubation (the true incubation time of the samples will be 10 min). The reaction is stopped by heating the rack for 20 min at 80°C in an oven.

In the meantime, a second Teflon rack is loaded with 1 μl of reagent B (Figure 14) containing:

Imidazole–HCl, pH 6.9	50 mM
Glycogen[3]	0.08 %
NADP	0.03 mM
5'-AMP	0.01 mM
EDTA	1 mM
MgCl$_2$	0.5 mM
Glucose-6-phosphate dehydrogenase[4]	1 μg/ml
Phosphoglucomutase	3 μg/ml
Glycogen phosphorylase[5]	35 μg/ml
Bovine serum albumin	0.05 %

Two hundred nanoliters of reagent A are pipetted into reagent B. The reagent B is then incubated at 37°C for 30–60 min. The duration of this incubation depends on how quickly reagent B recovers a certain amount of inorganic phosphate ($10^{-9} M$ P$_i$).

Reagent B is tested before use within a photometer cuvette the following way: 500 μl of reagent B are kept at 37°C. There are some modifications in the composition of reagent B: phosphorylase a is increased to 100 μg, glucose-6-phosphate dehydrogenase to 3 μg, and phosphoglucomutase to 10 μg; the concentration of NADP is 100 μM. Eight nanomoles of inorganic phosphate are added and the extinction is recorded.

Thereafter, 400 nl of incubated reagent B are added to 250 μl of 0.04 N NaOH and incubated for 10 min at 60°C to destroy excess NADP. Then, 6 μl of

---

[3] Glycogen (rabbit liver, Sigma) is prepared in an 0.8% solution (80 mg glycogen to 10 ml 0.02 N NaOH) and incubated 10 min at 60°C for aggregation. The glycogen solution is stable for 1 month. If the solution becomes opaque, the incubation procedure should be repeated.

[4] The stock glucose-6-phosphate dehydrogenase and phosphoglucomutase suspensions in (NH$_4$)$_2$SO$_4$ are centrifuged, and the supernatant fluids removed. The phosphoglucomutase and glucose-6-phosphate dehydrogenase are washed 3 times with 2 volumes of (NH$_4$)$_2$SO$_4$ of the same concentration as the original solution. Each enzyme is finally suspended in the original volume of (NH$_4$)$_2$SO$_4$.

[5] In every analysis the activity of phosphorylase a should be tested. Sometimes an activation of phosphorylase a becomes necessary: 2.8 mg of crystalline rabbit muscle phosphorylase a is centrifuged 3 times in 1 ml of an imidazole–HCl buffer of pH 6.9 in a 50 mM concentration. The washed enzyme is then dissolved in 1 ml of:

Imidazole–HCl, pH. 6.9	50 mM
Dithiothreitol	0.5 mM
5'-AMP	0.1 mM
EDTA	1 mM
Bovine serum albumin	0.02 %

and the enzyme preparation is incubated for 60 min at 37°C in a water bath and stored at 4°C. The activated phosphorylase a is stable for 1 week.

the incubated NaOH are pipetted into 25 μl cycling reagent (reagent C in Figure 14) containing:

Tris–HCl, pH 8.0	100 mM
Oxoglutarate	5 mM
Glucose-6-phosphate	1 mM
Ammonium acetate	20 mM
5'-ADP	300 mM
Glutamate dehydrogenase	150 μg/ml
Glucose-6-phosphate dehydrogenase	35 μg/ml
Bovine serum albumin	0.02 %

Reagent C without enzymes can be stored indefinitely at $-80°C$. At $-20°C$, there is some loss of oxoglutarate within 2 weeks (Lowry and Passonneau, 1972). The enzymes are added only before use and reagent C is kept at $0°C$. The glucose-6-phosphate dehydrogenase is washed 3 times in an ammonium acetate solution of a concentration in which this enzyme is usually kept.

After an incubation time of 60 min at $37°C$, the cycling reaction is stopped by boiling for 2 min.

In a last step, the formed 6-phosphogluconate is determined by adding 200 μl of indicator reagent (reagent D in Figure 14), containing:

Tris–HCl, pH 8.0	20 mM
EDTA	100 μM
Ammonium acetate	60 mM
MgCl$_2$	3 μM
NADP	100 μM
6-Phosphogluconate dehydrogenase	1 μg/ml
Serum bovine albumin	0.05 %

After an incubation time of 30 min at $37°C$, the volume is pipetted into a fluorometer tube and the reading is made with an excitation at 365 nm and an emission at 480 nm. Blanks and phosphate standards (5, 10, 15×10^{-12} mol P$_i$) are measured throughout the whole procedure.

The enzyme activity is expressed in moles of inorganic phosphate liberated per kilogram dry weight of tissue per hour at $37°C$ (MKH units).

5. Methodological Considerations

ATP Hydrolysis and Time of Incubation. Figure 16 shows the liberation of P$_i$ versus time in microdissected segments of the proximal convoluted tubule: linearity exists up to 30 min of incubation at $37°C$. Nevertheless, for the ATPase reaction, an incubation time of 5 min is sufficient. It is interesting that during the incubation time of 5 or 10 min the tubule segment remains visible within the reagent. This observation is in contrast to earlier assumptions according to which the freeze-dried tissue was believed to disintegrate rapidly when transferred into an aqueous phase.

Substrate Optimum. During an incubation time of 5 or 10 min, 3–14% of the

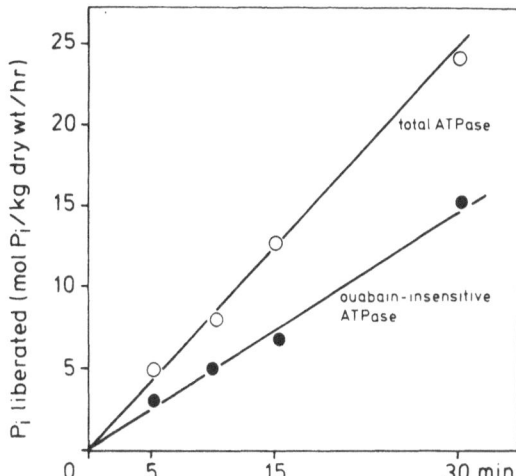

Figure 16. Time course of release of inorganic phosphate by the proximal convoluted tubule in the presence and absence of 2 mM ouabain, 55 mM Na, 5 mM K, 2 mM Mg, and 2 mM ATP (mean values from three experiments). ○, complete assay; ●, 2 mM ouabain added and K omitted.

excess ATP is hydrolyzed, depending on the tubule segment and amount of dry weight; i.e., the ATP concentration decreases from 2.2 mM to 1.8 mM maximally. Thus, an optimal substrate concentration is maintained throughout the reaction time. Kinetic studies have shown that an optimal velocity of the ATPase reaction is achieved when 2 mM ATP is added to the reagent, independent of whether 1 or 2 mM Mg is used (Schmidt and Dubach, 1971b; Schmidt and Habicht, 1976). This substrate concentration of 2 mM ATP is lower than the ATP concentration of 3–6 mM ATP which has been used by almost all investigators working with a purified Na–K-ATPase preparation (Skou 1965, 1975; Epstein, 1973). The ATP content of the tubular epithelial cell is probably not more than 2 mM *in vivo* (Urbaitis and Kessler, 1969; Kessler, 1970; Cohen and Barac-Nieto, 1973). Therefore, no more than 2 mM ATP are put into the ATPase reagent. Kinetic experiments in our laboratory have shown that this substrate concentration is also convenient for human and rabbit kidney ATPase.

Influence of Deoxycholate. As discussed in the introductory section, Na–K-ATPase activity is manifest only in part in membrane preparations from mammalian tissues. A substantial (sixfold) increase in activity can be observed after incubation with detergents like deoxycholate (Skou, 1965). Almost all investigators working with a membrane preparation, therefore, use deoxycholate in a millimolar concentration for unmasking the catalytic sites of the Na–K-ATPase.

In freeze-dried renal tissue, in contrast, deoxycholate in a concentration of 0.6 mg/ml increases Na–K-ATPase activity only slightly (Figure 17).

Sodium and Potassium. Many kinetic studies with a purified enzyme preparation revealed that sodium and potassium concentrations of 120 mM and 20–30 mM are necessary for optimal activation. In our assay conditions, the maximal activity of Na–K-ATPase occurs with 40–50 mM sodium (K_m 8 mM). Higher concentrations of sodium (above 120 mM) become inhibitory (Schmidt and Dubach, 1971b; Schmidt and Habicht, 1976). Increasing the potassium

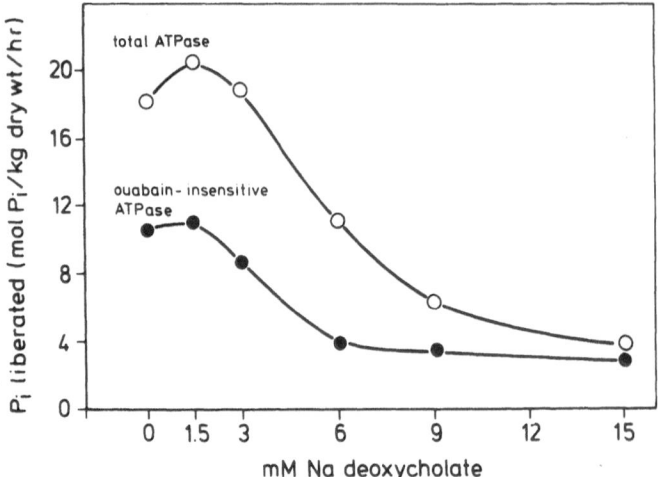

Figure 17. Effect of an increasing deoxycholate concentration on the release of inorganic phosphate by rat renal total ATPase and ouabain-insensitive ATPase at 20°C. Lyophilized homogenate corresponding to 400 ng dry weight was incubated in 1 ml with the indicated concentrations of deoxycholate, 2 mM EDTA, and 50 mM imidazole–HCl, pH 6.9, for 30 min. Five-microliter aliquots were transferred to test tubes (100 μl) containing the reagent for total ATPase and for ouabain-insensitive ATPase. The substrate concentration was 2 mM ATP (Na-salt).

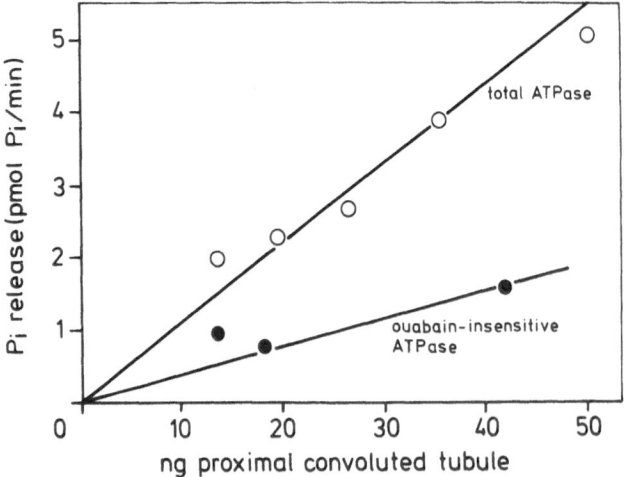

Figure 18. The rate of ATP hydrolysis in relation to the amount of proximal tubule dry weight. Each symbol represents one microdissected segment. The assay conditions are described in the text.

concentration to 3–5 mM (K_m 0.6 mM) results in a progressive increase in Na–K-ATPase activity; beyond this range a significant decrease in activity is observed when more than 30 mM potassium is present in the assay. In the living cell it seems that on the sodium site of the enzyme no more than 30 mM sodium is active and on the potassium site no more than 5 mM potassium. In our assay system (with freeze-dried renal tissue) with a sodium to potassium ratio of 50:5, the order of magnitude for Na–K-ATPase activity is as high as with a sodium to potassium ratio of 120:30. We prefer, however, cation concentrations closer to those occurring *in vivo*.

ATP Hydrolysis and Amount of Dry Tissue. Figure 18 reveals that the rate of inorganic phosphate formation is linear with respect to the amount of dry tissue in the range of 5–50 ng. This linearity is observed with segments of the proximal and distal tubule in the presence and absence of ouabain. The values for P_i at 13 ng in Figure 18 are above the regression lines. The reason for this observation is the amount of inorganic phosphate in the tubular segment without any ATPase reaction. In the proximal convoluted tubule, 1.2 pmol of P_i per 20 ng dry weight are measured. The ATPase activity, however, amounts to 13.4 pmol of P_i per 20 ng dry weight per 5 min incubation time at 37°C. Thus, about 10% of the liberated P_i is not formed by the ATPase reaction. For the segments of the distal tubule, a phosphate concentration of 0.3 pmol of P_i per 10 ng dry weight and a P_i liberation by the ATPase of 11 pmol per 10 ng dry weight per 5

Table IV. Na–K-ATPase activity (mol P_i/kg dry wt/hr) in Microdissected Segments of the Human, Rat, and Rabbit Nephron

Nephron segment[a]	Human	Rat	Rabbit A	Rabbit B
G_{SN}	0.02[b]	0.8	0	0
PCT_{SN}	2.1	1.8	2.4	3.3
PST_{SN}	0.2[b]	0.3[b]	c	c
G_{JM}	0.6[b]	0.6[b]	c	c
PCT_{JM}	4.1	3.8	4.47	6.32
PST_{JM}	0.3[b]	0.8[b]	0.6[b]	1.1
CTAL	5.6	6.7	6.6	12.10
MTAL	17.3	15.2	19.00	26.07
CCD	4.3	6.2	7.2	8.2
MCD	1.4	2.0	2.1	3.0

[a] Abbreviations: G, glomerulus; PCT, proximal convoluted tubule; PST, proximal straight tubule; CTAL, cortical thick ascending loop of Henle; MTAL, medullary thick ascending loop of Henle; CCD, cortical collecting duct; MCD, medullary collecting duct.
[b] Not significant.
[c] Not detectable in the total microdissected sample; A is from freeze-dried section, B from fresh section.

min are measured; 2% of inorganic phosphate is therefore not derived from ATP hydrolysis by the enzyme.

The small amount of tissue phosphate can be neglected in the calculation of Na–K-ATPase because its activity is derived from the difference between total ATPase and ouabain-insensitive ATPase.

The high sensitivity of Na–K-ATPase measurements which is achieved with the oil-well technique in combination with the enzymatic inorganic phosphate analysis allows measurement of this enzyme in one dissected segment of the proximal or distal tubule. For the proximal convoluted tubule, the minimal dry weight for ATPase determination is 20 ng; the segment is divided into two halves, one half of 10 ng serves for measuring total ATPase, the other half for ouabain-insensitive ATPase. For the distal tubule, a minimal dry weight of 10 ng is necessary: 5 ng for total ATPase and 5 ng for ouabain-insensitive ATPase.

Na–K-ATPase Profile Along the Nephron. Table IV lists the Na–K-ATPase activities in the different well-defined segments of the nephron from human, rat, and rabbit kidney. It can be recognized that each segment is clearly distinguished from the adjacent segment by its characteristic order of magnitude in enzyme activity. The Na–K-ATPase assay at the ultramicro level has the advantage that the microdissected tubular structures are transferred directly into the reagent without any disintegration throughout the incubation time. This may be the reason why the Na–K-ATPase works optimally in a reagent containing substrate and effectors (sodium, potassium) in concentrations similar to the living cell. The measured activity can also be related to tubule length; the single segment microassay, therefore, is a prerequisite for relating metabolic data to transport rates on the level of a nephron unit.

REFERENCES

Banerjee, S. P., Dwosh, I. L., Khanna, V. K., and Sen, A. K. 1970. Solubilization of guinea pig kidney Na^+, K^+-activated ATPase with Lubrol W and Triton x-100. *Biochim. Biophys. Acta,* *211:*345.

Bonting, S. L., Simon, K. A., and Hawkins, N. M. 1961. Studies on sodium-activated adenosine triphosphatase: I. Quantitative distribution in several tissues of the cat. *Arch. Biochem. Biophys., 95:*416.

Burg, M., and Green, N. 1973. Function of the thick ascending limb of Henle's loop. *Am. J. Physiol., 224:*659.

Burg, M., Grantham, J., Abramow, M., and Orloff, J. 1966. Preparation and study of fragments of single rabbit nephrons. *Am. J. Physiol., 210:*1293.

Cohen, J. J., and Barac-Nieto, M. 1973. Renal metabolism of substrates in relation to renal function. In: *Renal Physiology*, pp. 909–1001. Ed. by Orloff, J. and Berliner, R. W. Williams & Wilkins, Baltimore, Md.

Dörge, A., Rick, R., Bauer, R., and Thurau, K. 1976. Evidence for a syncytial Na transport compartment in frog skin epithelium. *Pflügers Archiv., 362:*R14.

Epstein, F. H. 1973. Role of sodium-potassium-ATPase in sodium reabsorption by the kidney. In: *Modern Diuretic Therapy in the Treatment of Cardiovascular and Renal Disease*, pp. 188–195. Excerpta Medica, Amsterdam.

Horster, M., and Thurau, K. 1968. Micropuncture studies on the filtration rate of single superficial and juxtamedullary glomeruli in the rat kidney. *Pflügers Archiv., 301:*162.

Horster, M., and Larsson, L. 1976. Mechanisms of fluid absorption during proximal tubule development. *Kidney Int., 10:*348.

Horster, M., Burg, M., Potts, D., and Orloff, J. 1973. Fluid absorption by proximal tubules in the absence of a colloid osmotic gradient. *Kidney Int., 4:*6.

Jacobson, H. R., and Kokko, J. P. 1976. Intrinsic differences in various segments of the proximal convoluted tubule. *J. Clin. Invest., 57:*818.

Jørgensen, P. L. 1974. Purification of (Na$^+$ + K$^+$)-ATPase: Active site determinations and criteria of purity. *Ann. N.Y. Acad. Sci., 242:*36.

Jørgensen, P. L. 1975. Isolation and characterization of the components of the sodium pump. *Quart. Rev. Biophys., 7:*239.

Jørgensen, P. L., and Skou, J. C. 1971. Purification and characterization of (Na$^+$ + K$^+$)-ATPase. I. The influence of detergents on the activity of (Na$^+$ + K$^+$)-ATPase in preparations from the outer medulla of rabbit kidneys. *Biochem. Biophys. Acta, 233:*366.

Kessler, R. H. 1970. The effects of glucose and inhibitor compounds on renal nucleotides *in vivo.* In: *Proc. 4th Int. Congr. Nephrol.,* Stockholm 1969, Vol. 2, pp. 137–143. Karger, Basel/München/ New York.

Kokko, J. P. 1970. Sodium chloride and water transport in descending limb of Henle, *J. Clin. Invest., 49:*1838.

Kokko, J., Burg, M., and Orloff, J. 1971. Characteristics of NaCl and water transport in the renal proximal tubule. *J. Clin. Invest., 50:*69.

Kriz, W. 1967. Der architektonische und funktionelle Aufbau der Rattenniere. *Z. Zellforsch., 82:*495.

Kriz, W., and Koepsell, H. 1974. The structural organization of the mouse kidney. *Z. Anat. Entwickl.-Gesch., 144:*137.

Kriz, W., Schnermann, J., and Koepsell, H. 1972. The position of short and long loops of Henle in the rat kidney. *Z. Anat. Entwickl.-Gesch., 138:*301.

Larsson, L., and Horster, M. 1976. Ultrastructure and net fluid transport in isolated perfused developing proximal tubules. *J. Ultrastr. Res., 54:*276.

Lowry, O. H., and Passonneau, J. V. 1972. *A Flexible System of Enzyme Analysis.* Academic Press, New York and London.

Schmidt, U., and Dubach, U. C. 1969. Differential enzymatic behaviour of single proximal segments of the superficial and juxtamedullary nephron. I. Alkaline phosphatase and Na–K-ATPase. *Z. Ges. Exp. Med., 151:*93.

Schmidt, U., and Dubach, U. C. 1971a. Sensitivity of Na K adenosine triphosphatase activity in various structures of the rat nephron: studies with adrenalectomy. *Europ. J. Clin. Invest., 1:*307.

Schmidt, U., and Dubach, U. C. 1971b. Quantitative Histochemie am Nephron. In: *Progress Histochem. Cytochem.,* Vol. 2, p. 185, Gustav Fischer Verlag, Stuttgart and Portland.

Schmidt, U., and Dubach, U. C. 1971c. Na–K-stimulated adenosine-triphosphatase: intracellular localization within the proximal tubule of the rat nephron. *Pflügers Arch., 330:*265.

Schmidt, U., and Dubach, U. C. 1974. Induction of Na–K-ATPase in the proximal and distal convolute of the rat nephron after uninephrectomy. *Pflügers Archiv., 346:*39.

Schmidt, U., and Habicht, A. 1976. Localization and function of Na–K-ATPase activity in various structures of the nephron (A review). In: *Membranes and Disease,* pp. 311–329. Ed. by Bolis, L., Hoffman, J. F., and Leaf, A. Raven Press, New York.

Schmidt, U., and Horster, M. 1977. Sodium-potassium-activated ATPase. Activity maturation in rabbit nephron segments microdissected *in vitro, Am. J. Physiol. 233:*755.

Schmidt, U., Schmid, H., Funk, B., and Dubach, U. C. 1974. The function of Na,K-ATPase in single portions of the rat nephron, *Ann. N.Y. Acad. Sci., 242:*489.

Schmidt, U., Schmid, J., Schmid, H., and Dubach, U. C. 1975. Sodium- and potassium-activated ATPase. A possible target of aldosterone. *J. Clin. Invest., 55:*655.

Schulz, D. W., Passonneau, J. V., and Lowry, O. H. 1967a. The measurement of pyridine nucleotides by enzymatic cycling. *J. Biol. Chem., 236:*2746.

Schulz, D. W., Passonneau, J. V., and Lowry, O. H. 1967b. An enzymatic method for the measurement of inorganic phosphate. *Annal. Biochem., 19:*300.

Skou, J. C. 1965. Enzymatic basis for active transport of Na and K across cell membrane. *Physiol. Rev., 45:*596.

Skou, J. C. 1971. Sequence of steps in the Na–K-activated enzyme system in relation to sodium and potassium transport. *Curr. Top. Bioenerget., 4:*357.

Skou, J. C. 1975. The Na–K-activated enzyme system and its relationship to transport of sodium and potassium. *Quart. Rev. Biophys., 7:*401.

Somogyi, J., Budai, M., Nyiro, L., Kaluza, G. A., Nagel, W., and Willig, F. 1969. Activity and structural changes in Mg^{++}-dependent and Na^+–K^+-activated adenosine triphosphatase prepared from rat brain following detergent treatment. *Acta Biochem. Biophys. Acad. Sci. Hung., 4:*219.

Urbaitis, B. K., and Kessler, R. H. 1969. Concentration of adenine nucleotide compounds in renal cortex and medulla. *Nephron, 6:*217.

Chapter **11**

Methodology for Enzymatic Studies of Isolated Tubular Segments: Adenylate Cyclase

François Morel, Danièlle Chabardès, and
Martine Imbert-Teboul

Laboratoire de Physiologie Cellulaire
Collège de France
Paris, France

I. INTRODUCTION

Adenylate cyclase (AC) is an ubiquitous enzyme present in the plasma membrane of most cell types; it plays a key role in hormonal control of cell function. At the level of the cell membrane, adenylate cyclase is involved in the transduction of the extracellular signal provided by the hormone for the intracellular production of cyclic AMP. In the cell interior, cyclic AMP is responsible for inducing the appropriate biological response, and was accordingly named "the second hormonal messenger." The specificity of hormone recognition, by the corresponding target cells, results from the presence of stereospecific hormone receptor sites located on the outer border of cell membranes. These receptor sites are coupled to the AC catalytic units facing the cell interior, so that hormone binding to the receptor results in enzyme activation (Figure 1). The nature of the response induced by cAMP depends essentially on the type of the target cell, i.e., on its specific differentiation, and is not directly related to the structure of the stimulating hormone itself.

Adenylate-cyclase activity, as well as its responsiveness to specific hormone stimulations, may readily be measured *in vitro*. It is generally measured in terms of the rate of $[^{32}P]cAMP$ generated from $\alpha[^{32}P]ATP$ precursor. The hormone receptor units and the catalytic units are accessible only from their

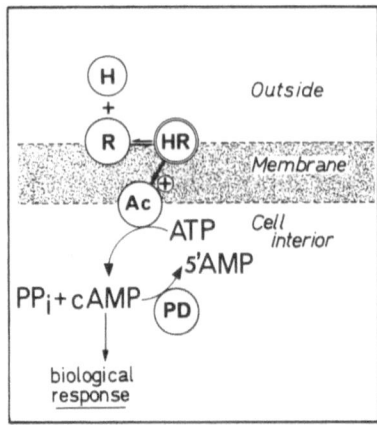

Figure 1. Schematic representation of the mechanism of hormone action via cyclic AMP generation. Within the membrane of the target cell for the hormone, the amplifying unit of the transducing system, i.e., adenylate-cyclase, converts ATP into cyclic AMP (cAMP) plus pyrophosphate (PP_i); cAMP, in turn, is responsible for inducing in the cell interior the response to the hormone input signal. H, hormone; R, receptor; Ac, adenylate-cyclase; PD, phosphodiesterase.

respective faces of the membrane. Since untouched cell membranes are normally impermeable to both nucleotides and polypeptidic hormones, AC activity measurements are generally performed by using either crude tissue homogenates, or membrane fractions prepared from such homogenates. In such conditions it is assumed that all cell membranes are disrupted or made permeable, and are therefore accessible to substrates from both sides.

It is now well established that homogenates prepared from kidney cortex and from kidney medulla contain adenylate cyclase which can be stimulated by different hormones, namely, vasopressin (Chase and Aurbach, 1968; Beck et al., 1971; Dousa et al., 1971; Forte, 1972; Neer, 1973), parathyroid hormone (PTH) (Chase and Aurbach, 1968; Melson et al., 1970; Beck et al., 1972; Kurokawa and Massry, 1973), calcitonin (Melson et al., 1970; Marx et al., 1972b; Marx and Aurbach, 1975), beta-adrenergic agonists (Melson et al., 1970; Marx et al., 1972a; Kurokawa and Massry, 1973; Bell, 1974), etc. This type of approach has been discussed by Dousa (1976) in Volume 4A of this series. It was observed that vasopressin-dependent AC is mainly located in kidney medulla, whereas PTH preferentially stimulated cortical AC; this observation demonstrates that the two hormones act at different sites along the kidney tubules (Chase and Aurbach, 1968). Homogenates form kidney medulla or cortex, however, are heterogeneous mixtures of membranes from all cell types present in the tissue, so that it is not possible to ascertain precise localization along the nephron for sites of hormone action by using such preparations. In order to overcome this major limitation, we developed a micromethod allowing AC measurements to be made on single pieces of kidney tubule, isolated by microdissection from collagenase-treated rabbit kidneys (Imbert et al., 1975a).

The detailed procedure used to prepare the samples and to measure their AC activity is described in this chapter. The results obtained are briefly summarized and the technique is discussed with respect to reliability, accuracy, reproducibility, as well as specificity and sensitivity to hormones.

II. NEPHRON MICRODISSECTION AND SEGMENT IDENTIFICATION

Single pieces of tubule can be microdissected directly from rabbit kidneys, as reported by Burg *et al.* (1966), but this is not easy or even possible from kidneys of other mammalian species. Burg *et al.* (1966) also reported that preincubation of the kidney tissue with collagenase must be avoided since it results in the lysis of peritubular basilar membranes. *In vitro* microperfusion of such tubules leads to the rupture of the wall. When enzyme activity measurements have to be performed in single tubules, disappearance of the basilar membrane is not *a priori* a problem. We have checked this point using homogenates of rat kidney medulla pretreated or not with collagenase and hyaluronidase. In comparing the responses of such homogenates to vasopressin, it appeared (Figure 2) that these enzymes induced no detectable damage to the AC system; indeed, both control and hormone-stimulated activities were actually enhanced to some extent. Similar observations were recently reported by Hanoune *et al.* using collagenase in other AC systems. In addition, the microdissection conditions of rabbit kidney are greatly improved if the tissue is preincubated in the presence of collagenase (see below): complete tubular structures can easily be isolated in large numbers. When using the conditions described here, three to four persons can routinely prepare in 1 day up to 200 samples, each containing a single, well-localized piece of tubule. Nearly all

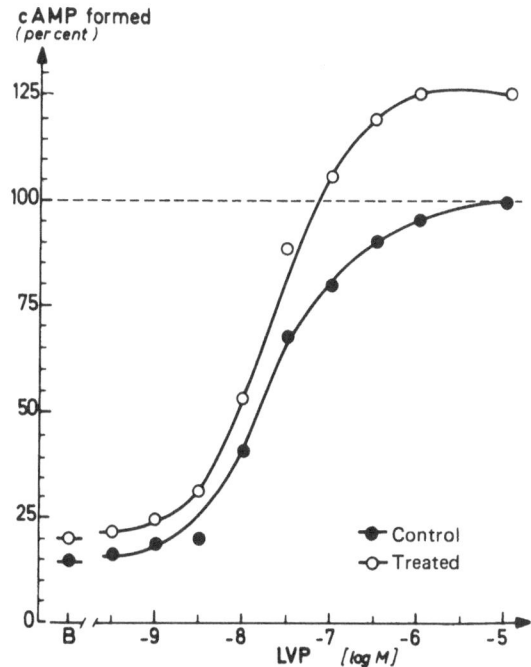

Figure 2. Effects of collagenase on vasopressin-dependent adenylate-cyclase in homogenates from rat kidney medula. A homogenate from rat kidney medulla was prepared and its AC activity measured as described by Rajerison *et al.* (1974). Preincubation in the presence (treated) or absence (control) of collagenase (0.1%) and hyaluronidase (0.1%) added into the medium. Abcissa: log of the lysine-vasopressin concentrations used. Ordinate: AC activity expressed as percent of the maximal stimulation obtained in the absence of added enzymes. Note that the collagenase enhanced to the same extent both control and vasopressin-dependent AC activities in this homogenate from rat kidney medulla.

segments from the nephron can be dissected from different zones of the rabbit kidney.

When applied to the rat kidney, this collagenase treatment allows microdissection of the tubular segments contained in the outer medulla (thin descending limb of the loop, thick portion of the ascending limb and medullary collecting tubules); the structures contained in the inner medulla are definitely more difficult to isolate from each other in the rat as well as in the rabbit. But microdissection of the rat cortex has, up to now, been completely unsuccessful in our laboratory. Various concentrations of collagenase, with or without hyaluronidase, have been checked at different temperatures and for different periods. The tubules were always found to disintegrate and no structure could be dissected, in sharp contrast to rabbit cortex where all segments of the nephron are generally easy to recognize and to separate.

The different portions of the rabbit nephron which can be localized and identified without ambiguity from simple stereomicroscopic observation of microdissected kidney tubules are depicted in a schematic way in Figure 3.

For proximal tubules, the initial part of the convoluted portion (PCT) is easy to recognize in those tubules which can be isolated with their glomerulus attached. Similarly, the terminal portion of the pars recta (PR) is easy to identify if it comes out of the outer medulla together with the thin descending limb attached. However, when pieces of proximal tubules with broken ends are isolated, no accurate localization along PCT is possible; such pieces should be used only with caution since, as will be discussed later, differences in AC activities exist between the convoluted and the straight portions of the proximal tubule (Chabardès *et al.*, 1975a).

As regards the thin segment of the loop, it is also important to separate the descending from the ascending limbs. When microdissected, however, these two portions are difficult to distinguish from each other by appearance only; but if they are isolated with either a pars recta or a thick ascending limb attached, then descending and ascending limbs are easily identified. If samples of thin descending limb from the inner medulla are required, a safe way to obtain them is to dissect very long descending portions starting with the pars recta. The tubules are then cut at a distance of about 1.5–2 mm from the end of the pars recta, the portion beyond the section site corresponding to the inner medulla.

The two end portions of the thick ascending limb, i.e., MAL and CAL, are easy to locate by the presence of either the thin ascending limb, or the macula densa. As in the case of the proximal tubules, when pieces of thick ascending limb are obtained with broken ends, they should be used only with caution, although the structure is easily recognized from its narrow diameter and typical appearance. Exact localization of the site where the samples are taken along the structure is needed since the hormone-dependent AC activity is different in MAL and CAL.

The so-called distal convoluted tubule (DCT), i.e., the nephron portion included between the macula densa and the first branching with another tubule, is probably the most heterogeneous segment of the rabbit nephron as regards morphological aspect under stereomicroscopic observation as well as AC

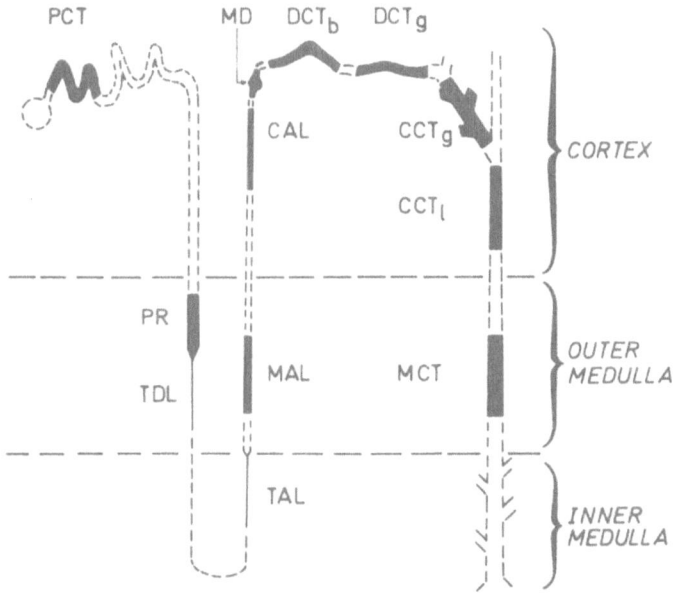

Figure 3. Segment location along microdissected rabbit nephron. This figure shows in a diagrammatic way a rabbit nephron, with the segments that can be easily located by microdissection indicated in black. PCT, proximal convoluted tubule (initial portion); PR, pars recta of the proximal tubule (terminal portion); TDL, thin descending limb of the loop of Henle (initial portion); TAL, thin ascending limb of the loop of Henle (terminal portion); MAL, medullary portion of the thick ascending limb of the loop; CAL, cortical portion of the thick ascending limb of the loop of Henle (terminal portion, located just before the macula densa); MD, macula densa; DCT, distal convoluted tubule, including (1) an inconstant DCTa portion resembling the CAL, but localized immediately beyond the macula densa; (2) a "bright" DCTb portion; (3) a "granulous" DCTg portion and (4) in a few instances, a terminal, light DCT1 portion. DCTa and DCT1 portions are not shown in this scheme. CCTg, granulous portion of the cortical collecting tubule; CCT1, light portion of the cortical collecting tubule; MCT, outer medullary portion of the collecting tubule. Note that the figure does not depict the relative length of the various segments.

activation by hormones (Morel *et al.*, 1976). Up to four different successive portions can be observed along some rabbit DCT; at least two distinct portions are always found (DCTb and DCTg, Figures 3 and 4); these portions are generally of short length (0.4 mm as an average value). Two photographic examples of DCT microdissected over their full length are shown in Figure 4.

The cortical collecting tubule (CCT), exhibits two distinct portions in the rabbit: these portions, which are likely to be of a different embryonic origin (Morel *et al.*, 1976), differ when observed under a microscope, the one being of "granular" appearance (CCTg), the other of "light" appearance (CCTl). We shall consider the differences in AC activities which were observed to be associated with such anatomical segmentation of the rabbit nephron later in this chapter. It is necessary first to describe in detail the procedure used to prepare the samples and to measure AC activities, and to discuss the reliability of the method.

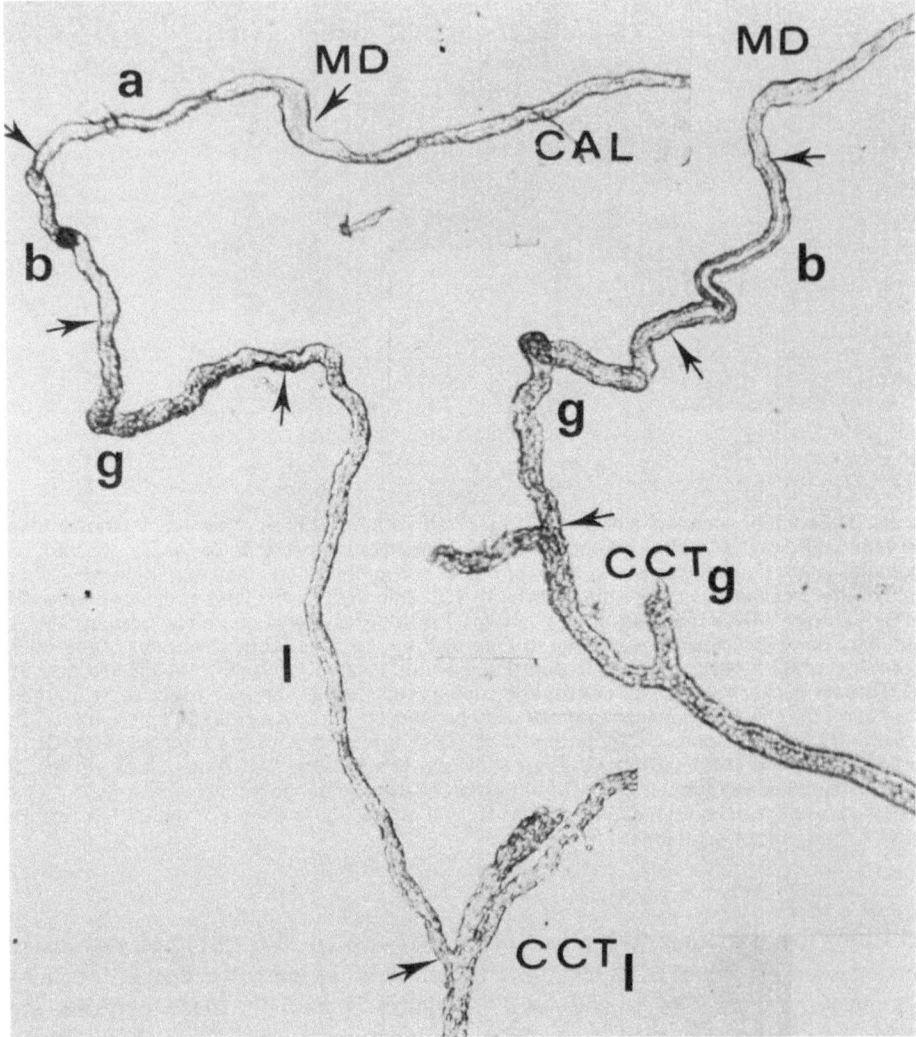

Figure 4. Segmentation of the rabbit distal convoluted tubule. Photographic picture of two rabbit distal tubules microdissected over their full length from the same rabbit kidney. Most rabbit DCT are short (about 1 mm) and include only a bright (b) and a granulous (g) portion, like the one shown in the right part of the figure. Many also include an initial (a) portion located just beyond the macula densa (MD) and resembling the cortical thick ascending limb (CAL). Finally, a few DCT are longer and end with a long and narrow "light" portion (DCTl). The second tubule shown on this figure represents an example of DCT including these four portions. The arrows indicate the limits between two successive portions. (For additional details, see Morel *et al.*, 1976.)

III. EXPERIMENTAL PROCEDURE

A. Preparation of Single Tubule Samples

New Zealand rabbits of about 1.5 kg body weight receive intravenously pentobarbital (Nembutal, about 40 mg/kg) and heparin (Liquemin, Roche). When anesthetized, the animals are bled from a section of the carotid artery, and the kidneys are quickly removed and immersed in ice-cold microdissection solution (see Section III-D for solution composition).

The renal artery is cannulated and the kidney perfused with about 10 ml chilled collagenase solution; when all the blood is drained, the renal vein is ligated, and an additional 10 ml collagenase solution is perfused until the (occasional) rupture of the kidney capsule. The kidney is then decapsulated and sliced parallel to the axis of the pyramid. The pieces of tissue are incubated in aerated collagenase solution for 35–45 min at 35°C. After two quick rinses, the pieces of tissue are transferred to petri dishes filled with ice-cold microdissection solution.

Microdissection is performed by hand with the help of thin steel needles under stereomicroscopic control. Large portions of nephron are isolated from the surrounding tissue, and the required segment(s) are cut over an appropriate length from each isolated structure, using the anatomical and morphological criteria described earlier. Each piece of tubule is then transferred together with a small volume of microdissection solution onto a sunken bacteriological glass slide. (In order to limit the area covered by the liquid over the glass, the slides are pretreated by liquid silicone and thereafter by putting, in the center, a drop (1 μl) of 0.05% bovine serum albumin (BSA) in distilled water, which is evaporated to dryness. The droplet of microdissection solution containing the sample of tubule is deposited onto this small disk of BSA.) Each sample is quickly photographed in order to determine the length of tubule used, by curvimeter measurement of a drawing made after constant magnification of the film. The glass slide is then tightly covered with another, Vaseline-coated glass slide, so as to maintain a watertight seal. The samples are stored at ice-cold temperature until use.

B. Pretreatment of the Samples

As already mentioned, cell membranes are only slightly permeable to polypeptide hormones and nucleotides. It is therefore necessary to make the tubule samples permeable to ATP, cAMP, and to the ATP regenerating system. It was found that a combination of two steps is necessary to fulfill this requirement—an osmotic shock plus a quick freezing.

When hypoosmotic solution was added to the samples, rapid swelling of proximal tubules was noted under stereomicroscopic observation, whereas swelling was limited or absent in the other portions of the nephron. In Figure 5, samples photographed before and after osmotic shock application are shown. The osmotic shock alone was not sufficient to ensure full permeabilization of all

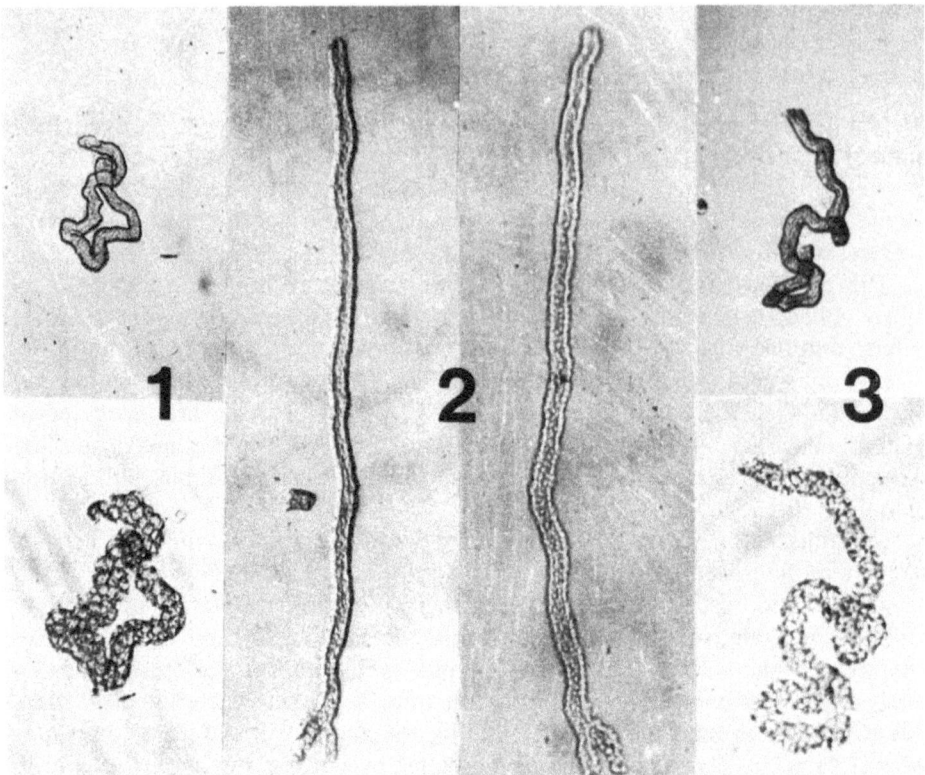

Figure 5. Effect of storage and osmotic shock on isolated microdissected tubules. (1) Microdissected rabbit proximal tubule (PCT) photographed just after microdissection and after 2 days of storage at 0°C in modified Hanks's solution. (2) Cortical collecting tubule (CCTI) of rabbit photographed before (left-side) and after (right side) applying osmotic shock as described in the text. (3) Microdissected proximal tubule (PCT) photographed before (upper part) and after (lower part) applying the osmotic shock. For each structure, the two photographs are presented at the same magnification. Length of the pieces of tubule before treatment: (1) 0.95 mm; (2) 1.43 mm; (3) 1.09 mm respectively. Note that both storage at low temperature and osmotic shock led to a large swelling in PCT. In contrast, swelling was much less pronounced in CCTI.

tubule segments. It is clear from the data of the experiment shown in Table I that AC activity measured in the presence of fluoride remained very low in certain segments, e.g., CAL and DCT, except when the samples were frozen for a short period in addition to osmotic shock application.

The permeabilization procedure is performed as follows: Excess microdissection solution contained in each sample is carefully aspirated under microscopic control by using thin glass tubing connected to a mouthpiece; 0.5 μl ice-cold hypoosmotic solution is then delivered to each sample. The hormone, where required, is present in the hypotonic medium at a concentration fivefold that necessary during the incubation period since addition of the incubation medium results in a fivefold dilution of the samples. After they are covered, the samples are kept at ice-cold temperature for about 30 min. Then each sample is

Table I. Effect of Sample Freezing on Adenylate-Cyclase Activity[a]

| Segment | cAMP formed (fmol/mm/30 min) | | p | Frozen/nonfrozen |
	Without freezing	With freezing		
PCT	393 ±54 (3)[b]	555 ±43 (3)[b]	Not significant	1.4
CAL	6 ±2 (2)	245 ±27 (3)	<0.01	40.0
DCT	34 ±1 (2)	1.045 ±16 (2)	<0.001	30.3
CCTl	146 ±19 (3)	380 ±19 (3)	<0.001	2.6

[a] In all samples. AC activity was measured in the presence of NaF, 5 mM. The way in which part of the samples were frozen is given in the text. PCT, proximal convoluted tubule; CAL, cortical portion of the thick ascending limb; DCT, distal convoluted tubule; CCTl, "light" portion of the cortical collecting tubule. An osmotic shock was applied to all samples; note that without freezing the AC activity was extremely low in CAL and DCT. (From Imbert *et al.*, 1975a.)
[b] Number of replicates in parentheses.

quickly and deeply frozen for a few seconds by putting the glass slide into contact with dry ice at the location of the sample droplet.

C. Incubation of the Samples

Incubation starts with the addition of 2 μl incubation solution to each sample. This is done by using a motor-driven Hamilton microsyringe. Mixing of the incubation solution with the hypotonic solution is ensured by flushing water-saturated chilled air over the surface of the droplet. Once tightly covered again, each sample is immersed into a water bath regulated at 30°C. Thirty minutes were chosen as the incubation time since AC activity was observed to increase almost linearly over 60 min under the conditions of these experiments as illustrated by Figure 6.

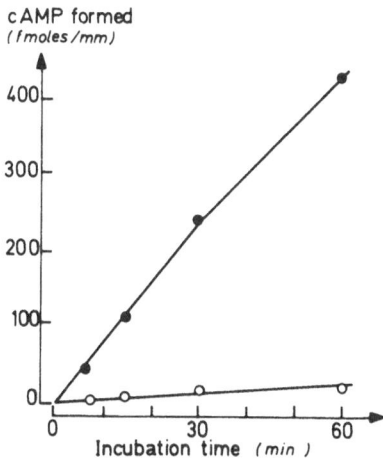

Figure 6. cAMP generation as a function of incubation time. Abscissa: incubation time at 30°C. Ordinate: amount of cAMP per millimeter of tubular length. All samples were cortical collecting tubules (CCTl) microdissected from the same rabbit kidney. Each point represents the mean value of two to four replicate samples. Open circles, AC activity measured without hormone added; filled circles, AC activity measured in the presence of arginine-vasopressin 10^{-6} M in the incubate. Other conditions as described in the text. (Redrawn from Imbert *et al.*, 1975a.) Note that the reaction was nearly linear throughout the 60-min period.

The incubation is terminated by adding 150 μl stopping solution to each sample; this solution contains a large excess of cold ATP and cAMP; the ATP specific radioactivity, therefore, abruptly drops by dilution and formation of [^{32}P]cAMP is stopped; on the other hand, the excess cAMP added prevents [^{32}P]cAMP from degrading into 5′-AMP by phosphodiesterase. The stopping solution also contains [^{3}H]cAMP as a tracer, so that, after extraction, the yield of cAMP recovery can be calculated for each sample. The mixture (2.5 μl incubate plus 150 μl stopping solution) is either delivered directly on the top of a dry aluminum oxide microcolumn if cAMP chemical extraction is performed in one step, or delivered into a glass tube containing 1 ml distilled water, if the two-step extraction procedure is used.

1. [^{32}P]cAMP Chemical Extraction

The ^{32}P-labeled cAMP formed during the incubation period has to be separated from the α[^{32}P]ATP precursor and from the other [^{32}P]nucleotides formed, before its radioactivity can be measured. This separation must be highly efficient, since the fraction of the ATP radioactivity converted into cAMP during the incubation period generally represents much less than one per thousand.

We have successfully used two different methods among those reported in the literature. Since we used these methods under nearly the same conditions as those described in details in the original papers, they are only briefly recalled here.

1. The first method allows the separation of cAMP from the other nucleotides in one step by using a dry aluminum oxide microcolumn, as reported by Ramachandran (1971) and described by Bockaert et al. (1972). Each column (a Pasteur pipet, 0.6 cm inside diameter, 15 cm in length) contains 1 g dry aluminum oxide; the incubation mixture is deposited on the top of the column, followed by twofold 1 ml of Tris–HCl buffer solution (50 mM, pH 7.6). The effluent is collected directly into plastic counting vials. Bray solution (8 ml) (Bray, 1960) is used as the scintillation medium. This method is very efficient and simple insofar as the [^{32}P]ATP used is of high radiochemical purity. Otherwise blank controls may have a relatively high value (compared with true background samples); since ^{32}P blank radioactivity has to be substracted from the overall ^{32}P counting of all samples, high blank values obviously decrease the sensitivity and the accuracy of the method; this is particularly true in the case of samples containing a short piece of tubule and when the AC activity is measured in the absence of hormonal stimulation (basal activity). The one-step method has another limitation. The yield of cAMP recovery may vary highly from one batch of aluminum oxide to another (for example, from 20 to 80%), so that several batches often must be checked before a good one is obtained.

2. The second method, the one we use now, has been described by Salomon et al. (1974) and includes two steps: the samples are first passed through a cation-exchange resin, i.e., AG^{R} 50 W-X8 Dowex columns 200–400 mesh, H^{+}. Each column consists of a glass tube, 0.7 cm inside diameter, 20 cm length, containing about 1 g dry Dowex. The column is washed with 2 or 3 ml

distilled water, and the corresponding effluent which contains more than 99% of the ^{32}P radioactivity is discarded. Four or 5 ml distilled water are again added to the columns and the effluents are directly collected on the second, alumina columns. The alumina columns are of the same size as the Dowex columns and contain 1 g dry neutral alumina (previously equilibrated by passing 8 ml imidazole–HCl 0.1 M solution, pH 7.5). This effluent is discarded as well as the effluent resulting from washing the column with 1 or 2 ml of the imidazole solution used for column equilibration.[1] The cAMP adsorbed on the column is then eluted by adding 4 ml of the same imidazole solution, and by collecting the effluent directly into counting vials containing 5 ml scintillation solution (Unisolve, Koch-Light Laboratories Ltd., Coinbrook, Bucks, England). The vials have to be thoroughly stirred and cooled for about 5 hr before radioactivity measurements.

D. Composition of the Solutions Used

Microdissection Solution. This is a modified Hanks (Hanks and Wallace, 1949) solution of the following composition: NaCl, 137 mM; KCl, 5 mM; Mg SO$_4$, 0.8 mM; Na$_2$HPO$_4$, 0.33 mM; KH$_2$PO$_4$, 0.44 mM; MgCl$_2$, 1 mM; Tris–HCl, 10 mM; CaCl$_2$, 0.25 mM; pH 7.4.

Collagenase Solution. This is of the same composition as the microdissection solution except that calcium concentration is 1 mM; it also contains 0.1% beef serum albumin and, for the rabbit, collagenase Sigma, type 1, added up to a final concentration of 0.1%. For the rat, we used 0.07% Worthington collagenase from *Clostridium histolyticum*, type CLS II, together with 0.1% hyaluronidase (Calbiochem, enzyme from bovine testis).

Hypoosmotic Solution. This solution always contains EDTA, 0.25 mM; MgCl$_2$, 1 mM; BSA, 0.1%; Tris–HCl, 1 mM; pH 7.4. When the effects of hormones or fluoride are to be tested, they are added to this solution up to a concentration fivefold that required in the final incubate, since the addition of the incubation solution to the samples results in a fivefold dilution of the hypoosmotic solution.

Incubation Solution. $\alpha[^{32}P]ATP$ (Saclay, France, or Nen, U.S.A.) of high specific activity is diluted with cold ATP up to a specific activity ranging between 1.5 and 2 Ci per mM; ATP concentration, 0.35 mM; 2 μl of incubation solution (the volume delivered to each sample) therefore contain about 1 μCi ^{32}P. Cold cAMP, 1.25 mM; EDTA, 0.325 mM; MgCl$_2$, 5 mM; phosphocreatine, 25 mM; creatine-kinase, 1.25 mg/ml; Tris–HCl, 125 mM; pH 7.4. Grade 1 reagents are used; ATP was purchased from Sigma (St. Louis, Mo.), cAMP, creatine-kinase, and creatine-phosphate were purchased from Boehringer (Mannheim). During the incubation period, the composition of the incubate corresponds to a 1.25-fold dilution of this incubation solution, since 2 μl were added to the 0.5 μl hypoosmotic solution contained in each sample.

---

[1] The exact volume of distilled water and imidazole solution to be used varies with the amount of Dowex and must be determined experimentally for each set of new columns. Both the Dowex and the alumina columns can be reused many times.

Stopping Solution. This contains: ATP, 3.3 mM; cAMP, 5 mM; [³H]cAMP as a tracer (about 30,000 CPM/ml); Tris–HCl, 50 mM; pH 7.6.

E. Calculation of the Results

Using either one of the two methods for cAMP separation, the following control and reference vials must be prepared and measured. Several blank samples (samples which contain no kidney tubule) are introduced all along the series of experimental samples; they are treated exactly as the other samples in any respect. Reference samples of stopping solution are prepared, in order to measure yields of [³H]cAMP recovery, and incubation solution samples of an appropriate dilution are prepared in order to determine α[³²P]ATP specific radioactivity. The ³H and ³²P radioactivities are measured in all vials under optimal discrimination conditions, and for at least two 10-min periods.

Under the experimental conditions reported in this paper, each sample contains about 1 μCi ³²P, i.e., 10^6 to 1.5 10^6 CPM, and a total amount of ATP equal to 0.7×10^6 fmol (namely, 2×10^{-6} liters, volume of incubation solution times $0.35 \times 10^{-3}M$, ATP concentration). This corresponds to about 1.5 to 2 CPM per femtomole ATP over blank sample radioactivity; this value is also the ³²P specific radioactivity of the cAMP formed during the incubation period. From this value and from the blank sample total radioactivity in the ³²P channel (25–30 CPM as a mean value), the sensitivity limits of the technique can be estimated. According to Poisson's law, and if all samples are counted for 20 min, such ³²P counting rates would allow 2 fmol cAMP per sample to be detected, 10 fmol to be measured with an average accuracy of about ±25%, and 100 fmol to be measured with an accuracy better than ±5%. By using the two-step extraction technique, the yield in cAMP recovery generally ranges between 60 and 70%.

The adenylate cyclase (AC) activity of the samples is expressed as femtomoles (i.e., 10^{-15} mol) cAMP formed per 30 min incubation time per millimeter tubular length; it may be calculated by using the formula

$$AC = (Q/L) \times {}^{32}P[(x - B_1)/R_i]/{}^3H(x/R_s)$$

where Q is the total amount of ATP per sample (femtomoles); L is length of the piece of tubule (mm); ³²P is total ³²P radioactivity counted in the unknown sample (x), the blank samples (B_1) and 2 μl incubation solution (R_i) respectively; and ³H is total ³H radioactivity counted in the unknown sample (x) and 150 μl stopping solution (R_s) respectively.

IV. DISCUSSION OF THE METHOD

The discussion of the described technique will be focused mainly on the special problems concerned with development of a micromethod for AC activity measurements in single pieces of tubules. Special attention will be paid to the conditions chosen for dissection of the tubules and pretreating the samples. It should be stressed from the beginning that when AC activity is measured *in vitro*, by the rate of conversion of added [^{32}P]ATP into [^{32}P]cAMP, the conditions are necessarily very different from those existing *in vivo*. As mentioned in the introduction to this paper, the two main membrane components, namely the receptor sites for the hormone and the cyclase units, must be freely accessible to their respective substrates or ligands, when added to the system. Since the hormone acts on the cell membrane from outside, whereas ATP reaches the catalytic site from the cell interior, the cells must be made permeable to nucleotides, regenerating system, etc. In other words, the chemical asymmetry between intracellular and extracellular media, proper to the living situation, is no longer a condition in which to measure AC activity. Thus, the best *in vitro* conditions may be quite different from those leading to the optimal stimulation of the system by a given hormone. It may well be, for example, that a high calcium concentration (similar to that prevailing in extracellular fluid) is sometimes required for optimal hormonal binding, although such Ca^{2+} concentrations are known to almost completely inhibit the catalytic AC unit (Bockaert *et al.*, 1972).

Since the conditions to be used are of necessity very different from the physiological ones, it is clear that absolute values of AC measurements remain of limited significance. As a consequence, if the method is used in order to analyze the pattern of AC hormone dependency in different cell types, the sensitivity of the enzyme is better judged in terms of hormone concentration inducing threshold responses rather than of maximal effects induced by high hormone concentrations. Such a criterion can be adopted to decide whether or not the hormone used is physiologically active on the segments tested.

A. Effect of Collagenase on AC Activity

The technique must be discussed in relation to the use of collagenase, since available collagenase preparations are known to contain proteolytic enzymes and proteolytic enzymes may have considerable effect on AC activity and its sensitivity to hormones. The following direct and indirect evidence suggests that collagenase does not lead to such deleterious effects under the conditions described in this paper. (a) As already mentioned (Figure 2), AC activation by vasopression in rat kidney homogenate exhibited no loss of sensitivity or intensity when the tissue was pretreated by collagenase and hyaluronidase. (b) When the results obtained with the single tubule technique and the current homogenate technique are compared, it appears that the hormonal concentrations inducing half-maximal AC stimulations are similar for vasopressin (Imbert *et al.*, 1975c). For parathyroid hormone (Chabardès *et al.*, 1975a), catecholamines (Chabardès *et al.*, 1975b), and calcitonin (Chabardès *et al.*, 1976), they are definitely lower in the isolated responsive portions of microdissected nephrons than in kidney homogenates untreated with collagenase. The same holds true when the results are expressed as the lowest hormone concentration inducing a significant AC stimulation (threshold response). Finally, in spite of the use of collagenase, microdissected structures exhibited a higher sensitivity to hormones than homogenates, at least for some of the hormones tested. This may indicate that the biochemical integrity of the receptor-transducer-enzyme membrane system is better preserved under the conditions described in this paper than when the homogenization procedure must be applied to the tissue. It is interesting to note that this difference exists in spite of the fact that collagenase apparently destroys peritubular basal membranes, as already mentioned.

B. Storage of the Samples

It is well known that homogenates from kidney tissue, unless stored frozen at very low temperature, have to be used within a few hours of preparation, so

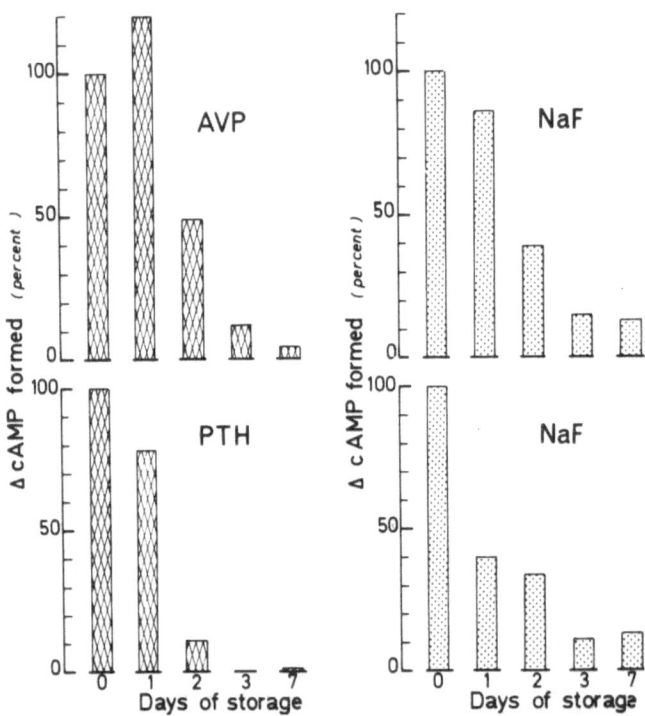

Figure 7. Effect of sample storage on AC activity. Samples of single proximal tubule (lower part of figure) or of cortical collecting tubule (upper part of the figure) were prepared from different rabbit kidneys on different days, and then stored at 0°C for various periods before AC activity measurements. All samples were incubated at the same moment and under the same conditions except for hormones. The collecting tubule samples were incubated in the presence of either arginine-vasopressin (AVP) 10^{-6} M, or NaF, 5 mM, whereas proximal tubule samples received parathyroid hormone (PTH, 1–34 synthetic bovine fragment, 1 U/ml) or NaF. Each bar corresponds to the mean value of at least four replicates. Ordinate: the AC activities were calculated as increases in cAMP generation in response to hormone or NaF (stimulated minus control activities, femtomoles cAMP/millimeter tubule/30 min) and expressed as percent of the results obtained in the absence of storage. Abcissa: duration of sample storage (days). Zero corresponds to samples which were dissected and incubated on the same day (samples used as reference). In the case of collecting tubule samples, no loss of activity was noticed after 1 day of storage and about 50 percent of the initial activity was still measured after 2 days. The loss in AC activity was faster in the case of samples from proximal tubules.

as to avoid a rapid drop in AC activity. Samples of microdissected tubule differ from homogenates, since they can be stored unfrozen at a temperature close to 0°C for much longer periods. This is illustrated in Figure 7, which shows that hormone and fluoride AC activation, in the collecting tubule, remained nearly unchanged after a day of storage. In proximal convoluted tubule samples, the loss in AC activity was faster. When a large number of samples from distal segments have to be prepared from the same kidney, one full day can be devoted to microdissection. The incubation can be postponed until the following day, provided that the samples are stored at 0°C.

Bicarbonate buffered solutions are generally used when metabolic studies have to be carried out using surviving tissue slices or suspension of tubules. AC activity in isolated tubules was therefore measured in Krebs's bicarbonate buffer solution instead of the modified Hanks's solution, which is used to prepare both the collagenase solution and the microdissection solution. As shown in Figure 8, no difference was noticed between the two types of buffer.

C. Permeabilization Procedure

When microdissected tubules were incubated without receiving any specific pretreatment to increase their cell permeability, the results varied according to

Figure 8. Effect of microdissection medium composition on AC activity. In the experiment shown here, Hanks's solution or bicarbonate Krebs's solution (gassed with O_2 95%/CO_2 5%) were used for preparation of the collagenase medium as well as the microdissection medium. One type of solution was used for one kidney and the second type for the other kidney from the same rabbit. AC activities were measured on the day of sample preparation as usual, or after 3 days of storage at 0°C in the two respective microdissection media. The samples were either collecting tubules stimulated by vasopressin or proximal tubules stimulated by parathyroid hormone as indicated in the legend for Figure 7. AC activities were calculated as increases in cAMP production (stimulated minus control activities) and expressed on the ordinate as percent of the results obtained with nonstored samples treated with Hanks's buffer. Right-hand columns: Krebs's bicarbonate; left-hand columns: Hanks's solution. No statistically significant difference was observed between these two conditions.

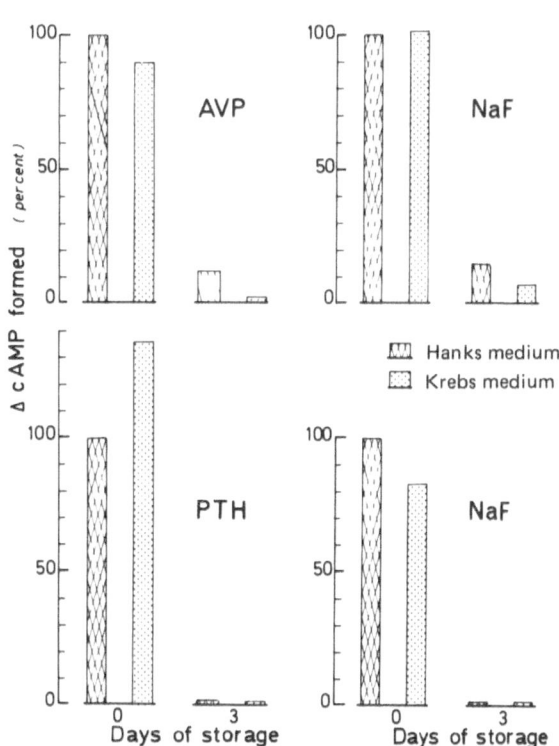

the type of segment used. In the case of samples from proximal tubule, almost maximal AC responses could be elicited by PTH or fluoride without applying osmotic shock and/or freezing procedures. In the case of collecting tubule, an osmotic shock was required in order to obtain clear-cut AC responses to AVP or fluoride, but higher responses were obtained when both osmotic shock and freezing were applied. With samples from the thick portions of the ascending limb and from distal convoluted tubule, both osmotic shock and freezing must be applied, since when the freezing step was omitted AC activity measured in the presence of fluoride was rather low. The reason for such differences in properties from segment to segment is not clear. The fact that an osmotic shock was not required with PCT is unlikely to indicate an enhanced permeability in this segment resulting from some cell damage, since a large and rapid swelling of the structure was always observed in response to the addition of hypoosmotic solution. This observation suggests that most cell membranes maintain their semipermeable properties. In contrast, collecting tubules which require an osmotic shock for $[^{32}P]ATP$ entry into the cell, do not swell in hypoosmotic media as much as proximal portions (Figure 5).

It is difficult to ascertain whether or not the permeabilization procedure used: (a) maintains an unchanged AC sensitivity to hormones and (b) renders the cell membranes for all structures fully permeable to nucleotides ($[^{32}P]ATP$, cAMP). As indirect evidence concerning this point, we may recall that a very high AC sensitivity to hormones was measured using this technique. (Imbert *et al.*, 1975c, Chabardès *et al.*, 1975a,b); in addition, maximal stimulation factors up to thirty to fortyfold control activities were obtained in various structures (see Table VI). Such hormonal responses could not have been elicited if the rate of ATP entry into the cells (or of cAMP exit) acted as a limiting factor in the reaction. In the few segments in which maximal stimulation ratios of a lower magnitude were obtained, very high AC control activities were measured. Such segments are the granular portions of CCT and DCT in which AC activity was stimulated about sixfold by catecholamine (Chabardès *et al.*, 1975b) and PTH (Morel *et al.*, 1976); refer also to Table V.

D. Effects of Incubation Conditions on AC Activity

Incubation should be discussed in relation to temperature, duration, ATP concentration, ionic composition of the medium, and phosphodiesterase inhibition. We have not systematically investigated the effects produced by changes in ATP concentration, pH, temperature, and ionic composition of the medium. The conditions adopted are those originally reported by others to be optimal for AC measurements in whole tissue homogenates (Bockaert *et al.*, 1972). We have only increased magnesium concentration from 1 to 3.8 mM in the incubate, which resulted in an increase in control and stimulated AC activities in some but not all structures (Table II). Increment of basal AC activities was desirable because the accuracy of the method is rather poor when ^{32}P measurements in the samples are close to background activity (see above), a situation which is sometimes encountered with proximal tubule.

Table II. Effect of Mg Concentration on Adenylate-Cyclase Activity[a]

Segment	Condition	fmol cAMP/mm/30 min		Ratio	p
		1 mM Mg	3.8 mM Mg		
PCT	Control	3.5	6.3	1.8	<0.01
	PTH (1 μ/ml)	260	468	1.8	<0.01
	NaF (5 mM)	169	322	1.9	<0.01
CCT	Control	11.2	12.1	1.1	Not significant
	AVP ($10^{-6}\,M$)	243	235	0.9	Not significant
	NaF (5 mM)	343	257	0.7	Not significant

[a] Mg concentration in the incubate was either 1 mM or 3.8 mM. PCT, proximal convoluted tubule; CCT, cortical collecting tubule. Note that enhancement of Mg concentration resulted in an increase in control and stimulated AC activities on PCT but produced no change in CCT. (From Imbert *et al.*, 1975a.)

As exemplified by the results shown in Figure 6, cAMP formation per millimeter of tubule increases proportionally with the incubation time, for at least an hour. Such a linear dependence was found in proximal tubule samples (controls and PTH stimulated) and in collecting tubule samples (controls and AVP stimulated) (Imbert, 1975a).

The catalytic conversion of ATP into cAMP will not proceed at a constant rate for an hour unless the ATP concentration is maintained constant at the site of the enzyme. As the piece of tubule certainly contains ATPase activity in much greater amount than adenylate cyclase activity, it must be concluded that the [^{32}P]ADP formed in the tissue is continuously and efficiently reconverted into ATP by the ATP regenerating system (phosphocreatine-creatine kinase) present in the incubation medium.

No linearity in [^{32}P]cAMP accumulation would be observed if a large fraction of the [^{32}P]cAMP formed was converted into 5'-AMP by phosphodiesterase. In the presence of a large excess of cold cAMP (1 mM in the incubation solution), the total cAMP concentration is likely to remain constant—or even to decrease—with time. [^{32}P]cAMP specific activity must therefore increase as a function of time. If the rate of cAMP degradation by phosphodiesterase remains constant, then the amount of [^{32}P]cAMP destroyed per unit of time would progressively increase and [^{32}P]cAMP accumulation would tend to saturate. Since such a tendency was not noted, it is concluded that the rate of cAMP degradation is indeed very low. We therefore thought it not necessary to add phosphodiesterase inhibitors such as theophylline in the incubation medium. Indeed, theophylline has been reported sometimes to interact with AC itself.

Finally, the observed linearity indicates that the AC enzyme system, the hormone receptor system, and their coupling mechanism are not inactivated to a significant extent during the incubation itself. The fact that the technique avoids cell destruction by mechanical means may explain why structures are well preserved. If less proteolytic and other enzymes are released from lysosomes and related organelles into the incubate, rapid inactivation of added hormones (PTH, for example) would be prevented and this could account for the observed high sensitivity of isolated tubule AC to hormones.

E. Tubular Length as a Reference Standard

In most publications, AC activities are expressed per milligram protein content in the incubate. Reference to protein content is not possible in our case, since (a) each sample contains a different tissue quantity, and (b) their protein content, in any case, is far below the sensitivity limits of the current techniques for protein assay (Lowry *et al.*, 1951). Tubular length was therefore used as a reference unit (Imbert *et al.*, 1975a); as shown by the example given in Figure 9, it is clear that definite normalization of the data among replicates resulted from dividing overall cAMP production by the length of the corresponding segment. Thus, reference to the unit of tubular length appears to be a simple and appropriate procedure, although it is of a limited accuracy in at least two cases: (a) when samples of proximal convoluted tubule are so twisted that their length is difficult to measure from the photographic picture; (b) when the diameter of the structure under consideration varies to a large extent from one sample to another. This may be observed in the case of collecting tubules, which are quite variable in diameter even when compared at the very same level along the kidney pyramid, and is most marked in the papilla.

Finally, this reference standard is open to criticism, when the responses of different segments of the nephron to the same stimulus have to be compared. It is quite obvious that AC activities per unit tubular length are expected to be different in two structures such as the proximal convoluted tubule and the thin segment of the loop of Henle, for example. However, in such cases, it is not clear that reference to protein content, to fresh or dry weights, would be more

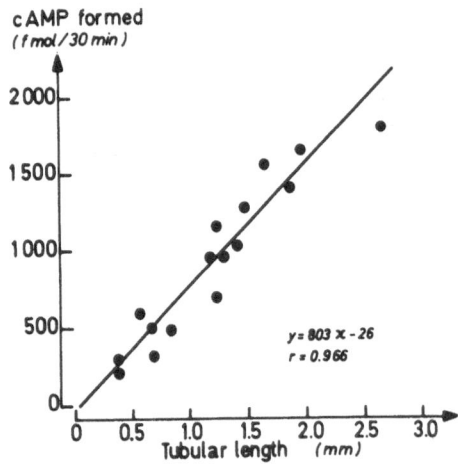

Figure 9. cAMP generation as a function of tubular length. Single microdissected portions of cortical collecting tubules (CCTl) from the same rabbit kidney were incubated for 30 min under the conditions given in the text and in the presence of AVP, $10^{-6}\,M$. For each sample, adenylate-cyclase activity is plotted on the ordinate as a function of the length of the corresponding tubule on the abcissa. Linearity is obvious. (Redrawn from Imbert *et al.*, 1975a.)

Table III. Protein Content in Various
Portions of the Rabbit Nephron[a]

Segment	Protein content (µg/mm)
PCT	0.25
PR	0.23
TDL	0.02
MAL	0.09
CAL	0.06
CCTl	0.15

[a] Whole protein content was measured in different tubular segments according to Lowry *et al.* (1951) by pooling in one sample 20–50 measured, microdissected pieces of each structure.

justified. These parameters are proportional to tissue volume, whereas what is needed is a reference proportional to membrane surface, since AC is a membrane enzyme. Even if such a reference were available and easy to measure, it still would be questionable, as long as we do not know in which cell membrane portion hormone-dependent AC activity is precisely located. In contrast, reference to the unit of length is an acceptable way of expressing data when AC activities of the same structure have to be compared in different conditions; for example, when hormonal effects are measured or when dose-response curves are established, etc.

In order to make comparisons possible with the data in the literature, we measured the protein content of some of the main segments of the rabbit nephron; this was achieved for a given structure by pooling a large number of tubules from different nephrons, by measuring the lenth of each of them, and by measuring the total protein content by the Lowry method (Lowry *et al.,* 1951) in the corresponding pooled sample. Table III gives the results obtained for six different segments of the nephron. The data are expressed as micrograms whole protein content per millimeter tubular length, and can be used to compare with data reported in the literature for kidney homogenates. It should be mentioned that even when made in this way, such comparisons are not fully valid, since whole protein content is given here for tubules, whereas in the case of tissue homogenates, the protein content is determined in the fraction which is used for AC activity measurements, namely, after partial purification of the membranes by centrifugation.

F. Reliability and Accuracy of the Method

The reliability of a technique can be discussed on theoretical grounds or judged experimentally after a sufficient period of experience. We shall focus on this second aspect.

The technique described here can be expected, *a priori*, to display lower accuracy and less reproducibility than those using whole tissue homogenates. There are two reasons for such an expectation. The first is technical and results from miniaturization, which always leads to some loss of accuracy. The second is biological and inherent to the method itself. No true replicate measurements were performed here, as with homogenates. Although several replicate samples may be prepared, they contain of necessity a homologous portion but from different nephrons; or, alternately, they may contain a portion of tubule from the same nephron, and even from the same segment, but from a different locality along the structure. It is not known at present whether or not AC activity and its hormone dependency (a) are uniformly distributed over the full length of a given nephron segment, and (b) have the same absolute magnitude in corresponding portions from different nephrons. Biological fluctuations, at least, must be expected; but systematic variations could also be present.

In order to estimate the accuracy of the method described here, we decided to adopt the following procedure. A series of nine experiments recently performed in the rat was selected for these statistical calculations. All these experiments included a large number of AC measurements from only two different segments [thick ascending limb (MAL) and medullary collecting tubules (MCT)] under a variety of vasopressin concentrations. More precisely, these experiments included 150 groups of four to six replicate samples (690 samples altogether), each group corresponding to AC measurements made on the same type of structure, from the same rat kidney, and under the same experimental conditions as regards hormone concentration. For each group, a mean value (fmol/mm per 30 min) and a standard deviation, S.D., were calculated. The 150 groups were then subdivided into three classes according to their mean value: (a)

Table IV. Accuracy of Adenylate Cyclase Measured in Single Tubule Samples[a]

Class	AC mean activity	Number of Groups	Mean relative S.D. ($\pm$S.E.M.)
A	25.5	36	33.4 ($\pm$2.5)
B	135.4	50	32.5 ($\pm$2.3)
C	650.0	64	29.6 ($\pm$1.7)
Total	328.4	150	31.5 ($\pm$1.2)

[a] 150 groups of 4 to 6 replicate samples from 9 experiments in the rat were subdivided into three classes according to the AC mean value obtained in each group; class A: AC activities lower than 50 fmol/mm/30 min; class B: AC activities ranging from 50 to 250 fmol; class C: AC activities higher than 250 fmol. For each group, the standard deviation (S.D.) was expressed as percent of the mean (relative S.D.); the table gives the relative S.D. mean value ($\pm$S.E.M.) for each class. No difference in relative S.D. was noted among the three classes, indicating that in practice the reproducibility between replicates is limited by biological and experimental factors other than statistical fluctuations in ^{32}P counting rate; otherwise, relative S.D. of class A should be higher than those of the two other classes.

those with a mean value less than 50 fmol/mm per 30 min; (b) those with a mean value between 50 and 250, and finally, (c) those with a mean value higher than 250 fmol/mm per 30 min. Such a subdivision should result in larger relative S.D. among the first class compared with the others, if part of the scatter resulted from a poor accuracy when AC activity was low. In order to make comparisons easier, all S.D. values were expressed as percent of the corresponding mean values.

The relative scatter of data was about the same for each class since the average value for relative S.D. was similar in the three cases, as shown in Table V. This observation demonstrates that AC activities below 50 fmol were measured with the same accuracy as the higher AC activities. It follows from the results given in Table IV that, when quadruplicate samples are prepared, the value of the mean can be measured with an average accuracy (S.E.M.) of about ±16% (relative S.D. = 32%; S.E.M. = S.D./$\sqrt{N}$).

Although the distribution of relative S.D. among the 150 groups is not gaussian but exhibits some degree of asymmetry (Figure 10, it is nevertheless of interest to calculate how large the difference between the mean values of two experimental groups must be in order to reach statistical significance. Figure 11 gives the limits of $\bar{m}_2$ (expressed as a multiple of $\bar{m}_1$), beyond which p for the difference is either <0.05 or <0.01, as a function of the number of replicates used per group (N). These curves confirm our empirical observation that when the mean values of two groups of four replicates differ by a factor of two or more, then their difference is generally statistically significant. In order to render significant differences of a lower magnitude, it is necessary to increase the number of replicates.

It must be concluded that the present micromethod is less accurate than techniques using homogenates. The main cause of the scatter in the results is of

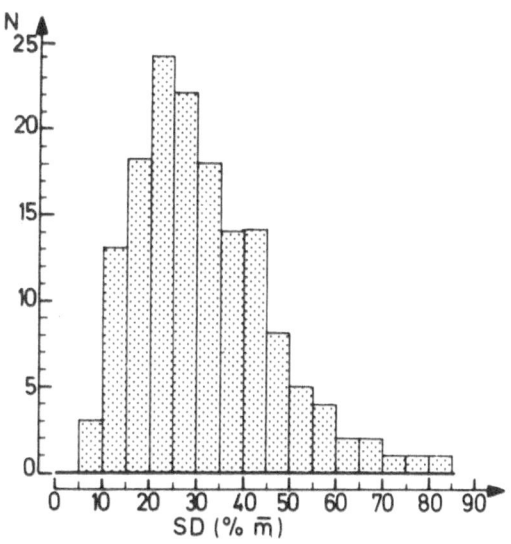

Figure 10. Reproducibility among replicate samples. The figure depicts the histogram corresponding to a series of 150 groups of replicate samples (each group including four to six samples; refer to the text and to Table IV). In each group, the scatter among measurements was expressed as percent of the mean (relative S.D.). The figure gives the number of groups (N, ordinates) per step of 5% variation in relative S.D. (abcissa). It is obvious that the distribution of variances is widely scattered and asymmetric. However, the relative S.D. of 90% of the groups is lower than 50%; this indicates that as an average and for groups of four replicates, 9 out 10 mean value determinations are obtained with an accuracy equal to or better than 25% (S.E.M. = relative S.D./$\sqrt{N}$).

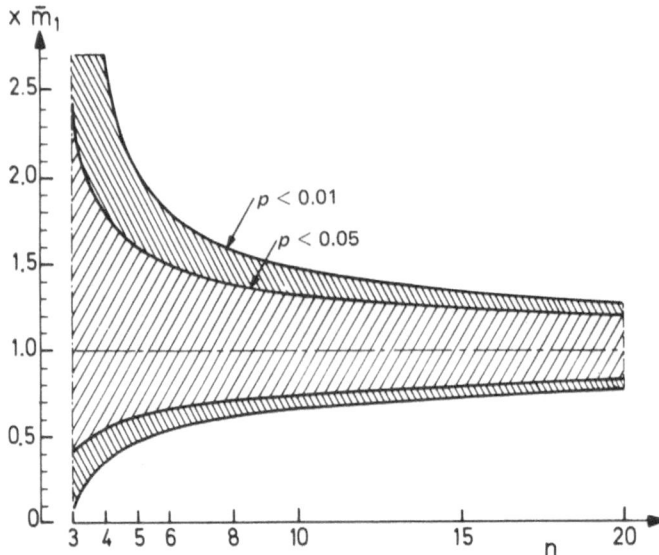

Figure 11. Accuracy of the method as a function of the number of replicate samples used. This graph sets the limits beyond which statistical significance is reached, when the mean values of two groups of replicate samples are compared. The curves depicted on the figure were computed from the data of Table IV. Ordinate: the mean value of group 2 ($\bar{m}_2$), expressed as a fraction of the mean value of group 1 ($\bar{m}_1$). Abcissa: N, the number of replicate samples in each of the two groups. Any point on the figure located outside the interval limited by the two external curves corresponds to a $\bar{m}_2$ mean value statistically different from $\bar{m}_1$ at the level $p < 0.01$; any point located outside the interval limited by the two inner curves is different from $\bar{m}_1$ at the level $p < 0.05$.

biological origin and can be accounted for by the fact that no true replicate samples can be used for comparison.

1. Biological Data

We will summarize here the results obtained using this micromethod insofar as they concern the reliability, specificity, and sensitivity of the method, in respect to hormone action. The different hormones which were tested—vasopressin (Imbert *et al.*, 1975c) PTH (Chabardès, 1975a), catecholamines (Chabardès, 1975b), calcitonin (Chabardès *et al.*, 1976)—were all observed to stimulate cyclase activity in several, specific segments. The pattern of activation was reproducible from one experiment to another and quite specific for each hormone. Dose-response curves were established on the main responsive segments, which always indicated high hormonal sensitivity. Figure 12 shows as an example the average dose-response curve which was obtained for vasopressin in the cortical collecting tubule of the rabbit. In Table V we have summarized the mean values of the control activities as well as hormone-stimulated activities measured in some of the segments depicted in Figure 3. The results are expressed both as femtomoles cAMP formed/millimeter of tubule per 30 min and

Table V. AC Maximal Responses to Hormones in Various Segments of the Rabbit Nephron[a]

Segment	Condition	N[b]	cAMP formed[c]		
			fmol/mm/30 min	pmol/mg/10 min	Stimulated/Control
PCT	Control	60	12.4	16	—
	PTH	47	490.0	653	39.5
TDL	Control	55	8.1	135	—
	AVP	19	13.6	227	1.7
TAL[d]	Control	12	9.1	155	—
	AVP	12	82.6	1,377	8.9
MAL	Control	40	10.7	40	—
	PTH	15	19.1	71	1.8
	AVP	30	122.8	455	11.5
	SCT	19	389.9	1,444	36.4
CAL	Control	65	8.7	48	—
	PTH	55	131.4	730	15.1
	AVP	47	37.9	211	4.4
	SCT	12	92.9	516	10.7
CCTg[e]	Control	29	91.2	203	—
	PTH	26	605.3	1,345	6.6
	Iso	15	494.2	1,098	5.4
	AVP	37	182.3	405	1.9
	SCT	3	98.8	220	1.1
CCTl	Control	96	33.1	74	—
	PTH	45	30.9	69	0.9
	Iso	21	178.6	397	5.4
	AVP	59	694.5	1,543	21.0
	SCT	7	31.1	69	0.9

[a] Note that differences in hormone responsiveness were observed (a) in the thin ascending limb (TAL) compared with the thin descending limb (TDL) of the loop; (b) in the cortical (CAL) compared with the medullary (MAL) portions of the thick ascending limb; (c) in the "granular" (CCTg) compared with the "light" (CCTl) portions of the cortical collecting tubule. Data calculated from Imbert et al. (1975b,c); Chabardès et al. (1975a,b); Morel et al. (1976); Chabardès et al. (1976).

[b] N: total number of samples used for calculating the mean values given. Segment symbols correspond to those defined in the legend of Figure 3.

[c] The results are expressed as femtomoles cAMP formed per millimeter of tubule per 30 min incubation time on one hand and as picomoles cAMP formed per milligram protein content per 10 min incubation time on the other. The hormones used were: PTH: 1–34 synthetic fragment of bovine PTH, Beckman, 1U/ml; AVP: arginine-vasopressin 10^{-6} M; Iso: isoproterenol, 10^{-6} M; SCT: synthetic salmon calcitonin, Sandoz, 100 ng/ml.

[d] The protein content measured in TDL samples (Table III) was used to calculate TAL results.

[e] The protein content measured in CCTl samples was used to calculate CCTg results.

as picomoles cAMP formed/milligram protein content per 10 min using the data given in Table III. It is clear that a functional segmentation of AC sensitivity to hormone is superimposed on the anatomical segmentation of nephron. A difference in vasopressin sensitivity is observed between thin ascending and thin descending limbs of the loop. Regarding the thick portions of the ascending limb, it should be stressed that qualitative and quantitative differences in AC respon-

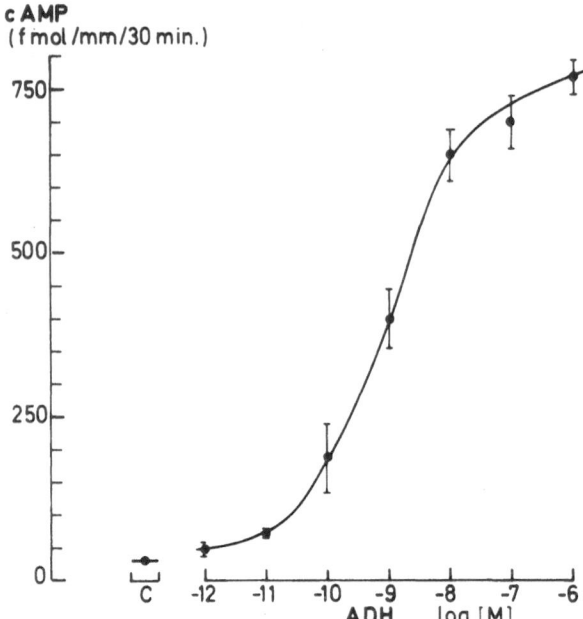

c AMP
(f mol /mm/30 min.)

Figure 12. AC dose-response curve to AVP in the rabbit cortical collecting tubule. Ordinate: AC activities are expressed as femtomoles cAMP generated per millimeter of tubule length per 30 min incubation time. Abcissa: AVP concentrations used, molar log scale. Each point is the mean value ±S.E.M. from several experiments, each including three to six replicate samples per AVP dose. Note that a highly statistically significant increase in AC activity was obtained with 10^{-11} M AVP concentration, and that half-maximal stimulation corresponded to about 10^{-9} M AVP. (Recalculated from Imbert et al., 1975c.)

siveness were also noted between the two end portions of this structure. The outer medullary portion (MAL) is sensitive to AVP and SCT whereas the cortical portion close to the macula densa (CAL) is mainly sensitive to PTH and only to a small extent to AVP and SCT. How and where transitions from one of these patterns of AC sensitivity to the other are distributed along the full length of the thick ascending limb remains to be established.

The so-called distal convoluted tubule, DCT, is probably the most heterogeneous segment of the nephron as regards AC activation by hormones; up to four successive portions with a different pattern of AC activation can be found along some DCT; two of them are always present (Morel et al., 1976).

As shown by Table V, the granulous, CCTg, and the light, CCTl, portions of the cortical collecting tubule also exhibit different and typical hormone dependence. The first portion is stimulated by PTH and isoproterenol but not by AVP. The second portion is stimulated by AVP and, to a less extent, by isoproterenol, whereas PTH is completely inactive.

Table V calls for another comment. None of the hormones tested up to now stimulated AC in thin descending limb, which nonetheless contains fluoride-sensitive AC (Imbert et al., 1975a). The tubular segments of the inner medulla are physiologically placed in an environment of high osmotic pressure; although MCT and MAL exhibited high and specific hormone responses, it may well be that the incubation conditions used to measure AC activity were not optimal in the case of TDL. It is also possible that the presence of factors or agents like prostaglandins act normally as modulators of the enzyme or its coupling to hormone receptor sites. All these factors and parameters still have to be carefully studied.

V. CONCLUSION

The biological results which were obtained using the technique described in this paper support the conclusion that the method is able to achieve its purpose. Some loss in reproducibility was noted compared with techniques using homogenates, but this limitation was fully counterbalanced by a gain in stimulation factors induced by hormone and fluoride. As regards hormone activation, the requirements for specificity and sensitivity are satisfactory and the technique allowed localization of the sites of action of different hormones along the nephron. This has not been possible by means of any other available technique. Among such techniques, cytochemical localization of AC activity was proposed by Jande and Robert (1974). The results they obtained leave uncertainty regarding the reliability of the technique since (a) PTH-dependent AC activity was associated with brush borders, and (b) fluoride did not reveal any AC activity in the CCT.

We would like to emphasize the fact that if the technique described in this paper was developed for measuring AC activity in isolated kidney tubules, it could be applied without much modification to many other biological systems, especially those in which the cell heterogeneity present in homogenates can be overcome by using appropriate cell type separation methods.

It should also be stressed that a further increase in sensitivity of about one order of magnitude could be achieved without loss in accuracy simply by using $\alpha[^{32}P]ATP$ of high specific radioactivity (now easily available) without dilution with cold ATP; if the incubation volume were reduced proportionally to the increase in ATP specific activity, the amount of radioactivity used per sample, as well as ATP concentration, could be kept unchanged. It is expected that the AC activity could then be measured in samples containing a single cell, at least if relatively large cells are used, such as some types of nervous cells.

REFERENCES

Beck, N. P., Kaneko, T., Zor, U., Field, J. B., and Davis, B. B. 1971. Effects of vasopressin and prostaglandin E1 on the adenyl cyclase-cyclic 3',5'-adenosine monophosphate system of the renal medulla of the rat. *J. Clin. Invest.*, *50:*2461.

Beck, N. P., Derubertis, F. R., Michelis, M. F., Fusco, R. D., Field, J. B., and Davis, B. B. 1972. Effect of prostaglandin E1 on certain renal actions of parathyroid hormone. *J. Clin. Invest.*, *51:*2352.

Bell, N. H. 1974. Evidence for a separate adenylate cyclase system responsive to beta-adrenergic stimulation in the renal cortex of the rat. *Acta Endocr. (Kbh)*, *77:*604.

Bockaert, J., Roy, C., and Jard, S. 1972. Oxytocin-sensitive adenylate cyclase in frog bladder epithelial cells. *J. Biol. Chem.*, *247:*7073.

Burg, M., Grantham, J., Abramow, M., and Orloff, J. 1966. Preparation and study of fragments of single rabbit nephrons. *Am. J. Physiol.*, *210:*1293.

Bray, G. A. 1960. A simple efficient liquid scintillator for counting aqueous solutions in a liquid scintillation counter. *Anal. Biochem., 1:*279.

Chabardès, D., Imbert, M., Clique, A., Montegut, M., and Morel, F. 1975a. PTH-sensitive adenyl cyclase activity in different segments of the rabbit nephron. *Pflügers Arch., 354:*229.

Chabardès, D., Imbert-Teboul, M., Montegut, M., Clique, A., and Morel, F. 1975b. Catecholamine-sensitive adenylate cyclase activity in different segments of the rabbit nephron. *Pflügers Arch., 361:*9.

Chabardès, D., Imbert-Teboul, M., Montegut, M., Clique, A., and Morel, F. 1976. Distribution of calcitonin-sensitive adenylate-cyclase activity along the rabbit kidney tubule. *Proc. Nat. Acad. Sci. (USA), 73:*3608.

Chase, L. R., and Aurbach, G. D. 1968. Renal adenyl-cyclase: anatomically separate sites for parathyroid hormone and vasopressin. *Science, 159:*545.

Dousa, T. 1976. Drugs and other agents affecting the renal adenylate activity, In: *Methods in Pharmacology,* Vol. 4A, *Renal Pharmacology,* p. 293. Ed. by Martinez-Maldonado, M., Plenum Press, New York.

Dousa, T., Hechter, O., Schwartz, I. L., and Walter, R. 1971. Neurohypophyseal hormone-responsive adenylate cyclase from mammalian kidney. *Proc. Nat. Acad. Sci. (U.S.), 68:*1693.

Forte, L. 1972. Characterization of the adenyl cyclase of rat kidney plasma membranes. *Biochim. Biophys. Acta (Amst.), 266:*524.

Hanks, J. H., and Wallace, R. I. 1949. Relation of oxygen and temperature in the preservation of tissue by refrigeration. *Proc. Soc. Exp. Biol. (N.Y.), 71:*196.

Hanoune, J., Sengel, D., Lacombe, M. L., Coudrier, E., and Feldmann, G. Submitted. Proteolytic activation of rat liver adenyl cyclase by contaminant of crude collagenase of *Clostridium histoliticum.*

Imbert, M., Chabardes, D., Montegut, M., Clique, A., and Morel, F. 1975a. Adenylate cyclase activity along the rabbit nephron as measured in single isolated segments. *Pflügers Arch., 354:*213.

Imbert, M., Chabardes, D., Montegut, M., Clique, A., and Morel, F. 1975b. Présence d'une adenyl-cyclase stimulée par la vasopressine dans la branche ascendante des anses des néphrons du rein de lapin. *C.R. Acad. Sci. Paris, 280:*2129.

Imbert, M., Chabardes, D., Montegut, M., Clique, A., and Morel, F. 1975c. Vasopressin-dependent adenylate cyclase in single segments of rabbit kidney tubule. *Pflügers Arch., 357:*173.

Jande, S. S., and Robert, P. 1974. Cytochemical localization of parathyroid hormone activated adenyl cyclase in rat kidney. *Histochemistry, 40:*323.

Kurokawa, K., and Massry, S. G. 1973. Evidence for two separate adenyl cyclase systems responding independently to parathyroid hormone and beta-adrenergic agents in the renal cortex of the rat. *Proc. Soc. Exp. Biol. (N.Y.), 143:*123.

Lowry, O. H., Rosebrough, N. J., Farr, A. L., and Randall, R. J. 1951. Protein measurement with the Folin phenol reagent. *J. Biol. Chem., 193:*265.

Marx, S. J., and Aurbach, G. D. 1975. Renal receptors for calcitonin: coordinate occurrence with calcitonin-activated adenylate-cyclase. *Endocrinology, 97:*448.

Marx, S. J., Fedak, S. A., and Aurbach, G. D. 1972a. Preparation and characterization of a hormone-responsive renal plasma membrane fraction. *J. Biol. Chem., 274:*6913.

Marx, S. J., Woodard, C. J., and Aurbach, G. D. 1972b. Calcitonin receptors of kidney and bone. *Science, 178:*999.

Nelson, G. L., Chase, L. R., and Aurbach, G. D. 1970. Parathyroid hormone-sensitive adenyl cyclase in isolated renal tubules. *Endocrinology, 86:*511.

Morel, F., Chabardes, D., Imbert, M., Montegut, M., and Clique, A. 1976. Functional segmentation of the rabbit distal tubule by microdetermination of hormone-dependent adenylate cyclase activity. *Kidney Intern., 9:c*264.

Neer, E. J. 1973. The vasopressin-sensitive adenylate cyclase of the rat renal medulla. *J. Biol. Chem., 248:*4775.

Rajerison, R., Marchetti, J., Roy, C., Bockaert, J., and Jard, S. 1974. The vasopressin-sensitive adenylate-cyclase of the rat kidney: effect of adrenalectomy and corticosteroids on hormonal receptor-enzyme coupling. *J. Biol. Chem., 249:*6390.

Ramachandran, J. 1971. A new simple method for separation of adenosine 3',5'-cyclic monophosphate from other nucleotides and its use in the assay of adenyl-cyclase. *Anal. Biochem., 43:*227.

Ramachandran, J., and Lee, V. 1970. Divergent effects of *o*-nitrophenyl sulfenyl ACTH on rat and rabbit fat cell adenyl cyclase. *Biochem. Biophys. Res. Commun., 41:*358.

Salomon, Y., Londos, C., and Rodbell, M. 1974. A highly sensitive adenylate-cyclase assay. *Anal. Biochem., 58:*541.

Chapter **12**

Methodology for Study of Kidney Intermediary Metabolism

Saulo Klahr

Renal Division, Department of Medicine
Washington University School of Medicine
St. Louis, Missouri

I. INTRODUCTION

A great variety of methods are available for the study of renal metabolic processes and it is necessary to have some idea of their applicabilities and limitations. No attempt will be made in this chapter to compile a list of all the methods that are or have been used, or to cover all the range of techniques which can be utilized to study the nonexcretory functions performed by the kidney. It has become evident in the past two decades that the kidney, in addition to its well-known excretory functions, possesses an active metabolic machinery that is involved in the production of certain hormones or enzymes: renin, 1,25-dihydroxy vitamin D_3, erythropoietin, prostaglandins, etc. (Mulrow, 1976), as well as the removal or degradation of other hormones: insulin (Katz and Rubenstein, 1973), parathyroid hormone (Hruska et al., 1975), glucagon (Sherwin et al., 1976), etc. While these functions are now well recognized, their relation to some of the functional excretory parameters of the kidney is not immediately evident. Most of the material covered in this chapter is concerned with those parameters of intermediary metabolism that may in some way be related to the main functional excretory task performed by the kidney, that is, the reabsorption of salt and water from the glomerular filtrate. In this respect, techniques dealing with the utilization of substrates by the kidney, the rates of oxidation, and possible interconversion of different substances which subserve the generation of high-energy bonds necessary for reabsorption and active transport of NaCl will be considered. Recent reviews on this subject have been published (Cohen and Barac-Nieto, 1973; Cohen and Kamm, 1976; Klahr, 1976).

Since the major source of energy in mammals is the aerobic oxidation of substrates, the rate of O_2 uptake by the kidney should provide a gross estimate of total energy production by this organ. However, in addition to aerobic oxidative reactions, other mechanisms such as glycolysis and anaerobic oxidative decarboxylations have been shown to provide significant quantities of energy for renal function (Cohen and Barac-Nieto, 1973; Cohen and Kamm, 1976). The consumption of O_2 by the kidney *in vivo*, per unit weight, is one of the highest in the organism. Although the weight of the kidney is approximately 0.5% of total body weight, it accounts for approximately 10% of the total O_2 consumption by the body under basal conditions. In addition, the mammalian kidney demonstrates a considerable substrate specificity in that it selectively utilizes certain substrates from arterial blood. The uptake of substrates by the kidney is not always related to their concentrations in blood. For example, there is very little net uptake of glucose across the kidney despite a blood concentration of glucose of approximately 5 mM. In contrast, the kidney takes up considerable amounts of lactate and glutamine despite the fact that under most circumstances the concentrations of lactate and glutamine in blood are of the order of 1 and 0.5 mM, respectively (Pitts, 1972). While total O_2 consumption by the kidney may provide a measurement of total renal energy production and requirements, the rate of substrate uptake and the metabolic pathways by which a particular substrate is utilized may yield information about the mechanisms by which cellular metabolism and cellular functions are coupled. Reabsorption of NaCl is quantitatively, by far, the most important transport function of the renal tubules. It seems well established that the reabsorption of NaCl by the kidney is an active process, which requires the bulk of the O_2 consumed by the kidney.

II. OXYGEN CONSUMPTION

A. Studies In Vivo

Renal O_2 consumption *in vivo* can be divided into a small but constant basal O_2 uptake and a variable suprabasal or functional O_2 uptake (Lassen *et al.,* 1961). The basal O_2 consumption is defined as the O_2 uptake of the nonfiltering and hence nonreabsorbing kidney. It has been measured during marked hypotension and has been found to amount to approximately 1 μmol of oxygen per gram kidney per minute. The suprabasal or functional O_2 consumption is defined as the total O_2 uptake minus the basal. It has been measured on normally functioning kidneys and it has been found to correlate closely with the quantity of sodium reabsorbed. Different methods have been used to evaluate the relation of sodium reabsorption to O_2 consumption by the kidney *in vivo* and these include: hypotension due to hemorrhage; carotid occlusion; aortic compression; osmotic diuresis; pentobarbital anesthesia; diuretic agents and other metabolic inhibitors; partial ureteral occlusion; spontaneous changes in renal blood flow, etc. (Kessler *et al.,* 1964; Kiil *et al.,* 1961; Kjekshus *et al.,* 1969; Knox *et al.,*

1966; Thurau, 1961). Most studies have utilized the dog, although some studies have been done in the rabbit kidney (Torelli *et al.*, 1966).

For the determination of O_2 consumptions *in vivo*, dogs are anesthetized either with Nembutal or inactin, and oxygen may or may not be administered. The abdomen is opened through a medial incision and suitably large catheters are tied into both ureters, one femoral artery, and the right renal vein. Simultaneous clearances of inulin or exogenous creatinine and PAH to determine glomerular filtration rate and renal blood flow are performed. Blood pressure can be monitored by a mercury manometer or by direct intraarterial recordings using a catheter placed in the femoral artery. Clearance periods are obtained and in the middle of each period blood should be drawn simultaneously from the femoral artery and the renal vein and examined for hematocrit, O_2 content, O_2 saturation, plasma inulin, plasma PAH, and plasma sodium. The correct position of the catheter is verified at autopsy and the kidneys weighed after removal of the capsule, pelvic fat, and large vessels.

1. Analytical Methods and Calculations

Blood O_2 content can be measured manometrically as described by Van Slyke and Neill (1924) or by an O_2 electrode. The analysis should be completed within 30 min after a sampling and values can be compared to results of simultaneous duplicate photoelectric measurements of the oxygen saturation. Renal plasma flow (RPF) in milliliters per gram tissue per minute can be calculated for each dog as the mean value of the plasma flow in the different clearance periods. Similar calculations can be carried out for hematocrit (H), arterial renal venous oxygen difference $(A - R)O_2$ in μmoles per milliliter, the glomerular filtration rate (GFR) in milliliters per gram per minute, the plasma sodium concentration in microequivalents per milliliter, and the urinary excretion rate of sodium ($U_{Na}V$) in microequivalents per gram per minute. From these values several parameters can be calculated:

sodium reabsorption = GFR × plasma sodium − U_{Na} × V (μEq/g/min)
total renal oxygen uptake(Q_{O_2} total) = RPF/1 − H) × $(A - R)O_2$ (μmol/g per min)
net renal oxygen uptake (Q_{O_2} net) = Q_{O_2} total − oxygen uptake of the nonfiltering kidney
Na/net O_2 ratio or number of sodium equivalents reabsorbed per mole oxygen = sodium reabsorption/Q_{O_2} net

B. Oxygen Consumption by Kidney Slices or Isolated Tubules *In Vitro*

It has been known for a number of years that the metabolism of the renal cortex differs significantly from that of the renal medulla (Gyorgy *et al.*, 1928; Dickens and Weil-Malherbe, 1936). Studies conducted in rats revealed that the rate of O_2 consumption by slices of renal cortex was 3 to 4 times higher than for slices of inner medulla. On the other hand, the medulla was abundantly capable of glycolysis; by contrast, the cortex had a more limited glycolytic activity.

Similar observations have also been made in the guinea pig. Studies of dog kidney slices, incubated in a medium with an osmolality of 300 mOs*m*, revealed that O_2 consumption by the cortex was 6 to 7 times higher than that for the medulla per unit of dry weight (Kean *et al.*, 1961).

1. Technique—Kidney Slices

Kidneys obtained from rats, rabbits, and dogs are removed rapidly and placed in 0.15 *M* NaCl chilled to about 2°C. Slices of cortex or medulla about 0.3–0.4 mm thick can be made in a Stadie–Riggs microtome, after separating cortex and medulla, and kept in chilled 0.15 *M* NaCl. (A detailed description of the method and its limitation is presented in Section III-B.) No more than approximately 20 min should elapse from the time the animal is killed until the slices are completed. The tissues can be leached of substrate by incubating them for 1–3 hr at room temperature with the solution being aerated by a continuous stream of air and mixed by a slow-speed mechanical stirrer. They are then placed in a small volume of chilled 0.15 *M* NaCl and kept at about 2°C until the time of study 30 or so minutes later. Or they can be used after being incubated in the cold. The tissues are transferred to Warburg vessels which had been previously chilled in cracked ice. Approximately 50–100 mg of tissue are placed in 2.7 ml of suspending medium in the main compartment of each vessel. The suspension medium used has the following composition: KCl, 10 mEq/liter; Na phosphate buffer (pH 7.4), 3.7 mmol/liter; $CaCl_2$, 0.7 mmol/liter; and NaCl, 133 mEq/liter. Upon the addition of other compounds, either electrolytes or nonelectrolytes, the concentration of NaCl can be adjusted to provide a constant total osmotic pressure of 300 mosmol/liter. When organic acids are used as substrates they can be added as the sodium salt. The center well of each vessel should contain 10% KOH. The gas space is filled with O_2. The cups then can be shaken in a constant temperature bath at the temperature at which the rate of O_2 consumption is going to be studied and at a given number of cycles per minute. The tissues are then incubated for 20–40 min to allow for equilibration and then O_2 consumption can be measured at 20-min intervals by following the changes in pressure of the manometer for the next 1–2 hr. At the end of the incubation the vessels are removed from the bath in pairs and the tissues are promptly removed from the cups, blotted on filter paper, and weighed. A critical analysis of the tissue slice method in manometric experiments has been presented by Laser (1942) and Umbreit (1972).

2. Technique—Kidney Tubules

Renal tubules are prepared as described elsewhere (see Section III-B). Approximately 5–10 mg of protein of a tubule suspension are added to 3 ml of potassium phosphate Ringer's solution placed in a Warburg flask. Oxygen consumption can then be determined as described for renal slices. Oxygen consumption can also be determined using a Clark electrode (Haglhare, 1961) with continuous charting on a Varian G-11 or another recorder of similar type. With the electrode, measurements can be accomplished in 5–10 min.

3. Technique—Kidney Mitochondria

Kidneys from rabbits or rats are decapsulated after being quickly removed (Case *et al.*, 1973). The cortex is separated from the medulla and immediately placed in iced oxygenated 0.25 M sucrose containing 1–2 mmol/liter of EDTA and adjusted to pH 7.2 by the addition of Tris buffer. The tissue is homogenized in a Potter–Elvehjem apparatus (glass-Teflon) for about 60 sec, in a solution containing 0.25 M sucrose and 1 mM EDTA. The resulting suspension is centrifuged at 0°C at 800g for 10 min and the supernatant is respun at 8,500g for 10 min. After the supernatant is discarded, the walls of the centrifuge tubes are wiped clean of residual fat. The pellet is then resuspended in 2 ml of the sucrose–EDTA solution per original gram of kidney and spun at 8,500g at 0°C for 10 min. Two more identical washings are performed and the mitochondrial pellet is suspended in a volume of 0.25 M sucrose to give a final protein concentration of around 20 mg/ml as determined by the Lowry method (Lowry *et al.*, 1951). Oxygen consumption can be measured using standard manometric techniques. Approximately 5 mg of mitochondrial protein are added to the main well of a respirometer flask containing (at final concentration) 10 mM KCl, 10 mM MgCl$_2$, 5 mM KPO$_4$ buffer (pH 7.2), 10 mM Tris buffer (pH 7.2), 10 mM glucose, and 200 mM sucrose. Sidearms of the flasks may contain substrates, 26 mg of hexokinase, and 5 mM ADP (by converting the ATP formed by oxidative phosphorylation to glucose-6-phosphate, the hexokinase trap would prevent ATP inhibition of mitochondrial respiration). All flasks are aerated and preincubated at 25°C for 30 min. The incubation is initiated by tipping the contents of the sidearm into the main flask. The other setup that can be used for the measurement of pO$_2$ consists of a Clark electrode (platinum-silver) with a Teflon membrane, a nano amperemeter amplifier and a potentiometric recorder. For calibration, mixtures of N$_2$ and O$_2$ are used, the O$_2$ content of which may be analyzed. This latter method allows the recording of rapid changes in mitochondrial oxygen consumption.

4. Manometric Techniques

The actual procedure in setting up systems for the measurements of respiration of living cells varies widely. A common procedure is as follows:

a. Add materials (except cells) to the main compartment of clean dry Warburg flasks having a center well.
b. Add materials (if subsequent additions are contemplated) through the sidearm.
c. Place 0.2 ml of 10% KOH in the center well, after greasing upper rim of well.
d. Grease attachment joint on manometer and grease and insert plug for sidearm.
e. Add tissue slices, homogenates, tubules, etc.
f. A strip of filter paper is added to the KOH in the center cup (this is important for absorption of CO$_2$).
g. Attach flask to manometer and place in constant temperature bath.

h. Adjust and tighten flask after shaking in bath for 5 min (this is done since sometimes the grease becomes softer and the flask tends to creep slightly).

i. Allow to equilibrate with shaking for 15–20 min. After this, adjust manometer fluid to reference point on close side of manometer with stopcock open. Close stopcock and begin readings.

Limitations. The limitations of the methods are as follows: (1) the gases exchanged must be only O_2 and CO_2. In most cases, these conditions are not difficult to meet since in the majority of tissues these are the only gases involved. (2) The atmosphere in the flask must be free from carbon dioxide. For some tissues this is of no consequence. They respire at the same rate and utilize the same metabolic pathways whether CO_2 is present or not. But for other tissues this is not the case. Carbon dioxide may inhibit, may stimulate, or may alter the path of metabolism of a given cell. Hence, measurements in the absence of CO_2 may not give a reasonable estimate of the reactions occurring in its presence. (3) The rate of O_2 uptake and CO_2 liberation and absorption must be between a particular range so that the assumptions of the method hold; that is, the fluid is always saturated with O_2 gas (or air) and the pressure of CO_2 in the gas phase approximates zero.

III. RENAL METABOLISM OF CARBOHYDRATES

Although renal tissue contains all the enzymes necessary for the phosphorylation of glucose and its metabolism by the glycolytic pathway, by the hexose monophosphate shunt, and by other metabolic pathways, no detectable net uptake or production of glucose by the intact kidney can be demonstrated, under most conditions, *in vivo* (Costello *et al.*, 1967; Dies *et al.*, 1970; McCann *et al.*, 1961). A precise understanding of the disposition of glucose in the functioning kidney *in vivo* is hampered because (1) the chemical measurements are not precise enough to determine the exact rate of net glucose utilization or production, (2) renal glucose utilization using radiolabeled compounds has been examined only under conditions of metabolic acidosis and alkalosis (Pitts and MacLeod, 1975), and (3) measurements of the conversion of glucose to lactate are complicated by the simultaneous high rate of renal lactate utilization. The principal fates of the glucose utilized by the kidney (as established by *in vitro* studies) are oxidation to CO_2 (Lee *et al.*, 1962; Lee and Peter, 1969; Pitts and MacLeod, 1975) and conversion to lactate via glycolysis (Lee *et al.*, 1962; Hems and Gaja, 1972). Glucose is converted to lactate by renal medullary slices and to a much lesser extent by renal cortical slices (Lee *et al.*, 1962; Pashley and Cohen, 1973). In addition, it has been demonstrated using the isolated perfused rat kidney that when glucose is the only substrate present, lactate is a major end product of its metabolism. However, in the intact kidney *in vivo*, there is no net production of lactate (Levy, 1965; Leaf-Pinto *et al.*, 1973; Brand *et al.*, 1974) due to the simultaneous oxidation of lactate to CO_2 and possibly its conversion to alanine. In addition, the kidney (particularly the cortex) is capable of synthesizing glucose *de novo* (gluconeogenesis).

A. Renal Glycolysis

The glycolytic capacity of the kidney has been studied using the isolated perfused rat kidney (Hems and Gaja, 1972), renal cortical or medullary slices (Underwood and Newsholme, 1967), and isolated tubules or membrane-free preparations obtained from renal cortex or medulla (Klahr *et al.*, 1971).

1. Glycolysis in the Isolated Perfused Rat Kidney

The methodology for this preparation is described in detail elsewhere in this book (see Chapter 15). Hems and Gaja (1972) studied the production of lactate from glucose by the isolated perfused kidney of the rat under aerobic and anaerobic conditions. A bicarbonate–albumin–saline perfusion medium was used. The gas phase was N_2 plus CO_2 (95:5) in anaerobic experiments and O_2 plus CO_2 (95:5) in aerobic experiments. Potassium cyanide, 1 mM, was added immediately before anaerobic perfusions. Bicarbonate was 25 mM in the medium at pH 7.4 and about 10 mM at pH 7.1. The time course of aerobic lactate formation by the isolated perfused kidney was linear for 1–2 hr and the rate was about 130 μmol per hour per gram dry weight of kidney. In aerobic perfusions, the glucose removed from the medium approximately corresponded to the lactate formed. Pyruvate also appeared regularly in the medium and the ratio of lactate to pyruvate was about 12 at all glucose concentrations during perfusions of kidneys from fed rats. The formation of lactate from glucose was linear with time for at least 2 hr in anaerobic perfusions with KCN. If cyanide was not present, the initial rate was slower and increased during perfusion presumably as anaerobiosis became complete. Anaerobic lactate production was dependent on glucose concentrations over the range of 0 to 10 mM. The maximal observed rate of lactate formation was in the order of 411 μmol/hr/g dry weight of kidney. In anaerobic perfusions, glucose removal from the medium was faster than under aerobic perfusions and again corresponded to the amount of lactate formed. Under anaerobic conditions, pyruvate formation was negligible and the ratio of lactate to pyruvate in the medium was greater than 50.

2. Glycolysis in Renal Slices

Renal slices are obtained as described elsewhere in this chapter. About 50 mg of slices are incubated in 4.0 ml of bicarbonate-buffer saline in 25-ml conical flasks in a Dubnoff metabolic incubator and shaken at 90–100 oscillations/min at 37°C. The flasks can be gassed with either N_2 plus O_2 (95:5) (aerobic) or N_2 plus CO_2 (95:5) (anaerobic) by blowing the stream of the relevant gas into the flask for about 45 sec and then sealing it with a bung as tightly as possible. Anoxic incubations are conducted in flasks with center wells which contain yellow phosphorus to remove the last traces of O_2 from the experimental atmosphere.

Slices are incubated usually for 2 hr when studying glucose uptake. At the end of this time, the flasks are cooled in ice and the slice removed and discarded. The medium is deproteinized with perchloric acid (final concentration 2%) and the protein precipitate is removed by centrifugation. A concentration of 2 mM glucose in the medium can be used for experiments in which glucose uptake is measured because at this concentration the rate of glucose uptake can be satisfactorily measured. At higher concentrations, differences in extinction or fluorescence between control and experimental flasks may be too low to be measured accurately. It is observed in glucose uptake experiments that glucose is released into the medium for the first 20 min of incubation, after which glucose uptake is linear for about 2 hr. Therefore, in most experiments in which glucose uptake is studied, slices should be incubated for 20 min without substrate and then transferred to another flask with medium containing 2 mM glucose. Glucose disappearance can be estimated by the hexokinase method (Lowry *et al.*, 1964). Lactate formation can be estimated by measuring lactate fluorometrically (Lowry *et al.*, 1964).

3. Renal Glycolysis in Membrane-Free Preparations

The use of membrane-free preparation avoids the problem of possible effects of substances tested on the transport of the substrate into slices or isolated tubules. In these latter two systems, decreased glycolysis may be observed if the transport of the substrate is decreased by the substance under study. The description that follows relates to the use of membrane-free preparations for the study of renal glycolysis. Rats or rabbits are killed by a blow to the head and the kidneys are rapidly removed and placed in an ice-cold solution of 175 mM KCl. Renal cortex and medulla are dissected and separated using a blade and the tissues are then blotted and weighed. The tissues are cut into small pieces and homogenized in 10 volumes (w/v) of 175 mM KCl. The homogenized tissue is then centrifuged at 50,000g for 30 min at 4°C. The resulting supernatant or soluble fraction should be a membrane-free preparation. Microscopic examination can be used to corroborate the lack of membranes in this supernatant.

Glycolysis is measured as the rate of lactate production from different substrates: fructose-1,6-diphosphate, glucose-6-phosphate, or 3-phosphoglycerate. Incubations are performed at 37°C and a pH of 7.8 using air as the gas phase. A 1-ml final volume of a medium containing the following, as final concentrations, is used: phosphate, 40 mM (consisting of a mixture of 5 parts of disodium to 1 part of monosodium phosphate); nicotinamide, 60 mM; ATP, 1.5 mM; NAD, 0.8 mM; MgCl$_2$, 5 mM; and fructose-1,6-diphosphate or glucose-6-phosphate, 7.5 mM. When 3-phosphoglyceric acid is used, 15 mM final concentration of the sodium salt and 1 mM NADH are added to the incubating medium. The reaction is started with the addition of 500 μl (0.5–2 mg protein) of membrane-free preparation. Exactly 30 min later, the reaction is stopped by adding 50 μl of 6.1 N trichloroacetic acid. Incubations can be carried out in the absence of inhibitors and in the presence of different concentrations of substances to be studied. Test substances usually should be in solution before addition to the incubation medium.

After acidification with trichloroacetic acid, the samples are cooled in ice water and neutralized with 7 M KOH. The amount of lactate produced during incubation is then measured enzymatically by fluorometric techniques (Lowry *et al.*, 1964). Blanks consist of tubes in which trichloroacetic acid is present prior to the addition of the membrane-free preparation. Protein can be measured by the method of Lowry *et al.* (1951).

Precautions. Mitochondrial contamination of the membrane-free preparation can be determined by studying the fate of pyruvate added to the system. When 1 mM pyruvate is added to such a system with NADH, 70% of the amount of pyruvate is usually recovered in the form of lactate and another 20–25% is found to be present as unchanged pyruvate after 30 min of incubation. Another way of assessing possible mitochondrial contamination is to check the effects of KCN addition to the incubation medium on the rate of lactate production from fructose diphosphate.

B. Renal Gluconeogenesis

The term gluconeogenesis indicates the formation of carbohydrate from any noncarbohydrate precursors (Krebs *et al.*, 1963). Such precursors include the glucogenic amino acids as well as the intermediates of the tricarboxylic acid cycle, glycerol, propionate, pyruvate, and lactate. Gluconeogenesis is known to occur both in liver and kidney cortex. As an experimental tissue for the study of gluconeogenesis, the kidney has some advantages over the liver. The content of preformed carbohydrate is much lower in kidney than in the liver. Liver of well-fed rats may contain more than 10% (weight/wet weight) of glycogen and more than 0.5% (weight/wet weight) of glucose. The corresponding values for rat kidney are 0.01% of glycogen and 0.05% of glucose (Krebs *et al.*, 1963). Thus, it is difficult to measure in the liver the net carbohydrate increases which occur after incubation for 1 or 2 hr with precursors, even when the preformed total carbohydrate has been reduced by starvation. By contrast, the increment of carbohydrate in kidney on incubation is relatively large. The end product of gluconeogenesis in kidney is glucose rather than glycogen because the quantities of glycogen which can be stored in the kidney are very small. It has been shown that the renal content of glycogen of normal rats rose from 0.48 mg/g wet weight to 1–1.5 mg/g wet weight after continued glucose infusion into the bloodstream. Under the same conditions, the liver glycogen value rose from 22 mg/g wet weight to 106–137 mg/g. Per unit of weight, therefore, the liver stored about 100 times as much glycogen as kidney. Renal gluconeogenesis has been studied in isolated perfused kidney (Bowman, 1970), kidney cortex slices (Klahr *et al.*, 1972, 1973; Schoolwerth et al., 1974), and in isolated kidney tubules (Gordon and deHartog, 1973; Guder and Wieland, 1972; Nagata and Rasmussen, 1970; Kurakawa and Massry, 1973).

1. Gluconeogenesis in the Isolated Perfused Rat Kidney

Elsewhere in this book Bowman describes the techniques for studies using the isolated perfused rat kidney. Bowman (1970) has used this preparation to study gluconeogenesis. The rate of glucose formation from pyruvate was linear and in excess of 1 μmol/min per g of tissue. Glucose production from L-lactate was less than that from pyruvate (0.5 μmol/min/g of tissue), and the uptake of lactate was also less. Fructose was converted to glucose more readily than was dihydroxyacetone, and at approximately the same rate as pyruvate. Glucose production from L-glutamate proceeded at about the same rate as that from L-lactate. L-Alanine produced no glucose, and no alanine uptake could be detected. A mixture of amino acids, pyruvate, L-lactate, and glycerol at normal plasma concentrations supported gluconeogenesis at an initial rate of about 0.6 μmol/min/g of kidney.

The rate of gluconeogenesis was found to be sensitive to small changes in the pH of the perfusate. With either lactate, pyruvate, glutamine, or a substrate mixture of predominantly amino acids, glucose production was greater at pH 7.23 than at pH 7.64. Conversely, gluconeogenesis from glycerol and fructose was inhibited by a pH of 7.23 and increased by pH 7.64. Addition of cyclic AMP to the perfusate stimulated gluconeogenesis from lactate, pyruvate, and amino acids, but not from glycerol. Neither glucagon, epinephrine, parathyroid extract, nor vasopressin altered the rate of gluconeogenesis in the isolated perfused kidney of the rat.

C. Kidney Slices

The use of tissue slices was introduced by Warburg (1923) as a method for studying *in vitro* the metabolism of tissue which has not been extensively disrupted and is still capable of metabolic activity similar to that which it would perform *in vivo*. Slices should be thin enough to allow O_2 from the surrounding medium to reach the innermost layers, but thick enough that the proportion of cells disrupted by the slicing would be a small proportion of the total. The slices are suspended in appropriate medium in a vessel containing a suitable gas mixture and incubated with shaking, usually at 37°C.

1. Preparation of Kidney Slices

Kidneys should be excised immediately after the animal is killed or under anesthesia and preparation of slices should start at once. If delay is unavoidable, the tissue should be kept cold in ice-cold Ringer's solution. Cortical slices of approximately 0.3–0.4 mm thickness can be prepared using a Stadie–Riggs microtome (Stadie and Riggs, 1944) which is a very satisfactory instrument for preparing slices of uniform thickness. A block of kidney of convenient size is placed on a piece of moist filter paper on the microtome pedestal (the paper prevents the tissue from slipping). The microtome is held over the tissue with enough pressure to cause a little flattening of the tissue block, and the slices cut by a to-and-fro movement of the blade. The cut slice lies between the blade and the top section of the microtome. Sliding the blade backward and forward usually leads to slices adhering to the top section, free of the blade so that they can be lifted off. Cutting slices is easier if the kidney and instrument have been moistened with a saline medium. The Stadie–Riggs microtome gives slices of fairly constant thickness. The thickness can be varied by using top sections with depressions of different depths. In the case of kidneys, some observers prefer not to use the outermost cortical slice. Caution also should be used when trying to study cortical versus outer medullary tissue. A definite change in color (red medulla) will be observed during slicing when most of the cortex already has been removed. Slices should be handled with fine forceps. Slices may be stored for short periods of time in a suitable cold saline medium, if possible the same medium as that in which they are to be incubated and containing glucose or other suitable substrates. Slices are rapidly weighed on a small aluminum weighing pan with a torsion balance. Slices which are being cut and stored wet must be drained first. The slice is best introduced into the incubation vessel by pushing it from the weighing pan onto the edge of the vessel and then pushing it down by means of any thin, slightly curved instrument. If slices have stuck together or become folded, it is advisable to swirl the vessel until the slices are open and separate.

The solution to be used as incubation medium depends upon the problem under study. Rates of metabolism are affected considerably by the inorganic as well as the organic composition of the medium. The media used commonly consist of a saline mixture of osmotic pressure and organic composition similar to that of serum.

2. Gluconeogenesis by Renal Cortical Slices in Vitro

Slices prepared as described above are transferred to an Erlenmeyer flask containing substrate-free Ringer's solution of the following composition in millimoles per liter: sodium, 130; potassium, 4; calcium, 1; magnesium, 1.4; chloride, 136; and phosphate, 2.4. The slices are incubated at 37°C for 1 hr in an effort to deplete them somewhat of endogenous substrate and then approximately 60–80 mg of wet tissue weight are added to each incubation flask containing 10 ml of Ringer's solution. Flasks would contain Ringer with either no substrate or 10 mM final concentration of the substrate under investigation (pyruvate, α-ketoglutarate, glutamine, etc.). Although these concentrations of substrates are higher than those in normal serum, only a few experiments are available in the literature on renal gluconeogenesis that use more physiologic concentrations of these gluconeogenic precursors. The pH of the incubation medium is adjusted to 7.4 with 0.1 N sodium hydroxide. Flasks are kept in ice until the beginning of incubation. Flasks containing no test substances serve as controls. The test substance under investigation for its effects on gluconeogenesis can be added to the remaining flasks at different concentrations. Every condition should be run in duplicate. Initial aliquots of the Ringer's solutions are obtained for the determination of glucose and thereafter the flasks are placed in a Dubnoff metabolic shaker and incubated for periods of 30, 60, or 90 min. The incubations are carried out at 37°C using 100% oxygen as the gas phase. After incubation, the flasks are transferred immediately to an ice bath, and aliquots for the determination of glucose are again obtained. Then the slices are removed, blotted on Whatman No. 1 filter paper, and weighed on watch glasses.

Glucose concentration in the Ringer's solution can be determined enzymatically with hexokinase and glucose-6-phosphate dehydrogenase by measuring fluorometrically the appearance of reduced triphosphopyridine nucleotide (Stein, 1962).

Calculations. Glucose production in each flask can be calculated as micromoles of glucose produced per unit wet weight of tissue per unit time. Corrections are usually not made for small changes in glucose content of the slices which could have occurred during incubation since glucose content of the slices is extremely small compared with total glucose in the medium. Usually values for glucose production in the absence of substrate are subtracted from glucose production in the presence of substrate. The results have been expressed in terms of the weight found when the tissue is removed at the end of the experimental period, drained, and dried at 100–110°C, to constant weight. This may not represent a satisfactory basis, because fragments of the slice, and materials leached out of the slice, are not accounted for, and results per unit weight are therefore falsely high. Another way of obtaining the weight is to add trichloroacetic acid to the medium. The slice, fragments, and precipitate are collected and washed on a centered glass filter. On drying the filter, the trichloroacetic acid is decomposed and volatilized and the complete dry weight is obtained. Also, it may be more convenient to obtain the initial weight before the slices are added to the incubation flasks and express the results per initial weight.

Precautions. Under certain conditions, when compounds other than substrates are being tested for their effects on gluconeogenesis, it may be important to exclude the influence of these test compounds on the transport of substrates from the external medium into the cell interior. The experiments on gluconeogenesis should then be conducted also by preloading the cortical slices with a given substrate using high concentrations of that substrate (Klahr and Schoolwerth, 1972). For example, concentrations of 50 mM α-ketoglutarate can be employed for preloading rat renal cortical slices for a period of 30–60 min. The slices can then be reexposed in a substrate-free medium to different concentrations of the test substance, and control flasks without test substance are run simultaneously. These types of experiments would reveal any influence of test substances on transport as a possible contributing factor in their effects on gluconeogenesis.

The kidney slice technique provides an overall picture of metabolism rather than information concerning single reactions and enzymes. However, certain limitations should be considered. The slice has no capillary circulation and all exchange between the tissue and the incubation medium must occur by diffusion through distances up to half the thickness of the slice. To maintain an adequate O_2 tension in the innermost layer of an actively respiring slice, an abnormally high and actually toxic concentration of O_2 has to be in contact with the outer layers. Similarly, the concentration of any rapidly utilized substrate provided in the medium has to be higher than the likely physiological level. The concentration of a substrate added to the medium does not represent the concentration within the slice; this will vary with the depth in the slice and the rate of consumption. The CO_2 tension, the H^+ concentration, and the concentrations of lactic acid and other metabolically produced substances tend to be significantly higher within the slice than in the surrounding medium.

D. Isolated Renal Cortical Tubules

Most of the studies of renal intermediary metabolism have employed either homogenates or renal cortical slices. Studies using slices may be inaccurate due to problems with diffusion and changes in the concentrations of intermediate metabolites caused by variable thickness and interstitial fluid content of slices. Many of these difficulties may be circumvented by employing isolated renal tubules. Isolated renal cortical tubules can be prepared from adult rats using a mixture of collagenase and hyaluronidase (Burg and Orloff, 1962, and Nagata and Rasmussen, 1970). Adult rats weighing between 150 and 300 g may be either anesthetized with urethane (0.16–0.2 g/100 g body wt.) or stunned by a blow to the head. The abdominal aorta is exposed through a midline incision and the celiac artery, abdominal aorta, and inferior vena cava are all ligated just below the diaphragm. The kidneys are then perfused via the abdominal aorta with 10 ml of a calcium Krebs–Ringer's phosphate buffer, pH 7.4, containing 40 mg of collagenase and 100 mg of hyaluronidase. Following the perfusion, the kidneys are rapidly removed and placed in ice-cold calcium-free Krebs–Ringer's phosphate, pH 7.4. The medulla is excised and the cortex from four to six perfused kidneys can be combined, minced finely with surgical scissors, and suspended in 10 ml of the same Ringer's enzyme solution and incubated in an Erlenmeyer flask at 37°C under O_2:CO_2 (95:5, by volume) for 30–60 min with shaking in a metabolic shaker at a rate of 60–70 oscillations per minute. At the end of incubation, the tubules are dispersed by gentle pipetting with a broad-tipped 10-ml serological pipet. The tubules are then filtered through two layers of fine surgical gauze and washed with 50 ml of calcium-free Krebs–Ringer phosphate, pH 7.4. The filtrate is then centrifuged at 90g for 90 sec at 4°C in a Sorvall centrifuge (Model RC2B). The supernatant is removed by suction and the resulting loose pellet is resuspended and washed twice with cold calcium and glucose-free Ringer phosphate and centrifuged at 30g for 60 sec. The final loosely packed pellet contains approximately 60–70 mg of protein per milliliter and is a preparation that can be used for *in vitro* studies. The entire procedure should require approximately 1 hr and the tubules should be utilized without delay. Microscopy indicates that both proximal and distal tubules contribute to the preparation. Proximal tubular elements represent 80% of the total preparation. It has been shown that both amytal or ether anesthesia may depress the respiratory activity of the isolated tubules. To test the functional intactness of the tubule preparations, two kinds of measurements can be made: (1) the rate of glucose production from α-ketoglutarate and (2) levels of adenine nucleotides, particularly ATP. The rate of glucose formation should be linear for periods up to 90 min and the ATP concentrations are usually maintained during this same interval in adequate preparations. Experiments lasting more than 90 min cannot be conducted using this preparation.

For the study of renal gluconeogenesis and its ionic and hormonal control, the buffer usually used is bicarbonate rather than phosphate and the medium should contain 2% bovine serum albumin and 0.5 mM palmitate. While the standard Krebs–Ringer's buffer employs 2.5 mM $CaCl_2$, it has been shown by Rasmussen (1975) that 1 mM $CaCl_2$ is a more physiological concentration for *in vitro* studies. This is of particular importance in studies of gluconeogenesis since glucose production by the tubules is sensitive to changes in extracellular calcium. Incubations can be carried out using $O_2:CO_2$ gas mixtures for 5–20 min at 37°C with constant shaking. All substrates are neutralized to pH 7.4 before addition to the incubation medium. The rate of gluconeogenesis is dependent upon the specific precursor added to the isolated tubules. In the absence of added substrate, there may be a small but detectable formation of glucose during a 15-min incubation period. The endogenous substrate for gluconeogenesis is probably derived from a pool of free amino acids or from amino acids derived from protein catabolism. Succinate and α-ketoglutarate are the most effective precursors for glucose formation in this system. Malate, glutamate, glutamine, lactate, and pyruvate are less effective and alanine, oxaloacetate, and glycerol are quite ineffective. At the end of the incubation, either trichloroacetic acid or perchloric acid extracts are prepared. Duplicate flasks should be run. In one set, the trichloroacetic acid or perchloric acid is added to the total contents of the flask. In the other, the contents of the flask are first subjected to centrifugation for 1 min at 600g or filtered through fine (0.5 mol pore size) Millipore filters and the acids are added to the supernatant or pellet. In this way the total amount of various intermediates or their concentrations in the medium can be determined. Glucose and most other metabolites can be assayed on perchloric acid extracts using fluorometric enzymatic methods (Lowry and Passonneau, 1972). Protein can be determined by the method of Lowry *et al.* (1951) and cyclic AMP by the method of Gilman (1970). These tubular suspensions have been shown to respond to parathyroid hormone and epinephrine as well as changes in calcium concentration in their rates of glucose production (Nagata and Rasmussen, 1970; Guder and Wieland, 1972; Kurakawa and Massry, 1973). Slices also increase their gluconeogenic rate in response to prostaglandin E_1 (Morrison *et al.*, 1976).

IV. UPTAKE AND METABOLIC FATE OF SUBSTRATES IN THE KIDNEY

A. Measurement of Substrate Oxidation by the Kidney *in Vivo*

Several techniques have been used to quantify the renal oxidation of substrates: (1) The single-pass indicator-dilution technique designed to determine the net uptake and metabolic fate of a substrate after a single injection of the radiolabeled substrate into the renal artery (Chinard *et al.*, 1959, 1962). This technique may underestimate substrate oxidation rate if the injected ^{14}C-labeled substrate or its products have a slow turnover rate in the kidney. Since this technique involves a short observation period (less than 1 min), the ^{14}C-labeled products may not leave the kidney in the renal venous blood during this interval. Thus, if large intrarenal pools of the compound or its derivatives exist, it may result in an apparent underestimation of the metabolism of the particular substrate.

2. A constant intravenous infusion of small amounts of ^{14}C-labeled compounds (Leal-Pinto *et al.*, 1973; Park *et al.*, 1974; and Pitts *et al.*, 1972). The

specific activities both in artery and renal venous blood are measured and the $^{14}CO_2$ production rate by the kidney is also measured. This technique may overestimate the renal oxidation of substrates considerably, especially if there is significant recycling of the administered ^{14}C into other substrates which are also oxidized by the kidney. This is especially true if the substrate is administered intravenously. This allows interconversion at different sites before it reaches the kidney and considerable rates of substrate oxidation may be observed.

3. Infusion of trace amounts of ^{14}C-labeled substrate directly into one renal artery (Brand and Cohen, 1972; Garza-Quintero et al., 1975). For accurate measurements of the oxidation to CO_2 of a substrate, the $^{14}CO_2$ production rate by the contralateral kidney (which represents the $^{14}CO_2$ produced from recycled ^{14}C) are subtracted from the $^{14}CO_2$ produced by the kidney receiving the infusion of the ^{14}C-labeled substrate. This technique is the most reliable one for quantifying the renal decarboxylation rate of a substrate.

1. Technique—Metabolism of Glutamine

Pitts and his co-workers (1972, 1975) have utilized the kidney of the dog *in vivo* to study the metabolic fate of a series of substrates. In brief, their methods consist of catheterizing the ureters of a dog separately to permit collection of urine from the two kidneys. A retention needle is inserted into the femoral artery to sample blood entering the kidney. A radiopaque catheter is inserted into the right renal vein to sample blood leaving the kidney. The essential features of these experiments consist of an intravenous infusion of a single ^{14}C uniformly labeled metabolite in tracer amounts, quantification of the label and its parent metabolite, and determination of the ^{14}C-labeled products added to venous blood by the kidney. Blood concentration of the metabolite is not appreciably changed by infusion of minute amounts of tracer of high specific activity. Renal blood flow, measured by clearance and extraction of PAH, and glomerular filtration rate, measured by creatinine clearance, are completely normal. These studies have been conducted in dogs in chronic metabolic acidosis induced by ammonium chloride and in chronic metabolic alkalosis. The fate of glutamine, lactate, palmitate, sterate, oleate, citrate, and glucose have been studied using this or similar methodology. The following is a detailed description of the method used by Pitts et al. (1972). Dogs weighing between 18 and 26 kg have been used. They are lightly anesthetized with intravenous pentobarbitol. Chronic acidosis was induced by adding 10–15 g of ammonium chloride in the food for 3 or 4 days before an experiment. Chronic alkalosis is induced by adding 10–20 g of sodium bicarbonate in the food for a similar perod of time. During the experiments, *p*-aminohippurate (PAH) and creatinine are infused intravenously for the measurement of renal blood flow and glomerular filtration rate, respectively. GFR is only used in these experiments to assess normality of renal function. Another infusion containing a total of 83 μCi of [^{14}C]glutamine uniformly labeled with high specific activity was given as a prime and thereafter at a constant rate for 20 min before and through the 45 min of a three-period clearance experiment. No cold glutamine is given. Blood glutamine concentrations represent normal endogenous levels. Since the excretion of glutamine is negligible even at greatly elevated plasma levels, glutamine and radioactivity of glutamine in urine are negligible. From arterial and renal venous blood glutamine concentrations and renal arterial and renal venous blood flows, the extraction of glutamine by the kidney can be calculated in terms of micromoles per min. From counts per minute per minute of glutamine extracted calculated in a similar fashion, a specific activity can be calculated. Dividing counts per minute per minute of any product added to renal venous blood by the specific activity of the glutamine extracted yields the micromoles per minute of product produced by the kidney. The products that can be studied include ^{14}C-labeled glucose, ^{14}C-labeled CO_2, and ^{14}C-labeled glutamate in the case of glutamine. Total CO_2 produced by the kidney can be measured by the Van Slyke manometric technique using whole blood (Van Slyke and Neill, 1924). Dividing micromoles of CO_2 derived from glutamine by total CO_2 produced by the kidney yields the proportion which originated from glutamine. Experimental technique includes catheterization of the ureters separately through a low abdominal incision, introduction of a retention needle into the femoral artery and the insertion of a radiopaque catheter into the right renal vein under fluoroscopic guidance. Other veins are catheterized for administration of the two intravenous infusions. Arterial and renal venous blood samples are collected over timed intervals of 2 min at the middle of each 50-min urine collection period. All analyses except those of creatinine can be performed on whole blood. Creatinine can be analyzed in plasma. Renal arterial blood inflow to the kidney can be calculated from the clearance and extraction of PAH by the Wolf equation (Wolf, 1941). Renal venous blood outflow from the kidney can be estimated as arterial inflow minus urine flow. The product of concentration in micromoles per milliliter or counts/minute/milliliter of any component of arterial blood and the rate of arterial inflow is equal to the quantity entering the kidney each minute. Similarly, micromoles per milliliter or counts per minute per milliliter of any component of renal venous blood multiplied by renal venous outflow is equal to the quantity leaving the kidney each minute. The difference between the quantities entering and leaving constitutes the quantity extracted by, or produced in the kidney each minute. Glutamine and other neutral and acidic amino acids can be separated by column chromatography of picric acid filtrates of whole blood by the method of Moore and Stein (1954) and they can be analyzed in an automatic amino acid analyzer. Pitts et al. (1972) interposed a Nuclear Chicago liquid flow scintillation analyzer between the column and the ninhydrin portion of the amino acid analyzer to quantify ^{14}C activity of glutamine and certain of its metabolites. Evidence presented by Pitts indicates that the first two peaks immediately following the column volume represent ^{14}C-labeled glucose. $^{14}CO_2$ activity in whole blood was measured in a Packard liquid scintillation counter by a modification of the method of Passman et al. (1956). In order to convert counts per minute in the Packard liquid scintillation system to that in the Nuclear Chicago liquid flow scintillation system, Pitts et al. (1972) utilized portions of a mixture of cold and ^{14}C-labeled glutamate uniformly labeled and chromatographed and counted in the flow system. Other portions can be treated with an excess of ninhydrin to liberate the α-carboxyl CO_2 and then can be analyzed by the Passman *et al.* method in the Packard counter. The assumption made is that since one-fifth of the carbons of glutamate appear as CO_2 when treated with an excess of ninhydrin, a conversion factor relating the two systems can be calculated. [^{14}C]Glutamine is not used because liberation of the α-carboxyl carbon as CO_2 by ninhydrin is incomplete.

2. Technique—Metabolism of Lactate

The general principles are those described for glutamine. In this case 100 μCi of uniformly labeled [^{14}C]sodium lactate (30–40 μCi/mol) are dissolved in 41 ml of isotonic saline and infused at 0.5 ml/min into a radial vein. Leal-Pinto *et al.* (1973) began the infusion 40 min before starting the experiment and continued it throughout the first 40 min of a three-period clearance experiment lasting 45 min. That is, the infusion was continued until the last blood sample was collected. Less than 4 μmol of lactate were given as isotope over the period of 80 min, a dose that is relatively small. Lactate and [^{14}C]lactate can be measured in perchloric acid filtrates of whole blood by the methods of Marbach and Weil (1967) and of Von Korff (1969), respectively. PCA can be removed by adding KOH to pH 7.6–7.8. The portion to be analyzed for [^{14}C]lactate can be evaporated to dryness at 37°C with a flash evaporator and kept in a freezer. The portion to be analyzed enzymatically for "cold" lactate was frozen as the acid PCA filtrate and neutralized with KOH immediately before analysis. The dried and frozen residue containing [^{14}C]lactate can be diluted with 5 ml of deionized water prior to analysis. [^{14}C]Lactate can be separated from other ^{14}C-labeled metabolites by chromatographing 2 ml of the above-mentioned dilution (equivalent to a 2.5–3.0 ml aliquot of blood) on a 17 × 1 cm column of Dowex 1AG10X. A gradient of HCl varying from 0 to 0.01 N can be established for elution by pumping fluid from a 250-ml tubulated Erlenmeyer flask initially filled with water. Fluid can be pumped through the column at a flow rate of 1 ml/min. Hydrochloric acid, 0.01 N, entered the flask through the tubulation to replace the fluid pumped into the resin column. The effluent from the column is passed through a Nuclear Chicago liquid scintillation flow counter. The flow counter types a series of 2-min counts on a tape. Those contained in the glucose peak which was eluted at column volume and those on the lactic acid peak which came off at 2.5–3 hr are individually summed. The calculations for specific activity and the other calculations in terms of the contribution of lactate to CO_2 as a portion of total CO_2 are done as described in the method for glutamine.

B. Measurement of Substrate Oxidation by the Kidney *in Vitro*

Cortical slices, medullary slices, or isolated tubules can be incubated in Krebs–Ringer phosphate, pH 7.4, containing 135 mM Na, 5 mM K, 1.5 mM Ca, 2.0 mM phosphorus, and 0.5 mM magnesium. In these experiments the ^{14}C-labeled substrate to be used is added to each flask. After gassing with 100%

oxygen, the flasks are sealed with rubber serum stoppers. The amount of $^{14}CO_2$ produced can be determined as follows:

Ten minutes before the end of incubation, 0.25 ml of 1 M hyamine is injected through the rubber stopper onto a strip of filter paper 20 × 18 mm in a hanging well. Ten minutes later, 0.1 ml of 2 N H_2SO_4 is injected into the incubation medium and the flasks allowed to sit at room temperature for another 30 min. This will result in release of $^{14}CO_2$ from the medium and trapping in the center well. The filter paper and the fluid of the center well are then transferred quantitatively to a vial with scintillation fluid and counted in a liquid scintillation counter. The amount of radioactive substrate added initially is determined in aliquots obtained from the medium at zero time in control flasks, added to scintillation fluid, and then counted. From the concentration of "cold" substrate and the radioactivity added initially, the specific activity of the substrate in the medium can be calculated and the amount of CO_2 evolved can therefore be calculated in micromoles or other such units for amount of tissue added per time of incubation. Oxygen consumption and oxidation of substrates can be measured simultaneously using Warburg type flasks. In these experiments 2 ml of a buffer, pH 7.4, containing 10 mM Tris, 135 mM Na, 5 mM K, 1.5 mM Ca, 2 mM phosphorus, and 0.4 mM Mg are added to the flasks. Slices from either the cortex or outer medulla weighing 15–20 mg are added to 2 ml of medium. The flasks are then flushed with 100% oxygen and mounted in a Warburg or Gilson respirometer at 37°C and shaken at a rate of 140 oscillations/min. The slices can be incubated for a certain period of time, usually 3 hr, without exogenous substrate in the media in an effort to deplete them of endogenous substrate. Uniformly ^{14}C-labeled substrate can be used as radioactive tracer. Both unlabeled substrate to achieve the desired final concentration and radioactive tracer can be added simultaneously from one of the sidearms of the Warburg-type flasks. Incubations can then be continued for an additional 2 hr with measurements of oxygen consumption at 30-min intervals. At the end of the incubation, 10 N H_2SO_4 is added from the second sidearm of the Warburg flask to stop the reaction. The resulting $^{14}CO_2$ is trapped in 10% KOH placed in the center well. Aliquots of the solution of the radiolabeled substrates, the incubation medium, and the KOH are then counted in a liquid scintillation spectrometer. From specific activities, the amount of $^{14}CO_2$ evolved can be calculated. These values can then be compared with the simultaneously measured rates for O_2 consumption.

Using isolated tubules in suspension, substrate decarboxylation can also be estimated by measuring the rate of decarboxylation of specifically labeled compounds. $^{14}CO_2$ is collected and counted by the method of Fain et al. (1962).

V. METABOLISM OF LIPIDS BY THE KIDNEY

The oxidation of free fatty acids by the kidney has been considered to be a major source of energy for support of renal transport. However, in vivo studies in the dog have revealed that oxidation of free fatty acids can account for only 10–20% of the total renal CO_2 production.

A. Metabolic Fate of Palmitate in the Dog Kidney *in Vivo*

Studies have been performed on anesthetized dogs with catheters placed in the right renal vein and artery (Barac-Nieto and Cohen, 1971). The injection solution contains 4.5% albumin complexed to palmitate-1-^{14}C (100 μCi/ml, specific activity 44 μCi/mol), T 1824, 4 mg/ml, Krebs–Ringer's bicarbonate solution, and red cells. The hematocrit of the solution is adjusted to equal that of the animal's blood. The solution is equilibrated with 5% CO_2 in O_2 and warmed to 37°C. An aliquot of the solution is taken for analysis and 1 ml is injected in a calibrated syringe. Two seconds before injection, a collection of the entire renal blood flow from the experimental kidney is initiated. Thus, no recirculation of injected [^{14}C]palmitate or its metabolites will occur. The blood volume of the animal can be maintained by pumping blood into the jugular vein from a reservoir at a rate equal to the renal blood flow of the experimental kidney. Aliquots of renal venous blood are collected anaerobically at 2–3 sec intervals during the first 58 sec after injection using an automatic sampler. The remaining and major portion of the renal venous effluent during the first 60 sec is allowed to drain by gravity into an iced plastic bottle. After completion of the collections during the first minute period, the entire renal venous effluent can be collected in iced plastic bottles for three to four additional timed 1-min periods. Aliquots of blood from the large collection bottles are immediately pipetted into chloroform–methanol (2:1, v/v) for lipid extraction. Aliquots of the anaerobic samples can be used for $^{14}CO_2$ analysis (Passman *et al.*, 1956), T 1824 analysis (Chinard and Enns, 1954), and for lipid extraction with chloroform–methanol (Folch *et al.*, 1957). Upon completion of the collections, the right kidney is quickly excised, frozen in liquid nitrogen within 15 sec of excision, and pulverized in a stainless steel mortar while still frozen. It is then homogenized in chloroform–methanol. The radioactivity in the lipids of the washed chloroform–methanol extracts of tissue and blood samples is determined by liquid scintillation counting after separation of lipid classes on silica gel-impregnated paper (Marinetti, 1965). The radioactivity in the free fatty acid spot can be assumed to be entirely in [^{14}C]palmitate. Aliquots of arterial and renal venous blood are also obtained at 1 min before and at 2 and 3 min after the [^{14}C]palmitate injection for the determination of the arterial venous difference of endogenous palmitic acid across the kidney. Lipid extracts of whole blood samples rather than plasma are prepared since it has been shown that a significant fraction of the free fatty acid in blood is bound to the red cells. The lipids in the washed methanol–chloroform extract are then separated on silica gel-impregnated paper. The lipid spots on the paper can then be identified with rhodamine 6G under UV light. The paper containing the free fatty acid fraction is cut and immersed in BF 3-methanol reagent for esterification (Metcalff *et al.*, 1966). The methyl esters of the fatty acids are then chromatographed. Appropriate fatty acid standards are also chromatographed. Aliquots of the upper phase of the chloroform–methanol extracts are counted after acidification to determine the radioactivity in the nonvolatile water-soluble products of palmitate metabolism in the kidney. Of the [^{14}C]palmitate taken up, only a small fraction, 5–10%, is oxidized to $^{14}CO_2$ while significant amounts of ^{14}C-labeled cholesterol, cholesterol esters, phospholipid, triglycerides, or water-soluble products appear in the renal venous blood during the first 60 sec after the intraarterial injection. Thus, under the conditions of these experiments, palmitate does not undergo complete oxidation in the kidney; instead, it is incorporated into several products of incomplete oxidation.

B. Palmitate Utilization by the Kidney *in Vitro*

Tissue slices weighing 150–180 mg are incubated in 25-ml Erlenmeyer flasks with 5 ml of 154 mM Krebs–Ringer's phosphate buffer containing 0.5% bovine serum albumin, 28 μmol glucose, and 4 μmol palmitic acid, including 0.25 μCi of 1-[^{14}C]palmitic acid (Heinemann *et al.*, 1975). The flasks are gassed for 10 min with 100% O_2, placed in a Dubnoff metabolic shaker at 37°C, capped with rubber apron stoppers with attached center wells, gassed for an additional 2 min with O_2 and then sealed. At the completion of incubation, usually 1 hr, 0.5 ml of a 1:1 dilution of hyamine hydroxide with counting solution (0.5% diphenyl oxazole, 0.03% dimethyl POPOP in toluene) is introduced into the center well by needle puncture; 1 ml of 0.2 N sulfuric acid is added to the medium, and the flasks shaken for an additional 30 min. The hyamine mixture, which traps the CO_2 in the center well, is transferred to counting vials. Aliquots of the medium are counted to determine the specific activity of palmitate. To remove palmitic acid loosely attached to the tissue, slices are transferred after incubation into flasks containing 3% albumin for two successive 5-min periods. To establish esterification of palmitate, the slices are extracted with 2:1 chloroform–methanol (20:1, volume/wet weight), filtered, and washed once with 1/5 volume 0.05 M KCl to remove nonlipid components (Folch *et al.*, 1957). The chloroform phase is assayed for radioactivity and individual lipids are separated by thin-layer chromatography. Individual lipids can then be separated on silica gel H using a solvent 70:30:2, *n*-hexane, diethyl ether, glacial acetic acid. The component spots can be identified by comparison of R_f values with known standard mixtures. After visualization with iodine vapor, they can be identified, circumscribed, and when the iodine disappears they can be scraped and transferred to scintillation vials and radioactivity assayed in a scintillation counter (Snyder and Stephens, 1962).

VI. METABOLITE CONCENTRATIONS IN WHOLE KIDNEY, CORTICAL SLICES, AND ISOLATED TUBULES

A comparison has been made between the amount of adenine nucleotides, Krebs cycle intermediates, and glycolytic intermediates found in whole kidney quickly forzen *in vivo* and cortical slices or tubules incubated *in vitro* (Rasmussen, 1975). Marked differences in the concentration of Krebs cycle and glycolytic intermediates between whole organ and tubules has been observed. Slices had intermediate values. However, the values of adenine nucleotides are comparable in the three preparations. It has been suggested that the explanation for the marked differences between these preparations depends upon the following factors: (1) the different experimental protocols used to obtain the three different preparations; (2) the manner in which the data are reported; and (3) the difference in the ability of phosphorylated and nonphosphorylated intermediates to diffuse into and out of renal cells. It has been shown that a striking feature of the renal tubule preparations is their great permeability to Krebs cycle intermediates and to pyruvate, lactate, glutamate, aspartate, and glutamine. In contrast, glycolytic intermediates and adenine nucleotides do not permeate easily. In the case of whole kidney, the tissue is rapidly frozen between precooled aluminum tongs upon evulsion of the organ from the animal. In the kidney, the total intracellular fluid volume is probably on the order of 50% of the total tissue volume. In the case of kidney slices, they are removed from the incubation vessels, blotted, and then frozen and extracted. The total intracellular fluid volume is probably 30–40% of tissue volume. In the case of the renal tubules, tissue plus medium is treated with acid and the entire extract is analyzed. The total intracellular fluid volume is approximately 2.5% of the total volume analyzed, approximately 26 μl per 7 mg of tubular protein in a total volume of 1.1 ml.

All the data for concentrations of intermediates in tubules have been reported in terms of micromoles/milligram protein because of the difficulty of obtaining exact measures of intracellular fluid volume in this preparation. Therefore, the concentrations are not exactly equivalent to those obtained in preparations with a variable ratio of intra to extracellular fluid, unless all the intermediates are confined only to the intracellular space. This seems to be the case with adenine nucleotides and the phosphorylated glycolytic intermediates, but not with pyruvate, lactate, and the Krebs cycle intermediates. In fact, it has been shown that these latter intermediates appear in the medium. It has also been suggested that the distribution of the Krebs cycle intermediates in tubular preparations is the same in the medium and intracellularly and that equilibration is rapid, within 1 min or so. Therefore, it may be possible to measure concentrations of intermediates in the total incubation flask rather than separating the tubule from the medium, using [^{14}C]inulin to estimate extracellular water contained in the tubule pellet, and measuring only intermediate concentrations in the tissue itself.

A. Methodology: Content of Metabolites in Fresh Tissue

Adult rats are killed either by cervical dislocation or anesthetized with phenobarbital (175 mg/kg i.p.). In one method (Needleman *et al.*, 1968) the kidneys are rapidly removed and plunged within 1–2 sec into Freon-12 (CCl_2F_2) chilled to the freezing point ($-150°C$) in liquid nitrogen. Section of the kidney is carried out at $-20°C$ in a cold room with a razor blade (Waldman and Burch, 1963). Consecutive sections of approximately 1 mm thickness can be taken, two from cortex and two or more from the outer medulla. The frozen sections are then weighed at $-20°C$ and ground in absolute methanol containing 0.1 N HCl and extracted at 0°C with 0.3 M perchloric acid (containing 1 mM EDTA). After centrifugation (10 min at 10,000g), the supernatant is decanted and neutralized and the precipitate, which contains the glycogen, is solubilized by heating briefly with KOH. Glucose, lactate, ATP, glucose-6-phosphate, creatine phosphate, and glycogen can then be measured by enzymatic methods based on changes in pyridine nucleotide fluorescence (Lowry *et al.*, 1964; Passonneau *et al.*, 1967).

In the other method (Hems and Brosnan, 1970), the left kidney can be pulled free of vessels at the hylum and freeze clamped *in situ*. To study the effects of ischemia on metabolites, the right kidney can be separated from its blood supply and left *in situ* for variable periods of time (30–120 sec) before freeze clamping. Again, separation of cortex and medulla is important to evaluate concentrations of metabolites in these two different areas of the kidney. Frozen tissue can then be ground with a pestle and mortar. The powder is weighed into a centrifuge tube (cooled in liquid nitrogen) and homogenized in 4 volumes of 6% (wt/volume) of perchloric acid. After 30 min at 0°C, extracts are centrifuged at 35,000*g* for 15 min at 0°C. Supernatants are decanted and neutralized with a measured volume of 30% KOH. After a further 30 min at 0°C, potassium perchlorate is removed by centrifugation and the supernatant is used for determination of metabolites.

In the experiments on the distribution of glucose and related metabolites in rat kidney (Needleman *et al.*, 1968) it was observed that a glucose gradient was present, with highest levels in the outer cortex and lowest in the inner medulla. A threefold glycogen gradient was found running in the opposite direction to the glucose gradient. ATP and creatine phosphate were uniformly distributed. Lactate levels were low, with medullary levels slightly higher than cortical levels. After treatment with phlorizin, there was an increase in medullary glucose which reversed the normal gradient. Glucose loading also increased glucose concentrations in all layers but no changes in glycogen, ATP, creatine phosphate, or lactate were observed. Cutting off the blood supply to the kidney resulted in a precipitous fall in cortical ATP, whereas in the medulla the fall was much slower, apparently because of the higher rate of glycolysis. This method also can be used after manipulation of physiologic or metabolic conditions *in vivo* followed by acute freeze clamping to study the effects of such maneuvers on metabolites within the kidney.

B. Content of Metabolites in Slices or Tubules

Slices or tubules can be properly immersed in liquid nitrogen or in Freon at the intervals and under the metabolic conditions to be studied and treated similarly to the tissues obtained *in vivo*.

ACKNOWLEDGMENTS

The original portion of this work was supported by U.S. Public Health Service NIAMD grant AM-09976.

The author wishes to express his appreciation to Mrs. Patricia Verplancke for her assistance in the preparation of this chapter.

REFERENCES

Barac-Nieto, M., and Cohen, J. J. 1961. The metabolic fates of palmitate in the dog kidney *in vivo*. Evidence for incomplete oxidation, *Nephron, 8:*488.

Bowman, R. H. 1970. Gluconeogenesis in the isolated perfused rat kidney. *J. Biol. Chem., 245:*1604.

Brand, P. H., and Cohen, J. J. 1972. Effect of renal arterial infusion rate on distribution of radioisotopes in kidney. *J. Appl. Physiol., 33:*627.

Brand, P. H., Cohen, J. J., and Bignall, M. C. 1974. Independence of lactate oxidation from net Na^+ reabsorption in dog kidney *in vivo*. *Am. J. Physiol., 227:*1255.

Burg, M. B., and Orloff, J. 1962. Oxygen consumption and active transport in separated renal tubules. *Am. J. Physiol., 203:*327.

Case, D. B., Gunther, S. J., and Cannon, P. J. 1973. Ethacrynate-induced depression of respiration in transport systems and kidney mitochondria. *Am. J. Physiol., 224:*769.

Chinard, F. P. and Enns, Th. 1954. Transcapillary pulmonary exchange of water in the dog. *Am. J. Physiol., 178:*197.

Chinard, F. P., Taylor, W. R., Nolan, M. F., and Enns, T. 1959. Renal handling of glucose in dogs. *Am. J. Physiol., 196:*535.

Chinard, F. P., Enns, T., and Nolan, M. F. 1962. Indicator dilution studies with "diffusible" indicators. *Circ. Res., 10:*473.

Cohen, J. J., and Barac-Nieto, M. 1973. Renal metabolism of substrates in relation to renal function. In: *Handbook of Physiology*, pp. 909–927. Ed. by Orloff, J. and Berliner, R. W. American Physiological Society, Washington, D.C.

Cohen, J. J., and Kamm, D. G. 1976. Renal metabolism: relation to renal function. In: *The Kidney*, Vol. 1, p. 126. Ed. by Brenner, B. M. and Rector, F. C. Saunders, Philadelphia.

Costello, J., Scott, J. M., Wilson, P., and Bourke, E. 1973. Glucose utilization and production by the dog kidney *in vivo* in metabolic acidosis and alkalosis. *J. Clin. Invest., 52:*608.

Dickens, F., and Weil-Malherbe, H. 1936. Metabolism of normal and tumour tissue XIV. A note on the metabolism of kidney. *Biochem. J., 30:*659.

Dies, F., Herrera, J., Matos, M., Avelar, E., and Ramos, G. 1970. Substrate uptake by dog kidney *in vivo. Am. J. Physiol., 218:*405.

Fain, J. N., Scow, R. O., and Chernick, S. S. 1962. Effects of glucocorticoids on metabolism of adipose tissue *in vitro. J. Biol. Chem., 238:*54.

Folch, J., Lees, M., and Sloane, Stanley, G. H. 1957. A simple method for the isolation and purification of total lipids from animal tissues. *J. Biol. Chem., 226:*497.

Garza-Quintero, B., Cohen, J. J., Brand, P. H., and Kook, Y. J. 1975. Steady-state glucose oxidation by dog kidney *in vivo*. Relation to Na^+ reabsorption. *Am. J. Physiol., 228:*549.

Gilman, A. G. 1970. A protein binding assay for 3',5'-cyclic monophosphate. *Natl. Acad. Sci. U.S., 67:*305.

Gordon, E. E., and deHartog, M. 1973. Gluconeogenesis in renal cortical tubules: Effect of phenformin. *J. Am. Diab. Assn., 22:*50.

Guder, W. G., and Wieland, O. H. 1972. Metabolism of isolated kidney tubules: Additive effects of parathyroid hormone and free fatty acids on renal gluconeogenesis. *Eur. J. Biochem., 31:*69.

Gyorgy, P., Keller, W., and Brehme, T. 1928. Nierenentwicklung. *Biochem. Z., 200:*356.

Haglhare, B. 1961. Techniques for the application of polarography to mitochondrial respiration. *Biochim. Biophys. Acta, 46:*134.

Heinemann, H. O., Wagner, M., and Frederiksen, A. 1975. Palmitic acid utilization by the renal cortex of the rat. Symposium on Renal Metabolism. In: *Medical Clinics of North America*, Vol. 59, p. 699, Ed. by Baruch, S. Saunders, Philadelphia.

Hems, D. A., and Brosnan, J. T. 1970. Effects of ischaemia on content of metabolites in rat liver and kidney *in vivo. Biochem. J., 120:*105.

Hems, D. A., and Gaja, G. 1972. Carbohydrate metabolism in the isolated perfused rat kidney. *Biochem. J., 128:*21.

Hruska, K. A., Kopelman, R., Rutherford, W. E., Klahr, S., and Slatopolsky, E. 1975. Metabolism of immunoreactive parathyroid hormone in the dog: The role of the kidney and the effects of chronic renal disease. *J. Clin. Invest., 56:*39.

Katz, A. I., and Rubenstein, A. H. 1973. Metabolism of proinsulin, insulin and C-peptide in the rat. *J. Clin. Invest., 52:*1113.

Kean, E. L., Adams, P. H., Winters, R. W., and Davies, R. E. 1961. Energy metabolism of the renal medulla. *Biochim. Biophys. Acta, 54:*474.

Kessler, R. H., Weinstein, S. W., Nash, F. D., and Fujimoto, M. 1964. Effects of chlormerodrin *p*-chloromercuribenzoate and dichlorphenamide on renal sodium reabsoption and oxygen consumption. *Nephron, 1:*221.

Kiil, F., Aukland, K., and Refsum, H. E. 1961. Renal sodium transport and oxygen consumption. *Am. J. Physiol., 201:*511.

Kjekshus, J., Aukland, K., and Kiil, F. 1969. Oxygen cost of sodium reabsorption in proximal and distal parts of the nephron. *Scan. J. Clin. Lab. Invest., 23:*307.

Klahr, S. 1976. Effects of diuretics on kidney intermediary metabolism. In: *Methods in Pharmacology,* Vol. 4A. Ed. by M. Martinez-Maldonado, pp. 167–197, Plenum Press, New York.

Klahr, S., and Schoolwerth, A. C. 1972. Renal gluconeogenesis. Effects of quinolinic acid. *Biochim. Biophys. Acta, 279:*157.

Klahr, S., Yates, J., and Bourgoignie, J. 1971. Inhibition of glycolysis by ethacrynic acid and furosemide. *Am. J. Physiol., 221:*1038.

Klahr, S., Schoolwerth, A., and Bourgoignie, J. J. 1972. Relation of gluconeogenesis to ammonia production in the kidney. *Am. J. Physiol., 222:*813.

Klahr, S., Nawar, T., and Schoolwerth, A. C. 1973. Effects of catecholamines on ammoniagenesis and gluconeogenesis by renal cortex *in vitro. Biochim. Biophys. Acta, 304:*161.

Knox, F. G., Fleming, J. S., and Rennie, D. W. 1966. Effects of osmotic diuresis on sodium reabsorption and oxygen consumption of kidney. *Am. J. Physiol., 210:*751.

Krebs, H. A., Bennet, D. A. H., De Gasquet, P., Gascoyne, T., and Yoshida, T. 1963. Renal gluconeogenesis: The effect of diet on the gluconeogenic capacity of rat kidney cortex slices. *Biochem. J., 86:*22.

Kurakawa, K., and Massry, S. G. 1973. Evidence for stimulation of renal gluconeogenesis by catecholamines. *J. Clin. Invest., 52:*961.

Laser, H. 1942. A critical analysis of the tissue slice method in manometric experiments: Effect of variations in O_2 and CO_2 tension. *Biochem. J., 36:*319.

Lassen, N. A., Munck, O., and Thaysen, J. H. 1961. Oxygen consumption and sodium reabsorption in the kidney. *Acta Physiol. Scand., 51:*371.

Leal-Pinto, E., Park, H. C., King, F., MacLeod, M., and Pitts, R. F. 1973. Metabolism of lactate by the intact functioning kidney of the dog. *Am. J. Physiol., 224:*1463.

Lee, J. B., and Peter, H. M. 1969. Effect of oxygen tension on glucose metabolism in rabbit kidney cortex and medulla. *Am. J. Physiol., 217:*1464.

Lee, J. B., Vance, V. K., and Cahill, G. F., Jr. 1962. Metabolism of ^{14}C-labelled substrates by rabbit kidney cortex and medulla. *Am. J. Physiol., 203:*27.

Levy, M. N. 1965. Lactate uptake by the intact kidney. *Ann. N.Y. Acad. Sci., 119:*1029.

Lowry, O. H., and Passonneau, J. V. 1972. *A Flexible System of Enzymatic Analysis,* Academic Press, New York.

Lowry, O. H., Rosebrough, N. J., Farr, A. L., and Randall, R. J. 1951. Protein measurement with the Folin phenol reagent. *J. Biol. Chem., 193:*265.

Lowry, O. H., Passonneau, J. V., Hasselberger, F. X., and Schultz, D. W. 1964. Effect of ischemia on known substrates and cofactors of the glycolytic pathway in brain. *J. Biol. Chem., 239:*18.

Marbach, E. P., and Weil, M. H. 1967. Rapid enzymatic measurements of blood lactate and pyruvate. Use and significance of metaphosphoric acid as a common precipitant. *Clin. Chem., 13:*314.

Marinetti, G. V. 1965. Chromatographic separation, identification and analysis of phosphatides. *J. Lipid Res., 6:*315.

McCann, W. P., Gulati, O. D., and Stanton, H. C. 1961. Renal glucose metabolism during diuresis induced by infusions of hypotonic saline. *Bull. Johns Hopkins Hosp., 108:*36.

Metcalff, L. D., Schmitz, A. A., and Pelka, J. R. 1966. Rapid preparation of fatty acid esters from lipids for gas chromatographic analysis. *Anal. Chem., 38:*514.

Moore, S., and Stein, W. H. 1954. Procedures for chromatographic determination of amino acids on four percent cross-linked sulfonated polystyrene resins. *J. Biol. Chem., 211:*895.

Morrison, A. R., Yates, J., and Klahr, S. 1976. Effect of prostaglandin E_1 on the adenyl cyclase-cyclic AMP system and gluconeogenesis in rat renal cortical slices. *Biochim. Biophys. Acta,* 421:203.

Mulrow, P. 1976. Renal hormones. In: *The Kidney,* Vol. 1, p. 477. Ed. by Brenner, B. M. and Rector, F. C., Saunders, Philadelphia.

Nagata, N., and Rasmussen, H. 1970. Renal gluconeogenesis: Effects of Ca^{++} and H^+. *Biochim. Biophys. Acta, 215:*1.

Needleman, P., Passonneau, J. V., and Lowry, O. H. 1968. Distribution of glucose and related metabolites in rat kidney. *Am. J. Physiol., 215:*655.

Park, H. C., Leal-Pinto, E., MacLeod, M. B., and Pitts, R. F. 1974. CO_2 production from plasma free fatty acids by the intact functioning kidney of the dog. *Am. J. Physiol., 227:*1192.

Pashley, D. H., and Cohen, J. J. 1973. Substrate interconversions in dog kidney cortex *in vitro. Am. J. Physiol., 225:*1519.

Passmann, J. M., Radin, N. S., and Cooper, J. A. D. 1956. Liquid scintillation technique for measuring carbon-14-dioxide activity. *Anal. Chem., 28:*484.

Passonneau, J. V., Gatfield, P. D., Schulz, D. W., and Lowry, O. H. 1967. An enzymic method for measurement of glycogen. *Anal. Biochem., 19:*315.

Pitts, R. F. 1972. Metabolic fuels of the kidney. In: *Proc. 5th Internat. Cong. Nephrology,* Vol. 2, pp. 2–15. Ed. by Villarreal, H., S. Karger, Basel.

Pitts, R. F., and MacLeod, M. B. 1975. Metabolism of blood glucose by the intact functioning kidney of the dog. *Kidney Internat., 7:*130.

Pitts, R. F., Pilkington, L. A., MacLeod, M. B., and Leal-Pinto, E. 1972. Metabolism of glutamine by the intact functioning kidney of the dog. Studies in metabolic acidosis and alkalosis. *J. Clin. Invest., 51:*557.

Rasmussen, H. 1975. Isolated mammalian renal tubules. In: *Methods in Enzymology,* p. 11. Ed. by Hardman, J. C. and O'Malley, B. W., Academic Press, New York.

Schoolwerth, A. C., Blondin, J., and Klahr, S. 1974. Renal gluconeogenesis. Influence of diet and hydrogen ions. *Biochim. Biophys. Acta, 372:*274.

Sherwin, R. S., Bastil, C., Finkelstein, F. O., Fisher, M., Black, H., Hendler, R., and Felig, P. 1976. Influence of uremia and hemodialysis on the turnover and metabolic effects of glucagon. *J. Clin. Invest., 57:*722.

Snyder, F., and Stephens, N. 1962. Quantitative carbon-14 and tritium assay of thin-layer chromatography plates. *Anal. Biochem., 4:*128.

Stadie, W. C., and Riggs, B. C. 1944. Microtome for the preparation of tissue slices for metabolic studies of surviving tissue *in vitro. J. Biol. Chem., 154:*687.

Stein, M. W. 1963. D-Glucose determination with hexokinase and glucose-6-phosphate dehydrogenase. In: *Methods of Enzymatic Analysis,* p. 117. Ed. by Bergmeyer, H. V., Academic Press, New York.

Thurau, K. 1961. Renal Na-reabsorption and O_2-uptake in dogs during hypoxia and hydrochlorothiazide infusion. *Proc. Soc. Exp. Biol. Med., 106:*714.

Torelli, G., Mella, E., Faelli, A., and Constantini, S. 1966. Energy requirements for sodium reaborption in the *in vivo* rabbit kidney. *Am. J. Physiol., 211:*576.

Umbreit, W. W. 1972. Constant volume manometry—the "Warburg." In: *Manometric and Biochemical Techniques,* pp. 1–19. Ed. by Umbreit, W. W., Burris, R. H., and Staufer, J. F., Burgess, Minneapolis.

Underwood, A. H., and Newsholme, E. A. 1967. Control of glycolysis and gluconeogenesis in rat kidney cortex slices. *Biochem. J., 104:*300.

Von Korff, R. W. 1969. Ion-exchange, chromatography of citric acid cycle components and related compounds. In: *Methods in Enzymology,* p. 425. Ed. by Lowenstein, J. M., Academic Press, New York.

Van Slyke, D. D. and Neill, J. M. 1924. The determination of gases in blood and other solutions by vacuum extraction and manometric measurement. *J. Biol. Chem., 61:*523.

Waldman, R. H., and Burch, H. B. 1963. Rapid method for study of enzyme distribution in rat kidney. *Am. J. Physiol., 204:*749.

Warburg, O. 1923. Versuche an uberlebendem Carcinomgewebe. *Biochem. Z., 142:*317.

Wolf, A. V. 1941. Total renal blood flow rate at any urine flow or extraction fraction. *Am. J. Physiol., 133:*496.

Chapter **13**

Methodology for Study of Isolated Perfused Dog Kidney *in Situ*

George J. Kaloyanides

Chief, Division of Nephrology
UCLA San Fernando Valley Medical Program
Veterans Administration Hospital
Sepulveda, California

I. INTRODUCTION

Early in the history of renal physiology, investigators resorted to the isolated blood perfused kidney technique to try and unravel the complex determinants of renal function. The pump perfused isolated kidney technique of Richards and Drinker (1915) and the heart–lung–kidney preparation of Starling and Verney (1925) testify to the high level of sophistication and ingenuity in isolated organ perfusion achieved by investigators of that period. Considering the materials and equipment available, the limited success of these workers in attaining a viable isolated kidney preparation is all the more remarkable. Over the ensuing 50 years, the quest for developing an isolated perfused kidney preparation whose function approximates that of the normal kidney has continued with some, albeit incomplete, success. Nevertheless, the state of the art has reached the point where it is possible, using these techniques, to address certain questions pertaining to renal physiology that cannot be approached or totally resolved by study of the intact kidney. This chapter details three techniques of *in situ* isolated dog kidney perfusion, the functional characteristics of the preparation, and their experimental application. The term *in situ* is here broadly defined to include those techniques in which the circulation of the isolated kidney communicates directly or indirectly with the circulation of the dog.

II. TECHNIQUES OF ISOLATED DOG KIDNEY PERFUSION
IN SITU

In the intact animal, the renal vasculature constitutes one of multiple resistance circuits connected in parallel with the arterial circulation. Renal blood flow (RBF) is determined by the systemic arterial pressure, generated by the pumping of blood by the heart, and the resistance of the renal vascular bed. So long as renal arterial pressure is maintained within the autoregulatory range of 80–180 mm Hg, RBF is determined by intrarenal and extrarenal factors, which regulate renal vascular resistance (RVR).

There are two basic techniques for perfusing the isolated dog kidney *in situ*. One technique preserves the relationship of the renal vascular bed as a resistance circuit in parallel with the arterial circulation. Renal arterial pressure is the regulated variable and the heart serves as the pump for generating the arterial pressure. This technique is defined as pressure-regulated perfusion.

Isobaric perfusion is a variation of pressure-regulated perfusion in that the force for driving RBF is generated by the barometric pressure within a closed blood reservoir connected to the renal arterial circuit.

In the second technique, a mechanical pump is inserted in the arterial circulation between the heart and the kidney so that the renal vascular bed is converted to a resistance circuit in series with the mechanical pump. RBF is the regulated variable determined by the output of the pump, and renal arterial pressure is the dependent variable determined by the product RBF × RVR. This technique will be referred to as flow-regulated perfusion.

A. Pressure-Regulated Isolated Kidney Perfusion

A simple example of this technique is the regulation of renal arterial pressure by placing a clamp around the renal artery or the aorta. When combined with renal denervation, this technique provides a high degree of experimental control over hemodynamic and neurogenic influences on renal function (Schrier and Humphreys, 1971; Schrier *et al.*, 1971).

The upper range of renal arterial pressure control is restricted by the level of systemic arterial pressure. To overcome this limitation, Kaloyanides *et al.* (1971) modified a technique of isolated kidney perfusion first described by Semple and DeWardener (1959) which permits regulation of renal arterial pressure over a higher range of pressure than that usually seen in the intact dog.

The technique is illustrated in Figure 1. A kidney (7) is removed from a donor dog and perfused with blood from the femoral artery (1) of a second dog (perfusion dog) which provides the arterial pump. Renal venous blood (2) flows by gravity into a reservoir (4) from which it is pumped (5) to the femoral vein of the perfusion dog. The dog rests on an adjustable platform (6) and by raising or lowering the platform with respect to the level of the isolated kidney, a hydrostatic pressure can be added to or subtracted from the femoral arterial pressure of the dog, thereby permitting adjustment of the arterial pressure seen in the isolated kidney.

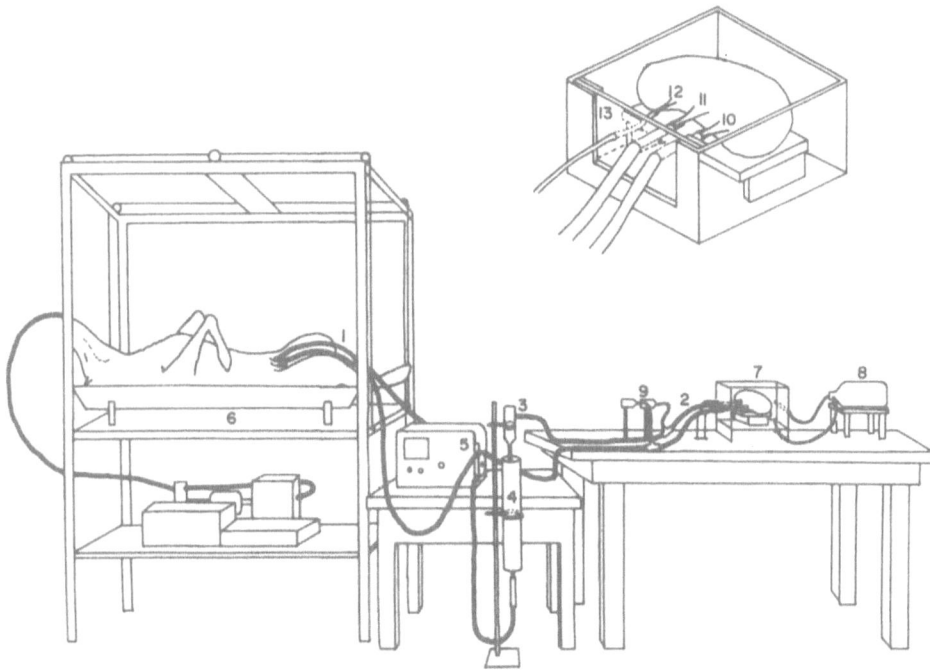

Figure 1. Diagram of pressure-regulated perfusion system. The isolated kidney is perfused with femoral arterial blood (1). Renal venous blood (2) flows by gravity into a double reservoir system (3,4) from which it is pumped (5) to the femoral vein of the dog. Arterial pressure of the kidney is regulated by adjusting the height of the platform (6) supporting the dog. The kidney (7) rests in a Lucite chamber through which a pump (8) recirculates 0.9% saline at 38°C. The insert illustrates the face of the Lucite chamber, which is removable and contains three holes to accommodate the catheters of the artery (10), vein (11), and ureter (12). Pressures are monitored by transducers (9) connected to the arterial and venous lines.

1. Methods

Equipment and Materials. The lift depicted in Figure 1 is constructed of aluminum and measures 213 × 152 × 76 cm. The double platform is suspended by wire cables attached to an electrically powered, reversible drive shaft mounted on top of the frame. The top platform supports the dog; the bottom platform supports the respirator and the infusion pumps. Although a powered lift with a variable speed control provides the greatest flexibility for adjusting renal arterial pressure, an alternative approach is to place the dog on a platform of sufficient height so as to provide the maximum hydrostatic pressure required during the study and to adjust renal arterial pressure with a screw clamp (Semple and DeWardener, 1959).

Silastic tubing (Dow Corning) of 0.48 cm internal diameter (i.d.) is used throughout. The plastic needle adaptor (0.3 cm i.d.) from a Plexitron R41 (Travenol) solution administration set is used as the cannula for the renal and femoral arteries. A 4-cm length of Tygon tubing (0.5 cm i.d.) is used to cannulate the renal and femoral veins. Polypropylene T-tubes are inserted approximately

10 cm from the end of the renal arterial and venous catheters to permit monitoring pressures. The distal end of the renal venous catheter inserts into the barrel of a 50-ml calibrated syringe (Figure 1, 3) which drains into a 1,000-ml polypropylene graduated cylinder (Figure 1, 4). Blood from the cylinder is returned to the femoral vein of the dog by a Holter roller pump (Figure 1, 5) (model RE 161, Extracorporeal Medical Specialties, Inc.). The extracorporeal circuit is rinsed with a silicone solution (Siliclad, Clay Adams Co.) before each experiment.

The isolated kidney rests in a Lucite chamber filled with 0.9% saline maintained at 38°C by continuous recirculation via a pump (Figure 1, 8) through tubing covered by an electrical heating tape. The front face (Figure 1, 13) of the Lucite chamber, which has three holes of appropriate size to provide a tight fit for the arterial and venous tubing and the ureteral catheter, is removable to facilitate catheterization of the renal vessels and ureter prior to placement of the kidney in the chamber.

Surgical Preparation. Choice of kidney for dissection is dictated by the requirement that the renal artery must have a common trunk of at least 1.5 cm. Whenever possible, the left kidney should be used because the dissection is easier and its longer renal vein facilitates connection to the extracorporeal circuit. The kidney is mobilized through a midline abdominal incision by double ligation and severing the peritoneal reflection and renal ligaments. Particular care should be taken to avoid cortical compression or rupture of perforating cortical vessels. The ureter is dissected free and severed, leaving a length of at least 6 cm for subsequent catheterization. Then the renal vein and artery are freed from the surrounding connective and adipose tissue, which is doubly ligated and severed. At this point the kidney, which should be totally free except for its vascular attachments, is returned to its normal position while preparation of the perfusion dog is completed.

The perfusion dog should be 5–10 kg heavier than the donor dog so as to minimize the cardiovascular stress imposed by the extracorporeal circulation. The femoral arteries and veins of the perfusion dog are exposed through small incisions. Complete hemostasis must be achieved because systemic heparinization can lead to significant blood loss during the course of the study. After the extracorporeal circuit is primed with heparinized saline, the arterial and venous limbs of the circuit are secured in a femoral artery and vein. Catheters are also placed in the remaining femoral artery and vein in order to monitor systemic pressures, infuse solutions, or withdraw blood samples. Immediately after the vessels are catheterized, the perfusion dog is given heparin, 200 units/kg body weight, intravenously and blood is allowed to circulate through the extracorporeal circuit to ensure proper function and to prime the renal arterial line. Then the lines are clamped until the kidney is connected to the circuit. Finally, the perfusion dog is raised to a height estimated to provide a head of pressure at the renal arterial cannula of 125 mm Hg.

The donor dog is given heparin, 200 U/kg body weight, immediately before removing the kidney. The renal artery and vein are occluded simultaneously with small clamps placed midway along the length of the vessels to keep the renal vasculature distended with blood. Vascular clamps are then placed on the renal artery and vein as close as possible to the aorta and inferior vena cava and the vessels are severed. Cannulation of the renal vessels is performed on a small table placed in front of the lucite chamber. The table has a hole in its center to accommodate a polypropylene funnel that is connected to the reservoir by Silastic tubing. After the renal artery is cannulated, the clamps on the vessels are removed and the arterial line is opened to restore blood flow. The renal vein is positioned over the funnel to return blood to the reservoir. Simultaneously, the pump is activated to return blood to the dog at a rate that maintains the level of the reservoir constant. By means of this technique the ischemia time, defined as the interval from the initial clamping of the vessels to the time when RBF is reestablished, routinely is less than 2.5 min. At this point the renal vein is cannulated so that venous blood now flows to the reservoir via the graduated syringe (Figure 1, 3). Next the ureter is catheterized, after which the kidney and tubing are maneuvered into position in the Lucite chamber. Finally the T-tubes are connected to the pressure transducers (Figure 1, 9). Renal arterial pressure is adjusted by raising or lowering the animal lift; renal venous pressure is adjusted by raising or lowering the level of the distal end of the venous line. RBF is measured by timing the venous flow into the calibrated syringe or alternatively an electromagnetic flow probe can be inserted in the renal arterial line to give a continuous recording of blood flow.

2. *Physiology of the Pressure-Regulated Isolated Perfused Dog Kidney*

Renal Hemodynamics. Glomerular filtration rate (GFR) determined by inulin clearance was found to average 0.56 ± 0.04 and 0.62 ± 0.04 ml/min per gram kidney weight (Kaloyanides and Azer, 1971), values which agree with data for the intact dog kidney (Smith, 1951). Renal blood flow (RBF) determined by direct measurement of renal venous outflow averages 4.2 ± 0.3 to 4.7 ± 0.3 ml/min per gram kidney weight, values somewhat higher than those quoted by Selkurt (1963). Over the course of 4 hr of perfusion, GFR remained stable whereas RBF decreased 15–20% below control levels, reflecting a spontaneous rise in RVR. The rise in RVR probably reflects the release of vasoconstrictor material from erythrocytes in contact with a foreign surface (Nizet, 1975).

The pressure-regulated isolated perfused kidney retains the capacity for autoregulating GFR and RBF. Kaloyanides *et al.* (1974a) found that renal autoregulation was 80% of that predicted for perfect autoregulation over the range of 75–150 mm Hg.

Distribution of cortical blood flow as determined by the radiolabeled microsphere technique parallels the pattern observed in the intact dog kidney. In response to drug-induced renal vasodilation, redistribution of flow to the inner cortex was noted (Kaloyanides *et al.*, 1973b) whereas redistribution of flow to the outer cortex was observed after inhibition of prostaglandin secretion (Kaloyanides *et al.*, 1976).

The clearance of p-aminohippurate (PAH) by the isolated kidney was similar to that of the perfusion dog's kidney after correcting for differences in kidney weight (Kaloyanides *et al.,* 1971). Moreover, PAH extraction averaged 0.77 ± 0.02, which is within the range reported for the intact dog kidney (Selkurt, 1963).

Sodium Metabolism. In the absence of experimental perturbation, sodium excretion by the isolated kidney remained stable for up to 4 hr (Kaloyanides and Azer, 1971). The level of sodium excretion depends on the prior natriuretic state of the donor and perfusion dog. When the isolated kidney was obtained from a donor dog fed a standard kennel ration and perfused with blood from a dog fed a similar diet, fractional sodium excretion was usually less than 2% of the filtered load (Kaloyanides *et al.,* 1971; DiBona *et al.,* 1972, 1973; Kaloyanides *et al.,* 1974c). In contrast, when the isolated kidney was perfused by blood from a salt-loaded dog, control fractional sodium excretion was usually greater than 2% of the filtered load (Kaloyanides and Azer, 1971; Kaloyanides and Azer, 1972; Kaloyanides *et al.,* 1975).

Sodium excretion parallels changes in renal arterial pressure. An increase in renal arterial pressure within the autoregulatory range in the absence of significant changes in GFR or RBF led to a significant increase in sodium excretion, indicating that the natriuresis was secondary to a decrease in tubule sodium reabsorption (Kaloyanides *et al.,* 1971). When renal arterial pressure was restored to normal, sodium excretion returned toward the baseline level. Saline loading of the perfusion dog promoted an increase in sodium excretion by the isolated kidney in the absence of a change in renal arterial pressure or GFR (DiBona *et al.,* 1972).

3. Experimental Application

Autoregulation of GFR and RBF. The pressure-regulated isolated perfused kidney technique is particularly suited for the study of autoregulation. In contrast to studies of autoregulation in the intact dog, this technique permits examination of the renal response to a standard pressure stimulus over a uniform range and excludes the possibility that extrarenal factors related to aortic constriction or carotid sinus stimulation, maneuvers commonly used to alter systemic arterial pressure in the intact dog, might influence the response. Semple and DeWardener (1959) used this technique to examine the influence of renal venous pressure on blood flow autoregulation. Kaloyanides *et al.* (1974a) used this technique to examine the autoregulatory capacity of the renin-depleted dog kidney and observed that renin depletion reduced the autoregulatory efficiency from 82 to 42% of that predicted for perfect autoregulation. These data imply a role for the renin–angiotensin system in renal autoregulation. It should be mentioned, however, that in a recent study Kaloyanides and DiBona (1976) found that infusing [1-sarcosine-8-alanine] angiotensin II, a specific inhibitor of angiotensin II, did not impair renal autoregulation.

The role of renal prostaglandins in renal autoregulation was also investigated in this model. In contrast to the study of Herbaczynska-Cedro and Vane (1973), who reported that inhibition of prostaglandin secretion abolished autoregulation in a pump-perfused kidney, Kaloyanides *et al.* (1976) found no significant impairment of autoregulation following indomethacin or meclofenamateinduced inhibition of prostaglandin synthesis. The latter observations are in agreement with those reported for the intact dog kidney (Venuto *et al.*, 1975; Anderson *et al.*, 1975).

Renal Arterial Pressure and Sodium Excretion. Because of the capability of regulating renal arterial pressure over a wide range, this technique also lends itself to the study of the relationship between renal arterial pressure and sodium excretion. McDonald and DeWardener (1965) observed that the natriuretic response of the isolated kidney following saline loading of the perfusion dog was directly correlated with renal perfusion pressure. Kaloyanides *et al.* (1971) observed that raising renal arterial pressure from 100 to 150 mm Hg caused an increase in sodium excretion of 110 $\pm$ 20 (S.E.M.) μmol/min without an associated change in GFR or RBF. Micropuncture experiments revealed no change in fractional or absolute reabsorption of filtrate along the accessible portion of proximal tubule, suggesting that the natriuresis induced by raising renal arterial pressure derived from a decrease in tubule sodium reabsorption at some distal segment (DiBona *et al.*, 1973).

Regulation of Renin Secretion. The pressure-regulated isolated perfused kidney has also proved useful in studying the influence of the baroreceptor and macula densa receptor in regulating renin secretion (Kaloyanides *et al.*, 1973a). Ureteral occlusion increased renin secretion in the isolated kidney, presumably by activating the macula densa receptor. However, when a pressure stimulus was superimposed on the stimulus of arterial occlusion, renin secretion was reduced to normal levels. In addition to providing evidence for the existence of a renal baroreceptor, these experiments demonstrate that the baroreceptor can override macula densa-mediated renin release.

In another study, no change in renin secretion was detected when [1-sarcosine-8-alanine] angiotensin II, a specific competitive inhibitor of angiotensin II, was infused at 1.9 μg/min into renal artery of the isolated kidney (Kaloyanides and DiBona, 1976). This dose was sufficient to completely block the vasoconstrictor action of exogenous angiotensin II infused at 1.15 μg/min. The failure of renin secretion to change during the infusion of the angiotensin II antagonist suggests that basal renin secretion in the isolated kidney is not influenced by angiotensin II operating via a negative feedback loop.

The Isolated Kidney as a Bioassay Organ. One of the earliest applications of the isolated kidney technique was to establish that vasopressin was secreted by the pituitary gland (Verney, 1926). In more recent times the isolated kidney technique has been used as a bioassay for "natriuretic hormone." Kaloyanides and Azer (1971) observed that volume expansion of the perfusion dog with equilibrated blood promoted an increase in sodium excretion by the isolated kidney. Since the natriuresis could not be explained by changes in renal hemodynamics or blood composition, it was postulated that blood volume expansion of the dog stimulated release of a humoral natriuretic factor which depressed tubule sodium reabsorption in the isolated kidney. Micropuncture experiments support the conclusion that the natriuresis derived from a decrease in tubule sodium reabsorption at some segment distal to the accessible portion of the proximal tubule (Kaloyanides *et al.*, 1975). In an attempt to identify the source of the postulated "natriuretic hormone," the effect of selected endocrine organ ablation on the natriuretic response the isolated kidney to blood volume expansion was examined. The findings that adrenalectomy, thyroparathyroidectomy or hypophysectomy did not abrogate the natriuresis in the isolated kidney argue against these glands as the source of the "hormone" (Kaloyanides et al., 1974b).

Renal Pharmacology. Renal vascular resistance and cortical distribution of blood flow change in parallel with renal perfusion pressure (McNay and Abe, 1970). Therefore, in order to accurately assess the effects of a vasoactive agent on renal hemodynamics and blood flow distribution, it is essential that renal arterial pressure be maintained constant, a requirement which cannot always be met in the intact dog if recirculation of the agent alters systemic hemodynamics. The capability of regulating renal arterial pressure in the isolated perfused kidney obviates this problem. Moreover, measurement of blood flow distribution using the radiolabeled microsphere technique is greatly simplified in that reproducible results can be obtained by injecting the spheres directly into the renal arterial cannula (Kaloyanides et al., 1974a).

Several studies illustrate the application of the isolated kidney technique to the study of renal pharmacology. Bastron and Kaloyanides (1972) demonstrated that infusing nitroprusside into the renal artery at a dose sufficient to cause systemic hypotension in the perfusion dog had little effect on RBF and RVR of the isolated kidney when renal arterial pressure was maintained constant. These results indicate that nitroprusside is a weak renal vasodilator. By means of a similar experimental design, it was found that [1-sarcosine-8-alanine] angiotensin II had no effect on renin secretion, sodium excretion, or renal hemodynamics in the isolated kidney, indicating that this angiotensin II antagonist is free of significant agonist properties (Kaloyanides and DiBona, 1976) whereas inhibition of prostaglandin secretion with indomethacin caused a marked decrease in RBF accompanied by redistribution of flow to the outer cortex and antinatriuresis (Kaloyanides et al., 1976). Stowe et al. (1973) used this technique to examine the effect of furosemide on sodium excretion and hemodynamics.

B. Isobaric Perfusion

In 1971, Seely and Boulpaep reported a technique of isobaric perfusion which eliminates arterial pulsation in the dog kidney, thereby allowing the study of surface nephrons by using micropuncture and electrophysiological techniques.

1. Methods

Figure 2 illustrates the technique of isobaric perfusion of the dog kidney. Blood flow from the carotid artery passes through a depulsator and then to the renal artery of the isolated kidney. The depulsator communicates with an air reservoir, the pressure of which is adjusted to maintain perfusion pressure slightly below that in the systemic circulation. Renal venous blood is returned to the jugular vein by a rotameter which continuously monitors RBF. The isolated

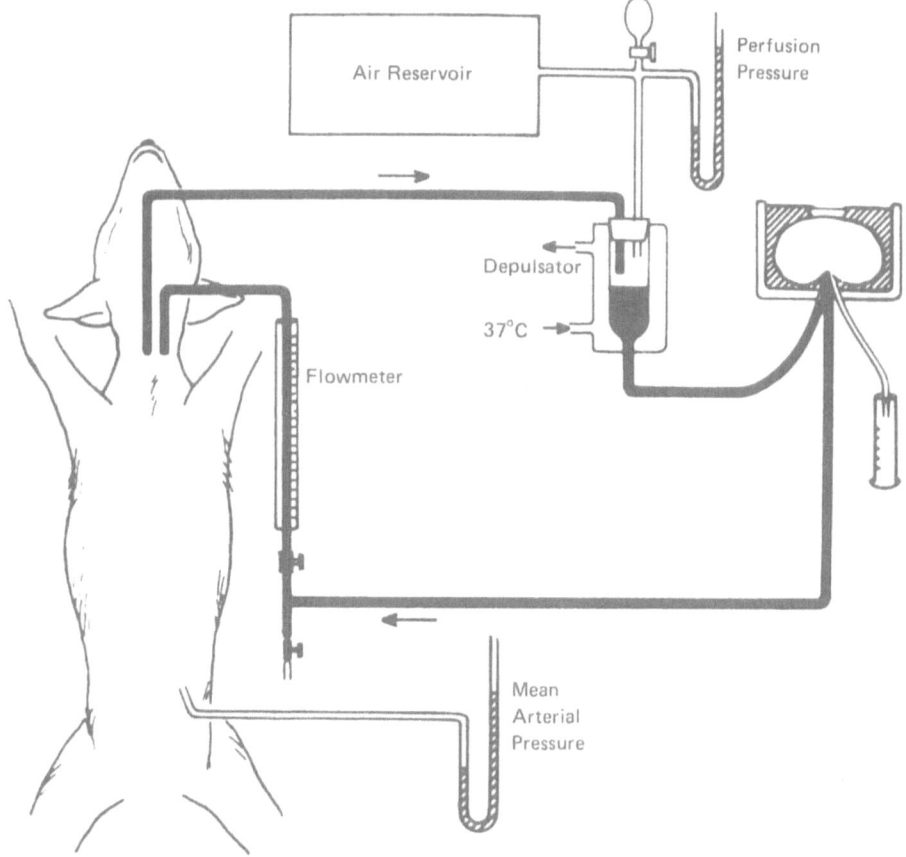

Figure 2. Diagram of circuit for isobaric perfusion of dog kidney. Arterial blood from carotid artery passes through depulsator at 37°C connected to a damping reservoir maintaining a constant perfusion pressure. Isolated kidney is imbedded with agar, leaving a small area on surface accessible for micropuncture. Renal venous blood returns through a rotameter to jugular vein. (From Seely and Boulpaep, 1971, with permission of the American Physiological Society.)

kidney is placed in a lucite chamber and immobilized by Tyrode-agar solution. Systemic heparin is used for anticoagulation. The combination of nonpulsatile blood perfusion plus fixation of the kidney in agar provides sufficient stability for free-flow micropuncture and electrophysiological measurements.

2. Physiology

Hemodynamic and Excretory Function. During the first hour of perfusion, RBF ranged between 3 and 5 ml/min per gram kidney weight but progressively declined to the lower limit of normal after 4 hr of perfusion due to a rise in RVR. GFR of the perfused kidney averaged 0.47 ml/min per gram kidney weight, a value significantly lower than that of the nonperfused kidney. Urine volume, osmolality, and sodium and potassium excretion by the perfused kidney tended to be lower than that of the nonperfused kidney although the differences were not statistically significant. Fractional water excretion and fractional sodium excretion by the perfused kidney averaged 2.19% and 1.37%, respectively.

Micropuncture Data. Proximal tubule transit time in the perfused kidney averaged 31.1 sec compared to 18.2 sec in the intact kidney. Transit time to the early distal tubule was also prolonged. TF/P inulin of proximal tubular fluid averaged 1.61 ± 0.07, indicating a fractional reabsorption rate of 35.2%. These values are similar to those obtained in the intact dog kidney (Dirks and Seely, 1970; Seely and Dirks, 1969). Similar to the intact kidney TF/P chloride of end proximal tubular fluid was greater than unity, signifying that fractional reabsorption of chloride was less than fractional reabsorption of water. Proximal tubule reabsorptive capacity, estimated by the Gertz technique, was similar to that reported for the proximal tubule of the intact dog kidney. Absolute reabsorptive rate determined from free-flow measurements of single nephron GFR and tubular fluid flow rates were not reported.

3. Experimental Application

The technique of isobaric perfusion was developed for the specific purpose of performing electrophysiological measurements in the dog kidney. Thus, Boulpaep and Seely (1971) were able to define for the first time the electrical driving forces mediating transepithelial transport in the dog kidney and to establish that the electrical properties of the dog proximal and distal tubule are similar to those of the rat. This study also provided additional evidence for the existence of a paracellular pathway for fluid and electrolyte transport across the proximal tubular epithelium. The potential of this technique for studying the renal action of drugs at the tubular level has not been explored.

C. Flow-Regulated (Pump) Perfusion

Flow-regulated (pump) perfusion has been the most commonly used technique for studying the isolated dog kidney *in situ* (Richards and Drinker, 1915; Brull, 1950; Selkurt, 1951; Shipley and Study, 1951; Miles *et al.*, 1954; Langston *et al.*, 1959; Hardin *et al.*, 1960; Gilmore, 1964; Zimmerman *et al.*, 1964; Selkurt *et al.*, 1965; Takeuchi *et al.*, 1965; Wolf *et al.*, 1969; and Humphreys *et al.*, 1975). The complexity of the various techniques ranges from simple pump perfusion via a cannula inserted into the renal artery *in situ* (Gilmore, 1964) to complete removal of the kidney with perfusion accomplished via a two-pump extracorporeal circuit connected to the arterial and venous circulation of the dog (Humphreys *et al.*, 1975).

The choice of technique will be dictated by the requirements of the experimental design as well as the functional characteristics and stability of the preparation. In the past, most studies of the pump-perfused isolated dog kidney have focused on hemodynamic parameters, with little assessment of renal excretory function. One exception is the pump-perfused *in situ* dog kidney preparation reported by Wolf *et al.* (1969) which is described below.

1. Methods

The basic technique involves perfusion of the left kidney through a specially designed aortic cannula illustrated in Figure 3. The cannula is made of an 11-gauge stainless steel tube fixed to a stainless steel collar (collar II). Blood enters through one end of the tube and exits through a side hole at the other end. The distal collar (collar I) is fitted with a Teflon ring through which a hole is drilled to permit the collar to slide along the cannula while maintaining a watertight fit. A second hole in the Teflon ring accommodates a small polyethylene catheter to monitor pouch pressure.

Figure 4 illustrates the technique for aortic cannula placement. The aorta is approached retroperitoneally through a flank incision and lumbar arteries in the area of the pouch are ligated. Sutures are loosely placed around the aorta as shown in step 1. Then the aorta is clamped below the renal arteries, the most distal suture is tied and the aorta is transected. In step 2 the cannula is inserted into the aorta and the distal collar is secured in place with a suture. In step 3 the clamp is removed and the cannula is advanced until the proximal collar is positioned between the renal arteries. During this time, flow around the collar

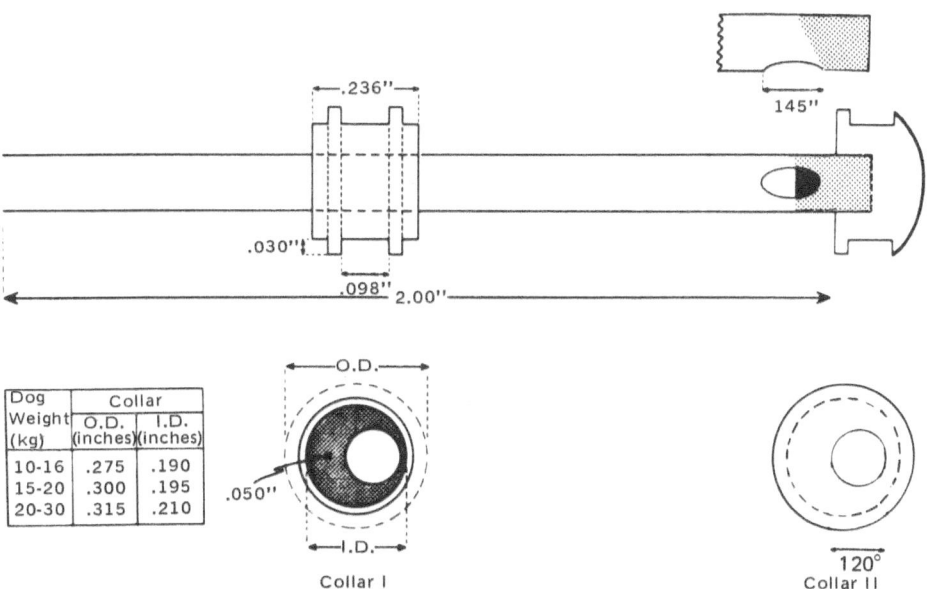

Figure 3. Design of aortic cannula. Cross-hatched pieces are of Teflon, remainder is stainless steel. Insert in lower left indicates diameter sizes used in dogs of various weight. (From Wolf *et al.*, 1969, with permission of the American Physiological Society.)

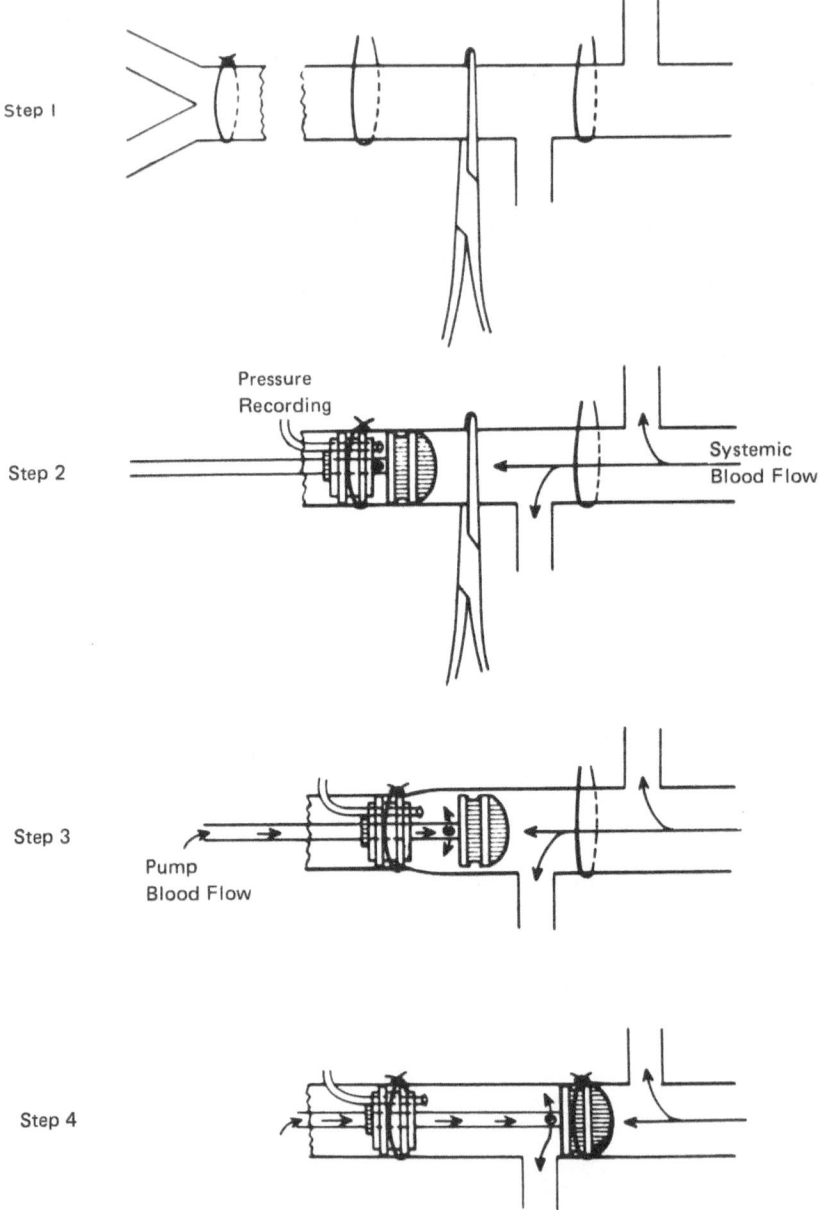

Figure 4. Installation of aortic cannula. Teflon core in collar I allows collars to be approximated for insertion in step 2. When clamp is released, full aortic pressure recorded from polyethylene tube in collar I indicates free flow of blood around collar II. Pump is turned on before completion of step 4. No ischemia is incurred by either kidney during cannula placement. (From Wolf et al., 1969, with permission of the American Physiological Society.)

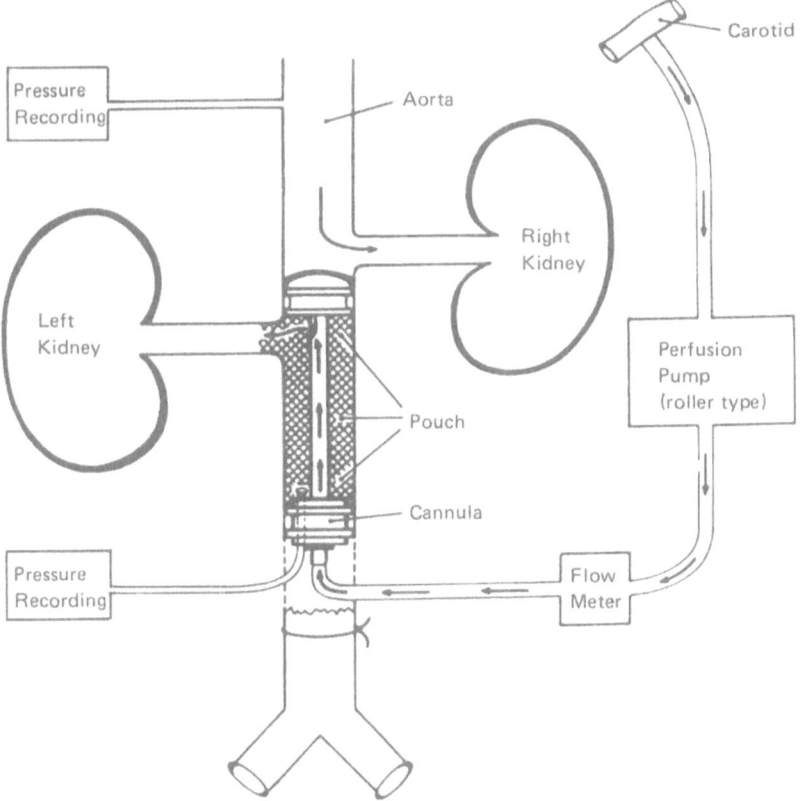

Figure 5. Aortic pouch perfussion model for differential right and left renal circulation. Surgical elimination of two pairs of lumbar arteries (not shown) leaves only left renal artery for outflow from aortic pouch. (From Wolf *et al.*, 1969, with permission of the American Physiological Society.)

maintains perfusion of the left kidney. Before the collar is secured in place, the pump is activated so that renal blood flow is not interrupted.

Figure 5 illustrates the completed procedure. The extracorporeal circuit which consists of Silastic tubing, a pump and an electromagnetic flow probe, delivers blood from the carotid artery to the aortic cannula. The authors report that priming the circuit with 200 U of heparin plus a constant heparin infusion of 12 U/min into the carotid arterial line is sufficient to prevent coagulation.

2. Physiology

This technique, similar to isobaric perfusion, allows comparison of function in the perfused and nonperfused kidneys (Table I). When renal perfusion pressure of the isolated kidney was within 15 mm Hg of the nonperfused kidney, there were no significant differences in GFR, C_{PAH}, filtration fraction, urine volume, or solute excretion. Fractional sodium reabsorption averaged 97.8% of the filtered load in the perfused kidney compared to 98.2% in the nonperfused

Table I. Comparison of Function of Perfused and Nonperfused Kidneys[a]

	PP (mm Hg)	C_{IN} (ml/min)	C_{PAH} (ml/min)	FF	UV (ml/min)	$U_{Na}V$ (μmol/min)	U_KV (μmol/min)	$U_{osm}V$ (μosmol/min)
Perfused	133	34	100	0.334	2.0	105	38	473
	±7	±4	±5	±0.026	±.24	±20	±4	±25
Nonperfused	135	36	103	0.355	2.0	89	35	475
	±5	±3	±5	±0.029	±.16	±15	±3	±25
p	>0.20	>0.05	>0.20	>0.05	>0.50	>0.10	>0.10	>0.10

[a] Data represent mean ± S.E. of 15 paired collections; PP, perfusion pressure, FF, filtration fraction. (From Wolf et al., 1969.)

kidney; $p > 0.5$. RBF averaged 3.44 ± 0.15 ml/min per gram kidney weight, which approaches the lower limit of normal for the dog kidney. GFR averaged 0.54 ml/min per gram. According to the authors, "the stability of the preparation at constant flow was excellent and adjustments in the pump rate were necessary only once or twice an experiment."

3. Experimental Application

Although autoregulation has been examined in the flow-regulated isolated kidney (Shipley and Study, 1951; Miles *et al.*, 1954, Langston *et al.*, 1959; Takeuchi *et al.*, 1965; Herbaczysnka-Cedro and Vane, 1973), the suitability of this technique for defining autoregulatory phenomena is open to question. The reversal of the normal pressure-flow relationship in the kidney dictates that blood flow must be increased in order to increase perfusion pressure. Out of necessity, therefore, autoregulation of RBF will be incomplete. Moreover, in some instances little or no autoregulation was evident in the flow-regulated kidney (Langston *et al.*, 1959; Herbaczynska-Cedro and Vane, 1973).

The reversal of the normal pressure–flow relationship also opens to question the suitability of the flow-regulated kidney for studying the influence of renal perfusion pressure on electrolyte and water excretion (Selkurt, 1951; Selkurt *et al.*, 1965; Langston *et al.*, 1959).

In contrast to pressure-regulated or isobaric perfusion, the renal nerves can be left intact in flow-regulated perfusion; thus, it is possible to study the influence of neurogenic stimuli on renal function during constant RBF or pressure (Gilmore, 1964).

One of the earliest applications of the flow-regulated isolated perfused kidney technique was to investigate the mechanism of drug action on the kidney (Richards and Plant, 1915). The study of renal pharmacology probably constitutes the most important application of this technique (Dluhy *et al.*, 1970). The potential for elucidating drug action at the tubular level by micropuncture under conditions of constant perfusion pressure or blood flow warrants investigation.

REFERENCES

Andersen, R. J., Taher, M. S., Cronin, R. E., McDonald, K. M., and Schrier, R. W. 1975. Effect of β-adrenergic blockade and inhibitors of angiotensin II and prostaglandin on renal autoregulation. *Am. J. Physiol., 229:*731.

Bastron, R. D., and Kaloyanides, G. J. 1972. Effect of sodium nitroprusside on function in the isolated and intact dog kidney. *J. Pharmacol. Exp. Therap., 181:*244.

Boulpaep, E. L., and Seely, J. F. 1971. Electrophysiology of proximal and distal tubules in the autoperfused dog kidney. *Am. J. Physiol., 221:*1084.

Brull, L. 1950. Mechanical heart with coagulable blood. *Arch. Internat. Physiol., 58:*8.

DiBona, G. F., Kaloyanides, G. J., and Bastron, R. D. 1972. Response of the isolated kidney to saline infusion. *Proc. Soc. Exp. Biol. Med., 140:*1405.

DiBona, G. F., Kaloyanides, G. J., and Bastron, R. D. 1973. Effect of increased perfusion pressure on proximal tubular reabsorption in the isolated kidney. *Proc. Soc. Exp. Biol. Med., 143:*830.

Dirks, J. H., and Seely, J. F. 1970. Effect of saline infusion and furosemide on the dog distal nephron. *Am. J. Physiol., 219:*114.

Dirks, J. H., Cirksena, W. J., and Berliner, R. W. 1965. The effect of saline infusion on sodium reabsorption by the proximal tubule of the dog. *J. Clin. Invest., 44:*1160.

Dluhy, R. G., Wolf, G. L., and Lauler, D. P. 1970. Vasodilator properties of ethancrynic acid in the perfused dog kidney. *Clin. Sci., 38:*347.

Gilmore, J. P. 1964. Contribution of baroreceptors to the control of renal function. *Circ. Res., 14:*301.

Hardin, R. A., Scott, J. B., and Haddy, F. 1960. Relationship of pressure to blood flow in the dog kidney. *Am. J. Physiol., 199:*1192.

Herbaczynska-Cedro, K., and Vane, J. R. 1973. Contribution of intrarenal generation of prostaglandin to autoregulation of renal blood flow in the dog. *Circ. Res., 33:*428.

Humphreys, M. H., Reid, I. A., Ufferman, R. C., Lieberman, R. A., and Earley, L. E. 1975. The relationship between sodium excretion and renin secretion by the perfused kidney. *Proc. Soc. Exp. Biol. Med., 150:*728.

Kaloyanides, G. J., and Azer, M. 1971. Evidence for a humoral mechanism in volume expansion natriuresis. *J. Clin. Invest., 50:*1603.

Kaloyanides, G. J., and Azer, M. 1972. Failure to demonstrate a humoral mechanism in the antinatriuresis of acute caval constriction. *J. Clin. Invest., 51:*1297.

Kaloyanides, G. J., and DiBona, G. F. 1976. Effect of an angiotensin II antagonist on autoregulation in the isolated dog kidney. *Am. J. Physiol., 230:*1078.

Kaloyanides, G. J., DiBona, G. F., and Raskin, P. 1971. Pressure natriuresis in the isolated kidney. *Am. J. Physol., 220:*1660.

Kaloyanides, G. J., Bastron, R. D., and DiBona, G. F. 1973a. Effect of ureteral clamping and increased renal arterial pressure on renin release. *Amer. J. Physiol., 225:*95.

Kaloyanides, G. J., Bastron, R. D., and DiBona, G. F. 1973b. Role of increased renal blood flow and blood flow distribution in the natriuresis of renal vasodilatation and elevated perfusion pressure. *Clin. Res., 21:*691.

Kaloyanides, G. J., Bastron, R. D., and DiBona, G. F. 1974a. Impaired autoregulation of blood flow and glomerular filtration rate in the isolated dog kidney depleted of renin. *Circ. Res., 35:*400.

Kaloyanides, G. J., Cohen, L., Bastron, R. D., and DiBona, G. F. 1974b. Effect of organ ablation on the natriuresis of extracellular volume expansion in the isolated kidney. *Clin. Res., 22:*533.

Kaloyanides, G. J., DiBona, G. F., and Bastron, R. D. 1974c. Response of the isolated kidney to acute volume expansion with equilibrated blood, *Proc. Soc. Exp. Biol. Med., 147:*619.

Kaloyanides, G. J., DiBona, G. F., and Bastron, R. D. 1975. Effect of blood volume expansion on tubule sodium transport in the isolated dog kidney. *Proc. Soc. Exp. Biol. Med., 148:*765.

Kaloyanides, G. J., Ahrens, R. E., Shepherd, J. A., and DiBona, G. F. 1976. Inhibition of prostaglandin E_2 secretion: failure to abolish autoregulation in the isolated dog kidney. *Circ. Res., 38:*67.

Langston, J. B., Guyton, A. C., and Gillespie, W. J., Jr. 1959. Acute effect of changes in renal arterial pressure and sympathetic blockade on kidney function. *Am. J. Physiol., 197:*595.

McDonald, S. J., and DeWardener, H. E. 1965. The relationship between the renal arterial perfusion pressure and the increase in sodium excretion which occurs during an infusion of saline. *Nephron, 2:*1.

McNay, J. L., and Abe, Y. 1970. Pressure dependent heterogeneity of renal cortical blood flow in dogs. *Circ. Res., 27:*571.

Miles, B. E., Ventom, M. G., and DeWardener, H. E. 1954. Observations on the mechanism of circulatory autoregulation in the perfused dog's kidney. *J. Physiol., 123:*143.

Nizet, A. 1975. The isolated perfused kidney: possibilities, limitations and results. *Kidney Internat., 7:*1.

Richards, A. N., and Drinker, C. K. 1915. An apparatus for the perfusion of isolated organs. *J. Pharmacol. Exp. Therap., 7:*467.

Richards, A. N., and Plant, O. H. 1915. Urine formation by the perfused kidney: preliminary experiments on the action of caffeine. *J. Pharmacol. Exp. Therap., 7:*485.

Schrier, R. W., and Humphreys, M. H. 1971. Factors involved in the antinatriuretic effects of acute constriction of the thoracic and abdominal inferior vena cava. *Circ. Res., 29:*479.

Schrier, R. W., Humphreys, M. H., and Ufferman, R. C. 1971. Role of cardiac output and the autonomic nervous system in the antinatriuretic response to acute constriction of the thoracic superior vena cava. *Circ. Res., 29:*490.

Seely, J. F., and Boulpaep, E. L. 1971. Renal function studies on the isobaric autoperfused dog kidney. *Am. J. Physiol., 221:*1075.

Seely, J. F., and Dirks, J. H. 1969. Micropuncture study of hypertonic mannitol diuresis in the proximal and distal tubule of the dog kidney. *J. Clin. Invest., 48:*2330.

Selkurt, E. E. 1951. Effect of pulse pressure and mean arterial pressure modification on renal hemodynamics and electrolyte and water excretion. *Circulation, 4:*541.

Selkurt, E. E. 1963. The renal circulation, In: *Handbook of Physiology,* Vol. II, *Circulation.* Ed. by Hamilton, W. F., pp. 1457–1516. American Physiological Society, Washington, D.C.

Selkurt, E. E., Womack, I., and Dailey, W. N. 1965. Mechanism of natriuresis and diuresis during elevated renal arterial pressure. *Am. J. Physiol., 209:*95.

Semple, S. J. G., and DeWardener, H. E. 1959. Effect of increased venous pressure on circulatory autoregulation of isolated dog kidneys. *Circ. Res., 7:*643.

Shipley, R. E., and Study, R. S. 1951. Changes in renal blood flow, extraction of inulin, glomerular filtration rate, tissue pressure, and urine flow with acute alterations of renal artery blood pressure. *Am. J. Physiol., 167:*676.

Smith, H. W. 1951. *The Kidney, Structure and Function in Health and Disease,* Oxford University Press, New York.

Starling, E. H., and Verney, E. B. 1925. Secretion of urine as studied on the isolated kidney. *Proc. Roy. Soc. Ser. B Biol. Sci., 97:*321.

Stowe, N. T., Wolterink, L. F., Lewis, A. E., and Hook, J. B. 1973. Diuretic and hemodynamic effects of furosemide in the isolated dog kidney. *Arch. Pharmacol., 277:*13.

Takeuchi, J., Tadashi, K., Sawada, T., Funaki, E., Sanada, M., Kitagawa, T., and Nakada, Y. 1965. Autoregulation of renal circulation. *Jap. Heart J., 6:*243.

Venuto, R. C., O'Dorisio, T., Ferris, T. F., and Stein, J. H. 1975. Prostaglandins and renal function. II: The effect of prostaglandin inhibition on autoregulation of blood flow in the intact kidney of the dog. *Prostaglandins, 9:*818.

Verney, E. B. 1926. The secretion of pituitrin in mammals as shown by perfusion of the isolated kidney of the dog. *Proc. Roy. Soc. Ser. B. Biol. Sci., 99:*486.

Wolf, G. L., Dluhy, R. G., and Lauler, D. P. 1969. Physiology of the pump-perfused *in situ* dog kidney. *Am. J. Physiol., 217:*1809.

Zimmerman, B. G., Abboud, F. M., and Eckstein, J. W. 1964. Effects of norepinephrine and angiotensin on total and venous resistance in the kidney. *Am. J. Physiol., 206:*701.

Chapter **14**

Methodology for Study of Isolated Perfused Dog Kidney *in Vitro*

Alphonse H. Nizet

Department of Medical Clinics and Semiology
Institute of Medicine
University of Liège, Belgium

I. INTRODUCTION

The first investigations with totally isolated, blood perfused kidneys are more than a century old (Löbell, 1849; Bidder, 1862; Ludwig, 1868–69; Bunge and Schmiedeberg, 1877). Jacobj (1890) utilized a pump-oxygenator system and defibrinated blood; although the urine secreted proved to be different from a transudate (Jacobj and Sobieranski, 1892), the functional performance was poor and the blood flow was very low because of an intense vasoconstriction. Similar observations were made by Pfaff and Vejnx-Tyrode (1903) and Pavy *et al.* (1903). A better renal blood flow was achieved by Bainbridge and Evans (1914) with a perfusion circuit including the heart, the lung, and the kidney; the urine volume was small. Improved results were obtained by Starling and Verney (1925) with freshly defibrinated blood; these authors encountered the same difficulties as their predecessors when they attempted to replace the heart by a mechanical pump and they concluded, "It seems that the defibrinated blood becomes detoxicated in the heart-lung preparation, presumably in the lungs." Hemingway (1931) observed the vasoconstrictor properties of defibrinated blood and introduced a lung in the perfusion circuit during the initial phase of the experiments. Pump-lung preparations were also utilized by Bickford and Winton (1937), Kramer and Winton (1939), and Bing (1941). Another attempt to solve the problem has been the addition to the blood of various drugs such as chloral, amyl nitrite (Pavy *et al.*, 1903), or ergot preparations (Heymans *et al.*, 1932; Bing, 1941). Bayliss and Ogden (1932–33) found that heparinized blood also develops vasoconstrictor properties within a few minutes; assuming that the blood should be "detoxicated" by the kidney itself, they worked with a very small volume of blood; however the renal blood flow did not exceed 50–75% of its normal values. The vasoconstrictor properties of heparinized blood were confirmed by Brull and Louis-Bar (1957). The active material is released by the red blood cells (Nizet *et al.*, 1957c; Lustinec, 1965).

A systematic approach to the problem led to the following conclusions (Nizet *et al.*, 1957c). (a) The vasoconstrictor material is detectable in the heparinized blood at 37°C as early as 3 min after storage; the vasoconstriction increases and reaches its maximum after 30–40 min. The active material is not serotonin (Cuypers *et al.*, 1957). The vasoconstriction, if not too prolonged, is reversible upon perfusion with fresh blood. (b) The release of this material cannot be lessened by the contact of the blood with nonwettable (siliconized) surfaces. (c) The development of vasoconstriction is considerably accelerated by hemolysis and by mechanical stirring of the blood with various types of pumps. Only one passage of fresh blood drawn from the carotid artery through a rotating or alternative piston pump reduces the renal blood flow to about 60% of its normal value. (d) At a constant mean arterial pressure, the renal blood flow does not depend on the presence or absence of pulsations. The vasoconstrictor effect is abolished by decalcification of the blood (Nizet *et al.*, 1957a). That the contact of the blood with abnormal surfaces is not primarily responsible is confirmed by the fact that heparinized blood stored within a large blood vessel develops vasoconstrictor properties as fast as in glass or Plexiglas containers (Nizet *et al.*, 1959). The vasoconstrictor material present in protein-free extracts from red blood cells as well as the whole blood is neutralized by the lung (Nizet *et al.*, 1957b). Moreover, the vasoconstriction is suppressed by passage of the blood through the liver and the kidney (Cuypers *et al.*, 1961).

A solution to the problem can be found on the basis of the above-mentioned results provided that a series of conditions are fulfilled, the final functional performances of the perfused organ depending on a series of technical requirements (Nizet and Cuypers, 1962):

1. The perfusion should start with blood withdrawn from the donor animal within a maximum delay of 3 min, that is, before the development of significant vasoconstrictor activity. Moreover, a short-acting vasodilating drug must be added at the beginning.
2. The mechanical stirring of the blood in oxygenator, pump, and tubing should be reduced as much as possible. The choice of nonwettable material is of much lesser importance.
3. The mean interval of time between two passages of the blood through the kidney should not exceed 3 min; in these conditions, the neutralization of the vasoconstrictor material by this organ is faster than its release into the blood. The total volume of blood should therefore not exceed 15 times the weight of the kidney.

We shall now consider the description of the equipment, the general pattern of one experiment, the behavior of the perfused kidney as concerns its basic functional parameters, and some technical solutions which may limit the drawbacks of the technique.

II. DESCRIPTION OF EQUIPMENT

A. Oxygenator

Any type of oxygenator, such as a bubble oxygenator, which induces intense stirring of the blood and the formation of foam, is to be excluded. Membrane oxygenators proved quite satisfactory (Berkowitz *et al.*, 1967, 1968). Another suitable solution is to put a thin film of blood in direct contact with the gaseous mixture. Our oxygenator is made of two concentric Plexiglas cylinders in a vertical position (Figures 1 and 2). The venous blood is distributed on the internal surface of the external cylinder and on the external surface of the internal cylinder by a disk rotating at a speed of 12 rpm. The total surface

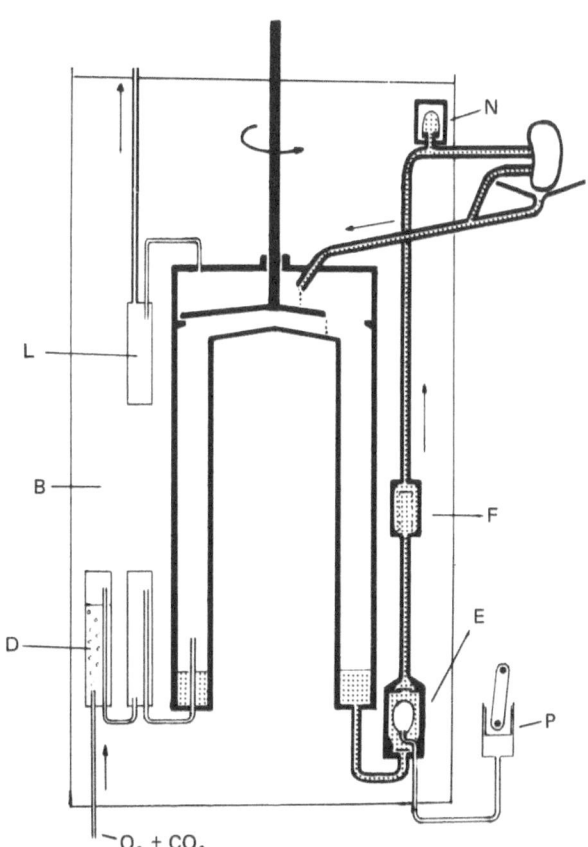

Figure 1. Schematic view of the double-cylinder oxygenator with rotating disk. B, thermostatic bath; E, Dale–Schuster pump; P, external, adjustable hydraulic control of the pump; F, filter; N, pulse damper; D, humidifier; L, trap for condensation water.

$O_2 + CO_2$

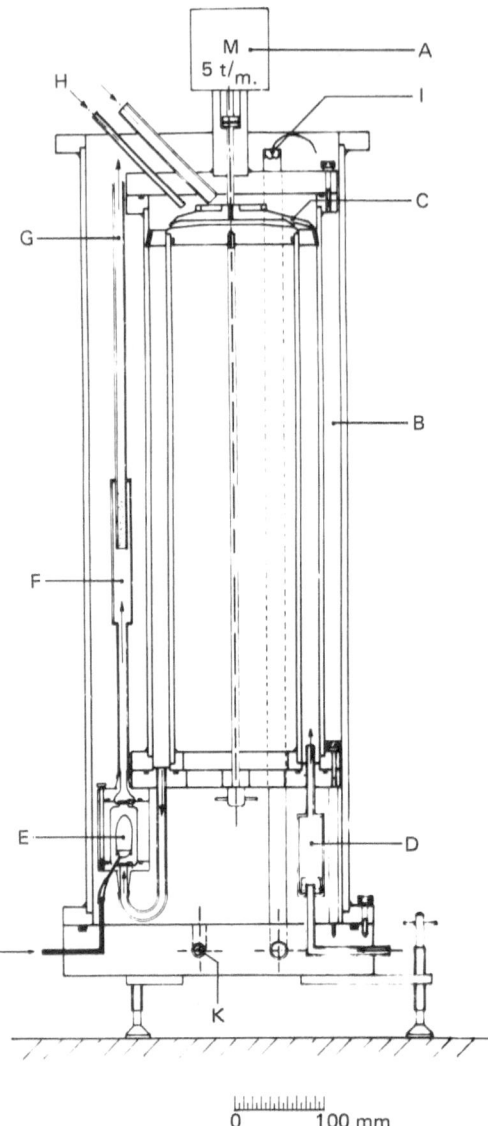

Figure 2. Detailed view of perfusion equipment. A, motor; B, thermostatic bath; C, rotating disk; D, gas humidifier; E, pump; F, filter; G, outlet of arterial blood; H, return of venous blood; I, outlet of thermostatic bath; K, inlet of thermostatic bath. (From Cuypers *et al.*, 1964, with permission.)

available for spreading out the blood film is about 0.6 m². The oxygenated blood is collected at the bottom of the space between the two cylinders. The oxygenator is contained in a thermostatic bath together with the pump and most of the tubing (Cuypers *et al.*, 1964). Waugh and Kubo (1969) successfully utilized a flat, filted Plexiglas surface of about 0.15 m² area, and 29 cm wide; an adjustable Plexiglas rod, 2 cm in diameter, ensures uniform repartition of the blood film. A gas mixture containing 95–97% oxygen and 3–5% carbon dioxide allows convenient oxygenation with stable pH and PCO_2 of the blood.

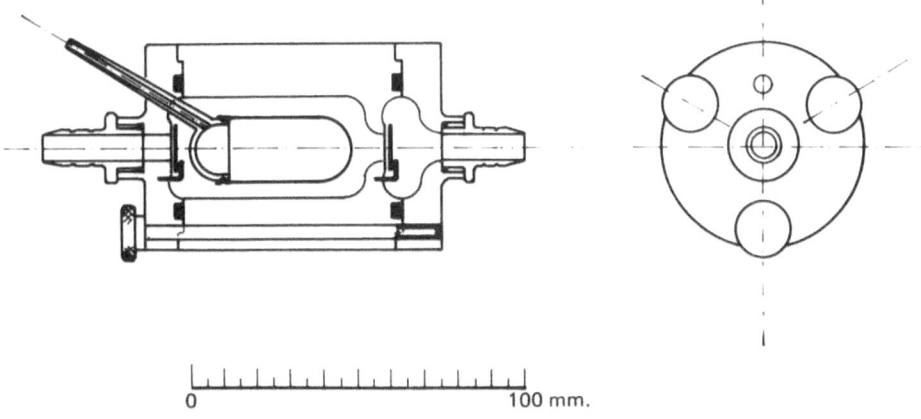

Figure 3. The pump is made of a Plexiglas cylinder fixed between two stainless steel disks. The piston is made of a dilatable tube such as a finger-stall and is controlled hydraulically. (From Cuypers *et al.*, 1964, with permission.)

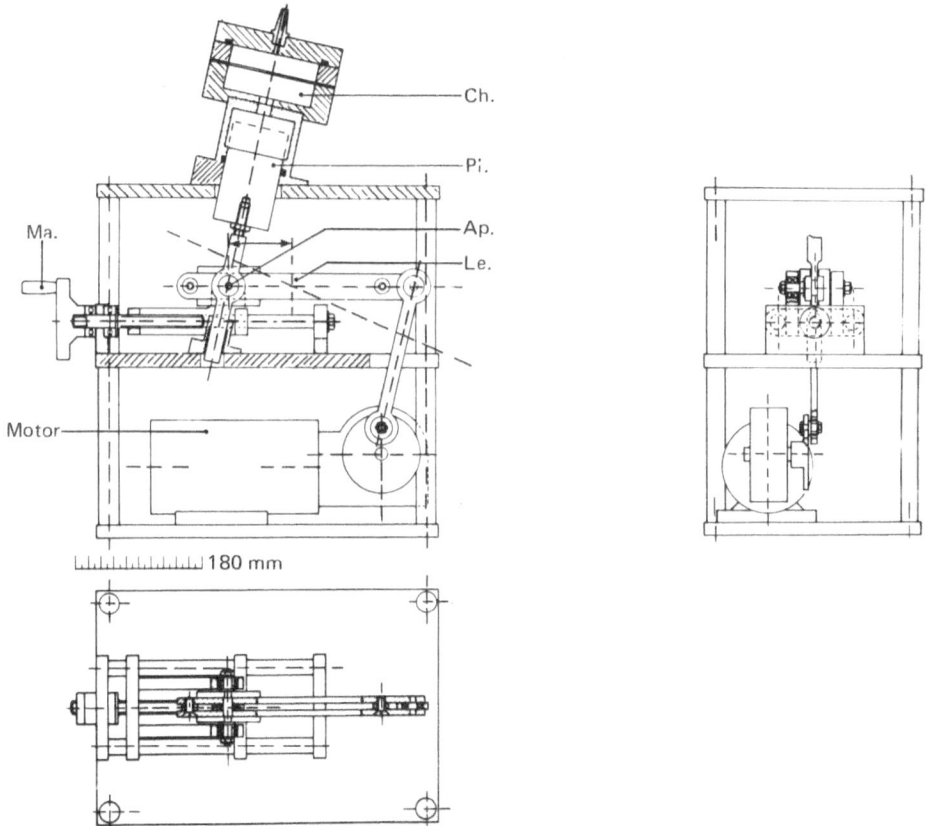

Figure 4. External control of the pump. Ch, chamber filled with water for hydraulic transmission; Pi, piston and cylinder; Ap., Le, rods and connections to the piston; Ma, crank connected to a screw and controlling the course of piston and systolic output. (From Cuypers *et al.*, 1964, with permission.)

B. Pump

Continuous flow, rotating type pumps and mechanical piston pumps are not suitable because of excessive hemolysis. Two types of pumps have proved to give good results. Waugh and Kubo (1969) utilized a 20-ml vinyl plastic ventricle with two bicuspid valves and compressed by an adjustable cam; similar pumps were included in the perfusion systems of Barkin *et al.* (1963) and Berkowitz *et al.* (1968). We choose a Dale-Schuster type pump with two light discoidal valves, controlled hydraulically by an independent motor-driven piston (Figures 1, 3, 4). The systolic volume can be adjusted continuously between 0 and 45 ml, the pulse rate being 2 per second. It is convenient to put a damping chamber with an air cushion between the pump and the kidney (Figure 1) (Cuypers *et al.*, 1964).

C. Heating

Two types of solutions can be retained. The first is represented by a heat exchanger consisting of parallel tubes immersed in a thermostatic bath at 39°C and located between the pump and the kidney (Waugh and Kubo, 1969). The second solution is to immerse oxygenator, pump, and most of tubing in a thermostatic bath at 37.5°C; only the kidney and the adjacent parts of tubing are out of the bath (Cuypers *et al.*, 1964).

D. Tubing

Tubing should be as short as possible, with gentle bents. Our equipment includes polyvinyl and glass tubes of about 20 mm internal diameter.

E. Filter

A filter should be put between the pump and the kidney; the filters included in blood transfusion sets are quite convenient.

F. Kidney Holder

Some degree of hemorrhage is unavoidable with heparinized blood. Two solutions can be chosen. In the first (Waugh and Kubo, 1969), the venous blood flows freely into a funnel; the total outflow can be measured with a graduated spout. The second solution (Figure 5) involves the cannulation of the renal vein or of the vena cava; only the blood lost by bleeding is collected by the funnel and is sent back into the oxygenator together with venous blood; an accurate measurement of renal blood flow is obtained by connecting a graduated pipet to the distal end of the vena cava (Cuypers *et al.*, 1964).

G. Building Material

According to our experience, building material does not represent a critical point. Stainless steel, Plexiglas, polyvinyl tubing are adequate; siliconization is

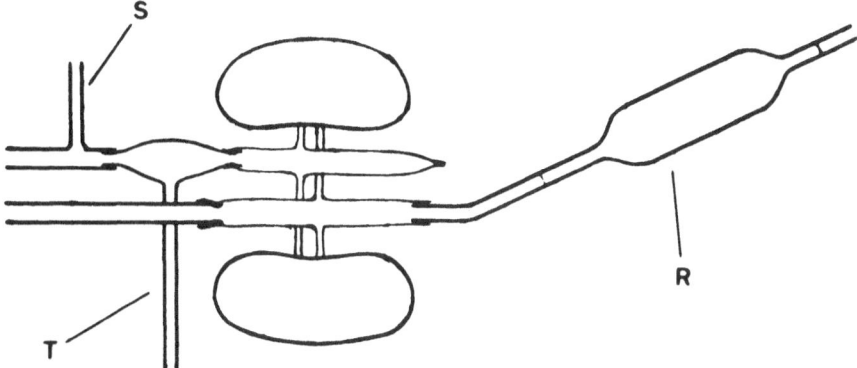

Figure 5. At left side, connections of the kidneys with the perfusion machine. The tubes S and T, on the arterial side, are connected to a manometer and allow the initial purging of air bubbles and blood sampling. The graduated pipet, R, allows an accurate measurement of blood flow during temporary clamping of venous return.

not necessary. Surfaces should be cleaned after use with pure water without detergents. New Plexiglas surfaces should be carefully rubbed with Vaseline before first use; the new material may release into the blood some toxic agents, inducing total anuria. A complete view of perfusion equipment is presented in Figure 6.

III. PLANNING AN EXPERIMENT

The same animal can serve as kidney and blood donor, one kidney only being perfused (Nizet *et al.*, 1967). It is also possible to utilize one dog as a blood donor and another dog as a kidney donor; moreover, such a procedure allows the simultaneous and independent perfusion of the two kidneys of the same pair by two machines (see below).

After narcosis (30 mg Nembutal/kg body weight), one carotid artery is cannulated for blood withdrawal and the kidney pair is dissected. Heparin is injected intravenously into the blood donor (1250 U/kg body weight). For a kidney weight between 30 and 60 g, 450 ml of arterial blood are collected and introduced immediately into the oxygenator. The kidneys are removed in the meantime after clamping aorta and vena cava; immediately before their connection to the perfusion machine, the pump is put into operation in order to fill tubing, filter, and damper with blood and to remove air bubbles. The interruption of renal blood flow should not exceed 5 min. A slight initial vasoconstriction can be avoided by addition of 25 mg promethazine to the blood or by a continuous intraarterial infusion of acetylcholine. Mean arterial pressure is adjusted to 110–140 mm Hg by control of the pump. A circulation of a humidified gaseous mixture containing 95% O_2 and 5% CO_2 is ensured throughout the experiment.

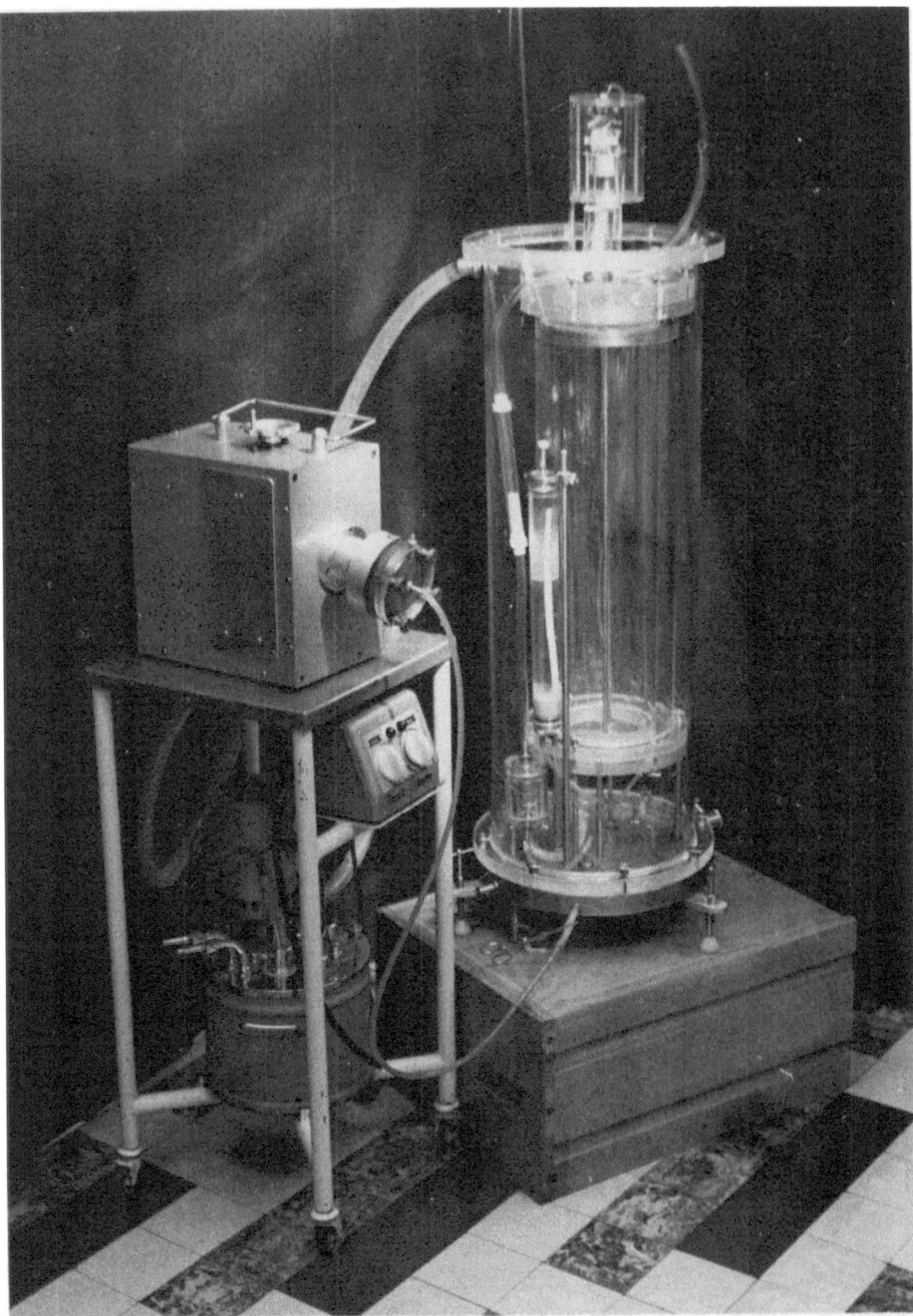

Figure 6. View of perfusion equipment. At left, control for pump and of thermostatic bath. Upper right: tubes for connection to the perfused organ.

Two procedures can be chosen for replacement of excreted water and solutes and of metabolic substrates.

1. If the total amount of excreted urine is collected, a continuous infusion is performed, at a rate of 6 ml/hr, of a solution containing 2 g glucose, 2 g urea, and 1.5 g potassium chloride per 100 ml of Ringer's fluid. In addition, urine is replaced periodically by equal volumes of Ringer's fluid, which should be diluted to one half if water diuresis is not avoided by supplementation with vasopressin.
2. The excreted urine is circulated back into the oxygenator and only small samples are collected at intervals. A steady state is reached and fluid replacement and infusion are performed as above but during collection periods only.

According to the experiments of Waugh and Kubo (1969), who obtained successful results with freshly defibrinated blood, the functional performance of the kidneys is improved by supplementation with additional substrates such as pyruvate, lactate, and citrate, and with proline; moreover, the embolization of fat droplets is minimized by addition to the defibrinated blood of pancreatic lipase or of an emulsifier such as Pluronic F-68. The total duration of one experiment should not exceed 5 hr, unless perfusion blood is periodically replaced.

IV. FUNCTIONAL BEHAVIOR OF THE KIDNEY

The same pattern of behavior has been observed by all recent investigators.

Renal blood flow. The renal blood flow remains stable at a normal value for about 1 hr. Afterward, it increases progressively and reaches abnormally high levels (Table I). This progressive vasodilatation seems to be related to the release of bradykininlike factors (Nizet *et al.*, 1967) and of prostaglandins (Vanherweghem *et al.*, 1975). A simultaneous and progressive loss of the autoregulation of renal blood flow is observed (Nizet, 1963; Berkowitz *et al.*, 1967; Waugh and Kubo, 1969). This loss of autoregulation parallels the depletion of angiotensinogen and might be the direct consequence of vasodilatation (Berkowitz *et al.*, 1967); it might also be related to a depletion of metabolic substrates (Waugh and Kubo, 1969). Together with the vasodilatation, there is some shift of blood flow from outer cortex toward inner cortex and medulla (Nizet *et al.*, 1967; Itskowitz *et al.*, 1973; Gagnon *et al.*, 1974). The extraction of *p*-aminohippurate is abnormally low (40–60%) (Schröder *et al.*, 1965; Waugh and Kubo, 1969); the tubular secretion of this substance is impaired (Fontaine *et al.*, 1969).

Glomerular filtration rate. Subnormal to normal values can be achieved (40–80 ml/min per 100 g) (Nizet *et al.*, 1967; Waugh and Kubo, 1969), followed by a progressive decrease after 2–4 hr. This impairment might be due partly to embolization of fat droplets in the glomeruli (Waugh and Kubo, 1969), partly to an increase of proximal intratubular pressure as a consequence of the interstitial

Alphonse H. Nizet

Table I. Renal Blood Flow and Glomerular Filtration Rate

Reference	Perfusion pressure (mm Hg)	Renal plasma flow (ml/min per g) and duration of perfusion	Glomerular filtration rate (ml/min per 100 g) and duration of perfusion
Schröder et al. (1965) Heparinized blood	90–120	3.07 ± 0.89 (15 min) 3.22 ± 1.07 (45 min)	26 ± 13 (15 min) 23 ± 9 (45 min)
Nizet et al. (1967) Heparinized blood	110	4.5 ± 0.7 (1 hr) 6 ± 1.2 (3 hr)	50.1 ± 6.9 (30 min) 50.1 ± 6.9 (2 hr)
Berkowitz et al. (1967) Heparinized blood	130	2.1 ± 0.5 (1 hr) 4.5 ± 1 (3 hr)	36 ± 9 (1 hr) 36 ± 9 (3 hr)
Waugh and Kubo (1969) Heparinized blood	100–120	4 ± 1.1 (0–1.30 hr) 6.5 ± 1.5 (3.30 hr–4.30 hr)	46 ± 7 (0–1.30 hr) 23 ± 10 (3.30–4.30 hr)
Defibrinated blood	100–120	4.7 ± 1 (0–1.30 hr) 7.4 ± 1.2 (3.30 hr–4.30 hr)	69 ± 9 (0–1.30 hr) 43 ± 8 (3.30–4.30 hr)

edema (Nizet *et al.*, 1967) which develops during the perfusion (Barkin *et al.*, 1963) (Table I).

Urine volume and concentration. A fairly high osmolality (800 mOsM) can be reached during the first hour of perfusion; later a typical water diuresis develops (60–150 mOsM) which is avoided by vasopressin supplementation (Nizet, 1963; Nizet *et al.*, 1967; Craig *et al.*, 1966; Berkowitz *et al.*, 1967; Kulatilake, 1967; Waugh and Kubo, 1969; Gagnon *et al.*, 1974). However, after 3–4 hr, the urine becomes uniformly isotonic. The loss of concentrating ability appears to be due to the washout of corticomedullary osmotic gradient by increased deep cortical and medullary blood flow (Nizet *et al.*, 1967; Gagnon *et al.*, 1974).

Sodium excretion. The fractional reabsorption of sodium depends on the previous dietary sodium balance of the kidney and blood donors (Table II). While it can reach normal values at the beginning, it decreases progressively after 2–3 hr; the impaired reabsorption of sodium might be the consequence of an accumulation of ammonia in the blood (Kulatilake, 1967; Waugh and Kubo, 1969). According to the experiments, of Waugh and Kubo (1969), the reabsorption of sodium is enhanced by supplementation with glucose, lactate, pyruvate, and proline.

Potassium excretion averages 30 μEq/100 g per min and is not clearly related to sodium excretion (Nizet *et al.*, 1967).

Acidification of urine. The isolated, blood perfused dog kidney is unable to secrete an acidic urine (Nizet, 1963; Kulatilake, 1967; Waugh and Kubo, 1969).

Urea, glucose, and phosphate excretion. Urea clearance represents about 60% of creatinine clearance (Nizet *et al.*, 1967). The T_m of glucose is proportional to the glomerular filtration rate and is not different from its values *in situ*; the T_m of phosphate is proportional to the filtered load of this ion and is considerably higher than *in situ* (Nizet, 1972).

Proteinuria. No abnormal proteinuria was observed by Waugh and Kubo (1969) or by us.

Changes in perfusion blood. In the above-mentioned experimental conditions involving oxygenation with a O_2/CO_2 gas mixture, replacement of urine, and continuous supplementation with water and solutes, the plasma concentra-

Table II. Overall Fractional Excretion of Sodium

Reference	Perfusion pressure (mm Hg)	Fractional excretion of sodium (% of filtered load) and duration of perfusion	
Schröder *et al.* (1965)	90–120	2.8 (15 min)	5 (30 min)
Nizet *et al.* (1967)			
Salt-depleted dogs	110		0.36 ± 0.09 (2 hr)
Salt-loaded dogs	110		2.50 ± 0.43 (1 hr)
Berkowitz *et al.* (1967)	130	4.90 ± 0.68 (1 hr)	11.50 ± 2.83 (3 hr)
Waugh and Kubo (1969)	100–120	0.90 ± 0.80 (0–1.30 hr)	4.10 ± 0.85 (3.30–4.30 hr)

tion of ions, solutes, and proteins as well as hematocrit, pH and pCO_2 can be kept practically constant (Nizet, 1963; Kulatilake, 1967; Waugh and Kubo, 1969). Some degree of mechanical hemolysis cannot be avoided; after 4 hr of perfusion the hemoglobin content of the plasma ranges between 80 and 200 mg/100 ml (Kulatilake, 1967; Berkowitz et al., 1967; Waugh and Kubo, 1969).

V. COMBINED PERFUSION EXPERIMENTS

Coupled experiments. A major limitation of the technique is the lack of stability of renal function during experiments, which complicates the interpretation of the results obtained during successive periods. This drawback can be overcome almost completely by coupled experiments: the two kidneys of the same donor are perfused simultaneously by two perfusion machines; the blood donor must be different from the kidney donor because of the large amount required. In order to avoid differences in blood composition occurring during blood withdrawal, the two machines must be filled alternately with fractions of the total volume. In such experimental conditions, one parameter only can be changed on one side, the other kidney serving as a permanent reference. This procedure proved quite adequate to demonstrate small changes; it has been applied in various investigations concerning water, sodium, urea and phosphate excretion, and renal circulation (Nizet et al., 1968, 1969, 1971; Tost and Nizet, 1973; Vanherweghem et al., 1975, 1976a,b). Differences of less than 1% in the fractional excretion of sodium can be demonstrated with a limited number of coupled experiments (Nizet et al., 1971).

Independent perfusion of two kidneys by the same blood pool. In order to investigate humoral interferences between two kidneys, two pumps can be connected to one oxygenator, thus allowing independent control of the perfusion and of the response of two kidneys, the same pool of blood being utilized (Tost and Nizet, 1973).

Comparative experiments with in vitro and in vivo perfused organs. In order to investigate the role of extrarenal humoral factors in kidney function, comparative experiments can be performed with kidney perfused with a machine or by a perfusor dog at identical arterial and venous pressures; in such conditions, there is no difference in surgical handling of the perfused organ, denervation, and disturbances of lymphatic circulation (Nizet, 1975, 1976), thus allowing adequate comparison of the responses.

VI. CONCLUSIONS

Provided that a series of requirements are fulfilled as concerns the perfusion equipment, primarily the type of pump and oxygenator, it is possible to obtain a reasonably good functional performance with subnormal or normal values adequate for pharmacologic and metabolic investigations. The major limitations of the technique are the disturbances of intrarenal circulation, the progressive impairment of sodium reabsorption and of concentrating ability, and the loss of urine acidification. These limitations can be partly overcome by the paired experiments which make possible the obtainment of accurate results and the detection of small differences. It should be emphasized that, although the principles of the technique are very simple, successful results depend entirely on the careful observance of the above-mentioned conditions and on the use of adequate mechanical equipment.

REFERENCES

Bainbridge, F. A., and Evans, C. L. 1914. The heart, lung, kidney preparation. *J. Physiol. (Lond.)*, 48:278.

Barkin, M., and Kerr, W. K. 1963. An aspect of the vascular role in the etiology of acute tubular necrosis. *Surg. Gynecol. Obstet.*, 116:673.

Barkin, M., Katz, S., D'Aloisio, J., and Kerr, W. K. 1963. Normothermic perfusion of the isolated dog's kidney on a pump-oxygenator system. *Surg. Gynecol. Obstet.*, 117:161.

Bayliss, L. E., and Ogden, E. 1932–33. "Vaso-tonins" and the pump-oxygenator kidney preparation. *J. Physiol. (Lond.)*, 77:34.

Berkowitz, H. D., Miller, L. D., and Itskowitz, H. D. 1967. Renal function and the renin-angiotensin system in the isolated perfused kidney. *Am. J. Physiol.*, 213:928.

Berkowitz, H. D., Miller, L. D., Itskowitz, H. D., and Bovee, K. C. 1968. Renal function in the isolated perfused kidney. *Surg. Gynecol. Obstet.*, 127:1257.

Bickford, R. G., and Winton, F. R. 1937. The influence of temperature on the isolated kidney of the dog. *J. Physiol.*, 89:198.

Bidder. 1862. Beiträge zur Lehre von der Function der Nieren. Diss. Dorpat. cit. by Jacoby, C., and Sobieranski, V., 1892. *Arch. Exper. Path.*, 29:25.

Bing, R. J. 1941. The effect of vasoconstrictor substances in shed blood on perfused organs. *Am. J. Physiol.*, 133:21.

Brull, L., and Louis-Bar, D. 1957. Toxicity of artificially circulated heparinized blood on the kidney. *Arch. Int. Physiol. Biochim.*, 65:470.

Bunge, G., and Schmiedeberg, O. 1877. Ueber die Bildung der Hippursäure. *Arch. f. Exp. Path.*, 6:233.

Craig, G. M., Mills, I. M., Osbaldiston, G. W., and Wise, B. L. 1966. The effect of change of perfusion pressure and haematocrit in the isolated perfused kidney. *J. Physiol. (Lond.)*, 186:113.

Cuypers, Y., Nizet, A., and Barac, G. 1957. Action directe de la 5-hydroxytryptamine de l'adrénaline, de l'artérénol et de l'histamine sur le débit sanguin rénal chez le chien. *Compt. Rend. Soc. Biol. (Paris)*, 151:1768.

Cuypers, Y., Köver, G., and Nizet, A. 1961. Neutralisation par différents organes de l'action vasoconstrictrice du sang hépariné et conservé. *Arch. Int. Physiol. Biochim.*, 69:213.

Cuypers, Y., Nizet, A., and Baerten, A. 1964. Technique pour la perfusion de reins de chien avec du sang hépariné. *Arch. Int. Physiol. Biochim.*, 72:245.

Fontaine, J. L., Mack, G., Geisert, J., Foucher, G., Negreras, L., and Fontaine, B. 1969. Perfusion du rein de chien: étude de quelques facteurs de variation de la résistance à l'écoulement de l'organe. *J. Urol. Néphrol.*, 75:507.

Gagnon, J. A., Grove, D. W., and Flamenbaum, W. 1974. Blood flow distribution and tissue solute content of the isolated-perfused kidney. *Pflügers Arch.*, 347:261.

Hemingway, A. 1931. Some observations on the perfusion of the isolated kidney by a pump. *J. Physiol. (Lond.)*, 71:201.

Heymans, C., Bouckaert, J. J., and Moraes, A. 1932. Inversion par l'ergotamine de l'action vasoconstrictrice des vasotonines du sang défibriné. *Arch. Int. Pharmacodyn.*, 43:468.

Itskowitz, H. D., Hebert, L. A., and McGiff, J. C. 1973. Angiotensin as a possible intrarenal hormone in isolated dog kidneys. *Circ. Res.*, 32:550.

Jacobj, C. 1890. Apparat zur Durchblutung isolierter überlebender Organe. *Arch. f. Exper. Path.*, *26*:388.

Jacobj, C., and Sobieranski, V. 1892. Ueber das Functionsvermögen der kunstlich durchbluteten Niere. *Arch. Exper. Path.*, *29*:25.

Kramer, K., and Winton, F. R. 1939. The influence of urea and of change in arterial pressure on the oxygen consumption of the isolated kidney of the dog. *J. Physiol.*, *96*:87.

Kulatilake, A. E. 1967. Isolated perfusion of canine and human kidneys. *Brit. J. Surg.*, *54*:877.

Löbell. 1849. De conditionibus quibus secretiones glandulis perficiuntur. Diss. Marburg: cit. by Jacobj, C., and Sobieranski, V., 1892. *Arch. Exper. Path.*, *29*:25.

Ludwig, C. 1868, 1869. *Arbeiten ausdem Physiol. Institut zu Leipzig.* p. 113.

Lustinec, K. 1965. Vasoconstrictor properties of blood in perfusion experiments. *Physiol. Bohemoslov.*, *14*:583.

Nizet, A. 1963. Recherches sur le rein isolé perfusé par un système artificiel. *Bull. Acad. Roy. Méd. Belg.* *3*(series 7):283.

Nizet, A. 1972. Excretion and tubular reabsorption of sodium, glucose and phosphate by isolated dog kidneys. Influence of blood dilution. *Pflügers Arch.*, *332*:248.

Nizet, A. 1973. The mechanism of fast renal compensation. *Pflügers Arch.*, *341*:209.

Nizet, A. 1975. The isolated perfused kidney: Possibilities, limitations and results. *Kid. Internat.*, *7*:1.

Nizet, A. 1976. Comparative evaluation of fractional excretion of sodium following saline infusion in transplanted kidneys and in isolated perfused kidneys in conditions of previous high or low dietary sodium intake. *Pflügers Arch.*, *361*:121.

Nizet, A., and Cuypers, Y. 1962. Perfusion prolongée de reins isolés de chien au moyen d'un dispositif artificiel utilisant du sang hépariné. XXII International Congress of Physiological Sciences. Leiden, 1962. Excerpta Medica, International Congress Series, *48*, Abst. 200.

Nizet, A., Cuypers, Y., and Massillon, L. 1957a. Neutralisation, par décalcification, des propriétés vasoconstrictrices du sang conservé. *Arch. Internat. Physiol. Biochim.*, *66*:454.

Nizet, A., Cuypers, Y., and Massillon, L. 1957b. Neutralisation par le poumon des facteurs vasoconstricteurs, extraits des hématies. *Compt. Rend. Soc. Biol.*, *151*:1982.

Nizet, A., Cuypers, Y., Massillon, L., and Lambert, S. 1957c. Mise en évidence de facteurs réduisant le débit sanguin rénal et libérés par les hématies. *Arch. Internat. Physiol. Biochim.*, *65*:568.

Nizet, A., Cuypers, Y., and Massillon, L. 1959. Sur les propriétés vasoconstrictrices du sang soumis à une stase intravasculaire. *Compt. Rend. Soc. Biol. (Paris)*, *153*:520.

Nizet, A., Cuypers, Y., Deetjen, P., and Kramer, K. 1967. Functional capacity of the isolated perfused kidney. *Pflügers Arch.*, *296*:179.

Nizet, A., Godon, J. P., and Mahieu, P. 1968. Quantitative excretion of water and sodium load by isolated dog kidney: Autonomous renal response to blood dilution factors. *Pflügers Arch.*, *304*:30.

Nizet, A., Godon, J. P., Mahieu, P., and Kramer, K. 1969. Autonomous response of dog kidney to increased blood pressure with and without saline loading. *Pflügers Arch. Ges. Physiol.*, *313*:245.

Nizet, A., Lefebvre, P., and Crabbe, J. 1971. Control by insulin of sodium, potassium and water excretion by the isolated dog kidney. *Pflügers Arch.*, *323*:11.

Pavy, F. W., Brodie, T. G., and Siau, R. L. 1903. On the mechanism of phlorhidzin glycosuria. *J. Physiol. (Lond.)*, *29*:467.

Pfaff, F., and Vejnx-Tyrode, M. 1903. Ueber Durchblutung isolierter Nieren und den Einfluss defibrinierten Blutes auf die Secretion der Nieren. *Arch. Exp. Path.*, *49*:324.

Schröder, E., Ochwadt, B., and Bethge, H. 1965. Herstellung und Funktion eines isolierten Nierenpräparates vom Hund. *Pflügers Arch.*, *286*:189.

Starling, E. H., and Verney, E. B. 1925. The secretion of urine as studied on the isolated kidney. *Proc. Roy. Soc.*, *97*:321.

Tost, H., and Nizet, A. 1973. Reduction of the glomerular filtration rate by the efferent blood from a kidney taken from a previously dehydrated dog. *Pflügers Arch.*, *345*:327.

Vanherweghem, J. L., Ducobu, J., and D'Hollander, A. 1975. Effects of Indomethacin on renal hemodynamics and on water and sodium excretion by the isolated dog kidney. *Pflügers Arch.*, *357*:243.

Vanherweghem, J. L., Ducobu, J., D'Hollander, A., and Toussaint, C. 1976a. Interactions between furosemide and vasopressin on hemodynamics and on water excretion by the isolated dog kidney. *Pflügers Arch., 362:*265.

Vanherweghem, J. L., Ducobu, J., D'Hollander, A., and Toussaint, C. 1976b. Effects of hypercalcemia on water and sodium excretion by the isolated dog kidney. *Pflügers Arch., 363:*75.

Waugh, W. H., and Kubo, T. 1969. Development of an isolated perfused dog kidney with improved function. *Am. J. Physiol., 217:*277.

Chapter **15**

Methodology for Study of Isolated Perfused Rat Kidney *in Vitro*

Roger H. Bowman

Veterans Administration Hospital and
Department of Pharmacology
State University of New York
Upstate Medical Center
Syracuse, N. Y.

I. INTRODUCTION

The advantages of isolated perfused organs for biological study are several. Delivery and removal of substrates and products via normal vascular channels, and the absence of modifying effects from other organs are primary benefits. In the case of the kidney, a further advantage accrues from the fact that transport events transpire while the perfused tissue is being studied. For an organ in which the major energy expenditure is believed to be for transport (a process that occurs to only a limited extent in slices and not at all in homogenates), this is an important consideration.

Depending on the conditions of perfusion, the isolated kidney can be variably suited for different types of physiological and biochemical study. Thus, under the proper conditions, a preparation can be obtained which will reabsorb 98% or more of filtered Na^+ for an hour or two of perfusion. With no special attention to detail, the perfused kidney will consistently display 85–90% of normal tubular transport activity, and this is probably adequate for most metabolic (Bowman, 1970; Coulson, 1976; Coulson and Bowman, 1974; Nishiitsutsuji-Uwo *et al.*, 1967; Walter and Bowman, 1973) and drug handling (Bowman, 1975b) studies.

II. METHODOLOGY

A. General Comment

Several methods of perfusing the rat kidney have been described (Bahlmann *et al.*, 1967; Bauman *et al.*, 1963; Nishiitsutsuji-Uwo *et al.*, 1967; Weidemann *et al.*, 1969; Weiss *et al.*, 1959; see also Ross, 1972). It is quite likely that, given the same perfusion medium and equal technical skill, all methods would yield comparable results. In essence, a workable method requires a procedure for rapidly introducing well-oxygenated perfusate into the renal artery, and a procedure for collecting, and in most instances reoxygenating and recirculating, the venous effluent. Temperature control is also required. In attempting to establish a method for kidney perfusion, we considered that the apparatus should be relatively simple in design and have the capacity for simultaneous multiple perfusions. The apparatus adopted (Bowman, 1970; Bowman and Maack, 1972) is essentially identical to that devised 20 years ago by Morgan *et al.* (1961) for rat heart perfusions.

In regard to the perfusion technique, itself, there are two major distinctions between the method described herein and methods of kidney perfusion which have been developed by others. First, the renal vein is not routinely cannulated in our procedure. Cannulation of the vein is an extra maneuver and allows the possibility of back-pressure if the cannula is not positioned with great care. Decreased flow and increased perfusion pressure, with time, may be results of this back-pressure. A second difference from other methods is that, in the present procedure, the chamber in which the kidney is housed during perfusion is also used as the oxygenator and perfusate reservoir. This greatly simplifies the apparatus.

B. Apparatus

The apparatus for perfusing the rat kidney is shown diagrammatically in Figure 1. It consists of two parts, (1) a gravity-feed system, and (2) the main recirculation apparatus. Figure 1(A) shows the gravity-feed arrangement used for preperfusion during the initial cannulation procedure. The drawing shows the kidney tied onto the arterial cannula, which in turn is attached to a three-way valve. The gravity-feed system and the recirculation system both are connected to this valve. An 18-gauge needle cut to a length of approximately 2.5 cm, slightly beveled and smoothed, is used as the arterial cannula. The recirculation system is depicted in Figure 1(B). It consists of the following parts: (1) A "fuljak" Allihn condenser (2.9 × 60 cm i.d.) with 29/42 standard taper ground joints serves as the kidney chamber, perfusate reservoir, and oxygenation chamber. A coarse-porosity sintered glass filter is fitted into the lower end of the Allihn condenser. The condenser (JC-5500) and the filter (JC-2350, 2A inner tube only) may be obtained from SGA Scientific, Inc. (2) Pump. (3) Flowmeter (A. H. Thomas 5083-D35). (4) Bubble trap. (5) Manometer.

We have had success with two styles of perfusion pump. One type (Model PA purchased without motor from New Brunswick Scientific Co.) is used in a

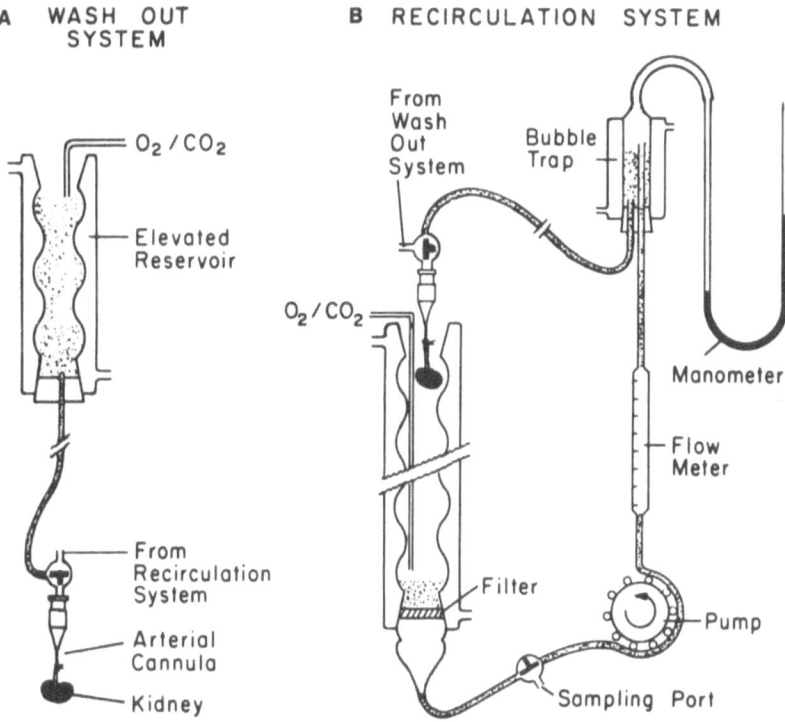

Figure 1. Schematic arrangement of apparatus for rat kidney perfusion. (A) System for initial washout of kidney vasculature, used during cannulation. The reservoir is elevated to a height of 100–120 cm above the rat. (B) System for perfusion by pump recirculation. See text for description of apparatus and procedure. (Modified and redrawn from Bowman, 1975a.)

series of several pumps mounted 12–18 inches apart, and driven by a common drive shaft from a single variable speed motor at 180 rpm. Control of flow is obtained by adjusting the yoke pressure against the tubing. A second type of pump which is satisfactory is Masterflex Model 7565 with No. 7014 pump head, purchased from Cole-Parmer Co. In choosing a pump, it is of importance to obtain one through which the flow of perfusate can be adjusted rapidly and with a fair degree of precision.

The bubble trap removes bubbles from the system prior to the arterial influent. Additionally, the upper part of the trap is connected to a manometer for recording the perfusion pressure. The bubble trap, which is double-walled, must be custom-made. Its outside dimensions are approximately 3 × 6 cm, with outlet and inlet ports for water circulation [see Figure 1(B)]. The inside diameter is about 1.5 cm, and should be made to accommodate a common-sized stopper, e.g., size "O." The inside section of the chamber is extended (unjacketed) through the top of the trap for 2 or 3 inches for connection by Tygon tubing to the manometer. Stainless steel tubing (approximately 13-gauge hypodermic needle) is used for the entrance and exit ports through the stopper at the bottom of the trap.

A three-way valve for perfusate sampling is inserted in the perfusion line between the kidney chamber and the pump. To avoid the formation of air bubbles in the perfusion line, fluid should be made to back up in the bulb of the glass filter before perfusion is begun.

The tubing used for the system is Tygon formulation S-50-HL (U.S. Stoneware, Inc.). The size of the main perfusion tubing is 0.093 × 0.156 inch (i.d. × o.d.), with other sizes used for making connections to the various parts of the apparatus. A finer diameter tubing, 0.05 × 0.08 inch (American Instrument Co., No. 5-8963), is used for gas delivery to the perfusion chamber [Figure 1(B)]. If care is taken not to allow the tip of this tubing to extend below the level of perfusate in the chamber, foaming usually can be avoided. Not shown in Figure 1(B) is a moistening chamber through which the O_2/CO_2 is passed prior to its delivery to the perfusion chamber.

The various pieces of glassware used for perfusion are attached by clamps to a scaffolding of lightweight rods mounted on the laboratory bench. Spring clamps (Arthur H. Thomas, 2835-LK15 or L20), which are used to hold the cannula and urine vials in place, are also secured to these supporting rods.

To summarize the sequence of flow through the apparatus: perfusate is drawn through the glass filter from the perfusion chamber and is pumped through the flowmeter and into the bubble trap. From the bubble trap the perfusate passes to the arterial cannula and enters the kidney vasculature. Perfusate leaves the cut end of the renal vein and flows down the sides of the chamber for reoxygenation and recirculation.

C. Perfusate

1. Basic Composition

The basic perfusion medium consists of Krebs–Henseleit bicarbonate buffer (Krebs and Henseleit, 1932) containing fraction V bovine serum albumin (see Section C-3 for choice of albumin concentration). The pH is adjusted to 7.45 after equilibrating the medium with O_2/CO_2 (95:5), and 30–50 ml is used for each perfusion. The particular preparation of fraction V albumin which is used appears to be of some importance. We originally used Armour Pharmaceutical Co. fraction V, but found that certain lots resulted in poor fluid reabsorption. More recently we have used Miles Laboratory's Pentex brand and believe that this gives more consistent results.

2. Preparation of Perfusate

Regardless of the source of fraction V albumin, it usually contains various small molecular weight substances which, in effect, contaminate the albumin. For experiments in which the investigator wants to be assured of the composition of the perfusate, it is necessary to dialyze the medium for 18–24 hr prior to its use. In addition to removing any impurities from the albumin, the dialysis step will also serve to equilibrate the perfusion medium with the ionic composition of the Krebs–Henseleit buffer. Dialysis against a tenfold excess of nonalbumin-containing buffer is satisfactory. (The dialysis tubing is boiled for a number of hours in frequent changes of distilled water before it is used. It is then stored in dilute HCl at 2°, and is well rinsed before filling with perfusate.) Following dialysis, the perfusate is removed from the dialysis tubing, and substrates or other substances are added. It is then equilibrated with O_2/CO_2, and the pH is adjusted. To assure that any small particulate matter is removed from the perfusate, it is finally filtered in two steps through 8 μm and 0.22 μm Millipore filters. Use of Millipore filtration device No. XX20 047 20 makes this procedure convenient and rapid.

3. *Choice of Albumin Concentration*

The albumin concentration which is used depends upon the renal process to be studied. Because of the high perfusate flow rate through the isolated kidney, the filtration fraction is abnormally low, and hence the postglomerular concentration of albumin is not appreciably elevated. An albumin concentration of 7.5 g/100 ml will approximate the normal efferent colloid concentration, and will yield a relatively high fractional fluid reabsorption without seriously reducing the filtration rate (Bowman and Maack, 1974). In some circumstances it may be desirable to have a larger output of urine (or tubular reabsorption and urine volume may not be critical) and in these circumstances less albumin can be employed. While learning the technique of perfusion it is not necessary to include albumin in the perfusate at all. Aside from the financial saving, the advantage of not using albumin is that urine collection is facilitated. This is due to the greatly reduced rate of tubular reabsorption and the consequent larger flow of urine.

4. *Choice of Ca^{2+} Concentration*

There has not always been consistency in the Ca^{2+} concentration used by investigators in *in vitro* incubation experiments (e.g., Ross *et al.*, 1973 vs. Silva *et al.*, 1975). Krebs–Henseleit buffer contains 2.5 mM Ca^{2+}, which is the normal plasma concentration, but since nearly one-half of plasma Ca^{2+} is protein-bound, it has not been unusual for experimenters to employ a half-normal concentration of Ca^{2+} (i.e., approximately 1 mM) in their solutions (Roobol and Alleyne, 1973, 1974; Schurek *et al.*, 1975; Silva *et al.*, 1975). For experiments in which the incubation medium does not contain protein, this is probably a reasonable approach to achieving the normal ionized calcium concentration. However, with perfusates containing 5–7.5 g/100 ml albumin, protein binding becomes a factor, and normal (2.5 mM) Ca^{2+} Krebs–Henseleit buffer would seem to be the physiologically appropriate solution to use. Nevertheless, for exactness, the specific albumin concentration and the ratio of perfusate to dialysate (if the medium is dialyzed) must be taken into account. For any particular perfusate constituency, some experimentation is necessary in order to establish the quantity of Ca^{2+} to be added for achievement of any desired final concentration of the ionized form.

D. Operative Procedure

The right renal artery of the rat leaves the aorta at a point approximately opposite the origin of the superior mesenteric artery. This anatomical arrangement permits insertion of a cannula into the mesenteric artery and subsequent passage of the cannula across the aorta and into the renal artery. Initiation of perfusion at the time the cannula enters the renal artery (see below) avoids any period of ischemia.

Male rats weighing 350–400 g are normally used as the kidney donors. After anesthesia is induced by sodium pentobarbital (approximately 5 mg/100 g body wt.), a midline incision is made and the renal segment of the aorta is exposed. By gentle dissection, the right renal artery and mesenteric artery are likewise exposed. A loose ligature is then passed around the right renal artery close to the aorta, and distal and proximal ligatures are placed around the mesenteric artery. It is important to contact the right renal artery as little as possible. To prevent leakage via the right adrenal artery, it may be ligated. However, in many instances the tip of the arterial cannula will extend beyond the origin of this branch vessel, and, if it is determined that this is routinely the case, ligation of the adrenal artery can be omitted. Note that, aside from optional ligation of the adrenal artery, the procedure employs only three ligatures.

To guard against clotting, and hence possible incomplete filling of the renal vasculature, we have injected heparin (approximately 200 units) via the left renal vein prior to manipulation of the renal and mesenteric arteries. This probably is of lesser importance after experience has been gained with the technique, and, for certain studies, heparin is not suitable.

If urine is to be collected, the ureter is catheterized with PE10 tubing. To avoid undue resistance to urine flow, the tubing should be kept as short as is feasible. After the kidney is suspended for perfusion (see below), urine is collected from the catheterized ureter into preweighed plastic vials (Scientific Products No. B2713-2 with caps). It is critical that the ureter not become twisted, and that the catheter be uniquely positioned for each kidney in order to obtain a free flow of urine.

E. Arterial Cannulation and Initiation of Perfusion

The foregoing procedure is carried out at some suitable worktable with the rat secured to a small operating tray. After preparation of the rat, the tray containing the animal is transferred to a surface adjacent to the perfusion apparatus. (We support the tray on a small pail which is topped with strips of plastic tape.) Before the renal artery is cannulated, air bubbles are eliminated from the section of tubing between the bubble trap and the cannula, and the pressure in the circulating system [Figure 1(B)] is brought to 120–140 mm Hg with zero flow. The three-way stopcock holding the cannula is then turned to allow flow from the overhead chamber, and after air bubbles are expelled from this tubing it is occluded with a hemostat. To prepare for cannulation, the distal ligature on the mesenteric artery is tied, and a small serrefine is placed on this vessel close to the aorta. A cut is then made in the mesenteric artery just proximal to the tied distal ligature, and the cannula is inserted into the artery up to the level of the serrefine; the serrefine is removed, and the cannula is manipulated across the aorta and into the renal artery. As the cannula enters the renal artery, the hemostat holding back the perfusate from the overhead reservoir is released, and kidney perfusion is begun. The proximal mesenteric ligature and the ligature around the renal artery are tied, securing the cannula in place. The inferior vena cava is rapidly severed, and the kidney is dissected free from the animal and trimmed of adhering tissue. During the time that the arterial cannula is being tied into place and the kidney trimmed, the gravity perfusion system serves to flush blood from the renal vessels and to maintain oxygen delivery to the tissue. This procedure takes about 1 min. Perfusate flow is then switched so as to be delivered from the recirculating system, the kidney is placed in the perfusion chamber, the cannula is secured in the spring clamp, and the perfusion pressure is adjusted. An enlarged view of the kidney in place during perfusion is shown in Figure 2.

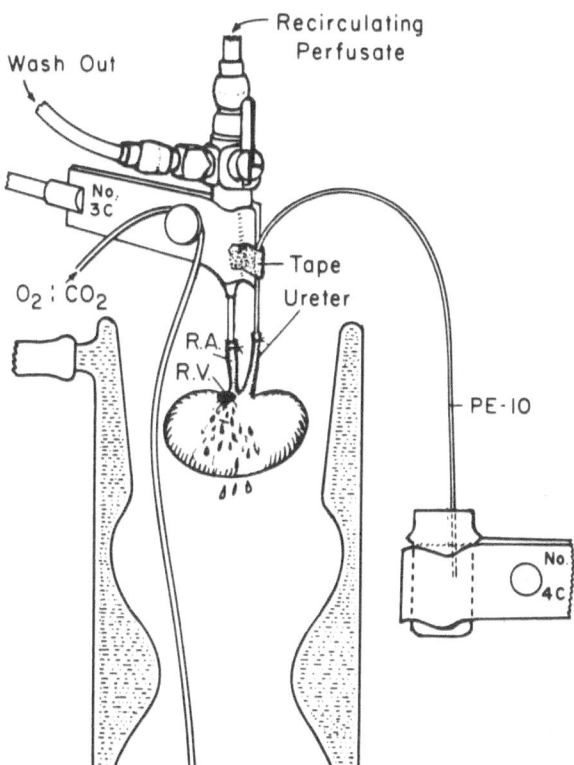

Figure 2. View of the kidney as it is positioned during perfusion. R.A., renal artery; R.V., renal vein. See text for description. (Redrawn from Bowman, 1975a).

III. OBSERVATIONS

A. Hemodynamic Behavior

A characteristic of the isolated perfused rat kidney is that it exhibits low resistance and high flow. Although this situation is opposite to that which was often found in earlier perfusion experiments (Bauman *et al.,* 1963; Weiss *et al.,* 1959), it is not a peculiarity of the present preparation and has been observed by Bahlmann *et al.* (1967), as well as by others (Nishiitsutsuji-Uwo *et al.,* 1967; Little and Cohen, 1974; Ross *et al.,* 1973; Schurek *et al.,* 1975). For most uses of the isolated kidney it is fortunate that the high flow exits, since it allows a very adequate oxygenation without the use of red cells.[1] Constitution of the perfusate is greatly simplified by not using red cells, and the problems of red cell metabolism and potential hemolysis are avoided. The major drawback to the rapid flow appears to be that the medullary solute concentration is diluted, and thus it is difficult to obtain urine with an osmolality much greater than that of the perfusate. In other words, the isolated kidney, perfused under the conditions described herein, will not "concentrate." The process of concentration must, of course, be distinguished from that of fluid reabsorption, which is discussed in a later section.

The maximal flow rate, 25–35 ml/min, is usually attained within a few minutes of the start of perfusion. A lower flow is most often due to constriction of the renal artery. An increase in pump pressure will, in most instances, overcome this vasoconstriction, and as dilation occurs the flow will increase and perfusion pressure will fall. Since oxygenation is dependent on a high flow, it is important to initially perfuse with as high a pressure as is required to give the desired flow. Fifteen ml/min is probably a minimal value. Our normally achieved relationship after 5–8 min of perfusion is a flow of approximately 30 ml/min at a pressure of 90–100 mm Hg. At this point, increasing the pressure further has little effect on perfusion flow. It may, however, decrease fluid reabsorption (see below), so that unless desired for some particular reason, it is best not to perfuse at a pressure much above 100 mm Hg (calculated at the tip of the cannula).

B. Tubular Function and Substrate Effects

1. Filtration and Reabsorption

Glomerular filtration rate (GFR) and fractional fluid reabsorption can be altered within fairly wide limits depending on the conditions of perfusion. In general, increasing the perfusion pressure (e.g., from 60 mm Hg to 90 mm Hg) will increase GFR, and increasing the concentration of oncotic material in the medium will decrease GFR. However, under any particular condition there is always some variability in GFR from kidney to kidney, and the quantitative

---

[1] When the perfusate is exposed to O_2/CO_2 (95:5) during perfusion, as described herein, the P_{O_2} of the arterial influent is approximately 500 mm Hg. The arterial–venous difference (P_{O_2}) is 60–200 mm Hg, depending on the perfusate flow rate. Addition of substrates (e.g., pyruvate) yields a larger oxygen extraction.

regulation of filtration remains a problem. Although a higher perfusion pressure usually will yield a greater filtration rate, the higher pressures mediate against fluid reabsorption. Therefore, if maximal percent reabsorption is desired, some compromise may have to be accepted for the filtration rate.

Regardless of perfusion pressure and GFR, the presence or absence of albumin in the medium has striking effects on fractional fluid reabsorption (Bowman and Maack, 1974; Little and Cohen, 1974). Nearly 50% of filtered fluid is excreted when albumin is omitted from the perfusate. This value diminishes linearly as albumin concentration is increased, and at 7.5 g/100 ml albumin (and no exogenous substrates) fluid excretion may be only 10–15% of the filtered load. Ten to 15% fluid excretion is a large amount compared with fractional excretion by the hydropenic kidney, but, under the circumstance, 85–90% reabsorption represents a reasonable approximation of renal physiology. This is especially so, since these are results which obtain in kidneys perfused without added substrate and without the antidiuretic, or other possibly involved hormones.

Excessive fluid excretion by the perfused kidney appears to be due predominantly to a distal (Henle's loop?) rather than proximal deficiency, and proximal tubular function, in general, appears to be less impaired by perfusion than are the more distal portions of the nephron (see Section III-B-4). It has been shown by Bowman and Maack (1972) that glucose fractional reabsorption is 98–99% at a perfusate glucose concentration of 100 mg/100 ml which is probably little different from that in the intact rat. Likewise, it is found that phosphate reabsorption is nearly complete in the perfused kidney (Bowman, unpublished data).

2. Substrate Effects on Fluid Reabsorption

A number of substrates have been tested for their ability to improve fluid reabsorption. Glucose (Ross *et al.*, 1973; Trimble and Bowman, 1973) and several amino acids (Maack *et al.*, 1974) are beneficial, and addition of vasopressin further improves reabsorption (Bowman and Maack, 1974; Ross *et al.*, 1973). A perfusate composition which in our hands will result consistently in 96–97% fluid reabsorption and 98–99% Na^+ reabsorption is as follows: glucose (5.5 mM); alanine (1 mM); glycine (1 mM); arginine (1 mM); and creatinine (4.5 mM). Filtration is measured with [^{3}H]polyethylene glycol. Results obtained with this perfusate are given in Table I.

It is not certain that the improvement in fluid reabsorption brought about by the above substrates is via their metabolism; in fact, for glucose the evidence is that its metabolism is not required (Trimble, 1975; but see Ross *et al.*, 1973). Rather, some form of cotransport with Na^+, or solvent drag, may be involved. The same may be true for the antinatriuretic effect of amino acids.

Fatty acids are believed to be important contributors to renal energy metabolism (e.g., Weidemann and Krebs, 1969), but exogenous fatty acids have only a small stimulatory effect on Na^+ reabsorption by the isolated kidney (Ross *et al.*, 1973; Trimble and Bowman, 1973). One reason for this may be that the endogenous lipid content of the kidney is high, and appears to be available for

Table I. Functional Parameters of the Isolated Perfused
Rat Kidney[a]

Parameter	Clearance periods (min of perfusion)		
	21–27	45–51	69–75
GFR (ml/min)	0.556	0.463	0.379
	±0.080	±0.071	±0.055
(U/P)[^{3}H]PEG	33.6	31.1	30.1
	±5.3	±5.4	±5.6
%Na$^+$ excreted	1.25	1.44	1.61
	±0.56	±0.46	±0.47
%K$^+$ excreted	25.5	36.9	49.9
	±7.5	±8.0	±13.9

[a] Values are means ± S.E.M. ($N = 7$). Values are for three clearance periods (6 min each) collected at the times shown during 75 min of perfusion. In these experiments, the perfusion pressure (at the tip of the cannula) ranged between 75 and 85 mm Hg, and this somewhat low pressure is responsible, at least in part, for the modest rates of filtration. The perfusate contained: glucose (5.5 mM); alanine (1 mM); glycine (1 mM); arginine (1 mM); and creatinine (4.5 mM). Filtration rate was measured with [^{3}H]polyethylene glycol.

Table II. In Vivo Labeling of Renal Lipids:
Comparison between Right and Left Kidney
Content of Lipid and of ^{14}C-lipids 20 min after i.v.
Injection of 5 μCi [U-^{14}C]Palmitate into
Functionally Hepatectomized Rats

Kidney	PL	NL	FFA
	μmol fatty acid/g dry weight		
Left	201 ± 11	23 ± 2	12 ± 1
Right	180 ± 9	29 ± 4	13 ± 1
	^{14}C DPM/g dry weight $\times$ 10^{-3}		
Left	332 ± 37	163 ± 15	24 ± 5
Right	284 ± 32	177 ± 14	23 ± 2

[a] Values are mean ± S.E.M. of eight kidneys. PL, phospholipid fatty acid; NL, neutral lipid fatty acid; FFA, free fatty acid; DPM, disintegrations per minute. Data are unpublished findings of M. E. Trimble. The right kidney was removed for perfusion after the 20-min labeling period. Perfusion was carried out in a closed system saturated with O_2/CO_2 (95:5). See text for observations, and Bowman (1966) for method of $^{14}CO_2$ analysis.

oxidation. Support for this view comes from two types of experiment. In the first, addition to the perfusate of α-bromopalmitate, an inhibitor of (endogenous) fatty acid oxidation, caused a decrease in fractional Na^+ reabsorption (Trimble and Bowman, 1973). In a second study the metabolism of endogenous renal lipid was investigated by prelabeling of the tissue (unpublished experiments of M. E. Trimble). In these experiments [^{14}C]palmitate was administered i.v. into functionally hepatectomized rats prior to removal of the kidneys for perfusion (Table II). More than 50% of the ^{14}C-label in the neutral lipid fraction disappeared during 2 hr of perfusion, and most of this was recovered as $^{14}CO_2$ when the kidneys were perfused without added substrate. With a mixture of exogenous substrates in the perfusing medium, the rate of $^{14}CO_2$ production was reduced by 70%.

3. Secretory Capacity

The isolated kidney lends itself well to studies of drug clearance and factors affecting such clearance. A low concentration (<10 μM) of *p*-aminohippurate (PAH) is cleared at a rate of somewhat more than 8 ml/min (Bowman, 1975b). This is 10 times its filtration rate, and indicates an active secretory component. However, PAH clearance in this preparation may well not represent total cortical flow, since it seems unlikely that the difference between measured total renal flow and PAH clearance (approx. 30 ml/min − 8 ml/min) could be entirely medullary. With such a rapid (cortical) flow rate, the maximum velocity of the secretory mechanism is probably exceeded.

Furosemide is secreted by the isolated kidney at about the same rate as is PAH. [^{35}S]Furosmide has been used in the presently described preparation to demonstrate that extensive protein binding of drugs may severely limit their renal clearance (Bowman, 1975b).

At least one substance [i.e., adenosine 3',5'-monophosphate (cAMP)] which was thought not to have any large secretory component in the kidney (Broadus *et al.*, 1970; Butlen and Jard, 1972), has been found by use of the isolated perfused preparation to be avidly extracted and degraded by kidney tissue (Coulson, 1976; Coulson and Bowman, 1974). The degradation is so rapid that urinary cAMP is only a fraction of that which is taken up peritubularly. The same is true for guanosine 3',5'-monophosphate. Other substances may be found to be handled similarly, and these data with the cyclic nucleotides (Coulson, 1976; Coulson and Bowman, 1974; Coulson *et al.*, 1974) serve to emphasize that the urinary content of any intracellularly appearing substance may be attenuated by metabolism. Failure of cAMP, for example, to appear in the urine of animals treated with antidiuretic hormone is not evidence that intracellular cAMP production has not been increased by the hormone.

4. Micropuncture Analysis of Tubular Function

Using the method described above (with slight modification of the kidney position), de Mello and Maack (1976) have studied the perfused kidney by

Table III. Concentration and Fractional Excretion of [³H]PEG, Na⁺, and K⁺ in Cortical Nephron Segments and Ureteral Urine of the Isolated Perfused Rat Kidney[a]

Nephron Segment	[³H]PEG (TF/P)	Na⁺(TF/P)	Na⁺/[³H]PEG (TF/P)	K⁺ (TF/P)	K⁺/[³H]PEG (TF/P)
End proximal	2.78 ± 0.16 (32)	0.98 ± 0.02 (14)	0.34 ± 0.01 (14)	0.78 ± 0.10 (7)	0.29 ± 0.05 (7)
Earliest distal	3.86 ± 0.57[b] (9)	0.88 ± 0.06[c] (8)	0.26 ± 0.04[c] (8)	1.11 ± 0.14[c] (7)	0.29 ± 0.06 (7)
Latest distal	5.97 ± 0.59[b] (10)	0.65 ± 0.10[c] (6)	0.12 ± 0.03[b] (6)	1.66 ± 0.22[c] (9)	0.24 ± 0.06 (6)
Ureteral urine	19.0 ± 3.1[b] (15K)	0.48 ± 0.05 (10K)	0.03 ± 0.01[b] (10K)	3.05 ± 0.40[b] (7K)	0.15 ± 0.02 (7K)

[a] Values are mean ± S.E.M. Number of samples are given in parentheses. K indicates number of perfused kidneys. (Data from de Mello and Maack, 1976.)
[b] $p < 0.01$ vs. value of preceding nephron segment.
[c] $p < 0.05$ vs. value of preceding nephron segment.

micropuncture. Single nephron filtration rate (SNGFR), intratubular hydrostatic pressures (IP), transit time (TT) and the reabsorption (R) of H_2O, Na^+, Cl^- and K^+ were measured in superficial proximal (PT) and distal (DT) tubules of the preparation. Mean SNGFR was 27.2 nl/min and 25.2 nl/min when measured in PT and DT, respectively, and remained nearly constant for the duration of the perfusion (120 min). The ratio GFR/SNGFR was lower than expected, indicating a greater depression of deeper nephron SNGFR. PT transport functions were well maintained throughout the perfusion (mean values were; IP, 14.3 mm Hg; TT, 17.7 s; fractional (F) R_{H_2O}, 64%; absolute R_{H_2O}, 15.4 nl/min; FR_{Na}, 66.5%; FR_K, 71% and tubular fluid to perfusate (TF/P) ratio of Cl^+, 1.37). Short loops of Henle reabsorbed less than 10% of the load of H_2O and Na^+ delivered to them, and TF/P's of electrolytes in the earliest DT segments were high (Na^+ TF/P = 0.88, Cl^- TF/P = 1.27 and K^+ TF/P = 1.11). This deficiency in Henle's loop function explains, at least in part, the degree of natriuresis of the preparation (overall FR_{Na} = 97.5%). TT to end DT was prolonged (82.3 s) and IP in DT elevated (14.9 mm Hg). Vasopressin decreased IP in DT to 10.8 mm Hg. The DT was able to compensate in part for the overload from Henle's loop by reabsorbing 32% of the fluid load and 57% of the Na^+ load delivered to it. A summary of some of the findings of de Mello and Maack is given in Table III. These micropuncture data should be of considerable value to persons employing the perfusion technique described in this chapter.

C. Biochemical Viability

1. Tissue Fixation

Either of two methods for rapidly freezing the perfused kidney is satisfactory. The most direct means is to clamp the kidney, while it is being perfused, in precooled Wollenberger tongs (Wollenberger *et al.*, 1960). A second and equally effective means is to sever a sagittal half of the kidney and allow it to drop into a mixture of dry ice and acetone. The second half (still being perfused) is then cut from the cannula and similarly frozen. Subsequent analyses of tissue components are carried out by a variety of previously published methods (Bowman, 1970; Bowman *et al.*, 1973).

2. Adenine Nucleotide Levels

The ATP content of renal tissue, *in situ,* is approximately 1.5 μmol/g wet tissue. A consideration of oxygen consumption, P:O ratio, and work performed (e.g., tubular transport; gluconeogenesis; and other synthetic processes) reveals that ATP must be regenerated numerous times each minute in order for the steady-state energy level to be maintained. Table IV lists values for ATP, ADP, and AMP in kidneys frozen without perfusion (Nishiitsutsuji-Uwo *et al.*, 1967) and in kidneys frozen after 1 hr of perfusion (Bowman, unpublished data). It is clear that the ATP-generating system is intact in the perfused kidney.

Table IV. Adenine Nucleotide Content of Perfused and Nonperfused Rat Kidneys

	ATP (μmol/g dry wt.)	ADP (μmol/g dry wt.)	AMP (μmol/g dry wt.)	Total (μmol/g dry wt.)
Nonperfused[a] (N = 4)	7.20 ± 0.38	2.66 ± 0.07	0.78 ± 0.10	10.69 ± 0.37
Perfused[b] (N = 4)	7.94 ± 0.25	3.56 ± 0.07	0.71 ± 0.09	12.21 ± 0.26

[a] Data from Nishiitsutsuji-Uwo et al. (1967).
[b] Kidneys frozen after 60 min of perfusion (Bowman, unpublished).

3. Metabolic Conversions

In addition to the studies with exogenous cyclic nucleotides (see above), we have investigated the metabolism of vasopressin and oxytocin in the isolated kidney (Walter and Bowman, 1973). Additionally, gluconeogenesis (Bowman, 1970; Nishiitsutsuji-Uwo, et al., 1967) and ammoniagenesis (Welbourne, 1974) have been studied. Numerous problems concerning the role of the kidney in the metabolism of plasma-borne substances remain to be examined. There is a real advantage to studying such processes in a functioning kidney which is, at the same time, separated from extrarenal influences. Reactions involving various hormones, vitamin D, and prostaglandins are a few of the problems that might be profitably investigated.

ACKNOWLEDGMENTS

The author's work discussed in this section was supported by the Public Health Service (AM-14401). Dr. Thomas Maack, Cornell University Medical College, was intimately involved in the improvement of the perfusion method for functional studies. Academic Press, copyright holder, generously granted permission for use of Figures 1 and 2, taken from Bowman (1975a).

REFERENCES

Bahlmann, J., Giebisch, G., Ochwadt, B., and Schoeppe, W. 1967. Micropuncture study of isolated perfused rat kidney. *Am. J. Physiol., 212:*77.

Bauman, A. W., Clarkson, T., and Miles, E. 1963. Functional evaluation of isolated perfused rat kidney. *J. Appl. Physiol., 18:*1239.

Bowman, R. H. 1966. Effects of diabetes, fatty acids, and ketone bodies on tricarboxylic acid cycle metabolism in the perfused rat heart, *J. Biol. Chem., 241:*3041.

Bowman, R. H. 1970. Gluconeogenesis in the isolated perfused rat kidney. *J. Biol. Chem., 245:*1604.

Bowman, R. H. 1975a. The perfused rat kidney. In: *Methods in Enzymology,* Vol. 39, pp. 3–11. Ed. by Hardman, J. G. and O'Malley, B. W. Academic Press, New York.

Bowman, R. H. 1975b. Renal secretion of [^{35}S]furosemide and its depression by albumin binding. *Am. J. Physiol., 229:*93.

Bowman, R. H., and Maack, T. 1972. Glucose transport by the isolated perfused rat kidney. *Am. J. Physiol., 222:*1499.

Bowman, R. H., and Maack, T. 1974. Effect of albumin concentration and ADH on H_2O and electrolyte transport in perfused rat kidney. *Am. J. Physiol., 226:*426.

Bowman, R. H., Dolgin, J., and Coulson, R. 1973. Furosemide, ethacrynic acid and iodoacetate on function and metabolism in perfused rat kidney. *Am. J. Physiol., 224:*416.

Broadus, A. E., Kaminsky, N. I., Hardman, J. G., Sutherland, E. W., and Liddle, G. W. 1970. Kinetic parameters and renal clearances of plasma adenosine 3′,5′-monophosphate and guanosine 3′,5′-monophosphate in man. *J. Clin. Invest., 49:*2222.

Butlen, D., and Jard, S. 1972. Renal handling of 3′,5′-cyclic AMP in the rat. *Pflügers Arch. Ges. Physiol., 331:*172.

Coulson, R. 1976. Metabolism and excretion of exogenous adenosine 3′,5′-monophosphate and guanosine 3′,5′-monophosphate: studies in the isolated perfused rat kidney. *J. Biol. Chem. 251:*4958–4967.

Coulson, R., and Bowman, R. Hn 1974. Excretion and degradation of exogenous adenosine 3′,5′-monophosphate by isolated perfused rat kidney. *Life Sci., 14:*545.

Coulson, R., Bowman, R. H., and Roch-Ramel, F. 1974. The effects of nephrectomy and probenecid on *in vivo* clearance of adenosine 3′,5′-monophosphate from rat plasma. *Life Sci., 15:*877.

de Mello, G., and Maack, T. 1976. Nephron function of the isolated perfused rat kidney. *Am. J. Physiol. 231:*1699.

Krebs, H. A., and Henseleit, K. 1932. Untersuchungen über die Harnstoffbildung im Tierkörper. *Z. Physiol. Chem., 210:*33.

Little, J. R., and Cohen, J. J. 1974. Effect of albumin concentration on function of isolated perfused rat kidney. *Am. J. Physiol., 226:*512.

Maack, T., Johnson, V., Tate, S. S., and Meister, A. 1974. Effects of amino acids on the function of the isolated perfused rat kidney. *Fed. Proc., 33:*305.

Morgan, H. E., Henderson, M. J., Regen, D. M., and Park, C. R. 1961. Regulation of glucose uptake in muscle. *J. Biol. Chem., 236:*253.

Nishiitsutsuji-Uwo, J. M., Ross, B. D., and Krebs, H. A. 1967. Metabolic activities of the isolated perfused rat kidney. *Biochem. J., 103:*852.

Roobol, A., and Alleyne, G. A. O. 1973. Regulation of renal gluconeogenesis by calcium ions, hormones, and adenosine 3′,5′-cyclic monophosphate. *Biochem. J., 134:*157.

Roobol, A., and Alleyne, G. A. O. 1974. Control of renal cortex ammoniagenesis and its relationship to renal cortical gluconeogenesis. *Biochim. Biophys. Acta, 362:*83.

Ross, B. D. 1972. *Perfusion Techniques in Biochemistry,* pp. 221–257. Clarenden Press, Oxford.

Ross, B. D., Epstein, F. H., and Leaf, A. 1973. Sodium reabsorption in the perfused rat kidney. *Am. J. Physiol., 225:*1165.

Schurek, H. J., Brecht, J. P., Lohfert, H., and Hierholzer, K. 1975. The basic requirements for the function of the isolated cell free perfused rat kidney. *Pflügers Arch. Ges. Physiol., 354:*349.

Silva, P., Ross, B. D., Charney, A. N., Besarab, A., and Epstein, F. H. 1975. Potassium transport by the isolated perfused rat kidney. *J. Clin. Invest., 56:*862.

Trimble. M. E. 1975. Effects of L-glucose on sodium reabsorption in the isolated perfused rat kidney. *Life Sci., 17:*1799.

Trimble, M. E., and Bowman, R. H. 1973. Renal Na^+ and K^+ transport: effects of glucose, palmitate, and α-bromopalmitate. *Am. J. Physiol., 225:*1057.

Walter, R., and Bowman, R. H. 1973. Mechanism of inactivation of vasopressin and oxytocin by the isolated perfused rat kidney. *Endocrinology, 92:*189.

Weidemann, M. J., Hems, D. A., and Krebs, H. A. 1969. Effects of added adenine nucleotides on renal carbohydrate metabolism. *Biochem. J., 115:*1.

Weidemann, M. J., and Krebs, H. A. 1969. The fuel of respiration of rat kidney cortex. *Biochem. J., 112:*149.

Welbourne, T. C. 1974. Ammonia production and pathways of glutamine metabolism in the isolated perfused rat kidney. *Am. J. Physiol., 226:*544.

Weiss, C., Passow, H., and Rothstein, A. 1959. Autoregulation of flow in isolated rat kidney in the absence of red cells. *Am. J. Physiol., 196:*1115.

Wollenberger, A., Ristau, O., and Schoffa, G. 1960. Eine einfache Technik der extrem Schnellen Abkühlung grosserer Gewebestück, *Pflügers Arch. Ges. Physiol., 270:*399.

Index